The Pharmacist's Expanded Role in Critical Care Medicine

Yasir Alzaidi • Mohamed Abdelzaher Gebily
Editors

The Pharmacist's Expanded Role in Critical Care Medicine

A Comprehensive Guide for Practitioners and Trainees

Volume I

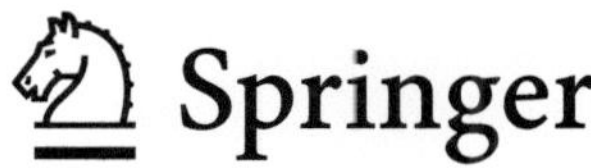 Springer

Editors
Yasir Alzaidi
Department of Pharmacy
Al Hada Armed Forces Hospital
Taif, Saudi Arabia

Mohamed Abdelzaher Gebily
Department of Intensive Care
Al Hada Armed Forces Hospital
Taif, Saudi Arabia

ISBN 978-3-031-77337-2   ISBN 978-3-031-77335-8   (eBook)
https://doi.org/10.1007/978-3-031-77335-8

This Springer imprint is published by the registered company Springer Nature Switzerland AG
The registered company address is: Gewerbestrasse 11, 6330 Cham, Switzerland

If disposing of this product, please recycle the paper.

Foreword

The role of the pharmacist in critical care medicine has become increasingly important and multifaceted in recent years. Critically ill patients are highly heterogeneous in terms of age, underlying comorbidities, prehospital medication usage, admission diagnoses, allergies, concurrent organ replacement therapies, and so on. The acute nature of their illness means that their condition and hence management can change rapidly during their stay, and the disease severity means that many will require multiple medications during, and after, their ICU stay. As integral members of the critical care team, ICU pharmacists have the essential training and knowledge to ensure that prescriptions are individualized such that each patient receives the best drug for them, at the optimal dose, with minimal adverse effects throughout their ICU and hospital stays. ICU pharmacists are also pivotal to successful antimicrobial stewardship programs and accurate interpretation of therapeutic drug monitoring, and their involvement in the diagnostic process and in identifying diagnostic, as well as medication, errors is increasingly encouraged.

Despite their increased presence on our ICUs and involvement in patient management, there are few textbooks aimed specifically at critical care pharmacists, particularly in terms of their potential role in diagnosis. Recognizing this important gap, the editors of this comprehensive book have gathered together 55 chapters that provide an overview of core aspects of critical care patient management from the pharmacist's perspective. The chapters, written by an international team of more than 100 experts, provide an important update on the physiological and pathological mechanisms of key areas of critical illness and the diagnostic and therapeutic approaches to these conditions for the pharmacist. There are chapters focusing on specific diseases or conditions, including shock, acute liver failure, acute kidney injury, delirium, and acute pulmonary embolism; chapters on interpretation of diagnostic tests, such as radiology and electrocardiography; chapters on therapeutic interventions, including mechanical ventilation, intravenous fluids, renal replacement therapy, ECMO, nutrition, and blood transfusion; and chapters on specific groups of ICU patients, including obstetric, oncology, transplant, and burn patients. Two of the chapters, on the approach to clinical reasoning in critical care and sustainable pharmacy practice in the ICU, are unique chapters to pharmacy education and training.

Providing an up-to-date overview of topics related to critical care and emphasizing the importance of correct diagnosis in providing appropriate and optimal treatment, this collection will help prepare ICU pharmacists for their multifaceted responsibilities as members of the ICU team, including an expanded role in limiting misdiagnosis. This book will serve as a useful resource for all pharmacists involved in the management of critically ill patients, whatever their level of experience and training, and I congratulate the editors on their achievement.

Université Libre de Bruxelles
Brussels, Belgium
Department of Intensive Care
Erasme University Hospital
Brussels, Belgium

Jean-Louis Vincent

Foreword

The critical care environment, encompassing the intensive care unit as well as critical care outreach to intermediate care units and the general ward in the form of rapid response systems and medical emergency teams, is tremendously challenging clinically and in terms of patient safety and quality. Pharmacists have a crucial and central role in ensuring the best quality of clinical care and promoting patient safety. Medication errors in these high-stress environments and situations are one of the most common patient safety and quality concerns, and pharmacists are the experts that intensivists, nurses, and respiratory therapists turn to for help in avoiding these types of medical errors. In addition, critically ill patients often receive a large number of medications and have deranged physiology and pharmacodynamics and pharmacokinetics that create a complicated milieu that needs to be carefully balanced to avoid complications and optimize outcome. Pharmacists enhance the quality of care by using their knowledge and education to guide the care team in making the best pharmacological choices for each patient. They also assist prescribers in making the most cost-effective choices, something that is crucial in the current healthcare environment where costs are a major concern. Their role, however, goes well beyond optimization of drug therapy and prevention of medication errors. In the ICU, pharmacists' role is increasingly underscored in ensuring precise diagnoses, a cornerstone for effective drug therapy. Notably, diagnostic errors in the ICU pose substantial concerns, as evidenced by a systematic review led by Winters et al. (2012), revealing alarming rates of errors, including those with lethal implications. Actively engaging in diagnostic deliberations, pharmacists leverage their extensive knowledge in pharmacotherapy to offer invaluable insights that either corroborate or challenge diagnoses. This interdisciplinary synergy is pivotal in aligning treatments with accurate diagnoses, thereby elevating the caliber of patient care.

This book aims to foster interdisciplinary team collaboration that cultivates a culture of safety and precision in patient care, essential for averting diagnostic pitfalls and ensuring therapeutic efficacy. The book contains chapters that enhance diagnostic reasoning and prevent diagnostic errors. In addition, the book provides a comprehensive state-of-the-art review of all topics related to critical care authored by experts from prestigious institutions. I congratulate Dr. Alzaidi on this achievement, and I hope that this book will inform administrators and providers as to the financial, safety, and quality benefits that pharmacists provide in the critical care environment and spur hospitals to make the central role of the pharmacist in the management of critically ill patients a universal reality that all intensive care units and their patients can enjoy and benefit from.

Department of Anesthesiology and Critical Care Medicine, Co-Director of the Johns Hopkins Hospital Surgical ICUs and the Bayview Medical Center Surgical and Burn ICUs, Core Faculty Armstrong Institute for Patient Safety and Quality The Johns Hopkins University School of Medicine, Baltimore, MD, USA

Bradford D. Winters

Foreword

The history of critical care pharmacists extends beyond 50 years, but the growth of services, personnel, research, and magnitude of impact has been exponential. Early in my critical care practice, the focus was on the recognition of our contributions and justification of our roles. While we created a ripple initially, the effect has magnified into a tidal wave of highly trained and engaged pharmacists providing comprehensive medication management for patients in a myriad of settings and with complex clinical problems and management programs.

Key milestones in the development of critical care pharmacists include organization as sections within professional organizations, description of our practice and services, Board Certification in 2012, expansion of critical care residency training programs, guideline and position paper authorship, leadership in influential multiprofessional organizations with active participation in committees, and ongoing documentation of our clinical and economic impact. While individuals are sometimes recognized, it is the influence of the whole that continues to build to tsunami levels.

This text provides a comprehensive view into the broad and expanding world of critical care pharmacy and pharmacologic challenges. I am consistently impressed and amazed by the dedication, knowledge, and creativity of my colleagues worldwide. We have come a long way from gentamicin dosing as a primary focus! The author list of this text includes an amazing group of contributors, and I congratulate them and the editors for comprehensive topics that illustrate current and future roles.

Importantly, the scope of contributions illustrates that we always have new areas to explore, new services to provide, and new growth opportunities. We will be challenged with tools like artificial intelligence or other new technologies, but I have faith that they will be harnessed to improve efficiency and processes. The ultimate reward will be the steadily improving care we provide, in conjunction with our critical care colleagues and teams.

At the same time, I feel that the million little things we do as pharmacists—consistently, every day (or night)—are the most important drivers for optimal patient outcomes (rather than the new and flashy). Additionally, the ability to admit when we are wrong (like my initial resistance to assuming responsibility for a valid medication history) is an important component of our growth as individuals and a professional.

Another important consideration is that while critical care pharmacists excel as entrepreneurs and love to develop new skills and services, a significant opportunity remains to ensure a consistent and standardized scope of practice that describes our foundation and commonalities of practice as a team of pharmacists. We need to ensure that other practitioners can understand and expect specific services, at a minimum. Other standardized tools that allow us to measure outcomes based on the severity of illness or complexity of therapeutics and care will strengthen our ability to document our impact as essential critical care team members.

The roles are limitless, and the tide is moving forward quickly.

Lebanon, IN, USA   Judith Jacobi

Contents of Volume I

Contents of Volume II

Contributors

Max W. Adelman Division of Infectious Diseases, Department of Medicine, Houston Methodist Hospital, Houston, TX, USA
Division of Pulmonary, Critical Care, and Sleep Medicine, Department of Medicine, Houston Methodist Hospital, Houston, TX, USA

Kathleen M. Akgün Yale University School of Medicine, Veterans Administration Connecticut Healthcare System, West Haven, CT, USA

Kaitlin M. Alexander University of Florida College of Pharmacy, Gainesville, FL, USA

Sajjadh M. J. Ali Beth Israel Deaconess Medical Center, Boston, MA, USA

Teresa A. Allison Department of Pharmacy, Memorial Hermann—Texas Medical Center, Houston, TX, USA

Yasir Alzaidi Department of Pharmacy, Al Hada Armed Forces Hospital, Taif, Saudi Arabia

Adrián Baranchuk Division of Cardiology, Queen's University, Kingston, ON, Canada

Nicholas Barker Cardiovascular Intensive Care Unit, Emory Saint Joseph's Hospital, Atlanta, GA, USA

Brooke Barlow Memorial Hermann-The Woodlands Medical Center, Houston, TX, USA

Erin F. Barreto Department of Pharmacy, Mayo Clinic Hospital—Rochester, Rochester, MN, USA

Christopher Bell Department of Pharmacy, Massachusetts General Hospital, Boston, MA, USA

Scott Benken Department of Pharmacy Practice, University of Illinois Chicago College of Pharmacy, Chicago, IL, USA

Karen Berger Nova Southeastern University, Fort Lauderdale, FL, USA
Broward Health Medical Center, Fort Lauderdale, FL, USA

Mauro Bernardi Department of Medical and Surgical Sciences, Alma Mater Studiorum—University of Bologna, Bologna, Italy

Sarah Bova University of Maryland Medical Center, Baltimore, MD, USA

Lauren R. Calnan Hillcrest Hospital South, Tulsa, OK, USA

Ryan Chaffee Department of Pharmacy, Massachusetts General Hospital, Boston, MA, USA

Cherylee W. J. Chang Department of Neurology, Duke University School of Medicine, Durham, NC, USA
Department of Neurosurgery, Duke University School of Medicine, Durham, NC, USA
Department of Medicine Division of Pulmonary, Allergy and Critical Care, Duke University School of Medicine, Durham, NC, USA

Lingye Chen Division of Pulmonary, Allergy, and Critical Care Medicine, Duke University School of Medicine, Durham, NC, USA

Michael Chen Anesthesiology, Perioperative and Pain Medicine, Stanford Hospital, Stanford, CA, USA

Sanjiv Chopra Beth Israel Deaconess Medical Center, Boston, MA, USA
Harvard Medical School, Boston, MA, USA

Aulina Chowdhury Boston Children's Hospital, Boston, MA, USA

Alana Ciolek New York-Presbyterian Hospital/Weill Cornell Medical Center, New York, NY, USA

Kevin G. Correa Division of Pulmonary, Allergy, and Critical Care Medicine, Stanford University, Palo Alto, CA, USA

Yuhamy Curbelo-Pena New York-Presbyterian Hospital, Columbia University Irving Medical Center, New York, NY, USA

Stephanie Davis Cardiovascular Surgical ICU and Clinical Nutrition, The Johns Hopkins Hospital, Baltimore, MD, USA

Michael A. DiCesare Department of Pharmacy, Hospital of the University of Pennsylvania, Philadelphia, PA, USA

Atul Dilawri Cardiothoracic Intensive Care, NewYork-Presbyterian Hospital, Columbia University Irving Medical Center, New York, NY, USA

Zachary Drabick Department of Pharmacy, University of Florida Health, Jacksonville, FL, USA

Amy L. Dzierba Department of Medicine, New York University Langone Health, New York, NY, USA

Lauren E. Eggert Division of Pulmonary, Allergy, and Critical Care Medicine, Stanford University, Palo Alto, CA, USA

Omar Elnaggar Anesthesiology, Perioperative and Pain Medicine, Stanford Hospital, Stanford, CA, USA

Annette Esper Division of Pulmonary, Allergy, Critical Care, and Sleep Medicine, Emory University School of Medicine, Atlanta, GA, USA

Alyson M. Esteves Dartmouth Hitchcock Medical Center, Lebanon, NH, USA

Hassan Farhan Anesthesiology, Perioperative and Pain Medicine, Stanford Hospital, Stanford, CA, USA

Juan M. Farina Division of Cardiothoracic Surgery, Mayo Clinic, Phoenix, AZ, USA

Nicholas Farina Michigan Medicine, Ann Arbor, MI, USA
College of Pharmacy, University of Michigan, Ann Arbor, MI, USA

Fionna Feller Division of Infectious Diseases, Vanderbilt University, Nashville, TN, USA

Fiorenza Ferrari Anestesia e Terapia Intensiva Adulti, Fondazione IRCCS Ca' Granda—Ospedale Maggiore Policlinico, Milan, Italy
International Renal research Institute of Vicenza (IRRIV), Vicenza, Italy

Jonathan Friedman Barnes Jewish Hospital, St. Louis, MO, USA

Lisa M. Gangarosa Division of Gastroenterology and Hepatology, Department of Medicine, UNC Chapel Hill School of Medicine, Chapel Hill, NC, USA

Sebastián Garcia-Zamora Coronary Care Unit, Delta Clinic, Rosario, Argentina

Ethan Garrigan Department of Anesthesiology, Duke University Medical Center, Durham, NC, USA

Jennifer A. Gass Ardent Health Services, Brentwood, TN, USA

Mohamed Abdelzaher Gebily, MD Consultant Intensivist, Director of Intensive Care Unit, Al Hada Armed Forces Hospital, Taif, Saudi Arabia
Former Director of ECMO program, KAMC, Jeddah, Saudi Arabia
Former Director of Critical Care Medicine Residency Program, KAMC, Jeddah, Saudi Arabia
Lecturer of Critical Care Medicine, Faculty of Medicine, Cairo University, Egypt

Gabrielle Gibson Barnes-Jewish Hospital Plaza, St Louis, MO, USA

Brian Gilbert Department of Pharmacy, Wesley Medical Center, Wichita, KS, USA

Neil Glassford Department of Intensive Care Medicine, Victorian Heart Hospital, Monash Health, Clayton, VIC, Australia
Department of Intensive Care Medicine, Monash Medical Centre, Monash Health, Clayton, VIC, Australia
Division of Acute and Critical Care, School of Public Health and Preventive Medicine, Monash University, Monash Health, Melbourne, VIC, Australia
School of Clinical Sciences, Monash University, Clayton, VIC, Australia

Lucas R. Goss Division of Pulmonary, Allergy, Critical Care, and Sleep Medicine, Emory University School of Medicine, Atlanta, GA, USA

Megan Grammatico Department of Internal Medicine, Yale School of Medicine, New Haven, CT, USA

Giacomo Grasselli Anestesia e Terapia Intensiva Adulti, Fondazione IRCCS Ca' Granda—Ospedale Maggiore Policlinico, Milan, Italy
Department of Pathophysiology and Transplantation, University of Milan, Milan, Italy

Traci M. Grucz Department of Pharmacy, The Johns Hopkins Hospital, Baltimore, MD, USA

Shyla Gupta Faculty of Medicine, University of Ottawa, Ottawa, ON, Canada

Kathleen M. Gura Department of Pharmacy, Division of Gastroenterology, Hepatology, and Nutrition, Boston Children's Hospital, Boston, MA, USA

Hala Halawi Houston Methodist Hospital, Houston, TX, USA

Brandy N. Hernandez Department of Pharmacy, Mayo Clinic Hospital—Rochester, Rochester, MN, USA

Lauren Kolodziej Barnes-Jewish Hospital Plaza, St Louis, MO, USA

Beth Hochman General Surgery & Critical Care Medicine, New York-Presbyterian Hospital, Columbia University Irving Medical Center, New York, NY, USA
Acute Care Surgery & Surgical Critical Care, NYU Langone Health, NYU Grossman School of Medicine, New York, NY, USA

GwangYee J. Hu Ernest Mario School of Pharmacy, Rutgers, the State University of New Jersey, Piscataway, NJ, USA
Robert Wood Johnson University Somerset, Somerville, NJ, USA

Nicole G. M. Hunfeld Department of Intensive Care Adults and Department of Hospital Pharmacy, Erasmus University Medical Center, Rotterdam, The Netherlands

Lauren A. Igneri Clinical Pharmacy Specialist, Critical Care, Department of Pharmacy, Cooper University Health Care, Camden, NJ, USA

Emaad J. Iqbal New York-Presbyterian Hospital, Columbia University Irving Medical Center, New York, NY, USA

Christine S. Ji Department of Pharmacy, Beth Israel Deaconess Medical Center, Boston, MA, USA

Heather Johnson University of Pittsburgh Medical Center, Pittsburgh, PA, USA University of Pittsburgh, Pittsburgh, PA, USA

Lesly V. Jurado Hernández Department of Pharmacy, Novant Health New Hanover Regional Medical Center, Wilmington, NC, USA

Ada Selina Jutba, PharmD, BCCCP Department of Pharmacy, Memorial Hermann Memorial City Medical Center, Houston, TX, USA

Nidhi Kataria Department of Laboratory Medicine and Pathology, Mayo Clinic, Rochester, MN, USA

Michael T. Kenes Michigan Medicine, Ann Arbor, MI, USA College of Pharmacy, University of Michigan, Ann Arbor, MI, USA

Soyoung Kristi Kim Clinical Pharmacy Specialist, Critical Care, Department of Pharmacy, Cooper University Health Care, Camden, NJ, USA

Bryan D. Kraft Division of Pulmonary, Allergy, and Critical Care Medicine, Duke University School of Medicine, Durham, NC, USA Division of Pulmonary and Critical Care Medicine, Washington University School of Medicine, Saint Louis, MO, USA

Justin Kreuter Department of Laboratory Medicine and Pathology, Mayo Clinic, Rochester, MN, USA

Caitlin E. Kulig Ernest Mario School of Pharmacy, Rutgers the State University of New Jersey, Piscataway New Jersey and St. Joseph's University Medical Center, Paterson, NJ, USA

Giovanna Landi Department of Cardio-Thoracic Surgery, Maastricht University Medical Centre (MUMNC+), Maastricht, The Netherlands

Grace Lee Los Angeles Medical Center, Kaiser Permanente, Los Angeles, CA, USA

Steven M. Lemieux Veterans Administration Connecticut Healthcare System, West Haven, CT, USA

Fanny Li Departments of Clinical Pharmacy and Pharmaceutical Services, University of California, San Francisco Health, San Francisco, CA, USA

Dusty Lisi Heart Failure, Emory Saint Joseph's Hospital, Atlanta, GA, USA

Natasha D. Lopez Department of Pharmacy, Massachusetts General Hospital, Boston, MA, USA

Uvette Lou Department of Pharmacy, Massachusetts General Hospital, Boston, MA, USA

Samantha Luk Department of Pharmacy, Massachusetts General Hospital, Boston, MA, USA

Fabio Macori Ospedale Santo Spirito Rome, Rome, RM, Italy

Kristin Madenci Brigham and Women's Hospital, Harvard Medical School, Boston, MA, USA

Ahmed A. Mahmoud Houston Methodist Hospital, Houston, TX, USA

Manu L. N. G. Malbrain First Department of Anaesthesiology and Intensive Therapy, Medical University Lublin, Lublin, Poland
Medical Data Management, Medaman, Geel, Belgium
International Fluid Academy, Lovenjoel, Belgium

Maricar Malinis Section of Infectious Diseases, Yale University School of Medicine, New Haven, CT, USA

Patrick Mazi Washington University in St. Louis, Barnes Jewish Hospital, St. Louis, MO, USA

Sharon L. McCartney Department of Anesthesiology, Pain, and Perioperative Medicine, University of Kansas, Kansas City, USA

Laura C. McNamara Department of Medicine, Beth Israel Deaconess Medical Center, Boston, MA, USA

Sachin Mehta Department of Anesthesiology, Pain, and Perioperative Medicine, University of Kansas, Kansas City, USA

Andres F. Miranda-Arboleda Brigham and Women's Hospital, Harvard Medical School, Boston, MA, USA

Alicia H. Muratore Division of Gastroenterology and Hepatology, Department of Medicine, UNC Chapel Hill School of Medicine, Chapel Hill, NC, USA

Andrea M. Nei Department of Pharmacy, Mayo Clinic Hospital—Rochester, Rochester, MN, USA

Haven Nisly Department of Medicine, Duke University School of Medicine, Durham, NC, USA

Cavan O'Kane Ernest Mario School of Pharmacy, Rutgers, the State University of New Jersey, Piscataway, NJ, USA
Penn Medicine Princeton Medical Center, Plainsboro Township, NJ, USA

Robert Olver Department of Intensive Care Medicine, Victorian Heart Hospital, Monash Health, Clayton, VIC, Australia
Department of Intensive Care Medicine, Monash Medical Centre, Monash Health, Clayton, VIC, Australia

Alejandro Narváez Orozco University of Antioquia, Medellín, Colombia

Alex Panuccio Los Angeles Medical Center, Kaiser Permanente, Los Angeles, CA, USA

Mona K. Patel Pulmonary, Critical Care & Sleep Medicine, NYU Langone Health, NYU Grossman School of Medicine, New York, USA

Tyler Peck Beth Israel Deaconess Medical Center, Harvard Medical School, Boston, MA, USA

Camille R. Petri Division of Pulmonary and Critical Care, Department of Medicine, Beth Israel Deaconess Medical Center, Harvard Medical School, Boston, MA, USA

Kayla Popova University of Michigan Health—Michigan Medicine, Ann Arbor, MI, USA

Andrew Posen Department of Pharmacy Practice, University of Illinois Chicago College of Pharmacy, Chicago, IL, USA

Leandro Luis Pozzer Section of Cardiac Electrophysiology, Buenos Aires Cardiovascular Institute, Buenos Aires, Argentina

Elias H. Pratt Division of Pulmonary Allergy, and Critical Care Medicine, Duke University School of Medicine, Durham, NC, USA

Malerie Pratt Brigham and Women's Hospital, Boston, MA, USA

Craig R. Rackley Division of Pulmonary Allergy, and Critical Care Medicine, Duke University School of Medicine, Durham, NC, USA

Lance Ray Department of Pharmacy, Denver Health Medical Center, Denver, CO, USA

Erin Reichert Department of Pharmacy, The Ohio State University, Wexner Medical Center, Columbus, OH, USA

Alyse Reichheld Department of Medicine, Beth Israel Deaconess Medical Center, Boston, MA, USA

Danilo Weir Restrepo Internal Medicine Resident, CES University, Medellín, Colombia

Adele Robbins Advanced Heart Failure and Transplant, Piedmont Hospital, Atlanta, GA, USA

Francisco Machiavello Roman Section of Infectious Diseases, Yale University School of Medicine, New Haven, CT, USA

Claudio Ronco International Renal research Institute of Vicenza (IRRIV), Vicenza, Italy

Mahmoud M. Sabawi Houston Methodist Hospital, Houston, TX, USA

Mehrnaz Sadrolashrafi Beth Israel Deaconess Medical Center, Boston, MA, USA

Ruben Santiago Department of Pharmacy, Jackson Memorial Hospital, Miami, FL, USA

Cina Sasannejad Department of Neurology, Duke University School of Medicine, Durham, NC, USA

Richard M. Schwartzstein Beth Israel Deaconess Medical Center, Harvard Medical School, Boston, MA, USA

Kristine N. Schwietz Department of Pharmacy, Massachusetts General Hospital, Boston, MA, USA

Yahya Shehabi Department of Intensive Care Medicine, Victorian Heart Hospital, Monash Health, Clayton, VIC, Australia
School of Clinical Sciences, Monash University, Clayton, VIC, Australia
Prince of Wales Clinical School of Medicine, University of New South Wales, Randwick, Sydney, NSW, Australia

Sheela V. Shenoi Yale University School of Medicine, Veterans Administration Connecticut Healthcare System, West Haven, CT, USA

Bethany R. Shoulders University of Florida College of Pharmacy, Gainesville, FL, USA

Sarah Matuszak Barnes-Jewish Hospital Plaza, St Louis, MO, USA

Chelsey Song University of Maryland Medical Center, Baltimore, MD, USA

Andrej Spec Washington University in St. Louis, Barnes Jewish Hospital, St. Louis, MO, USA

Katherine Spezzano University of Kentucky HealthCare, Lexington, KY, USA

Joanna L. Stollings Department of Pharmaceutical Services, Vanderbilt University Medical Center, Nashville, TN, USA
Critical Illness, Brain Dysfunction, and Survivorship (CIBS) Center, Vanderbilt University Medical Center, Nashville, TN, USA

David Sugrue Department of Pharmacy, UW Health, Madison, WI, USA

Lauren Sutton Barnes-Jewish Hospital Plaza, St Louis, MO, USA

Poornima Lakshmi Tamma New York-Presbyterian Hospital, Columbia University Irving Medical Center, New York, NY, USA

Erica Tavares Department of Pharmacy, Massachusetts General Hospital, Boston, MA, USA

Fernanda Tavares-Da-Silva Drug Safety, Organon BV, Brussels, Belgium

Seema S. Tekwani Division of Pulmonary, Allergy, Critical Care, and Sleep Medicine, Emory University School of Medicine, Atlanta, GA, USA

Hailey A. Thompson Department of Pharmacy, UW Health, Madison, WI, USA

Beverly Tomita Carle Illinois College of Medicine, University of Illinois, Urbana, IL, USA

Morgan Trammel Department of Pharmacy, Duke University Hospital, Durham, USA

Miguel H. Vicco Drug Safety Lead, Organon BV, Brussels, Belgium

Sybil E. Watkins Department of Internal Medicine, Vanderbilt University Medical Center, Nashville, TN, USA

Andrew J. Webb Massachusetts General Hospital, Boston, MA, USA

Dexter Wimer Departments of Clinical Pharmacy and Pharmaceutical Services, University of California, San Francisco Health, San Francisco, CA, USA

Adrian Wong Beth Israel Deaconess Medical Center, Boston, MA, USA

Nikitha Yagnala Department of Pharmacy, Hospital of University of Pennsylvania, Philadelphia, PA, USA

Giacomo Zaccherini Department of Medical and Surgical Sciences, Alma Mater Studiorum—University of Bologna, Bologna, Italy

Alberto Zanella Anestesia e Terapia Intensiva Adulti, Fondazione IRCCS Ca' Granda—Ospedale Maggiore Policlinico, Milan, Italy
Department of Pathophysiology and Transplantation, University of Milan, Milan, Italy

Part I
Clinical and Diagnostic Approach

Chapter 1
Approach to Clinical Reasoning in Critical Care

Yasir Alzaidi

1.1 Introduction

The diagnostic possibilities entertained in the critical care unit are limited in number versus other noncritical care settings. However, diagnostic errors are common. A study by Winters et al. identified 28% of autopsies as having at least one misdiagnosis, with potentially lethal misdiagnoses quantified at 6.3% [44]. A more recent study by Auerbach et al. reported similar findings, in which 23% of adult patients, who were transferred to the intensive care unit (ICU) or died in the hospital, had missed or delayed diagnoses [4]. In addition to being common, the unifying theme among all diagnostic errors is that they are largely preventable [45]. A major cause leading to diagnostic errors implicates cognitive bias, a flaw in judgment and decision-making [36]. Graber et al. in a study of diagnostic errors in internal medicine identified cognitive factors as being the leading cause of diagnostic errors, exceeding system-related factors [22]. More amenable environments to cognitive diagnostic errors are high-stress areas, including critical care units (CCUs). Accordingly, and in response to diagnostic errors being an urgent patient safety concern, the National Academy of Medicine's report, *"Improving Diagnosis in Health Care,"* outlined a set of recommendations to "improve diagnosis and reduce diagnostic errors," emphasizing the implementation of a collaborative, team-based approach to diagnosis, and the education and training of all healthcare professionals in the diagnostic process [5].

While pharmacists endeavor to ensure appropriate drug therapy in the ICU, it should be recognized that drug therapy cannot be appropriate unless related to the correct diagnosis. It has been said, and I agree, that "the two major products of clinical decision making are diagnoses and treatment plans. If the first is correct, the second has a greater chance of being correct too" [8]. Diagnostic errors, therefore,

Y. Alzaidi (✉)
Department of Pharmacy, Al Hada Armed Forces Hospital, Taif, Saudi Arabia

Y. Alzaidi, M. A. Gebily (eds.), *The Pharmacist's Expanded Role in Critical Care Medicine*, https://doi.org/10.1007/978-3-031-77335-8_1

3

Fig. 1.1 A collaborative approach to diagnosis and the role of the pharmacist clinician

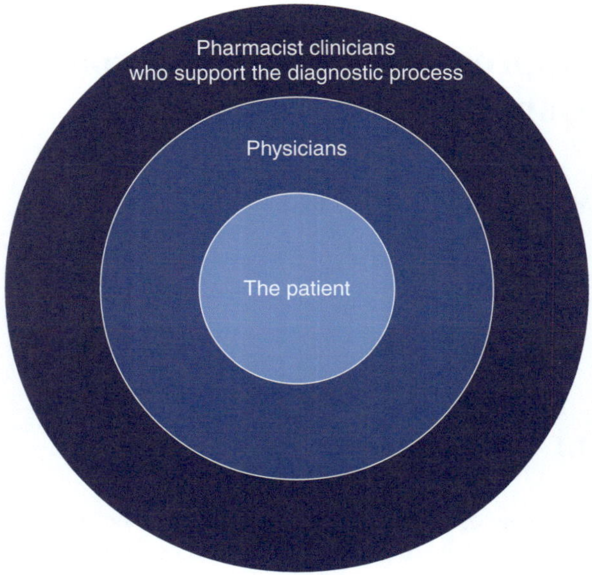

defy the best-intended efforts to improve drug therapy outcomes. Moreover, while misdiagnosis leads to wasteful or unnecessary treatments, it exposes patients to toxic medications, causes delay in treatment, and leads to failure in treating the correct underlying condition. The safe and effective use of drug therapy, therefore, mandates a collaborative, team-based approach to diagnosis, in which *the pharmacist clinician* plays an active role (Fig. 1.1). Graber et al. best described the collaborative approach to diagnosis as being a matter of "distributed cognition," to which pharmacist clinicians, I argue, contribute unique knowledge and perspective [23]. Specifically, pharmacists excel at checking for errors and would prove indispensable in preventing lapses in clinical reasoning. This "expanded role of the pharmacist" should not be perceived as nonessential or noncore to the pharmacy profession. In fact, the full potential of pharmacists' involvement in diagnostic safety has yet to be realized.

1.2 Cognitive Bias in Critical Care

Among important areas that are amenable to improvement in the ICU are the recognition and avoidance of diagnostic errors, of which cognitive biases constitute a principal cause [8]. In essence, what is referred to as cognitive biases are thought patterns that influence decision-making and subsequently set the stage for erroneous clinical judgment. Many types of cognitive biases are now appreciated, with the most commonly encountered types in the ICU are availability bias, confirmation bias, anchoring bias, framing effect, diagnostic momentum, and premature closure (Table 1.1; [26]).

Prevention of diagnostic errors due to cognitive factors relies on understanding how these errors occur. Flaws in clinical diagnostic reasoning contribute largely to diagnostic errors with knowledge deficits being less contributory [22]. One of the theories that explain diagnostic reasoning is the dual-process model, which theorizes two systems of thinking: the automatic thinking (System I) versus nonintuitive deliberate thinking (System II; [28]). These two systems of clinical reasoning markedly differ. System I thinking is fast and intuitive, relies on pattern recognition, and is automatic. In contrast, System II thinking is slow, effortful, analytical, and voluntary [28]. The majority of cognitive biases originate from the fast intuitive thinking of System I [9]. While System I thinking is error-prone, System II thinking—albeit imperfect—is error-resistant and less vulnerable to bias. Accordingly, it should be appreciated that clinical experience, per se, does not protect from cognitive bias. Expert clinicians are not immune from making cognitive errors, primarily because of their tendency to resort to System I thinking, opting for short-cuts, reflex assumptions, rules of thumb, and decision-making based on incomplete data. Notably, novices are not more likely to make diagnostic errors compared to expert clinicians [29]. All too often, novices default to the slow and deliberate System II thinking, and only make a 'working diagnosis' after having carefully analyzed all related data. It should be noted, however, that in the complex and fast-paced environment of critical care, it may be more difficult to resist System I thinking, mandating effective preventative strategies.

Strategies to prevent cognitive diagnostic errors include debiasing strategies and cognitive bias awareness, also known as metacognition [36]. Metacognition is increasingly adopted and involves self-reflection on the process of reasoning, employing System II problem-solving [36]. However, metacognition alone is likely to be insufficient and merits a synergistic approach. In addition to metacognition, external scrutiny of one's clinical diagnostic reasoning is proposed. A multidisciplinary approach to diagnosis, in which pharmacists play an active role, ensures

Table 1.1 Common cognitive biases in the ICU

Biases	Description
Anchoring bias	The tendency to fixate on initial impressions without adjusting to additional new information
Availability bias	The tendency to judge a diagnosis as more likely if it readily comes to mind
Confirmation bias	The selective search for evidence that supports the diagnosis
Diagnostic momentum	A diagnosis is accepted and passed on without supporting evidence
Base rate neglect	The tendency to neglect the true prevalence of a disease
Framing effect	The diagnosis is influenced by how the information is presented
Premature closure (or search satisficing)	The tendency to stop the search once the first plausible cause is identified
Commission bias	The tendency towards action in preference to inaction

sound clinical reasoning and prevents cognitive lapses leading to diagnostic errors. With the proper education on diagnostic reasoning, pharmacists are able to assist diagnosticians in avoiding diagnostic pitfalls, thus reducing diagnostic errors and improving drug therapy outcomes (Fig. 1.1).

1.3 The Art of Clinical Assessment in the ICU

The clinical assessment of a critically ill patient should follow a structured, systematic approach with careful attention to detail. The systematic approach should, preferably, begin with an independent review of systems—for example, the central nervous, respiratory, cardiovascular, gastrointestinal, genitourinary, and musculoskeletal systems (Table 1.2). The use of a mnemonic checklist as a supplement is of particular value. One of the most commonly used care bundle checklists in the ICU is the FASTHUG mnemonic [39]. Subsequently, the independent review of systems is then complemented by the documented patient-specific information, including history of present illness, past medical history, progress notes, clinical examinations, laboratory findings, medication history, etc. This sequential approach to patient assessment is proposed to ensure unbiased evaluation and to reconcile missing, discordant, or conflicting findings from the independent review of systems with that obtained from the documented patient-specific information. Drug therapy decisions can then be decided on the basis of findings from this assessment approach (Fig. 1.2).

Notably, an important element of clinical assessment in the ICU is sound clinical reasoning. As previously noted, a major cause of diagnostic errors implicates faulty clinical reasoning due to cognitive bias. Accordingly, sound clinical reasoning should incorporate debiasing strategies to counteract cognitive bias. For example, instead of searching for evidence that confirms the diagnosis, a sound clinical reasoning involves the search for evidence that is inconsistent with the diagnosis and always considers plausible alternative diagnoses. Specific questions to ask when evaluating the grounds for the initial diagnosis include the following: What finding does not fit with the proposed diagnosis? Is there an alternate cause that could satisfactorily explain the clinical presentation? If so, what additional causes might account for the clinical presentation, etc.? Importantly, when investigating several causes, a higher "diagnostic weight" should be assigned to the relatively more common cause (Table 1.3). "Common things occur commonly," and "uncommon presentations of common diseases are more common than common presentations of uncommon diseases." Failure to consider the base rate can result in diagnostic errors [3].

Table 1.2 Example of a structured review of systems

Organ system	Assessment
CNS	Brain imaging. Level of consciousness (LOC). Evaluation of pain, sedation, and delirium. Fever (grade, number of spikes, pattern, pulse-temperature relationship). External ventricular drains/VP shunts, etc. Penetrating head trauma/skull fracture.
Cardiovascular	Vital signs and tissue perfusion (skin, LOC, urine output, etc.). Electrocardiogram (ECG). Echocardiogram (ECHO). Central venous catheters (subclavian, internal jugular, femoral), PICC lines, chemo port, etc. Other intravascular devices (e.g., pacemakers, ICDs, LVADs).
Respiratory	Chest imaging. Pattern of breathing. Ventilation parameters. Arterial blood gas (ABG). Color, amount, and characteristics of sputum/endotracheal secretions. Chest drains/tubes, etc.
Gastrointestinal	Abdominal exam/imaging/intra-abdominal pressure (IAP). Oral/enteral/parenteral feeding. Bowel movements (frequency, size, consistency). Stress ulcer prophylaxis (if indicated). Gastric residuals. Operative notes. Abdominal drains, wounds, and stomas.
Genitourinary	Urine output. Inputs–outputs with balance. IV fluids. Indwelling Foley catheters, nephrostomy catheters, or suprapubic catheters.
Musculoskeletal	Bed sores. Hematomas. Skin and soft tissue infection. DVT prophylaxis, etc.

1.4   Approach to Common Clinical Presentations in the ICU

1.4.1   Sepsis

Septic shock is the commonest cause of circulatory failure in the ICU [7, 15]. Since common things occur commonly, the diagnostic approach to the patient with circulatory failure should always consider sepsis as one of the inciting causes. Sepsis requires *a porte d'entree* significant to overwhelm host defense mechanisms [13]. Without a significant source of infection, sepsis can be safely excluded [12]. Only few entry sources are implicated in sepsis. The four most common sources of sepsis in the ICU include pulmonary, gastrointestinal (GI), genitourinary (GU), and intravenous sources [12]. The pharmacist clinician should always assist in localizing the

Fig.
1.2 A stepwise approach for evaluating appropriateness of drug therapy in the ICU

Independent review of systems (e.g., CNS, CVS/respiratory, GI/GU, etc.)

Review of patient-specific information (e.g., initial history, progress notes, laboratory findings, medication history, etc.)

Reconcile missing/conflicting findings with the medical team

DRUG THERAPY DECISIONS

source of sepsis. The best approach to the septic patient is to systematically screen for the potential infection focus in order from most common to least common (Fig. 1.3). Notably, the source of sepsis is almost always a single source. Rarely, if ever, the septic patient has multiple sources of infection leading to sepsis at the same time.

Specific clinical and laboratory findings may aid the diagnosis. Common clinical signs associated with sepsis include acute encephalopathy, fever, tachypnea, and tachycardia. Fever is the most recognized sign of infection, defined in the ICU as a single temperature measurement greater than or equal to 38.3 °C [33]. However, not all causes of fever are of infectious origin. In the ICU, noninfectious causes are diverse and must be pursued only after careful exclusion of an infectious etiology. Notably, absence of fever does not rule out infection. Some patients in the ICU are unable to mount an immune response, characteristic of an ongoing infectious process. Immunocompromising factors leading to a blunted febrile response include older age, liver/renal disease, use of immunosuppressive agents (e.g., steroids), solid-organ transplant recipients, and hematological malignancies. In addition to clinical signs, nonspecific inflammatory markers, e.g., WBC, CRP, and ESR, are typically considered when trying to discern an infectious etiology. However, nonspecific inflammatory markers must be interpreted in the proper clinical context as undue reliance may lead to diagnostic errors. Without a source of infection, elevated inflammatory markers should not prompt initiation of antimicrobial therapy. In the ICU, the use of inflammatory markers, at best, is to complement rather than replace clinical judgment.

The therapeutic approach to the septic patient depends on the identification of the likely infection focus [13]. Localizing the site of infection determines the pathogenic flora that needs to be covered with empiric therapy. Antimicrobial therapy is,

Table 1.3 Example of diagnostic approach based on assigning a higher "diagnostic weight" to the more frequent cause(s)

Clinical findings/Dx.	Most common cause	Less common causes
ARDS [6]	Infection	Aspiration Noncardiogenic shock Trauma Pulmonary contusion Blood transfusion Acute pancreatitis Inhalation injury Drug overdose Pulmonary vasculitis Burn Drowning
Hypoglycemia	Insulin NPO status	Myxedema coma Adrenal insufficiency Liver disease Non-insulin drugs
Hypotension	Sepsis (+ source)	Hypovolemia Cardiogenic cause *Relatively less common causes:* Obstructive cause Adrenal insufficiency Anaphylaxis Drug-induced Myxedema coma
ICU-acquired diarrhea	Enteral feeding Laxatives	Drug-induced (e.g., tigecycline) *C. Difficile* (↑↑↑ watery diarrhea)
Polyuria	Excessive fluid administration Diuretics	Diabetes insipidus Cerebral salt wasting, etc.

therefore, appropriate only if based on source localization. Treating a presumed sepsis without source localization from the outset is the cause of needless, inappropriate therapy. A constellation of clinical signs, when present, can point to the potential source of infection (Table 1.4). Once the infection focus is discerned, treatment should be directed at the likely pathogenic flora. Examples of common pathogenic flora in the lower gastrointestinal tract infections are *B fragilis* and aerobic gram-negative bacteria, but not *Staphylococcus aureus*. Conversely, *Staphylococcus aureus* are usual pathogens in central line-related infections, but not *B. fragilis* [13]. Another notable example is *Candida* spp., which are pathogens in colonic perforation, but often nonpathogenic bystanders in pneumonia. The success of treating sepsis depends on early recognition, source control, and appropriate, timely antimicrobial therapy.

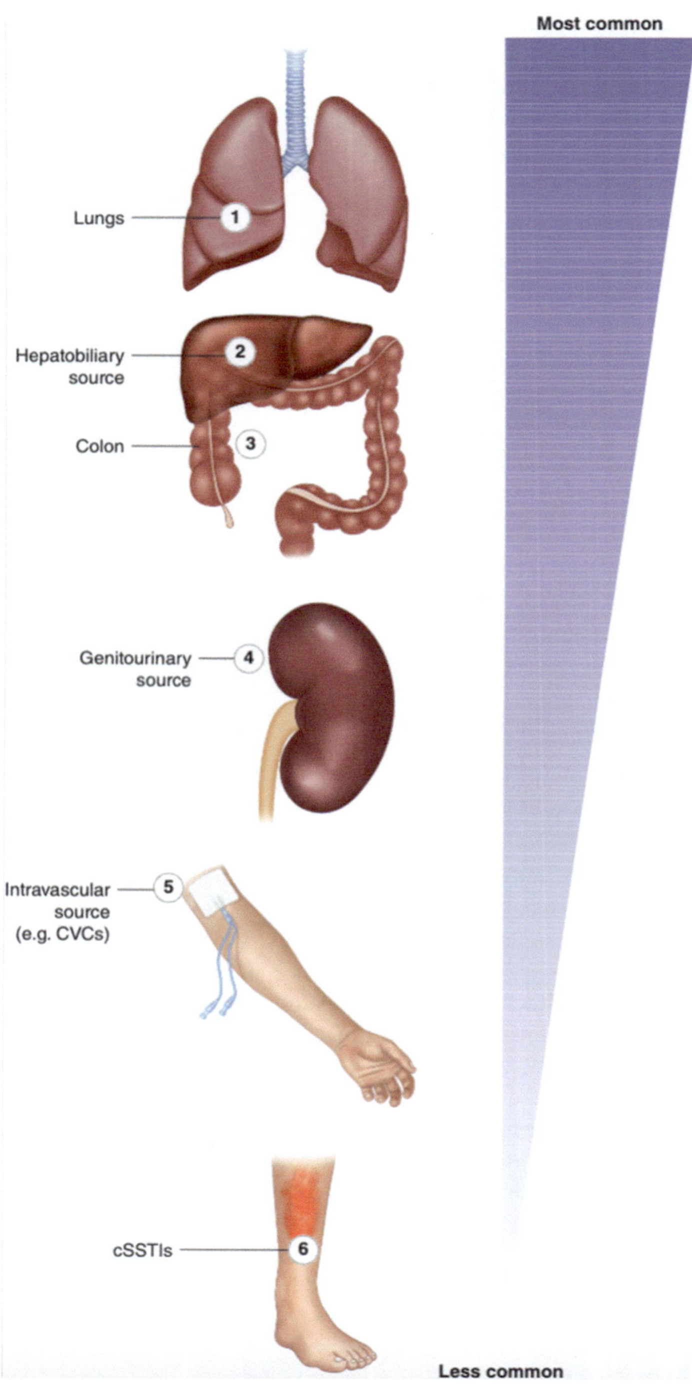

Fig. 1.3 A stepwise approach to screening for the source of sepsis

Table 1.4 Clinical signs commonly associated with each infection focus

Site of infection	Referable findings
Lungs	Infiltrates +/− fever with purulent secretions, new or increased oxygen requirements
Hepatobiliary (ascending cholangitis)	Increased liver function tests with cholestatic picture (e.g., elevated direct bilirubin)
Colon	Abdominal distention, severe abdominal pain, pneumoperitoneum, etc.
Genitourinary	Bacteriuria with pyuria plus local or systemic signs of infection
IV line infection	Evidence of infection around the site of insertion (not always present)
Complicated skin and soft tissue infections	Extreme pain, tenderness, warmth, swelling, redness, etc.

1.4.2   Acute Encephalopathy

Acute encephalopathy is a global disturbance of brain function, often in the absence of structural brain disease. Acute confusional state, acute brain dysfunction, acute brain failure, and altered mental status are non-preferred interchangeable terms [37]. The underlying mechanism is a pathobiological brain process expressed clinically as an acute change in baseline level of consciousness. The cause can be traced to either intracerebral or extracerebral origin (Table 1.5). The most common etiologies leading to acute encephalopathy may be conveniently divided into: toxic-metabolic, structural/primary CNS processes, and cardiovascular. Toxic-metabolic encephalopathy is most common, followed by primary CNS processes and cardiovascular conditions. The diagnostic approach to acute encephalopathy depends on the assessment of all potential causes, a focused history, and a physical examination to assess for localizing signs.

Toxic-metabolic encephalopathy (TME) is caused by sepsis, hepatic failure, renal failure, hypoxemia, hypercapnia, hyponatremia, hypoglycemia, hyperosmolar hyperglycemic state (HHS), hypercalcemia, toxins, drugs, and thiamine deficiency. These factors induce alterations in the normal brain milieu, leading to altered states of consciousness, going from delirium to coma [14]. Patients with delirium present with acute fluctuating attention, disorganized thinking, and altered arousal but are awake and responsive. In contrast, patients with coma are in a state of absent consciousness with no response to external stimuli. Although TME is reversible, severe or sustained insults may lead to neurological sequelae [14]. Identifying and reversing the cause of TME are, therefore, important. Diagnostically, the cause of toxic-metabolic encephalopathy may be evident from the predominant syndromic signs—e.g., hepatic encephalopathy is the cause of TME in patients with the signs of decompensated liver cirrhosis including asterixis, ascites, and esophageal varices. Septic encephalopathy is suspected in patients with a source of sepsis (e.g., indwelling CVCs) with systemic signs of infection. Although TME is the most common cause of encephalopathy in the ICU, the clinician should proceed in a

Table 1.5 Common causes of encephalopathy ("time CNS")

Toxic	Drug overdose or intoxication Withdrawal Drug-related causes
Infectious	Sepsis Urinary tract infection (elderly)
Metabolic	Electrolyte abnormalities Endocrine abnormalities Hepatic encephalopathy Uremic encephalopathy Wernicke's encephalopathy Hypoxia and hypercarbia
Epileptic	Nonconvulsive status epilepticus Postictal state
Cardiovascular	Arrhythmia Sustained hypotension Cardiac syncope
Neurodegenerative	Alzheimer's disease Lewy body dementia
Structural	Stroke with mass effect Thalamic hemorrhage Traumatic brain injury Encephalitis Cerebral vasculitis

diagnostic workup to rule out a structural/primary CNS-damaging process—if suspected.

Acute encephalopathy secondary to structural/primary CNS processes is caused, for example, by severe traumatic brain injury (sTBI), encephalitis/meningoencephalitis, nonconvulsive status epilepticus, stroke in the brainstem, and stroke with mass effect. Mass lesions or stroke confined to one hemisphere without mass effect, and without involving the brain stem, will not alter the level of consciousness. It is rather possible to differentiate structural from toxic-metabolic causes of acute encephalopathy on the basis of clinical examination [27]. Most notably, findings referable to structural damage include the presence of localizing signs (e.g., asymmetrical motor signs). The absence of localizing signs suggests alternate causes, most commonly toxic-metabolic. Specifically, toxic-metabolic encephalopathy causes a fluctuating level of consciousness, with an identifiable precipitant and without focal neurological deficits [27]. Additionally, involuntary limb movements (tremors, myoclonus, and asterixis), acid-base disturbances, and abnormalities of the respiratory patterns (hypoventilation or hyperventilation) are clues to a metabolic etiology [27].

The causes of acute encephalopathy attributable to the cardiovascular system include hypotension, syncope, and arrhythmia. Notably, syncope causes a drop in the level of consciousness that is transient, with rapid onset, short duration, and spontaneous recovery [31]. The cardiovascular causes of syncope include arrhythmia, structural heart disease, pulmonary embolus, acute aortic dissection, and pulmonary hypertension [31]. Syncope due to arrhythmia may not be a straightforward diagnosis. The clinical conundrum in the patient with recurrent, unexplained, brief episodes of loss of consciousness with spontaneous recovery can be resolved with the use of a Holter monitor (Fig. 1.4). Common cardiac arrhythmias leading to transient loss of consciousness include ventricular tachycardia, supraventricular tachycardia, sick sinus syndrome, and atrioventricular (AV) block [31].

1.4.3   Acute Stroke

Stroke encompasses ischemic and hemorrhagic stroke. The vast majority of strokes are ischemic. Stroke develops instantaneously and usually presents with asymmetric findings. The absence of localizing signs argues against the diagnosis of acute stroke. Ischemic stroke is classified according to the underlying etiology into cardioembolic, large-artery atherosclerotic, lacunar small-vessel disease, stroke of other determined etiology, and stroke of undetermined etiology [1]. The imaging modality most sensitive for the diagnosis of ischemic stroke is diffusion-weighted imaging (DWI) [21]. With DWI, the area of infarct appears hyperdense (bright) (Fig. 1.5). A non-contrast CT of the brain, however, remains the mainstay of

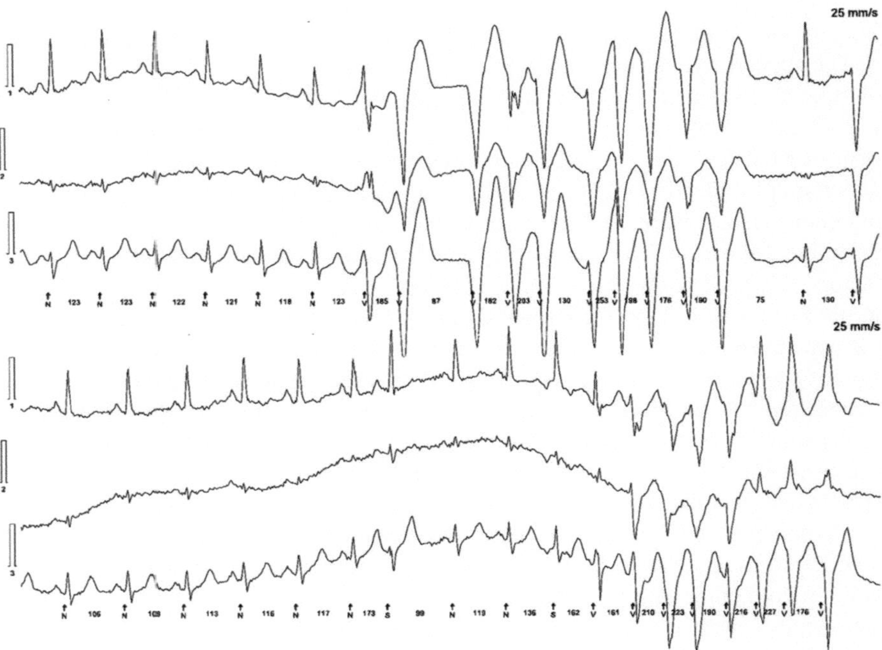

Fig. 1.4 Ambulatory 24-h Holter monitoring reveals episodes of polymorphic ventricular tachycardia [25]

Fig. 1.5 A diffusion-weighted scan reveals multiple infarcts (bright) in more than one territory, characteristic of a cardioembolic stroke

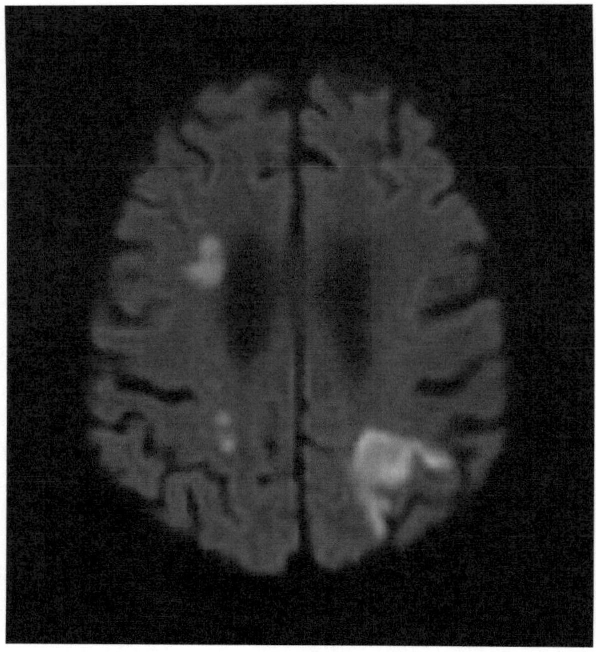

imaging because of speed, availability, and cost [43]. Unlike DWI, the infarct area on CT appears hypodense (dark) (Fig. 1.6).

Specific findings on DWI can help identify the source of ischemic stroke [42]. Most notably, a cardioembolic (CE) source causes multiple infarcts in more than one territory (Fig. 1.5). The commonest cause of CE strokes is due to non-valvular atrial fibrillation [16, 18, 19]. Atrial fibrillation originates in the atria causing hemostasis, hypercoagulability state, activation of platelets, and the subsequent thrombus formation. The risk of stroke from atrial fibrillation depends on specific factors, assessed using the CHA2DS2-VASc score. The most prominent site for thrombus formation is in the left atrial appendage, an anatomical structure originating from the main body of the left atrium. The gold standard for the diagnosis/exclusion of a left atrial appendage thrombus is transesophageal echocardiogram (TEE). In addition to atrial fibrillation, other 'high-risk' causes of CE strokes include left ventricular thrombus, dilated cardiomyopathy, infective endocarditis, and mechanical prosthetic valve [19]. When findings are suggestive of a specific subtype of ischemic stroke, the specific underlying etiology should be investigated.

Hemorrhagic stroke encompasses intracerebral hemorrhage (ICH) and subarachnoid hemorrhage (SAH). ICH is caused by hypertension, coagulopathy, and cerebral amyloid angiopathy, a form of angiopathy resulting from the accumulation of beta-peptide deposits in the walls of blood vessels in the leptomeninges, cerebral cortex, and cerebellar hemispheres [24]. Hypertension is the most common cause implicated in more than 50% of detectable hemorrhagic strokes [20, 32]. To some

Fig. 1.6 Axial CT image of the brain demonstrates, among other findings, a large cortical infarct (dark) with mass effect (arrow). Also noted, petechial hemorrhage within the area of infarct post-thrombolysis. This patient is likely obtunded

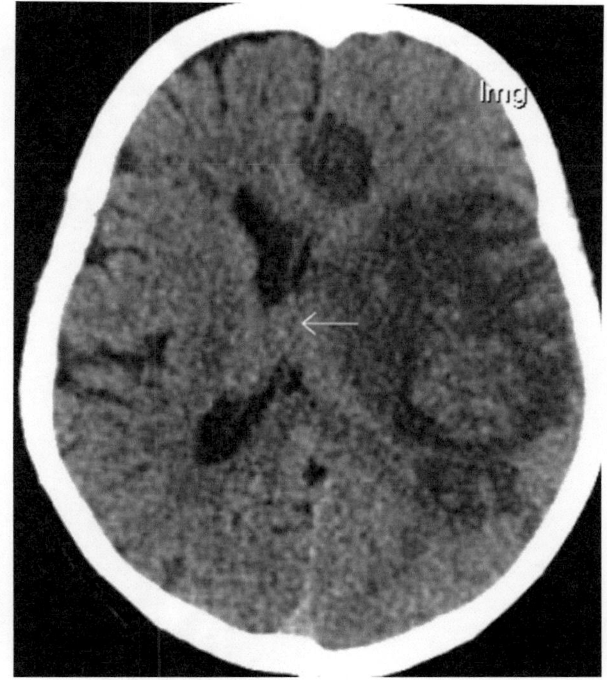

extent, the distribution of hemorrhage points to the inciting cause. ICH in the basal ganglion or thalamic region points to hypertension, while lobar hemorrhage is more suggestive of cerebral amyloid angiopathy (Fig. 1.7). The other less common type of hemorrhagic stroke is SAH, which causes hemorrhage in the subarachnoid space. The majority of SAH occurs in the context of aneurysmal rupture. In the setting of hemorrhagic stroke, a non-contrast-enhanced CT is commonly used. However, CT angiography is recommended to evaluate for an underlying vascular pathology in select patient populations [24, 43]. With CT, blood or bone structures (containing calcium) appear hyperdense (bright) (Figs. 1.8 and 1.7).

As previously noted, stroke limited to one hemisphere without mass effect, excluding stroke in the brainstem, will not affect the level of consciousness. This is in contrast to stroke with mass effect, stroke in the brainstem, or stroke affecting multiple territories in both hemispheres (Figs. 1.5 and 1.6). ICU management of patients with acute stroke, in addition to post-thrombolysis care, is centered on neuroprotective measures and prevention of secondary brain injury.

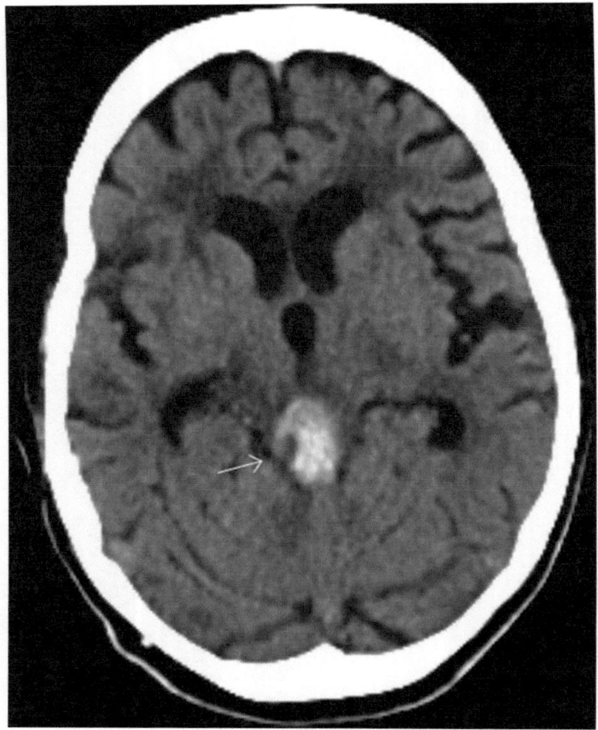

Fig. 1.7 Axial CT image of the brain demonstrates thalamic hemorrhage (arrow)

1.4.4   CNS Infection

CNS infection commonly seen in ICU patients are acute bacterial meningitis and acute viral encephalitis. TB Meningitis, Neurosyphilis, Toxoplasmosis Encephalitis, Cryptococcal Meningitis, etc. are less commonly encountered. The mode of pathogen acquisition may be natural or as a result of open head trauma or neurosurgical procedures. Notably, both immunocompromised and immunocompetent hosts can acquire CNS infection. A focused history, clinical presentation, cerebrospinal fluid (CSF) profile findings, CSF PCR, EEG, and radiological features, when combined, are helpful discriminants for the differential diagnosis.

Acute bacterial meningitis (ABM) is an infectious disease emergency demanding immediate diagnosis and treatment. The infection starts in the subarachnoid space and subsequently invades the brain parenchyma leading to severe neurological sequelae [14]. This is in contrast to viral meningitis/aseptic meningitis where the inflammation is confined to the subarachnoid space and presents with clear mentation [14]. The most common presenting symptoms of ABM include fever, headache, and nuchal rigidity. Severe headache is a characteristic finding in ABM due to the presence of nociceptive neurons in the meninges [14]. Other *less* sensitive meningeal signs referable to ABM include *Kernig's sign* (resistance to full extension of

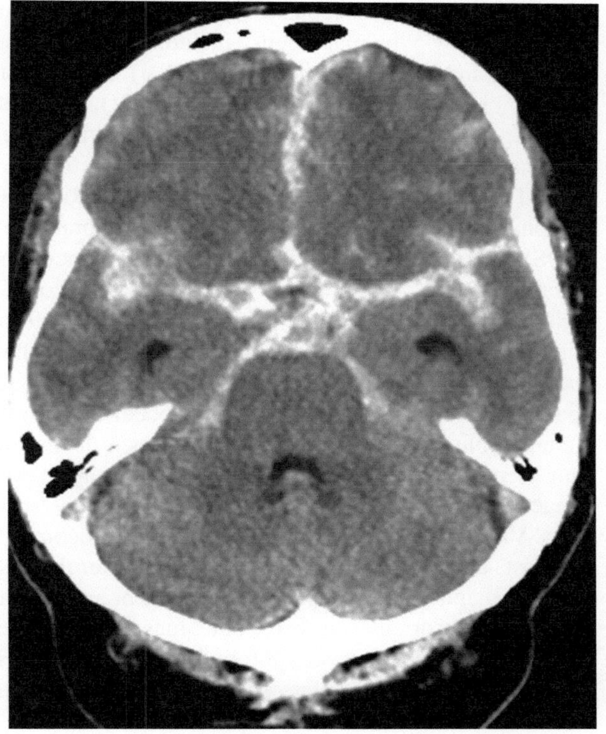

Fig. 1.8 Axial CT image of the brain demonstrates subarachnoid hemorrhage (SAH). Note the star shape, characteristic of SAH

the knee) and *Brudzinski's sign* (flexion of lower limb in response to passive flexion of the neck). Lumbar puncture (LP) is helpful in establishing the diagnosis, however, it should not delay treatment [38]. Relative contraindications to LP include increased intracranial pressure, coagulopathy, and suspected spinal epidural abscesses. A CSF consistent with ABM includes a high opening pressure, a neutrophil-predominant pleocytosis (usually WBC count > 1000/microliter), elevated protein concentration, a CSF to serum glucose ratio of less than 0.4, and low glucose [38]. The use of multiplex PCR panels can rapidly identify the implicated pathogen, with a special utility in cases where antibiotic administration preceded the LP. Only limited bacterial pathogens are implicated in ABM. *Streptococcus pneumoniae* is the predominant pathogen in community-acquired ABM. In contrast, hospital-acquired ABM is caused by *staphylococcus* species and gram-negative bacilli.

Encephalitis is an inflammatory process involving the brain parenchyma with associated neurologic dysfunction. Neurological findings, e.g., confusion, personality changes, seizure, focal deficits, speech or movement disorders, hemiparesis, flaccid paralysis, etc., are characteristic clinical features of encephalitis. An array of causes including infectious and non-infectious causes have been described. Non-infectious causes include acute disseminated encephalomyelitis (ADEM) and anti-NMDA receptor encephalitis, both of which are immune-mediated. The former is triggered by viral pathogens, including rubella, mumps, varicella, smallpox, influenza, and herpes simplex virus (HSV). In contrast, infectious encephalitis is caused by Herpes simplex virus (HSV), Varicella zoster virus (VZV), Cytomegalovirus (CMV), Human herpes virus type 6, West Nile virus, Enteroviruses, etc. The commonest viral cause of encephalitis is due to Herpes simplex virus-1 (HSV-1). HSV-1 has a specific neurotropism. Radiologically, the clue to HSV-1 encephalitis is enhancement of the medial temporal lobe (Fig. 1.9). The CSF typical of HSV-1 encephalitis includes a modest lymphocyte-predominant pleocytosis, an elevated protein concentration, and a normal glucose. The CSF PCR for HSV is highly sensitive and specific. Since the CSF is a distant mirror to the infection/inflammation at the brain parenchyma, care should be exercised when excluding viral encephalitis solely on the basis of negative CSF PCR [35] (Fig. 1.9). Specifically, false negative results may occur early in the disease process or when the tap is bloody. CMV encephalitis causes a distinct modest neutrophil predominant pleocytosis with periventricular white matter enhancement on T2 weighted images. CMV encephalitis is almost exclusively seen in immunocompromised hosts. VZV encephalitis can affect both immunocompromised and immunocompetent hosts and present preceding the rash or after the onset of rash by 6 months.

Early diagnosis and appropriate treatment are critical as delay in diagnosis can lead to complications and worse outcomes. In the ICU, a febrile patient with penetrating head trauma, post craniotomy/craniectomy, or with internal or external ventricular and lumbar catheters should be suspected to have a CNS infection until

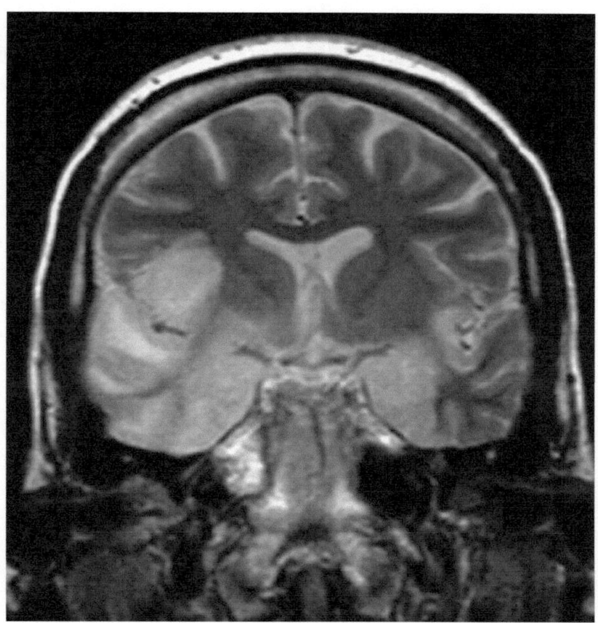

Fig. 1.9 Temporal lobe enhancement in coronal T2-weighted MR image. HSV PCR from cerebrospinal fluid was negative. PCR was repeated on a brain biopsy, which confirmed the diagnosis of HSV encephalitis. Source: http://www.radpod.org/2007/03/24/herpes-simplex-encephalitis/

proven otherwise. In general, treatment starts empirically then directed against a specific pathogen.

1.4.5 Severe Community-Acquired Pneumonia

Severe community-acquired pneumonia (sCAP) often requires ICU admission and, in some cases, ventilatory support. The severity of CAP depends on the immune status of the host and the baseline cardiopulmonary reserve [14]. In other words, patients with underlying immunocompromised conditions are likely to have a severe clinical course. Likewise, patients with cardiac or pulmonary dysfunctions at baseline are likely to decompensate following infection with a CAP pathogen. The pathogens implicated in CAP include bacterial, viral, and fungal pathogens. Specific clinical, laboratory, and radiological features are combined to discern the etiology of CAP.

Viral causes of CAP include influenza, SARS-CoV-2, respiratory syncytial virus (RSV), adenovirus, human metapneumovirus (hMPV), and cytomegalovirus (CMV). Viral pathogens are differentiated from other nonviral respiratory pathogens by means of imaging, clinical features, and laboratory findings. Classically, viral CAP presents on chest imaging as diffuse bilateral interstitial symmetrical infiltrates (Fig. 1.10). There are, however, other radiological mimics of viral CAP that are often missed, including infectious and noninfectious mimics. Noninfectious mimics of viral CAP include, among others, diffuse alveolar hemorrhage, cryptogenic organizing pneumonia, and drug-induced pneumonitis. Among the infectious mimics, *Pneumocystis jirovecii* (PJP) pneumonia is a notorious, nonviral mimic of viral CAP (Fig. 1.11). Laboratory findings are variably helpful for suspecting a viral etiology. Inconsistently, thrombocytopenia and lymphocytopenia may accompany

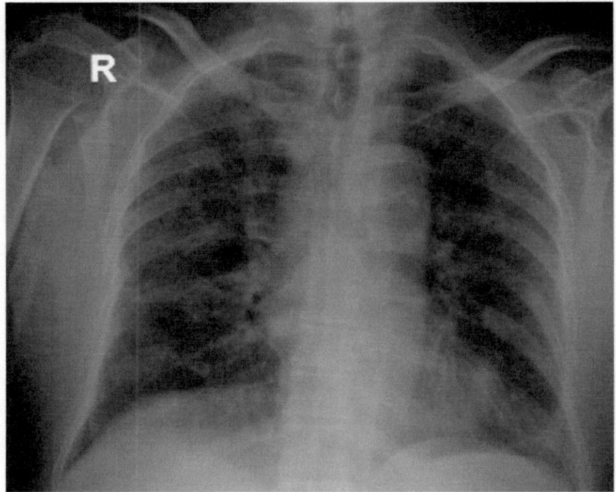

Fig. 1.10 Bilateral diffuse interstitial infiltrates in keeping with a likely viral etiology

Fig. 1.11 *Pneumocystis jirovecii pneumonia* with LDH >500 mg/dL

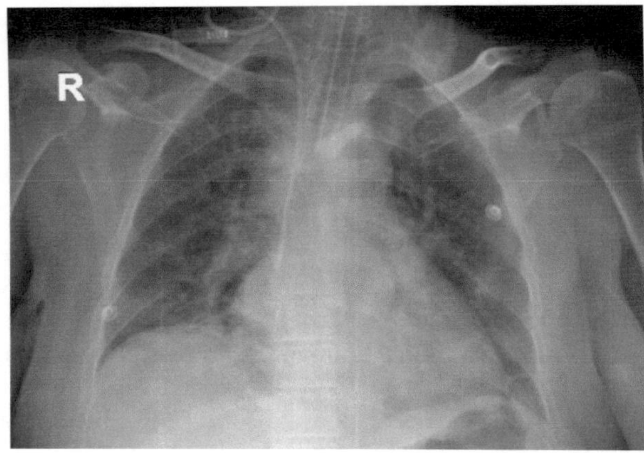

viral CAP; however, neither are sensitive nor specific [34]. Rarely, bacterial pathogens complicate viral CAP, resulting in co-bacterial or secondary bacterial infections.

Severe community-acquired pneumonia is also caused by fungal pathogens, of which *Pneumocystis jirovecii* deserves a special focus. *Pneumocystis jirovecii* is an intracellular opportunistic pathogen commonly associated with HIV, but it is a recognized pathogen in other immunocompromised hosts. The clinical presentation is distinct from viral CAP, in which patients with PJP pneumonia present subacutely (over several days to weeks) with symptoms of nonproductive cough and progressive exertional dyspnea [2]. Unlike viral CAP, extrapulmonary disease is rare with PJP pneumonia. Patients presenting to the ICU will typically have severe hypoxemia (PaO2 < 70 mmHg, Aa-gradient >35 mmHg). A clinically useful, albeit imperfect, clue to PJP pneumonia is the associated elevation in serum LDH (>500 mg/dL). The definitive diagnosis is based on histopathologic or cytopathogenic demonstration of the organism with appropriate staining [2]. Notably, bronchoscopy with bronchoalveolar lavage (BAL) has a lower sensitivity in non-HIV compared to HIV patients [2]. The diagnosis of PJP pneumonia relies on a high index of suspicion in the right patient population.

Bacterial CAP in immunocompetent hosts without an underlying cardiopulmonary dysfunction rarely leads to severe presentation mandating ICU care. The usual patients with severe bacterial CAP are immunocompromised hosts and/or those with low cardiopulmonary reserve [14]. Both typical and atypical bacteria are implicated in CAP. The typical respiratory pathogens include *Streptococcus pneumoniae, Haemophilus influenzae*, and *Moraxella catarrhalis*. In immunocompromised hosts and chronic alcoholics, *Klebsiella pneumoniae* is a recognized pathogen (Fig. 1.12). In cystic fibrosis, *Pseudomonas aeruginosa* is implicated. *Staphylococcus aureus* rarely complicates viral CAP and, if so, presents as cavitary pneumonia [10]. In addition to typical bacterial pathogens, other atypical non-zoonotic pathogens are causative including *Mycoplasma pneumoniae* and *Chlamydia pneumoniae*, and, rarely, *Legionella pneumophila* [10]. Specific to atypical CAP are the

Fig. 1.12 *Klebsiella pneumoniae* CAP in an immunocompromised host

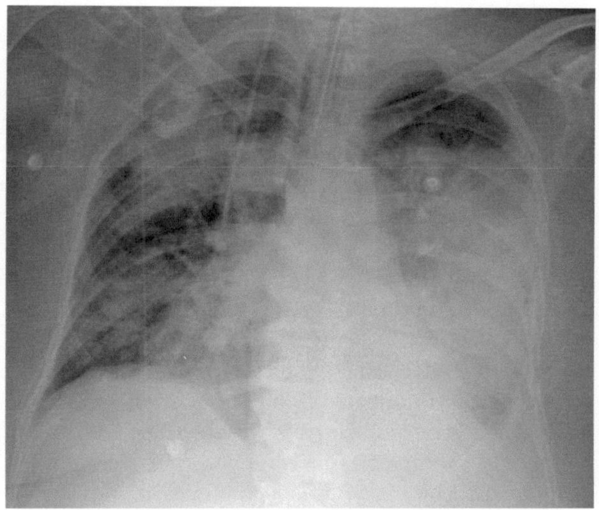

Fig. 1.13 *Mycoplasma pneumoniae* CAP in a severely hypoxic patient, presenting with extrapulmonary symptoms

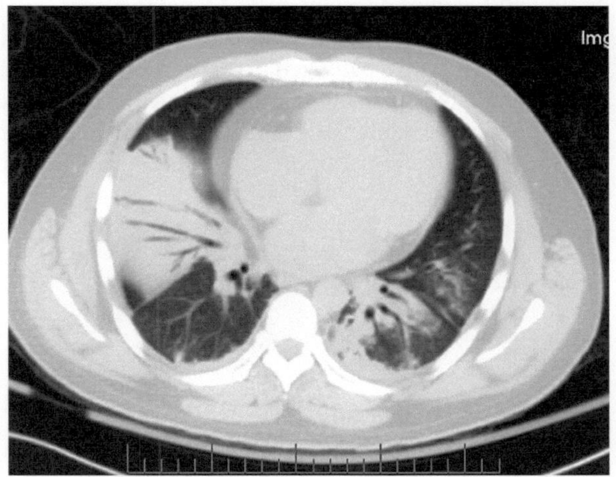

extrapulmonary manifestations, including gastrointestinal and neurologic symptoms. In fact, atypical CAP can be thought of as a systemic infection involving the lungs [10]. On chest imaging, bacterial CAP presents as alveolar airspace opacities with air bronchograms, thus differentiating bacterial CAP from viral CAP (Fig. 1.13).

1.4.6 Nosocomial Pneumonia

Nosocomial pneumonia (NP) including hospital-acquired pneumonia (HAP) and ventilator-associated pneumonia (VAP) is common in the ICU. The organisms most responsible for NPs are aerobic gram-negative bacilli. The clinical signs of pneumonia include increased colored secretions, pulmonary infiltrates, tachypnea, and new or increased oxygen requirements. The mere recovery of a pathogen without the accompanied clinical signs of infection should not prompt initiation of antibiotics. Radiological findings of bacterial NP typically include lobar or multilobar airspace alveolar opacities/consolidation with air bronchograms.

NP is usually caused by a single pathogen. Recovery of multiple organisms from the sputum/endotracheal aspirate is likely to represent colonization. The organisms typically implicated in NP are *Klebsiella pneumoniae*, *Pseudomonas aeruginosa*, and, less frequently, *Acinetobacter baumannii*. *Pseudomonas aeruginosa* commonly colonizes secretions of ventilated patients, and unless accompanied by characteristic findings, it should not be treated [14] (Fig. 1.14). Notably, *Staphylococcus aureus* is not a typical cause of NP [14]. In the setting of community-acquired pneumonia, *Staphylococcus aureus* rarely causes infection following viral pneumonia. The negative nasal MRSA PCR effectively rules out MRSA as a causative pathogen in suspected pneumonia. Not uncommonly, mechanically ventilated patients may develop ventilator-associated tracheobronchitis (VAT), which presents with clinical signs of pneumonia but without radiological evidence of infection. Importantly, when evaluating patients suspected of VAT,

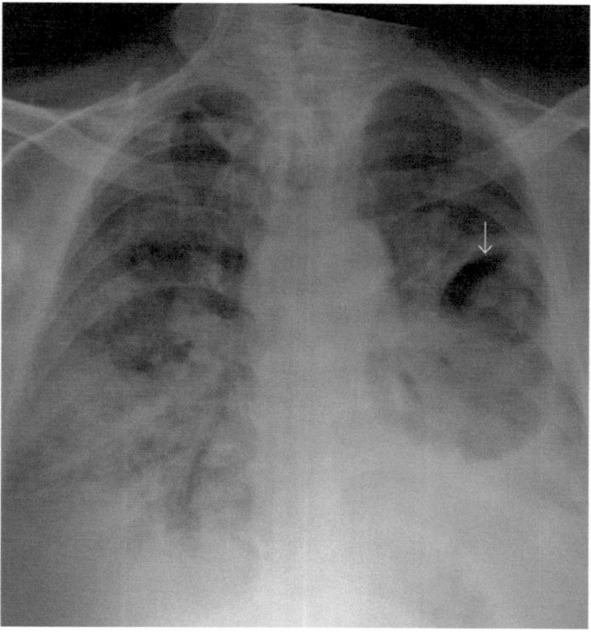

Fig. 1.14 Chest radiograph of nosocomial pneumonia caused by *Pseudomonas aeruginosa*. Note the cavitary lesion (arrow), hallmark of infection with *Pseudomonas aeruginosa*

other causes should be excluded including VAP which may not be apparent in portable chest radiographs (Fig. 1.15).

Herpes simplex virus (HSV) rarely causes nosocomial pneumonia in ventilated patients. HSV may be suspected as the cause of non-resolving VAP, manifesting clinically as failure to wean from the ventilator or, more typically, as severe hypoxemia requiring a high FiO2 [17]. Importantly, reactivation of HSV is common in mechanically ventilated patients and should be distinguished from true HSV pneumonia [30]. The mere detection of HSV from respiratory samples does not prove its etiologic role. The definitive diagnosis of HSV pneumonia is made with cytopathological evidence of invasion. In addition to HSV, other common respiratory viruses can be transmitted from healthcare staff to patients, especially during viral seasons, leading to nosocomial pneumonia.

1.4.7 Pulmonary Edema

Pulmonary edema develops secondary to cardiogenic and noncardiogenic causes, with cardiogenic pulmonary edema being the most common cause. Knowledge of the cause of pulmonary edema has important implications for management [41]. The differentiation of cardiogenic versus noncardiogenic pulmonary edema combines findings from history, clinical investigations, and, to some extent, radiological features. Substantial overlap between cardiogenic and noncardiogenic pulmonary edema, however, remains.

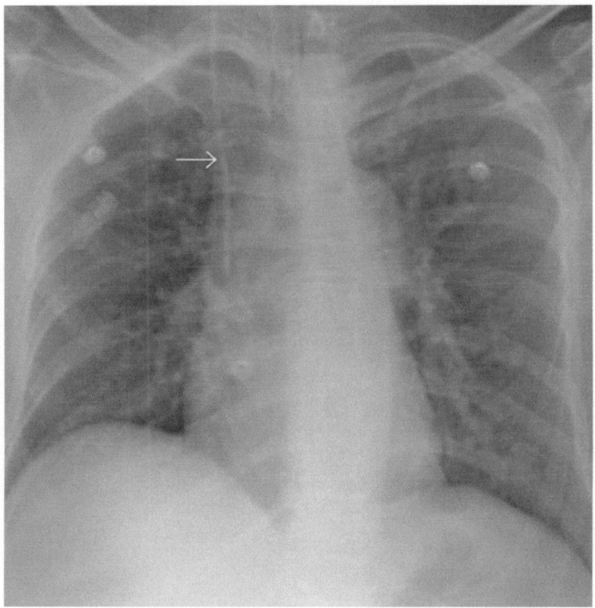

Fig. 1.15 A normal supine chest radiograph. The patient had purulent secretions with fever in keeping with VAT. What not to overlook is the central venous catheter (arrow), another potential source of fever

Cardiogenic pulmonary edema is caused by cardiac-related etiologies, most commonly seen in the setting of heart failure. The mechanism underlying cardiogenic pulmonary edema is increased pulmonary capillary pressure, transuding fluids first into the interstitium and later into the alveolar space [41]. Signs of interstitial edema include a centrally located, butterfly pattern of linear and reticular opacities. If progressed, a confluent airspace consolidation ensues, reflecting fluid accumulation in the alveolar space. These radiological findings, however, are common in both cardiogenic and noncardiogenic pulmonary edema. Associated findings that are characteristic, but not specific, for cardiogenic pulmonary edema include cardiomegaly with bilateral pleural effusions, more prominent in the right pleural cavity (Fig. 1.16). Notably, rapid regression of congestive signs with effective fluid removal and restoration of compensated state favors cardiogenic pulmonary edema.

Noncardiogenic pulmonary edema is caused by a multitude of factors, with acute respiratory distress syndrome (ARDS) being the most important cause in terms of severity. The mechanism underlying pulmonary edema in ARDS is increased alveolar-capillary permeability, leading to the influx of protein-rich fluids into airspaces [40, 41]. ARDS is caused by either pulmonary or extrapulmonary factors. Direct pulmonary insults include pneumonia, aspiration, radiation, inhaled toxins, and thoracic trauma. Extrapulmonary factors by contrast include sepsis, acute pancreatitis, burn, non-thoracic trauma, and blood transfusions. Certain features differentiate ARDS from that of cardiogenic pulmonary edema and include a known insult within 1 week of onset, noncardiogenic bilateral opacities on chest imaging, and refractory arterial hypoxemia [40] (Fig. 1.17).

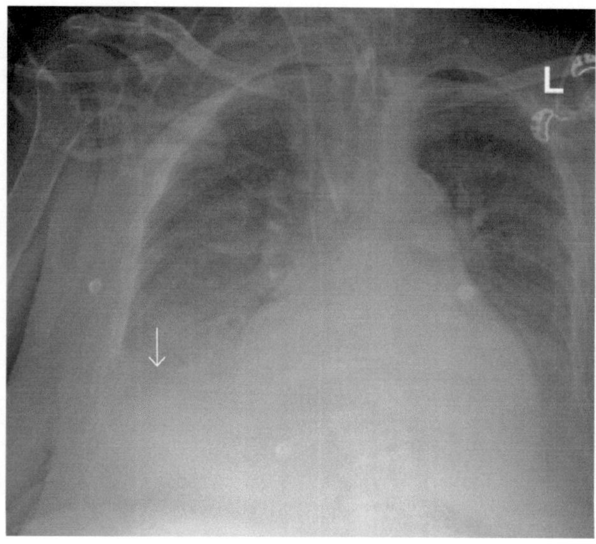

Fig. 1.16 Chest radiograph of cardiogenic pulmonary edema. Note the increased cardiac shadow with bilateral pleural effusions, more prominent in the right pleural cavity (arrow)

Fig. 1.17 Chest radiograph of noncardiogenic pulmonary edema. This patient had CMV pneumonitis with refractory arterial hypoxemia

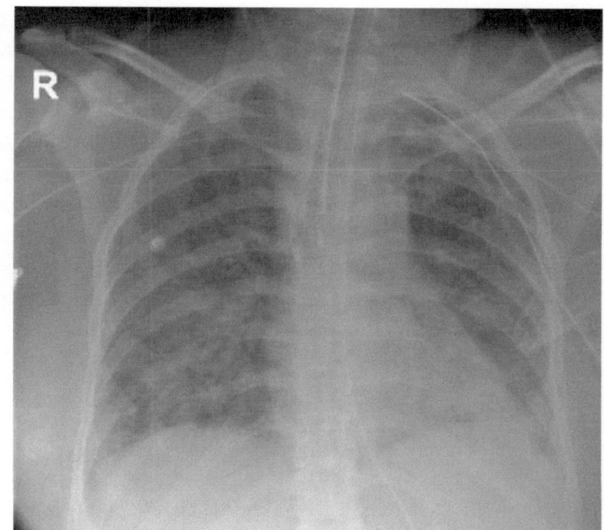

1.4.8   Fever

Fever ($\geq$38.3 °C) is common in ICU patients. The search for the cause of fever can be difficult, even for the experienced clinician. The approach to fever in the ICU is based on diagnostically discerning infectious from noninfectious fevers. In general, fever in a patient with a source of infection is an "infectious fever" until proven otherwise. This approach emphasizes the critical importance of early diagnosis and should not prompt initiation of antimicrobial therapy in otherwise stable patients unless an infectious cause is discerned. Notably, the source of infection can be overt or, in some cases, hidden. Hidden, or less apparent, infectious causes of fever include surgical site infections, acute acalculous cholecystitis, septic thrombophlebitis, intra-abdominal abscess collection, *C. difficile* colitis, sinusitis, and others. Each of these causes should be suspected in the right clinical context; for example, intra-abdominal abscess is suspected in patients with known risk factors, including a recent history of abdominal surgery, and acute acalculous cholecystitis presents with leukocytosis and abnormal liver tests. When all possibilities of an infectious etiology have been exhausted, a noninfectious cause should then be entertained. Fever of noninfectious origin in the ICU is caused by deep venous thrombosis, pulmonary embolism, myocardial infarction, central fevers, relative adrenal insufficiency, acute pancreatitis, gastrointestinal hemorrhage, atelectasis, transfusion of blood products, vasculitis, cryptogenic organizing pneumonia, and drugs [33].

Drug fever stands out as a unique cause of noninfectious fever with discernible clinical features. The pattern of drug fever is continuous or intermittent, usually high grade, and closely resembles fever of infectious origin. All too often, the diagnosis is made after a lack of response to the indiscriminate use of antimicrobial therapy. The associated clinical findings in drug fever reflect the likely underlying hypersensitivity reaction and include mild-to-moderate transaminitis, leukocytosis, eosinophilia, and elevated erythrocyte sedimentation rate (ESR) [11]. Important diagnostically, patients with drug fever will not appear in distress [11]. Skin rash may or may not accompany drug fever. However, the presence of a skin rash, per se, does not prove drug fever. It is common for clinicians to ascribe skin rash to drugs alone. Other febrile illnesses encountered in the ICU may present with skin manifestations, including various infectious diseases. Important of all, drug fever is a diagnosis of exclusion. If drug fever is suspected, the medication list should be scrutinized for potential culprits. The most common causes of drug fever are antimicrobial and antiepileptic agents. Once the inciting drug is discontinued, a rapid defervescence occurs, usually within 72 h.

References

1. Adams HP Jr, Bendixen BH, Kappelle LJ, Biller J, Love BB, Gordon DL, Marsh EE 3rd. Classification of subtype of acute ischemic stroke. Definitions for use in a multicenter clinical trial. TOAST. Trial of Org 10172 in Acute Stroke Treatment. Stroke. 1993;24(1):35–41.
2. AIDSinfo, Access. Guidelines for the prevention and treatment of opportunistic infections in adults and adolescents with HIV. 2019.
3. Aronowitz PB, Williams DM, Henderson MC, Winston LG. Mind the base rate: an exercise in clinical reasoning. J Gen Intern Med. 2019 Sep;15(34):1941–5.
4. Auerbach AD, Lee TM, Hubbard CC, Ranji SR, Raffel K, Valdes G, Boscardin J, Dalal AK, Harris A, Flynn E, Schnipper JL. Diagnostic errors in hospitalized adults who died or were transferred to intensive care. JAMA Intern Med. 2024;184(2):164–73.
5. Ball JR, Miller BT, Balogh EP, editors. Improving diagnosis in health care. Washington, DC: National Academies Press (US); 2015.
6. Bellani G, Laffey JG, Pham T, Fan E, Brochard L, Esteban A, Gattinoni L, Van Haren F, Larsson A, McAuley DF, Ranieri M. Epidemiology, patterns of care, and mortality for patients with acute respiratory distress syndrome in intensive care units in 50 countries. JAMA. 2016;315(8):788–800.
7. Cecconi M, De Backer D, Antonelli M, Beale R, Bakker J, Hofer C, Jaeschke R, Mebazaa A, Pinsky MR, Teboul JL, Vincent JL. Consensus on circulatory shock and hemodynamic monitoring. Task force of the European Society of Intensive Care Medicine. Intensive Care Med. 2014;40:1795–815.
8. Croskerry P. From mindless to mindful practice—cognitive bias and clinical decision making. N Engl J Med. 2013;368(26):2445–8.
9. Croskerry P, Singhal G, Mamede S. Cognitive debiasing 1: origins of bias and theory of debiasing. BMJ Qual Saf. 2013;22(Suppl 2):ii58–64.
10. Cunha BA. Community-acquired pneumonia: diagnostic and therapeutic approach. Med Clin North Am. 2001;85(1):43–77.
11. Cunha BA. Antibiotic selection in the penicillin-allergic patient. Med Clin North Am. 2006;90(6):1257–64.
12. Cunha BA. Infectious diseases in critical care medicine, vol. 27; 2007. p. 590.
13. Cunha BA. Sepsis and septic shock: selection of empiric antimicrobial therapy. Crit Care Clin. 2008;24(2):313–34.
14. Cunha CB, Cunha BA, editors. Infectious diseases and antimicrobial stewardship in critical care medicine. CRC Press; 2020 Jul 12.

15. De Backer D, Biston P, Devriendt J, Madl C, Chochrad D, Aldecoa C, Brasseur A, Defrance P, Gottignies P, Vincent JL. Comparison of dopamine and norepinephrine in the treatment of shock. N Engl J Med. 2010;362(9):779–89.
16. Dilaveris PE, Kennedy HL. Silent atrial fibrillation: epidemiology, diagnosis, and clinical impact. Clin Cardiol. 2017;40(6):413–8.
17. Eisenstein LE, Cunha BA. Herpes simplex virus pneumonia presenting as failure to wean from a ventilator. Heart Lung. 2003;32(1):65–6.
18. Ferro JM. Cardioembolic stroke: an update. Lancet Neurol. 2003;2(3):177–88.
19. Freeman WD, Aguilar MI. Stroke prevention in atrial fibrillation and other major cardiac sources of embolism. Neurol Clin. 2008;26(4):1129–60.
20. Gebel JM, Broderick JP. Intracerebral hemorrhage. Neurol Clin. 2000;18(2):419–38.
21. González RG, Schaefer PW, Buonanno FS, Schwamm LH, Budzik RF, Rordorf G, Wang B, Sorensen AG, Koroshetz WJ. Diffusion-weighted MR imaging: diagnostic accuracy in patients imaged within 6 hours of stroke symptom onset. Radiology. 1999 Jan;210(1):155–62.
22. Graber ML, Franklin N, Gordon R. Diagnostic error in internal medicine. Arch Intern Med. 2005;165(13):1493–9.
23. Graber ML, Grice GR, Ling LJ, Conway JM, Olson A. Pharmacy education needs to address diagnostic safety. Am J Pharm Educ. 2019;83(6):7442.
24. Greenberg SM, Ziai WC, Cordonnier C, Dowlatshahi D, Francis B, Goldstein JN, Hemphill JC III, Johnson R, Keigher KM, Mack WJ, Mocco J. 2022 guideline for the management of patients with spontaneous intracerebral hemorrhage: a guideline from the American Heart Association/American Stroke Association. Stroke. 2022;53(7):e282–361.
25. Han J, Lee J, Choi S, Lee H, Song YH. Case report: Myocarditis with nonsustained ventricular tachycardia following COVID-19 mRNA vaccination in a female adolescent. Front Pediatr. 2022;10:995167. https://doi.org/10.1016/j.jacc.2019.08.1061.
26. Hayes MM, Chatterjee S, Schwartzstein RM. Critical thinking in critical care: five strategies to improve teaching and learning in the intensive care unit. Ann Am Thorac Soc. 2017 Apr;14(4):569–75.
27. Howard RS. Coma and brainstem death. Medicine. 2012;40(9):500–6.
28. Kahneman D. Thinking, fast and slow. New York, NY: Farrar, Straus and Giroux; 2011.
29. Krupat E, Wormwood J, Schwartzstein RM, Richards JB. Avoiding premature closure and reaching diagnostic accuracy: some key predictive factors. Med Educ. 2017;51(11):1127–37.
30. Luyt CE, Forel JM, Hajage D, Jaber S, Cayot-Constantin S, Rimmelé T, Coupez E, Lu Q, Diallo MH, Penot-Ragon C, Clavel M. Acyclovir for mechanically ventilated patients with herpes simplex virus oropharyngeal reactivation: a randomized clinical trial. JAMA Intern Med. 2020;180(2):263–72.
31. Moya A, Sutton R. Guidelines for the diagnosis and management of syncope (version 2009): the task force for the diagnosis and management of syncope of the European Society of Cardiology (ESC). Eur Heart J. 2009;30(21):2631–71.
32. O'donnell MJ, Xavier D, Liu L, Zhang H, Chin SL, Rao-Melacini P, Rangarajan S, Islam S, Pais P, McQueen MJ, Mondo C. Risk factors for ischaemic and intracerebral haemorrhagic stroke in 22 countries (the INTERSTROKE study): a case-control study. Lancet. 2010;376(9735):112–23.
33. O'Grady NP, Alexander E, Alhazzani W, Alshamsi F, Cuellar-Rodriguez J, Jefferson BK, Kalil AC, Pastores SM, Patel R, Van Duin D, Weber DJ. Society of Critical Care Medicine and the Infectious Diseases Society of America guidelines for evaluating new fever in adult patients in the ICU. Crit Care Med. 2023;51(11):1570–86.
34. Raadsen M, Du Toit J, Langerak T, van Bussel B, van Gorp E, Goeijenbier M. Thrombocytopenia in virus infections. J Clin Med. 2021;10(4):877.
35. Roberts JI, Jewett GA, Tellier R, Couillard P, Peters S. Twice negative PCR in a patient with herpes simplex virus type 1 (HSV-1) encephalitis. Neurohospitalist. 2021;11(1):66–70.

36. Royce CS, Hayes MM, Schwartzstein RM. Teaching critical thinking: a case for instruction in cognitive biases to reduce diagnostic errors and improve patient safety. Acad Med. 2019;94(2):187–94.
37. Slooter AJ, Otte WM, Devlin JW, Arora RC, Bleck TP, Claassen J, Duprey MS, Ely EW, Kaplan PW, Latronico N, Morandi A. Updated nomenclature of delirium and acute encephalopathy: statement of ten societies. Intensive Care Med. 2020 May;46:1020–2.
38. Tunkel AR, Hartman BJ, Kaplan SL, Kaufman BA, Roos KL, Scheld WM, Whitley RJ. Practice guidelines for the management of bacterial meningitis. Clin Infect Dis. 2004;39(9):1267–84.
39. Vincent JL. Give your patient a fast hug (at least) once a day. Crit Care Med. 2005;33(6):1225–9.
40. Ware LB, Matthay MA. The acute respiratory distress syndrome. N Engl J Med. 2000;342(18):1334–49.
41. Ware LB, Matthay MA. Acute pulmonary edema. N Engl J Med. 2005;353(26):2788–96.
42. Wessels T, Wessels C, Ellsiepen A, Reuter I, Trittmacher S, Stolz E, Jauss M. Contribution of diffusion-weighted imaging in determination of stroke etiology. Am J Neuroradiol. 2006;27(1):35–9.
43. Wintermark M, Sanelli PC, Albers GW, Bello J, Derdeyn C, Hetts SW, Johnson MH, Kidwell C, Lev MH, Liebeskind DS, Rowley H. Imaging recommendations for acute stroke and transient ischemic attack patients: a joint statement by the American Society of Neuroradiology, the American College of Radiology, and the Society of NeuroInterventional Surgery. Am J Neuroradiol. 2013;34(11):E117–27.
44. Winters B, Custer J, Galvagno SM, Colantuoni E, Kapoor SG, Lee H, Goode V, Robinson K, Nakhasi A, Pronovost P, Newman-Toker D. Diagnostic errors in the intensive care unit: a systematic review of autopsy studies. BMJ Qual Saf. 2012;21(11):894–902.
45. Zwaan L, de Bruijne M, Wagner C, Thijs A, Smits M, van der Wal G, Timmermans DR. Patient record review of the incidence, consequences, and causes of diagnostic adverse events. Arch Intern Med. 2010;170(12):1015–21.

Chapter 2
Approach to ECG Interpretation in Critical Care

Miguel H. Vicco, Danilo Weir Restrepo, Shyla Gupta, Juan M. Farina, Leandro Luis Pozzer, Fernanda Tavares-Da-Silva, Sebastián Garcia-Zamora, Alejandro Narváez Orozco, Andres F. Miranda-Arboleda, and Adrián Baranchuk

2.1 Introduction

Since 2015, Advanced Cardiac Life Support guidelines have emphasized the importance of pharmacists being involved in cardiac emergencies to minimize the risk of medication-related errors, drug adverse reactions, and mortality [1, 2]. Based on

M. H. Vicco
Drug Safety Lead, Organon BV, Brussels, Belgium

D. W. Restrepo
Internal Medicine Resident, CES University, Medellín, Colombia

S. Gupta
Faculty of Medicine, University of Ottawa, Ottawa, ON, Canada

J. M. Farina
Division of Cardiothoracic Surgery, Mayo Clinic, Phoenix, AZ, USA

L. L. Pozzer
Section of Cardiac Electrophysiology, Buenos Aires Cardiovascular Institute, Buenos Aires, Argentina

F. Tavares-Da-Silva
Drug Safety, Organon BV, Brussels, Belgium

S. Garcia-Zamora
Coronary Care Unit, Delta Clinic, Rosario, Argentina

A. N. Orozco
University of Antioquia, Medellín, Colombia

A. F. Miranda-Arboleda
Brigham and Women's Hospital, Harvard Medical School, Boston, MA, USA

A. Baranchuk (✉)
Division of Cardiology, Queen's University, Kingston, ON, Canada
e-mail: Adrian.Baranchuk@kingstonhsc.ca

this, the Heart Rhythm Society's 2015 Statement on Clinical Cardiac Electrophysiology suggests that pharmacists should be trained in electrocardiogram (ECG) interpretation [2].

It is worth noting that not all pharmacists will practice in acute care settings. However, considering the growing involvement of pharmacists in the care of patients diagnosed with cardiovascular disease or at risk of developing it, understanding electrocardiograms (ECGs) is important. Moreover, given the relevance of drug-induced ECG alterations, pharmacists must be capable of independent ECG interpretation. The goal of this chapter is to provide a reference tool for pharmacists on ECG normal parameters and main ECG abnormalities concerning for the pharmacists involved in patient care in different settings.

2.2 Normal Conduction System and Physiology

To accurately interpret an ECG, it is imperative to have a comprehensive understanding of the heart's electrical system [3, 4].

Two key characteristics of the heart include its intrinsic capability to produce electrical impulses independently, a phenomenon known as automaticity, and its unique electrical structure, consisting of the sinoatrial (SA) node, the atrioventricular (AV) node, and the His-Purkinje system [3, 4]. Cardiac cells demonstrate a degree of specialization, with some cells being better at generating electrical signals (such as those in the SA and AV nodes), some being more conductive (like those in the His-Purkinje system), and some being primarily responsible for contraction (the muscular cells).

Typically, the cardiac cycle begins at the SA node, which acts as the pacemaker [3, 4]. From there, the electrical signal travels to the AV node, which serves as the only pathway for the impulses to reach the ventricles under normal circumstances. The AV node acts as a filter, preventing abnormal impulses from reaching the ventricles. Following the AV node, the His-Purkinje system takes over, specializing in the conduction of impulses. This system is divided into the right bundle branch and the left bundle branch. The left bundle branch splits into the anterior, septal, and posterior fascicles. Finally, the His-Purkinje system further divides into numerous microfibers, ensuring that the electrical impulse reaches the entire inner surface of the ventricles almost simultaneously.

The generation and propagation of electrical signals in cardiac cells are facilitated by their ability to control the opening and closing of numerous ion channels present in their membranes [3, 4]. The typical structure of a cellular membrane is composed of a lipid bilayer, which typically does not allow the passage of sodium, potassium, and calcium ions. As a result of the concentration differences of different electrolytes across the cellular membrane, an electrical gradient is formed. This creates a negatively charged interior environment within the cell and a positively charged exterior environment surrounding the cell. Depending on the specific type of cardiac cell, the ion channels possess a complex structure. These ion channels will exhibit distinct resting electrical gradients and properties (Table 2.1). However, despite these differences, they all share a common characteristic. When activated, they undergo a temporary alteration in the charge across their membrane, resulting in the generation of an action potential.

This normal action potential can be illustrated in five phases (Fig. 2.1):

- Phase 4—Resting membrane potential.
- Phase 0—Rapid depolarization.

Table 2.1 Types of ion channels and their function

Voltage-gated sodium channels (Na^+):
Predominantly found in cardiac myocytes.
During the initial phase of the cardiac cycle, voltage-gated sodium channels play a pivotal role in depolarizing cardiac myocytes.
Upon membrane depolarization, these channels rapidly open, allowing an influx of sodium ions into the cell (phase 0), resulting in the rapid upstroke of the action potential.
This depolarization phase initiates myocardial contraction and facilitates the propagation of electrical impulses throughout the heart.
L-type calcium channels (Ca^{2+}):
Expressed in cardiac myocytes and cardiac pacemaker cells.
L-type calcium channels are critical for sustaining myocardial contraction during the plateau phase of the action potential.
Upon activation by membrane depolarization, these channels facilitate calcium influx into cardiac myocytes (phase 2), leading to an increase in intracellular calcium concentration.
Elevated intracellular calcium triggers the release of additional calcium from the sarcoplasmic reticulum, facilitating excitation-contraction coupling and promoting myocardial contraction.
Voltage-gated potassium channels (K^+):
Abundantly present in cardiac myocytes.
Voltage-gated potassium channels are responsible for repolarizing cardiac myocytes during the latter phases of the cardiac cycle.
Following depolarization, these channels open, allowing potassium efflux from the cell, thereby restoring the negative resting membrane potential (phases 1, 2, and 3).
Repolarization of the cardiac myocytes enables myocardial relaxation and prepares the heart for subsequent contraction.
Inward rectifier potassium channels (Kir):
Predominantly expressed in cardiac pacemaker cells.
Inward rectifier potassium channels play a role in stabilizing the resting membrane potential and modulating pacemaker activity in cardiac pacemaker cells.
These channels permit potassium influx during membrane hyperpolarization, contributing to the maintenance of the resting membrane potential and the regulation of the pacemaker firing rate.
By modulating the excitability of pacemaker cells, inward rectifier potassium channels contribute to the initiation and regulation of the cardiac rhythm.
Ryanodine receptors (RyRs):
Ryanodine receptors are located on the sarcoplasmic reticulum in cardiac myocytes and play a crucial role in calcium-induced calcium release.
Activation of RyR channels leads to the release of calcium ions from intracellular stores in response to increased intracellular calcium concentration.
This calcium release mechanism facilitates excitation-contraction coupling, ensuring synchronized myocardial contraction and effective ejection of blood from the ventricles.

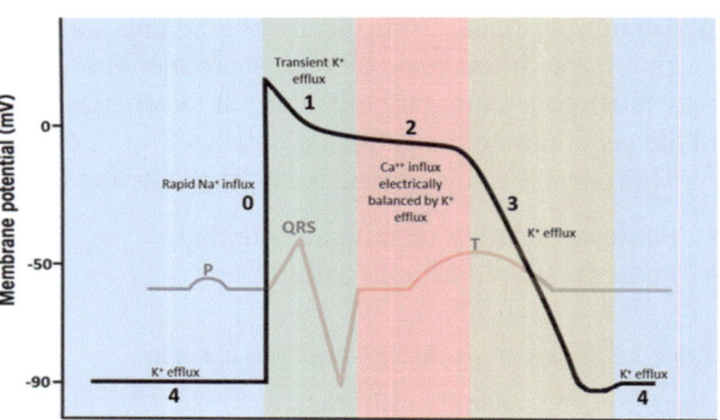

Fig. 2.1 Phases of the normal action potential and its correlation with the cardiac cycle in the ECG

- Phase 1—Early repolarization.
- Phase 2—Plateau.
- Phase 3—Rapid repolarization.

2.3 Formation of the 12-Lead ECG

The ECG is a visual representation detailing the spatial orientation and electrical activity produced during the depolarization and repolarization phases of the heart's atria and ventricles [3–5]. This electrical activity is captured by electrodes affixed to the skin. For example, if the electrical vector is approaching the electrode, this results in a positive deflection on the ECG. Inversely, if the electrical activity moves away from the electrode, this results in a negative deflection on the ECG. If the "observer" electrode is in the middle and first sees it approaching and then moving away, a signal will be drawn initially positive and then negative.

The conventional 12-lead ECG is obtained by placing 10 electrodes on the patient:

- Four limb electrodes (located in the vertical or frontal plane axis) are placed on the right arm (red), left arm (yellow), right leg (black), and left leg (green). These electrodes will give rise to six leads, i.e., I, II, and III (bipolar leads) and aVR, aVL, and aVF (unipolar leads).
- Six precordial electrodes (located in the horizontal plane axis) which will give rise to the precordial leads V1, V2, V3, V4, V5, and V6 (unipolar) are placed as follows:

  - V1: fourth intercostal space, right parasternal line.
  - V2: fourth intercostal space, left parasternal line.
  - V3: between V2 and V4.
  - V4: fifth intercostal space, left midclavicular line.
  - V5: fifth intercostal space, left anterior axillary line.
  - V6: fifth intercostal space, left midaxillary line.

Each of the 12 leads represents a particular orientation in space, to capture spatial information of the heart's electrical activity in three orthogonal directions, right to left and left to right; superior to inferior and inferior to superior; and anterior to posterior and posterior to anterior [3–5].

The horizontal plane is constituted by the unipolar precordial leads, consisting of a positive electrode that will show the posterior to anterior (V1, V2, and V3) or right to left-lateral (V4, V5, and V6) spatial information of the heart's electrical activity.

In the frontal plane, the 6 leads will constitute the hexaxial reference systems, which measures a copulate circle or 360 degrees around the heart. The hexaxial reference system is a geometric representation used to interpret the direction of the electrical vectors in this plane.

2.4 ECG Nomenclature

A normal ECG (Figs. 2.2 and 2.3) is comprised of the following elements [3–5]:

- Wave: A deviation (deflection) either above (positive) or below (negative) the baseline indicating a distinct electrical occurrence. The ECG depicts several waves, namely P, Q, R, S, T, and U waves.
- Interval: The duration between two ECG waves. Commonly assessed intervals include the PR, QRS (or QRS duration), QT, and RR.

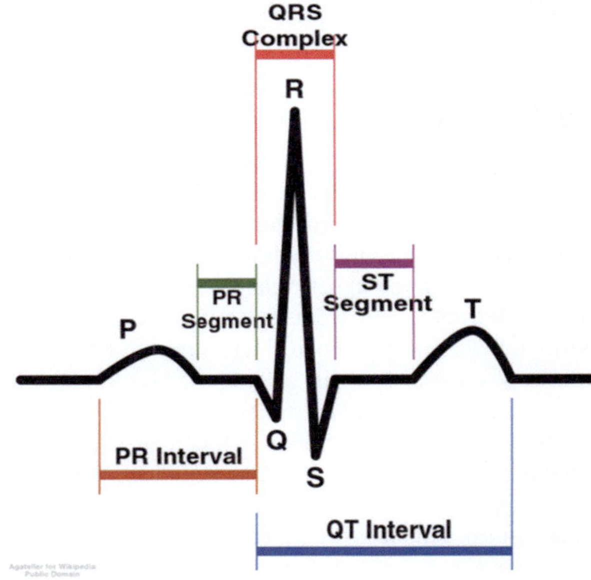

Fig. 2.2 Normal ECG nomenclature, waves, segments, and intervals

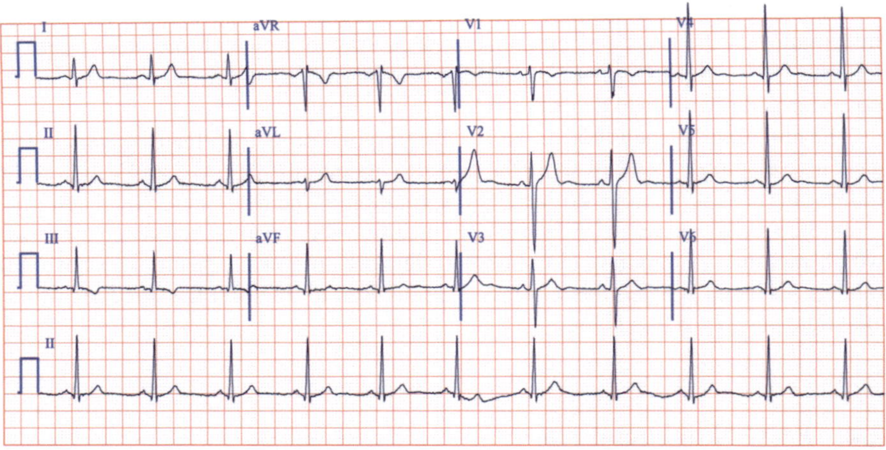

Fig. 2.3 Normal ECG. Nathanson LA, McClennen S, Safran C, Goldberger AL. ECG Wave-Maven: Self-Assessment Program for Students and Clinicians. http://ecg.bidmc.harvard.edu

- Segment: The length between two specific ECG waves that are expected to be at a baseline amplitude (neither positive nor negative). The main segments include the PR and ST segments.
- Complex: A cluster of multiple waves amalgamated together. The principal complex discernible on an ECG is the QRS complex.
- Point: Singularly identified as the J point, this point marks the transition from the QRS complex to the ST segment.

2.4.1 P Wave

The first element observed on an ECG during a normal cardiac cycle is the P wave [3–5]. The P wave represents atrial depolarization. Therefore, its presence indicates that the patient is in sinus rhythm. As a typical atrial impulse begins in the sinoatrial node, situated in the upper right region of the right atrium, the propagation of the activation front occurs from top to bottom and from right to left. This results in a positive P wave in lead I and II and a negative P wave in aVR. Usually, the P wave is also positive in lead III, aVF, and aVL, although this may differ based on the heart's orientation within the chest cavity.

Normal P waves typically last less than 100 ms and have a height of less than 2.5 mm (0.25 mV). Also, they may be bifid, mainly in the precordial leads, because of a slight asynchrony between the depolarization of the right and left atria. The peak-to-peak length is <1 mm, but if longer, this delayed conduction suggests a pathological condition, as the case of interatrial blocks.

2.4.2 PR Interval

The PR interval on an ECG represents the time interval from the beginning of atrial depolarization (start of the P wave) to the beginning of ventricular depolarization (start of the QRS complex) [3–5]. Thus, it reflects the time it takes for the electrical impulse to travel from the atria through the AV node to the Purkinje system, just before ventricular contraction.

The PR interval should not be confused with the PR segment, as the PR segment represents a period of electrical quiescence between atrial and ventricular depolarization. The PR segment extends from the end of the P wave to the beginning of the QRS complex.

The normal PR interval typically ranges from 120 to 210 ms; this duration can vary slightly based on factors such as age or heart rate.

It is important to note that typically, PR interval duration corresponds to the AV node. This is dependent on adrenergic tone, which can slow down or accelerate conduction. Thus, in the context of AV node dysfunction, or medications that alter the normal function of the AV node, the PR interval may also be prolonged.

2.4.3 QRS Complex

The next wave observed on the ECG is the QRS complex which provides information for understanding how electrical activity spreads through both ventricles (ventricular depolarization) [3–5].

The QRS complex represents a combination of three waves: Q for the first negative deflection, R for the first positive deflection, and S for the second negative deflection, with subsequent positive or negative deflections marked as R' or r' and S' or s'. A normal QRS complex can start with a Q wave that is not wider than 40 ms or 30% of the QRS height. A normal Q wave typically appears without notches and separates sharply from the baseline. The R wave is usually taller in limb leads compared to precordial leads. The characteristics of each wave constituting the QRS complex can be summarized as follows:

The QRS interval is usually narrow (<100 ms) due to rapid simultaneous activation of both ventricles. However, if there is a blockage in the conduction system, a myocardial scar, or other conditions, it may widen (>120 ms). Besides its length, it is important to determine its axis as it reveals crucial information regarding the orientation of cardiac electrical activity within the body. Deviations from the normal axis serve as pivotal indicators of diverse cardiac pathologies, including ventricular hypertrophy, bundle branch blocks, or myocardial infarction. Under normal circumstances, the normal axis falls between −15° and +105°. The QRS axis is calculated by examining the net direction of electrical depolarization in the heart during ventricular activation, which is primarily represented by the QRS complex on an ECG. There are several methods to determine the QRS axis; however, the most used ones are the following:

1. Quadrant method: This approach involves plotting the net QRS vectors from leads I and aVF on a graph with two axes, with one representing lead I and the other representing lead aVF. The intersection of these vectors indicates the approximate location of the QRS axis.
2. Isodirectional method: In this method, the leads showing the most isoelectric QRS complexes (neither predominantly positive nor negative) are identified. By determining the lead with the isoelectric QRS complex and observing its relation to other leads, the QRS axis can be estimated.

Abnormal axis deviation, indicating the underlying pathology, can be schematically divided into the following categories:

- Left axis deviation = QRS axis less than $-30°$.
- Right axis deviation = QRS axis greater than $+90°$.
- Extreme axis deviation = QRS axis between $-90°$ and $180°$.

In summary, understanding the characteristics of the Q, R, and S waves on an ECG is essential for accurate interpretation. While these waves often exhibit normal variations, pathological changes may indicate underlying cardiac abnormalities such as myocardial infarction, hypertrophy, or conduction disturbances.

2.4.4   J Point

The J point represents the junction between the termination of the QRS complex and the beginning of the ST segment [3–5]. It holds significant clinical relevance as it serves as a reference point for assessing myocardial depolarization and initiation of ventricular repolarization.

Under normal physiological conditions, the J point should be precisely aligned with the baseline (isoelectric), indicating that ventricular depolarization has been completed, and repolarization is commencing.

However, deviations from this normative pattern can occur, potentially indicating pathological processes, such as the following:

- ST-segment elevation: A J point that is elevated above the baseline by at least 1 mm (mV) in two contiguous leads (or 2.5 mm in V2–V3 in men under 40 years, or 2 mm in men over 40 years or in women) is indicative of ST-segment elevation. This finding is often associated with acute myocardial infarction (AMI) and requires urgent medical attention.
- ST-segment depression: Conversely, J point depression and an ST segment below the baseline may be considered pathological if it exceeds 0.5 mm in two contiguous leads. This finding can indicate myocardial ischemia and may be observed in conditions such as unstable angina or non-ST-segment elevation myocardial infarction (NSTEMI). ST-segment depression may also occur in other nonischemic conditions such as left ventricular hypertrophy or the digitalis effect.

Prompt recognition of ST-segment deviations is crucial for timely intervention and management to minimize myocardial damage.

It is imperative to meticulously identify deviations from the normal J point, as they may be crucial indicators of underlying cardiac pathology or ischemic events. Differential diagnoses should be considered based on the clinical context, accompanying symptoms, and additional ECG findings to determine appropriate management strategies and interventions.

2.4.5 ST Segment

The ST segment reflects the period between ventricular depolarization (end of the QRS complex) and repolarization [3–5]. It extends from the J point to the onset of the T wave. Understanding the normal characteristics and recognizing pathological changes in the ST segment are essential for accurate interpretation and diagnosis in clinical practice.

2.4.6 T Wave

T waves follow the QRS complex and reflect the electrical recovery of the ventricles as they prepare for the next cardiac cycle [3–5]. The T wave is typically a smooth, rounded waveform with upward deflection in most leads, though variations in morphology can occur. It corresponds to the phase of ventricular repolarization, during which potassium ions exit the cardiac myocytes. This leads to cellular relaxation and restoration of the electrical potential. Clinically, abnormalities in the T-wave morphology or duration can indicate underlying cardiac pathology or electrolyte imbalances.

The duration of the T wave is generally less than 0.2 seconds (or 200 ms), and its voltage varies widely among individuals and leads. A typical T-wave voltage range is 0.5–5 millivolts (mV), but higher voltages can be observed in certain pathological conditions such as ventricular hypertrophy.

Abnormalities such as flattening, inversion, or prominent peaked T waves may indicate underlying cardiac pathology, for example:

- T-wave inversion: Inverted T waves can be indicative of myocardial ischemia, injury, or infarction. They may also occur in the setting of electrolyte imbalances (e.g., hypokalemia), left ventricular hypertrophy, or conduction abnormalities.
- Peaked T waves: Tall, peaked T waves may suggest ischemia or hyperkalemia, especially in the setting of acute kidney injury or metabolic acidosis. Peaked T waves are considered a medical emergency and require immediate attention to prevent life-threatening arrhythmias.
- Flattened T waves: Flattened T waves may be nonspecific but can be associated with myocardial ischemia, electrolyte disturbances, or early repolarization patterns.

2.4.7　QT Interval

The QT interval on an ECG represents the duration of ventricular depolarization and repolarization [3–5]. It begins at the onset of the QRS complex and ends at the termination of the T wave, encompassing the total electrical activity of ventricular contraction and relaxation. Thus, it corresponds to the period when the ventricles contract (systole) and then relax (diastole) before the next cardiac cycle.

Normal QT intervals vary depending on age, sex, and heart rate. In adults, a normal QT interval is typically less than 450 ms for men and less than 460 ms for women, according to consensus when the heart rate (HR) is between 60 and 100 beats per minute. QT interval values outside this range may be considered abnormal and warrant further evaluation. Given the dependence of QT interval duration on heart rate, it is crucial to correct QT interval variations based on abnormal heart rates using formulas such as Bazett's, Fridericia's, or other validated methods. QT correction helps standardize QT interval interpretation across different heart rates.

Bazett's correction formula is still utilized by many clinicians worldwide; however, the formula is most accurate between the heart rates of 60 and 100 bpm. At heart rates of less than 60 bpm, the formula under-corrects the QTc value, while at HR values over 100 bpm, the formula overcorrects the QTc interval. Due to this limitation, other formulas have been proposed:

- Bazett's formula: $QTc = QT/[\sqrt{RR}$ in seconds] [6].
- Fridericia's formula: $QTc = QT/(RR\ 0.33)$ [6]
- Framingham's formula: $QTc = QT + 0.154(1 - RR)$ [6]
- Hodges's formula: $QTc = QT + 1.75(HR - 60)$ [6]

Prolongation of the QT interval can predispose individuals to life-threatening arrhythmias such as polymorphic ventricular tachycardia and ventricular fibrillation, increasing the risk of sudden cardiac death [7, 8]. The causes of QT prolongation include congenital long QT syndrome, electrolyte imbalances (e.g., hypokalemia and hypomagnesemia), certain medications (e.g., antiarrhythmics and psychotropic drugs), and myocardial ischemia (Table 2.2).

Table 2.2 Drugs associated with QTc prolongation and polymorphic ventricular tachycardia [7, 8]

Antiarrhythmics	Antimicrobials	Antidepressants	Antipsychotics	Others
Amiodarone	Levofloxacin	Amitriptyline	Haloperidol	Cisapride
Sotalol	Ciprofloxacin	Desipramine	Droperidol	Sumatriptan
Quinidine	Gatifloxacin	Imipramine	Quetiapine	Zolmitriptan
Procainamide	Moxifloxacin	Doxepin	Thioridazine	Arsenic
Dofetilide	Clarithromycin	Fluoxetine	Ziprasidone	Dolasetron
Ibutilide	Erythromycin	Sertraline		Methadone
	Ketoconazole	Venlafaxine		
	Itraconazole			

Conversely, shortening of the QT interval may occur in hypercalcemia, in hyperthyroidism, or following cardiac sympathectomy. The short QT syndrome is an inherited cardiac channelopathy much less common than the long QT syndrome. Regardless of its etiology, short QT syndrome is also associated with an increased risk of arrhythmias and sudden cardiac death.

2.4.8 U Wave

The U wave is a small, often subtle deflection, low in amplitude, seen following the T wave. It is most prominent in leads V2–V4 but may be present in other leads as well [3–5]. The precise physiological origin of the U wave is not fully understood, but it is believed to reflect the repolarization of the papillary muscles and Purkinje fibers of the ventricles. While the U wave is commonly observed in normal ECGs, its clinical significance is less well defined compared to other ECG components.

2.4.9 RR Interval

The RR interval represents the interval between consecutive R waves, reflecting the duration of one complete cardiac cycle. Its duration varies based on heart rate; shorter intervals correspond to faster heart rates, while longer intervals indicate slower heart rates [3–5]. In adults with a normal sinus rhythm, the RR interval typically ranges from 1000 to 600 ms (50–100 beats per minute).

2.5 Approach to ECG Interpretation Using the "Left-to-Right Approach"

Reading an ECG involves a systematic approach from left to right, examining various components to assess cardiac rhythm, conduction, and morphology [3–5].

The process begins by identifying the paper speed and calibration marks on the ECG strip. The standard paper speed is 25 mm/s horizontally and 10 mm/mV vertically. The calibration marks indicate the standardization of voltage measurements. Each small square typically represents 1 mm or 0.1 mV vertically, while each large square represents 5 mm or 0.5 mV.

After checking the speed and calibration, the initial focus lies on assessing technical aspects such as filters, patient's name, and lead placement. Then attention starts by focusing on rhythm and frequency. The normal rhythm is sinus rhythm, characterized by a regular RR interval and upright P waves preceding each QRS complex. Normal HR falls within the range of 60–100 bpm, although it can be higher in young children and lower in athletes or individuals with elevated vagal tone. It is calculated by measuring the distance between R waves (RR interval) with the formula:

- HR = 60/RR interval (in seconds).

For example, if the RR interval is 0.8 seconds, the HR would be calculated as:

- HR = 60/0.8; HR = 75 bpm.

Various drugs can inhibit or impair sinus node and conduction system function through various pharmacological mechanisms. Common drugs in critical care associated with bradyarrhythmia include opioid analgesics, anticonvulsants, antihistaminics, antipsychotics, benzodiazepines, steroids, and sedatives such as dexmedetomidine.

The next step is to determine if the electrical activation follows a normal pattern, which is done by assessing each of the elements that constitute the heart cycle. For this, the left-to-right approach can be used.

2.5.1 P Wave

When assessing the P wave, it is useful to consider if P waves are present, if the P wave originates from the sinus node, if there are multiple P wave morphologies, if the P waves are regular, and the P wave rate [3–5].

As the normal atrial impulse originates from the sinus node (located in the upper right part of the right atrium), the activation front will propagate downward and from right to left. Therefore, the P wave is usually positive in lead II, which is the best lead for assessing the presence of the P wave and its regularity on the ECG. If P waves are not visible, then it could be because they are absent or hidden (blended with other ECG waves).

Once the presence of P waves is determined, the wave should be analyzed to see if its origin is the sinus node. A P wave originating from the sinus node typically has a smooth, rounded morphology with a duration of ≤0.12 seconds (120 ms). Abnormalities in the left atrium, such as dilation, can sometimes be detected by assessing the morphology of the P wave. Lead V1 is particularly informative in evaluating the condition of the left atrium. In this lead, the P wave often exhibits a biphasic pattern, with the initial positive deflection originating from the right atrium.

The axis of the P wave (the direction of its electrical vector) can provide clues about its origin. A P wave with a normal axis (upright in lead II, biphasic, or inverted in lead aVR) is suggestive of a sinus node origin. Deviations from this axis may indicate ectopic atrial depolarization. In addition, the P wave precedes the QRS complex consistently. This reflects the physiological sequence of atrial depolarization preceding ventricular depolarization. Any variation from this pattern may indicate an abnormal atrial depolarization site.

2.5.1.1 Atrial Arrhythmias

Atrial Fibrillation

Atrial fibrillation (AF) (Fig. 2.4) is the most common sustained arrhythmia and can manifest as paroxysmal or persistent [9, 10]. In paroxysmal AF, the onset and termination of episodes may be visible on an ECG or more commonly on a Holter monitor. Within the atria, there is chaotic electrical activity, characterized by very rapid activations exceeding 300 cycles per minute. These impulses irregularly reach the AV node, which regulates their passage to the His-Purkinje system to safeguard ventricular hemodynamics. Consequently, the ventricular response appears irregularly irregular. While AF typically results in narrow QRS tachycardia, widened QRS complexes may occur due to bundle branch block or the presence of an accessory pathway.

In the absence of an accessory pathway, the number of impulses conducted to the ventricles depends on the "strictness" of the AV node, determined by its anatomical characteristics and medications. Agents such as beta-blockers and calcium channel blockers are primarily used to slow AV nodal conduction. Digoxin also affects AV nodal conduction but is considered a weaker agent. This approach, termed rate control strategy, manages the heart rate. Alternatively, the rhythm control strategy aims to restore and maintain sinus rhythm. Electrical cardioversion is the most effective method for restoring sinus rhythm, especially in unstable patients. Pharmacological agents (e.g., amiodarone, vernakalant, flecainide, or propafenone) may also be used, particularly for recent-onset AF, in stable patients.

Furthermore, several drug classes are linked to AF development, including inotropic agents (e.g., dobutamine, dopamine, and levosimendan), antiarrhythmics (e.g., adenosine, amiodarone, atenolol, digoxin, diltiazem, and verapamil), as well

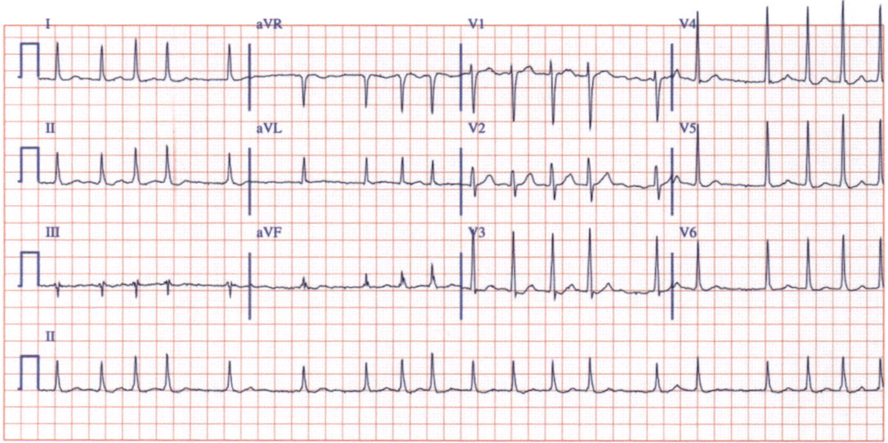

Fig. 2.4 Atrial fibrillation Nathanson LA, McClennen S, Safran C, Goldberger AL. ECG Wave-Maven: Self-Assessment Program for Students and Clinicians. http://ecg.bidmc.harvard.edu

as medications frequently used in critical care medicine (e.g., aminophylline, theophylline, albuterol, aformoterol, corticosteroids, fluticasone, ipratropium, pseudoephedrine, salmeterol, and atropine) [9, 10].

Returning to the ECG, while an irregularly irregular HR is typical of AF, other rapid atrial arrhythmias may produce a similar ventricular response pattern, such as atypical flutter, atrial tachycardias, or typical flutter in certain circumstances. Adenosine administration or carotid sinus massage may aid in clarifying the ECG by enhancing visualization of atrial activity and separating QRS complexes.

Atrial Flutter

Atrial flutter (AFL) (Fig. 2.5) is a supraventricular tachyarrhythmia characterized by regular atrial depolarizations at rates typically between 240 and 340 bpm [11]. AFL shares similarities with AF but differs in its distinct pattern of atrial activation. The underlying mechanism of AFL involves reentry circuits within the atria, most commonly revolving around the tricuspid annulus. Macro-reentry loops perpetuate rapid and organized atrial depolarizations, leading to the characteristic sawtooth pattern on ECG. Unlike the fibrillation waves in AF, flutter waves in atrial flutter have a more organized appearance.

Atrial Tachycardia

Atrial tachycardia (AT) is a common cardiac arrhythmia characterized by rapid, abnormal electrical activity originating from the atria, leading to an increased heart rate [12]. It poses significant clinical implications due to its association with symptoms such as

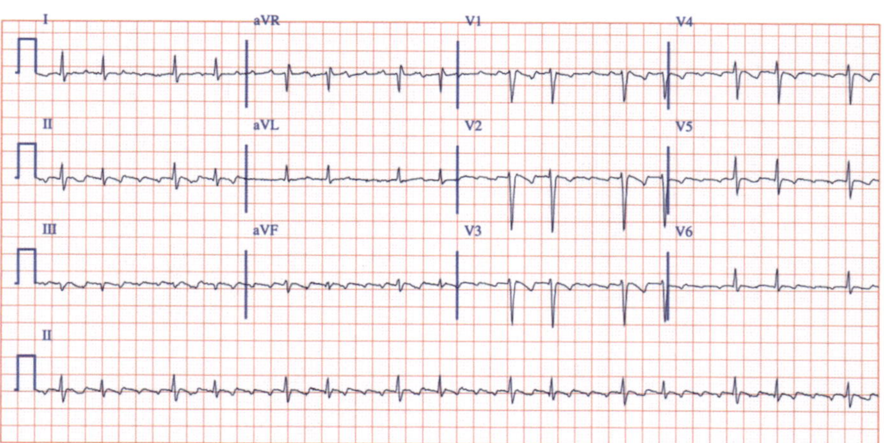

Fig. 2.5 Atrial flutter Nathanson LA, McClennen S, Safran C, Goldberger AL. ECG Wave-Maven: Self-Assessment Program for Students and Clinicians. http://ecg.bidmc.harvard.edu

palpitations, dyspnea, and potential hemodynamic compromise. Early and accurate diagnosis is essential for appropriate management and prevention of complications. AT typically arises from abnormal automaticity or triggered activity within the atrial myocardium. AT may also result from reentry circuits involving anatomical or functional abnormalities. Mechanisms underlying AT include enhanced automaticity of atrial cells, focal ectopic beats originating from specific sites, or micro-reentrant circuits within the atria. Factors such as sympathetic stimulation, electrolyte imbalances, structural heart disease, and ischemia can predispose individuals to AT.

The ECG serves as the foundation for diagnosing AT. Specific ECG criteria aid in distinguishing AT from other supraventricular arrhythmias. The following features are the characteristics of AT [3–5]:

- P-wave morphology: In AT, P waves may exhibit abnormal shapes, durations, and morphologies compared to sinus rhythm. Sometimes, P waves may blend into the preceding or following T waves, making them difficult to distinguish.
- Atrial rate: AT typically presents with a regular atrial rate ranging from 100 to 250 bpm.
- P-wave morphology in different leads: Variability in P-wave morphology across different leads indicates multifocal or chaotic atrial activity, characteristic of AT.

Multifocal Atrial Tachycardia

Multifocal atrial tachycardia (MAT) (Fig. 2.6) is a distinct form of supraventricular tachyarrhythmia characterized by irregular atrial activity originating from multiple ectopic foci within the atria [12]. Its diagnosis poses challenges due to its variable presentation and similarity to other atrial arrhythmias. The pathogenesis of MAT involves enhanced automaticity and triggered activity in atrial cells, often

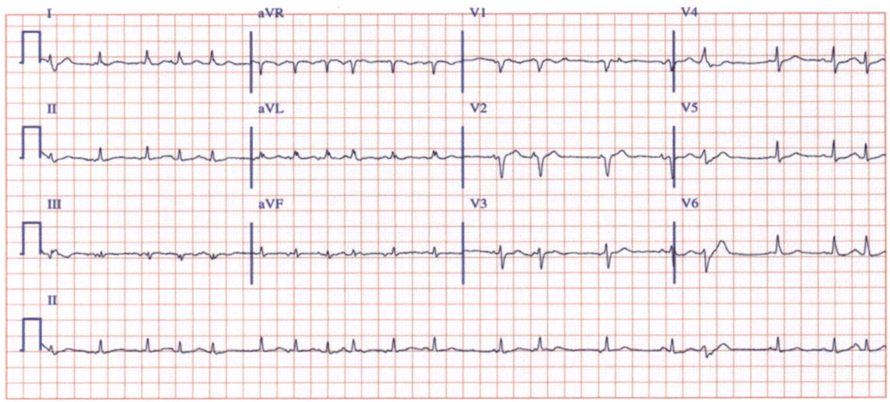

Fig. 2.6 Multifocal atrial tachycardia Nathanson LA, McClennen S, Safran C, Goldberger AL. ECG Wave-Maven: Self-Assessment Program for Students and Clinicians. http://ecg.bidmc. harvard.edu

exacerbated by underlying pulmonary or systemic disorders. Factors such as hypoxia, acid-base imbalances, sympathetic stimulation, and electrolyte disturbances contribute to the development of ectopic foci within the atria. These foci generate rapid and irregular atrial impulses.

The following electrocardiographic criteria aid in the identification of MAT:

- Irregular RR intervals: MAT is characterized by irregularity in the ventricular response due to the variable atrial depolarizations originating from multiple ectopic foci.
- Variable P-wave morphology: P waves in MAT exhibit diverse morphologies, amplitudes, and durations, reflecting the asynchronous atrial activity originating from different sites within the atria.

2.5.1.2 Interatrial Blocks

Interatrial block (IAB) is a distinct electrocardiographic pattern describing the conduction delay between the right and left atria, through Bachmann's bundle [13–17]. Because of the above, the ECG shows a P wave of $\geq$120 ms in leads II, III, and aVF (P wave must be measured from the earliest detection of the P wave in any lead [onset] to the last one [offset]).

Identification of IAB is important as different studies have demonstrated its association with the development of AF, stroke, cognitive impairment, and mortality. Of note, the association between IAB and SVT, particularly AF, has been named Bayes' syndrome. According to the duration and morphology of the P wave, it is classified into three groups:

Partial Interatrial Block (P-IAB)

This is also called first-degree IAB and manifests as a P-wave duration $\geq$120 ms without a negative terminal component in the inferior leads.

Intermittent Interatrial Block (I-IAB)

It is also known as second-degree IAB and represents an intermediate phase of IAB with variable transitions between normal and partial or advanced IAB. P-wave morphology changes may appear after a premature beat-induced pause (known as atrial aberrancy), suggesting a rate-dependent manifestation of IAB.

Advanced Interatrial Block (A-IAB)

This is also termed third-degree IAB and occurs because the sinus impulse is completely blocked in Bachmann's bundle, and therefore, the left atrium is depolarized retrogradely via muscular bundles located close to the AV junction. Therefore, P

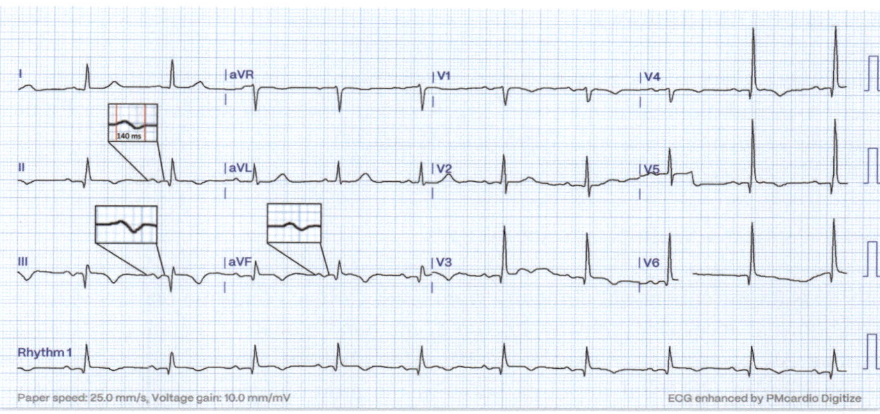

Fig. 2.7 Advanced interatrial block P-wave duration <120 ms with biphasic P wave in leads II, III, and aVF. Personal archive

wave is longer than 120 ms, and its morphology exhibits a biphasic configuration in the inferior leads (Fig. 2.7).

There are atypical patterns of A-IAB such as P-wave duration that is slightly shorter than 120 ms or P-wave morphology without the typical biphasic pattern in all inferior leads. Accordingly, it can be classified as follows:

2.5.2   P-QRS Ratio

After assessing the P waves, the next step is to determine the P-QRS ratio [18]. The P-QRS ratio provides valuable information about the conduction time between the atria and the ventricles in the heart. Normally, there is a consistent relationship between the duration of the P wave (atrial depolarization) and the duration of the QRS complex (ventricular depolarization), P-QRS = 1.

Abnormalities in the P-QRS ratio may indicate certain cardiac conditions or conduction disturbances:

2.5.2.1   Shortened P-QRS Ratio

A shortened P-QRS ratio (P-QRS < 1) may suggest ventricular rhythms because the electrical impulse originates from the ventricles and the QRS complex is often widened and prolonged [3–5]. As a result, the P-QRS index is less than 1, indicating a higher frequency of ventricular impulses compared to atrial impulses.

2.5.2.2 P-QRS Ratio = 1

Although P-QRS = 1 is a characteristic of the normal sinus rhythm; it can also be present in pathological conditions [18]. A special situation arises when a P-QRS ratio = 1 is accompanied by a shortened PR interval.

Wolff-Parkinson-White Syndrome (WPW)

WPW is an infrequent but clinically significant cardiac condition characterized by an abnormal accessory pathway, known as the bundle of Kent, which bypasses the normal AV conduction system [3–5, 19]. This aberrant pathway allows for rapid conduction of electrical impulses between the atria and ventricles, predisposing individuals to various arrhythmias, including supraventricular tachycardia and atrial fibrillation. The characteristics of ECG findings include a shortened PR interval, a widened QRS complex with a slurred initial upstroke called a delta wave, and a relatively short RR interval during tachyarrhythmias (Fig. 2.8).

Junctional Rhythm

In junctional rhythm, the electrical impulse originates from the AV junction (around the AV node or the bundle of His), bypassing the SA node. This leads to atrial depolarization and subsequent P wave being absent, or if present, it may appear retrograde (inverted) or buried within the QRS complex. The junctional impulse then directly activates the ventricles, resulting in ventricular depolarization (QRS complex). Again, due to the direct conduction from the AV junction to the ventricles,

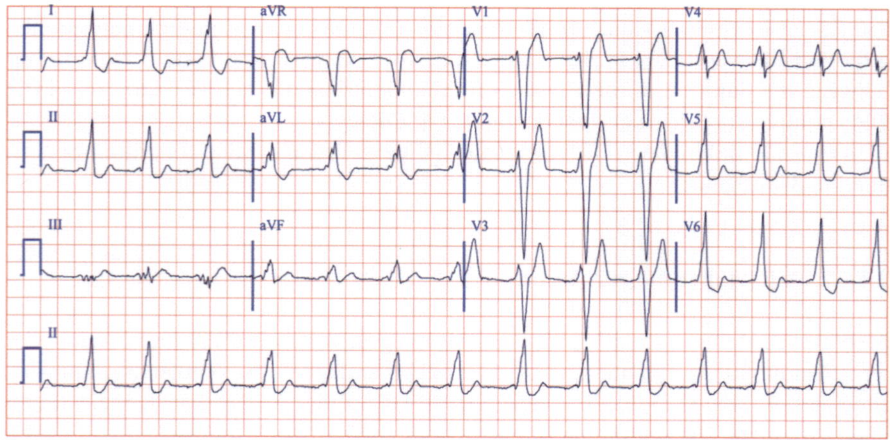

Fig. 2.8 Wolff-Parkinson-White. Nathanson LA, McClennen S, Safran C, Goldberger AL. ECG Wave-Maven: Self-Assessment Program for Students and Clinicians. http://ecg.bidmc.harvard.edu

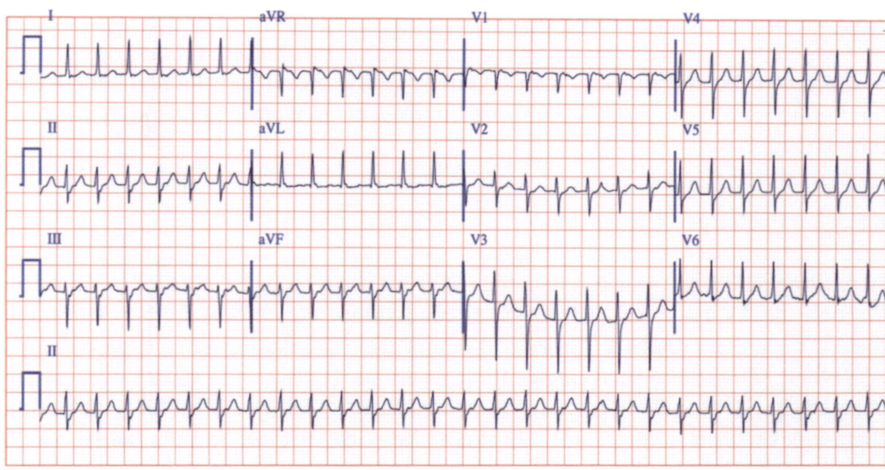

Fig. 2.9 Atrioventricular nodal reentrant tachycardia. Nathanson LA, McClennen S, Safran C, Goldberger AL. ECG Wave-Maven: Self-Assessment Program for Students and Clinicians. http://ecg.bidmc.harvard.edu

there is a 1:1 relationship between atrial (if present) and ventricular depolarization, resulting in a P-QRS index of 1.

Atrioventricular Nodal Reentrant Tachycardia (AVNRT)

AVNRT is a supraventricular tachyarrhythmia characterized by reentrant conduction within the AV node (Fig. 2.9). In AVNRT, there is typically a narrow QRS complex tachycardia with a regular rhythm and absent P waves or retrograde P waves occurring shortly after the QRS complex (RP interval < PR interval). Again, due to the rapid and direct conduction from the AV node to the ventricles, there is typically a 1:1 relationship between atrial and ventricular depolarization, resulting in a P-QRS = 1.

2.5.2.3 Prolonged P-QRS Ratio

Conversely, a prolonged P-QRS ratio (P-QRS > 1) may indicate delayed conduction through the AV node (see next section). This variability can provide additional diagnostic clues regarding the underlying rhythm disorder [20].

2.5.3 PR Interval

The PR interval on an ECG reflects the time it takes for the electrical impulse to travel from the atria through the AV node and into the ventricles. Variations in the PR interval indicate abnormalities in AV conduction. We can schematically divide it into the following [20].

2.5.3.1 Shortened PR Interval

A shortened PR interval (less than 120 ms) is indicative of accelerated conduction through the AV node, often seen in conditions such as Wolff-Parkinson-White syndrome (Fig. 2.8).

2.5.3.2 Prolonged PR Interval

A prolonged PR interval (greater than 200 ms) may suggest delayed conduction through the AV node. Overall, delayed conduction of electrical impulses through the AV node that creates a PR interval longer than 200 ms is known as first-degree AV block. This delay may arise due to various factors, including degenerative changes in the conduction system, medications affecting AV nodal conduction (beta-blockers, calcium channel blockers, digoxin), electrolyte imbalances, vagal stimulus, or myocardial ischemia.

2.5.3.3 Second-Degree AV Block

It represents a more advanced conduction abnormality. Second-degree AV block can be further divided into.

Mobitz Type I (Wenckebach)

There is a progressive prolongation of the PR interval until a P wave is not conducted. This is usually followed by a shorter PR interval, and the cycle starts over. On an ECG, there are a series of PR intervals that become progressively longer, while the RR interval becomes shorter until a QRS complex is dropped. This can be usually seen in normal hearts and does not necessarily imply a pathological finding [21].

Mobitz Type II

It is characterized by intermittent non-conducted P waves without progressive prolongation of the PR interval. This presents as regular PR intervals with occasional dropped QRS complexes (Fig. 2.10). This finding is almost always pathologic and deserves further investigation.

Advanced AV Block

This group encompasses the 2:1 AV block, where for every two P waves, only one is conducted to the ventricles [13–17]. This results in a 2:1 ratio of P waves to QRS complexes, and more extreme forms of AV block, where three or more P waves are observed for each QRS (i.e., 3:1, 4:1, 5:1 AV block), also known as high-degree AV

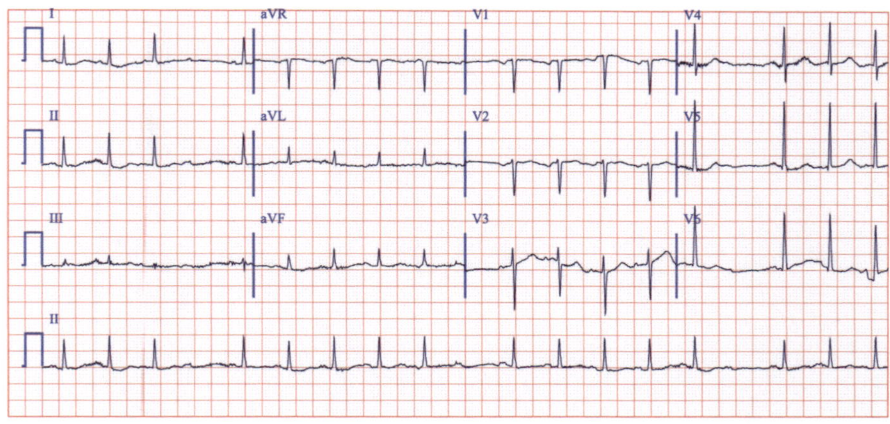

Fig. 2.10 Mobitz II second-degree AV block. Nathanson LA, McClennen S, Safran C, Goldberger AL. ECG Wave-Maven: Self-Assessment Program for Students and Clinicians. http://ecg.bidmc.harvard.edu

block. These types of blocks exhibit a great risk of progressing into a complete heart block.

Third-Degree AV Block (Complete Heart Block)

In third-degree AV block, there is complete dissociation between atrial and ventricular activity, which means that the atria activity is not conducted to ventricles. This implies that on the ECG, P waves occur at their own regular rate. Alternatively, QRS complexes (ventricular activity) occur at a slower rate, often regular but independent of atrial activity. Ventricular beats originate in the AV node (supra- or intra-Hisian), which causes the QRS to be narrow (Fig. 2.11), or below the AV node, which makes the QRS wide (the most frequent presentation in adults).

2.5.4   PR Segment

The PR segment, situated between the end of the P wave and the onset of the QRS complex on the ECG tracing, serves as a crucial interval for assessing AV conduction. Alterations in the PR segment, such as depression or elevation, can indicate underlying cardiac pathology.

2.5.4.1   PR-Segment Elevation

It is rare to observe in daily practice, but it can occur in the context of junctional rhythms or exceptional cases of atrial infarction. In acute pericarditis or Takotsubo syndrome, the PR segment can be elevated in aVR.

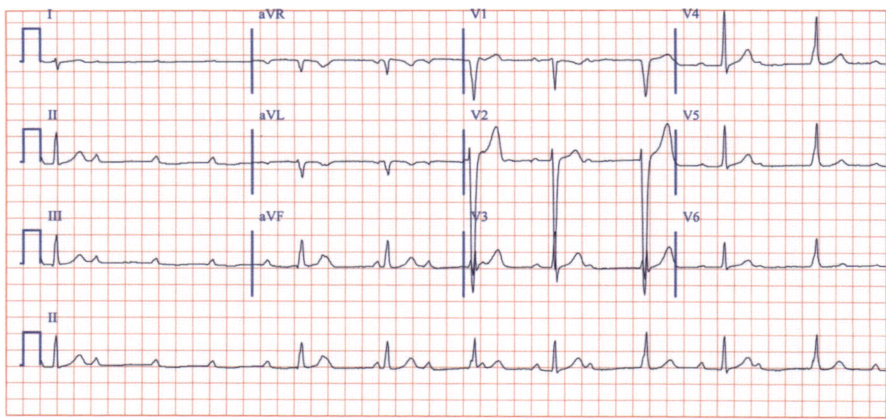

Fig. 2.11 Third-degree AV block with narrow QRS (supra-Hisian escape beats) Nathanson LA, McClennen S, Safran C, Goldberger AL. ECG Wave-Maven: Self-Assessment Program for Students and Clinicians. http://ecg.bidmc.harvard.edu

2.5.4.2 PR-Segment Depression

This refers to a downward displacement of the baseline following the P wave, typically observed in leads where the P wave is upright. Causes of PR segment depression include the following.

Acute Pericarditis

PR-segment depression is a characteristic of ECG findings in acute pericarditis, often described as a "saddleback" appearance. It results from inflammation and irritation of the pericardium, affecting atrial repolarization (Fig. 2.12). In addition, a widespread ST-segment elevation can be observed, typically seen in multiple leads and with a characteristic concave "upwards": morphology. This is due to inflammation-induced alteration in the transmural electrical gradient across the myocardium.

Digitalis Toxicity

Digitalis toxicity can manifest with various ECG changes, including PR-segment depression, due to its effects on atrial conduction and refraction.

Acute Myocardial Ischemia

PR-segment depression may occur in the setting of acute myocardial ischemia, reflecting impaired atrial repolarization due to inadequate blood supply to the myocardium.

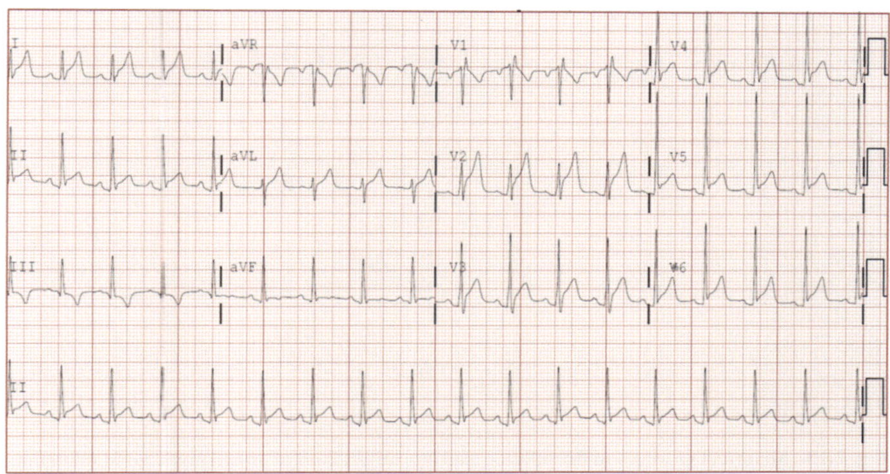

Fig. 2.12 Acute pericarditis. Nathanson LA, McClennen S, Safran C, Goldberger AL. ECG Wave-Maven: Self-Assessment Program for Students and Clinicians. http://ecg.bidmc.harvard.edu

2.5.5 Q Waves

While physiological Q waves are typically small and insignificant, pathological Q waves can signify myocardial damage or infarction [3–5]. Pathological Q waves are characterized by increased duration (>0.04 seconds), depth (>30% of the subsequent R-wave amplitude), and presence in specific leads indicative of myocardial territory (Fig. 2.13).

2.5.6 QRS Complex

A normal QRS complex typically lasts between 0.06 and 0.10 seconds (60–100 ms) [3–5]. A QRS complex is considered wide if its duration exceeds 0.12 seconds (120 ms). This can be indicative of various pathological conditions such as bundle branch blocks, ventricular hypertrophy, myocardial infarction, or electrolyte imbalances.

Bundle branch blocks (BBBs) are characterized by delayed or blocked conduction through one of the bundle branches (left or right). This delay results in widened QRS complexes. There are two main types:

1. Left Bundle Branch Block (LBBB) (Fig. 2.14): The QRS complex is widened due to delayed activation of the left ventricle. It typically presents as a broad, S wave in leads V1–V3 and a broad notched R wave in lateral leads.
2. Right Bundle Branch Block (RBBB): The QRS complex is widened due to delayed activation of the right ventricle. It typically presents as a broad S wave followed by a slurred R wave in leads V1 and V2, often described as an "rsR" pattern.

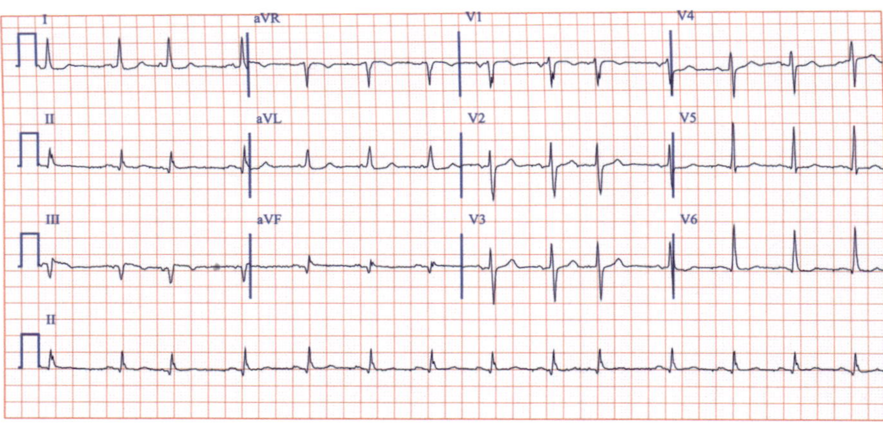

Fig. 2.13 Abnormal Q waves in the inferior lead a manifestation of an old myocardial infarction. Nathanson LA, McClennen S, Safran C, Goldberger AL. ECG Wave-Maven: Self-Assessment Program for Students and Clinicians. http://ecg.bidmc.harvard.edu

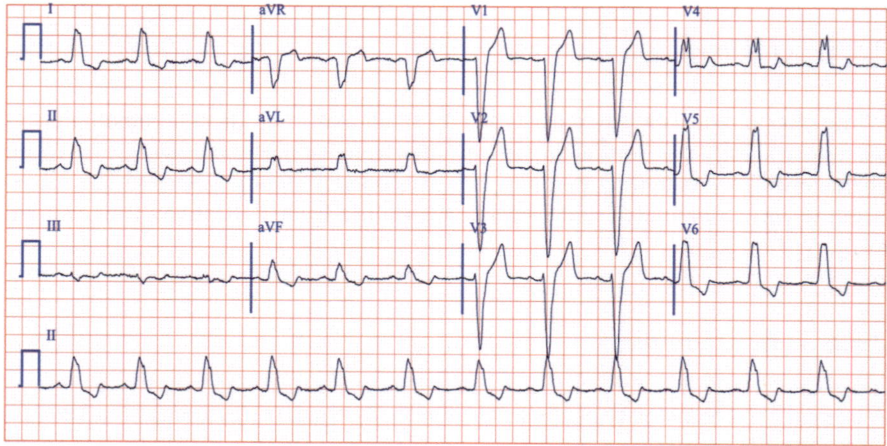

Fig. 2.14 Left bundle branch block (LBBB) Nathanson LA, McClennen S, Safran C, Goldberger AL. ECG Wave-Maven: Self-Assessment Program for Students and Clinicians. http://ecg.bidmc. harvard.edu

2.5.6.1 Heart Rate

The heart rate can be calculated based on the frequency of QRS complexes [3–5]. By counting the number of QRS complexes present in 10 seconds and multiplying by six, the number per minute can be calculated—because 10 seconds times six equals 60 seconds or 1 minute. One alternative method is based on identifying two consecutive R waves and counting the number of large squares between them. By dividing this number into 300 (remember, this number represents 1 minute), we can calculate a person's heart rate. Rate = 300/number of large squares between consecutive R waves.

When the rate exceeds 100 bpm, it indicates tachycardia. Furthermore, tachycardia can be categorized based on the duration of the QRS complex into narrow or wide QRS arrhythmias.

Causes of Narrow QRS Complex Tachycardia

Regular
- The possible diagnoses are sinus tachycardia, atrial tachycardia, atrioventricular nodal reentry tachycardia (AVNRT), orthodromic AV reentrant tachycardia (AVRT) via accessory pathway, and atrial flutter. Certain types of ventricular tachycardias may have a borderline narrow QRS complex (fascicular ventricular tachycardia).

Irregular
- The possible diagnoses are atrial fibrillation, multifocal atrial tachycardia (MAT), atrial flutter with variable AV conduction, and atrial tachycardia.

It is noteworthy that certain medications, including antiarrhythmics, beta-blockers, and calcium channel blockers, can influence AV nodal conduction, leading to irregular narrow QRS complexes. Additionally, abnormal levels of electrolytes, particularly potassium and magnesium, can disrupt atrial and AV nodal function, resulting in irregularities and narrow QRS complexes.

Causes of Wide QRS Complex Tachycardia

Regular
- Supraventricular tachycardia in the context of a bundle branch block or ventricular preexcitation syndromes.
- Ventricular tachycardia (VT): VT is a rapid rhythm originating from the ventricles. It can occur in the setting of structural heart disease (such as myocardial infarction or cardiomyopathy) or as an idiopathic condition. VT typically presents with wide QRS complexes (>0.12 seconds) with a regular or irregular rhythm (Fig. 2.15).
- Hyperkalemia: Elevated levels of potassium in the blood can affect myocardial conduction, leading to widened QRS complexes. Hyperkalemia can result from various causes, including renal failure, certain medications, and metabolic disorders.
- Ventricular preexcitation syndromes: These syndromes involve abnormal accessory pathways between the atria and ventricles, leading to early activation of ventricular tissue. Conditions such as Wolff-Parkinson-White (WPW) syndrome can result in widened QRS complexes during sinus rhythm or supraventricular tachycardia.

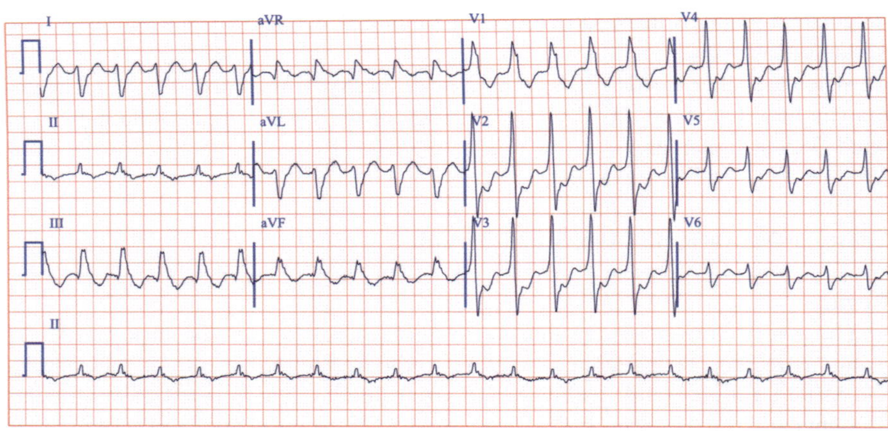

Fig. 2.15 Monomorphic ventricular tachycardia. Nathanson LA, McClennen S, Safran C, Goldberger AL. ECG Wave-Maven: Self-Assessment Program for Students and Clinicians. http://ecg.bidmc.harvard.edu

- Myocardial infarction: Acute myocardial infarction can disrupt normal myocardial conduction pathways, resulting in widened QRS complexes, particularly if the infarction involves the bundle branches or significant portions of the ventricular myocardium.
- Medications: Some medications, such as sodium channel blockers (e.g., flecainide, propafenone) or calcium channel blockers (e.g., verapamil, diltiazem), can delay ventricular conduction and widen QRS complexes, especially in overdose or in patients with underlying heart disease [22].
- Hypothermia: Severe hypothermia can affect cardiac conduction and lead to widened QRS complexes.

Irregular
- Ventricular fibrillation (VF): VF is a life-threatening arrhythmia characterized by chaotic and irregular ventricular electrical activity. It results in disorganized ventricular depolarization and wide irregular QRS complexes on the ECG. VF requires immediate defibrillation to restore normal cardiac rhythm.
- Polymorphic ventricular tachycardia (VT) (Fig. 2.16): Polymorphic VT, also known as torsades de pointes, is a type of VT characterized by a changing QRS morphology on the ECG. It often occurs in the setting of prolonged QT interval, electrolyte imbalances (such as hypokalemia or hypomagnesemia), or certain medications.
- Atrial fibrillation with aberrancy: In cases of atrial fibrillation (AF) with aberrancy or rate-dependent bundle branch block, irregular electrical impulses from the atria can lead to irregular and wide QRS complexes on the ECG.
- Ventricular premature complexes (VPCs) in bigeminy or trigeminy: Irregular occurrences of premature ventricular contractions (PVCs) in a pattern of bigeminy (every other beat) or trigeminy (every third beat) can result in irregular wide

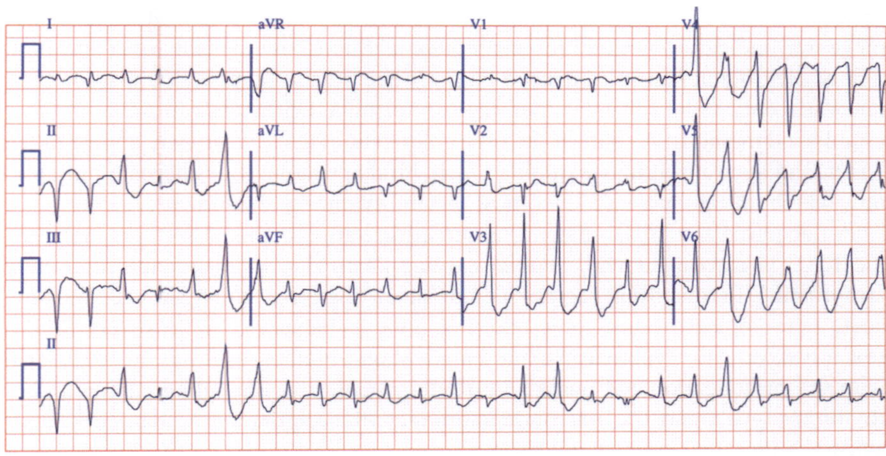

Fig. 2.16 Polymorphic ventricular tachycardia (TdP) Nathanson LA, McClennen S, Safran C, Goldberger AL. ECG Wave-Maven: Self-Assessment Program for Students and Clinicians. http://ecg.bidmc.harvard.edu

QRS complexes on the ECG. VPCs can occur in the setting of various cardiac conditions or as isolated events.

– Medication effects: Certain medications, such as antiarrhythmics, psychotropic drugs, or medications that prolong the QT interval, can lead to irregular wide QRS complexes as a side effect.
– Electrolyte imbalances: Severe electrolyte imbalances, particularly hypokalemia or hypomagnesemia, can disrupt normal ventricular conduction pathways and result in irregular wide QRS complexes on the ECG.
– BBB with variable conduction: Incomplete or intermittent BBB can lead to irregular wide QRS complexes on the ECG. These irregularities in conduction may be exacerbated by factors such as ischemia, electrolyte imbalances, or medication effects.

2.5.7 QT Interval

The following elements, the QT interval, ST segment, and T wave, are part of the "repolarization" assessment [3–5]. These elements should be considered highly as they are the most affected by factors influencing myocardial tissue repolarization. There are several causes of repolarization abnormalities, such as acute myocardial infarction, pericarditis, myocarditis, septic shock, and pulmonary embolism, among others, that will be commented on below.

Regarding the QT interval, its duration varies according to age, gender, and heart rate. In adults, a normal QT interval typically falls <450 ms for men and <460 ms for women, according to the AHA/ACC/HRS consensus, when the heart rate is between 60 and 100 beats per minute. QT interval values that deviate from this range may indicate abnormalities and require additional assessment. Since the duration of the QT interval is influenced by heart rate, it is important to adjust for heart rate variability using formulas like Bazett's formula, Fridericia's formula, or other established methods. As part of the QT prolongation, the T wave may appear taller, wider, and aberrant. It may exhibit a notch, bifid appearance, or alternate morphology, which reflects increased electrical instability during repolarization.

An acquired long QTc interval, observed in various clinical settings including the ICU, is associated with sudden cardiac death due to malignant ventricular arrhythmias. Predisposing factors include heart diseases, prolonged QTc interval, acute neurological events, ionic and metabolic imbalances, septic shock, female sex, advanced age, hypothermia, and intoxications. Numerous drugs are associated with QT prolongation and potential arrhythmogenic risk, including certain antiarrhythmics type I and III, macrolide antibiotics, fluoroquinolones, antidepressants, antipsychotics, and antihistamines.

Drew et al. recommend considering QTc values exceeding the 99th percentile as abnormally prolonged. This value is 470 ms for males and 480 ms for females in healthy postpubertal individuals. Values over 500 ms pose a high risk of developing arrhythmic events.

Prolongation of the QT interval on an electrocardiogram (ECG) can predispose individuals to a potentially life-threatening arrhythmia known as torsades de pointes (TdP). TdP is a type of polymorphic ventricular tachycardia characterized by a twisting or "twisting of the points" appearance on the ECG. It can degenerate into ventricular fibrillation and result in sudden cardiac death. Twisting QRS complexes are recognized by their unique morphology, where the QRS complexes appear to transition the QRS' axis around the baseline.

2.5.8   ST Segment

When the ST segment on an ECG appears depressed or elevated, it signifies an abnormality in myocardial repolarization [3–5]. As mentioned previously, the ST segment represents the interval between ventricular depolarization and repolarization. Normally, the ST segment is isoelectric.

2.5.8.1   ST-Segment Depression

This is diagnosed when the ST segment is observed to be below the baseline (isoelectric line) by at least 0.5 mm (or 0.05 mV) in leads with predominantly positive QRS complexes or 1 mm (or 0.1 mV) in leads with predominantly negative QRS complexes. Examples of causes of ST-segment depression are the following:

- Myocardial ischemia: It typically manifests as a horizontal or downward-sloping ST-segment depression. It is usually seen during exercise or periods of increased myocardial demand and may be transient.
- Hypokalemia: This causes diffuse ST-segment depression, often with a characteristic "sagging" appearance, T-wave flattening, or inversion.
- Hypoxia: Decreased oxygen supply to the myocardium, as seen in respiratory failure or severe anemia.
- Digitalis toxicity: Digitalis toxicity can cause down-sloping ST-segment depression, typically with associated T-wave flattening or inversion. It may also manifest as a "scooped" appearance of the ST segment.

2.5.8.2 ST-Segment Elevation

This is diagnosed when the ST segment is observed to be elevated above the baseline (isoelectric line) by at least 0.5 mm (or 0.05 mV) in leads with predominantly positive QRS complexes or 1 mm (or 0.1 mV) in leads with predominantly negative QRS complexes [3–5]. Examples of causes of ST-segment elevation are the following:

- Acute myocardial infarction (STEMI): STEMI (Fig. 2.17) is characterized by persistent ST-segment elevation (usually >1 mm in two contiguous leads) along with pathological Q waves (indicating myocardial necrosis) and T-wave changes (often inversion or hyperacute T waves).
- Pericarditis: Pericarditis (Fig. 2.12) typically presents with diffuse ST-segment elevation across multiple leads, often with concave upward morphology. The elevation is usually widespread and does not localize to specific coronary artery distributions.

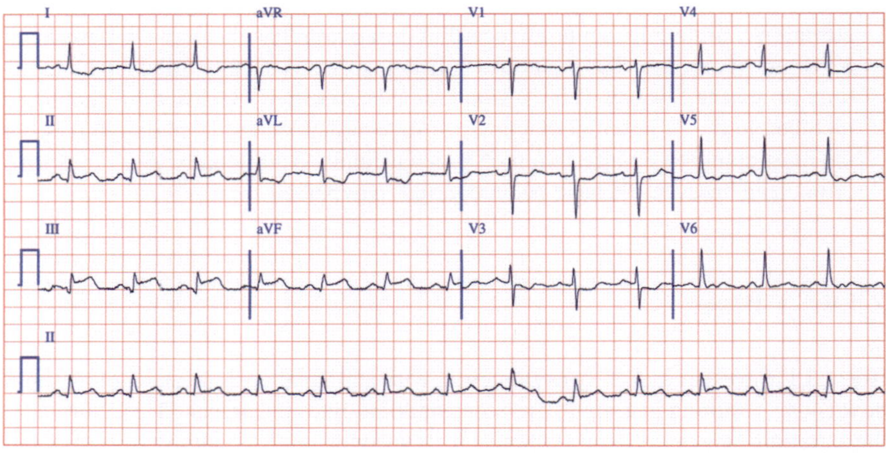

Fig. 2.17 Acute inferior STEMI Nathanson LA, McClennen S, Safran C, Goldberger AL. ECG Wave-Maven: Self-Assessment Program for Students and Clinicians. http://ecg.bidmc.harvard.edu

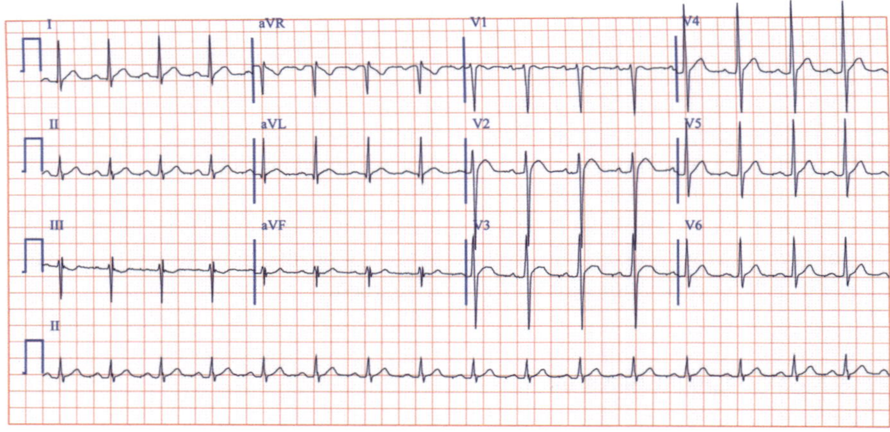

Fig. 2.18 Hypercalcemia, showing an ST-segment elevation with a scooped appearance. Nathanson LA, McClennen S, Safran C, Goldberger AL. ECG Wave-Maven: Self-Assessment Program for Students and Clinicians. http://ecg.bidmc.harvard.edu

- Myocarditis: Myocarditis can present with ST-segment elevation, like acute myocardial infarction. However, the elevation may be more diffuse and less pronounced compared to STEMI. ST-segment elevation may not meet the criteria for STEMI (>1 mm in two contiguous leads) but can still be present, along with T-wave changes and sometimes pathological Q waves.
- Prinzmetal's variant angina: Prinzmetal's angina is characterized by transient episodes of ST-segment elevation during angina attacks, typically occurring at rest and unrelated to exertion.
- Hypercalcemia: It can produce a wide range of ECG abnormalities, with shortening the c interval being the most common finding. However, a normal QTc interval is relatively common in mild-to-moderate hypercalcemia. ST-segment elevation mimicking acute myocardial infarction has been well described: ST-segment elevation has a scooped appearance and is usually followed by indistinct or absent T waves (Fig. 2.18). This false-positive ECG finding should be included in the differential diagnosis of myocardial ischemia, although it is not the most common manifestation of hypercalcemia. Additionally, sick sinus syndrome and bradycardia have been reported in hypercalcemia.

2.5.9 T Waves

Normal T waves are typically asymmetric, with a gradual upslope and a more rapid downslope, resulting in a slightly rounded or dome-like appearance [3–5]. Normally, the duration ranges between 0.08 and 0.10 seconds, and its amplitude varies but generally does not exceed 5 mm in limb leads or 10 mm in precordial leads. The polarity of the T wave is positive in most leads but may be negative in leads where the electrical vector is directed away from the electrode, such as in the aVR lead.

Pathological T waves are often categorized based on their morphology and can be broadly classified as peaked, flattened, biphasic, or inverted. Peaked T waves may indicate hyperkalemia or acute myocardial infarction, while flattened or inverted T waves may suggest myocardial ischemia, electrolyte disturbances, myocardial injury, or ventricular hypertrophy. Moreover, T-wave abnormalities can be transient or persistent, requiring careful evaluation to determine their clinical significance.

2.5.9.1 Inverted T Wave

- Left ventricular hypertrophy: Inverted T waves may be seen in leads with predominantly negative QRS complexes (e.g., V1–V3). The presence of LVH criteria, such as increased voltage in the QRS complexes or repolarization abnormalities, supports the diagnosis.
- Hypertrophic cardiomyopathy: Inverted T waves, often deep and asymmetric, may be present in leads facing the hypertrophied septum (e.g., V1–V3). Additional findings may include left atrial enlargement, left ventricular outflow tract obstruction, or dynamic left ventricular hypertrophy.
- Myocardial ischemia: Inverted T waves may appear in leads facing the ischemic region. Additionally, ST-segment changes (depression or elevation) and Q waves may be present, depending on the severity and chronicity of the ischemia or infarction (Fig. 2.19).
- Digitalis toxicity: Inverted T waves, often associated with ST-segment depression and a "scooped" appearance of the ST segment, may be present. Additional

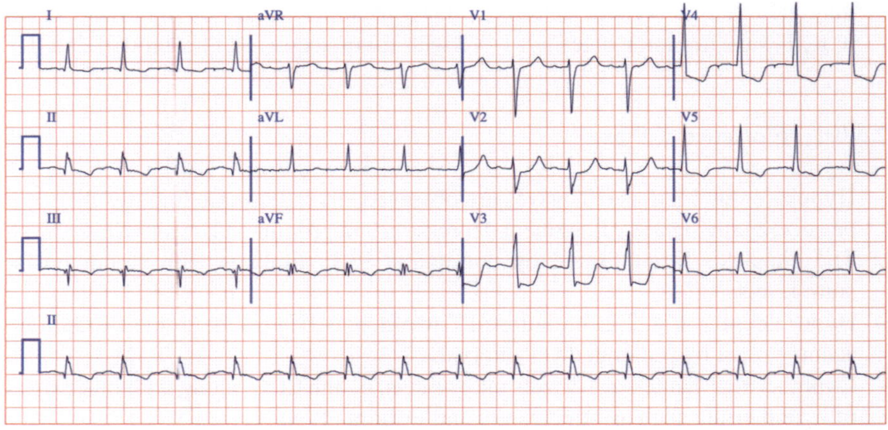

Fig. 2.19 T-wave inversion and ST-segment depression in precordial leads in the context of acute anterior ischemia. Nathanson LA, McClennen S, Safran C, Goldberger AL. ECG Wave-Maven: Self-Assessment Program for Students and Clinicians. http://ecg.bidmc.harvard.edu

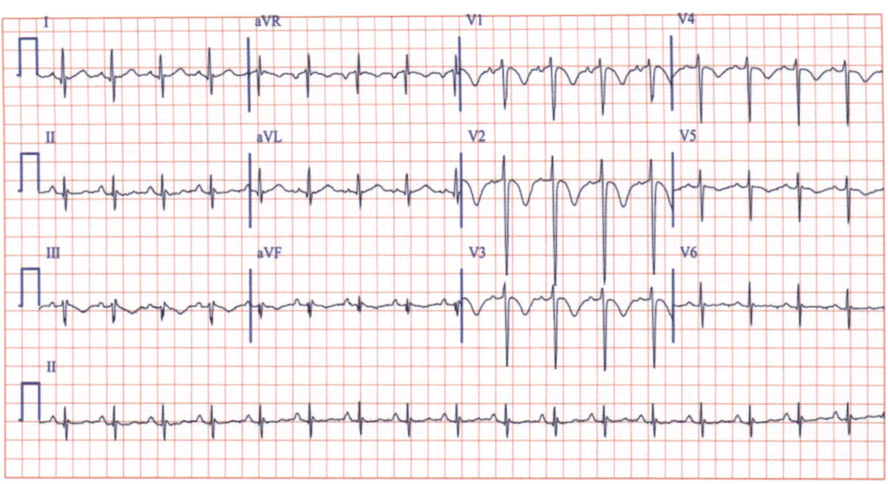

Fig. 2.20 Pulmonary embolism. Nathanson LA, McClennen S, Safran C, Goldberger AL. ECG Wave-Maven: Self-Assessment Program for Students and Clinicians. http://ecg.bidmc.harvard.edu

features of digitalis toxicity include bradyarrhythmias, AV block, or enhanced automaticity.

- Cerebrovascular events: Inverted T waves may occur as a secondary manifestation of neurogenic cardiac effects such as acute stroke or transient ischemic attack affecting the brain's autonomic control centers. Diagnosis involves correlating ECG findings with neurological symptoms and imaging studies to confirm the cerebrovascular event.
- Acute pulmonary embolism: Inverted T waves (Fig. 2.20) in leads reflecting right ventricular involvement (e.g., V1–V4) may be observed. Additional ECG findings may include right-axis deviation, S1Q3T3 pattern, or signs of right heart strain (e.g., T-wave inversion in leads V1–V3 with simultaneous ST elevation in lead III).

2.5.9.2 Flattened T Wave

- Hypokalemia: Flattened T waves are observed, and additional findings that may be accompanying are ST-segment depression and prominent U waves (Fig. 2.21). The diagnosis is confirmed by correlating ECG findings with serum potassium levels.
- Hypocalcemia (Fig. 2.22): Flattened T waves may be present on the ECG, often accompanied by prolonged QT intervals.
- Hypothermia: Flattened T waves may be seen on the ECG, along with other signs of hypothermia such as bradycardia and Osborn (J) waves.
- Acute myocardial ischemia/infarction: Flattened T waves may be observed in leads facing the ischemic region, along with other signs of ischemia such as ST-segment changes and chest pain.

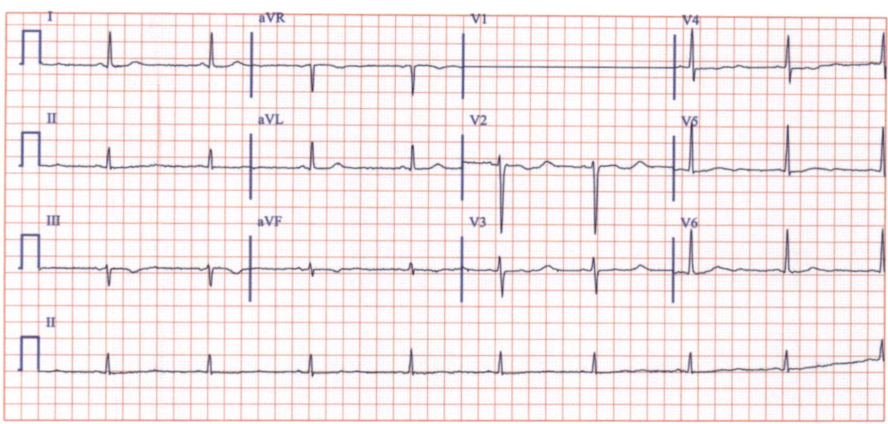

Fig. 2.21 Hypokalemia. Nathanson LA, McClennen S, Safran C, Goldberger AL. ECG Wave-Maven: Self-Assessment Program for Students and Clinicians. http://ecg.bidmc.harvard.edu

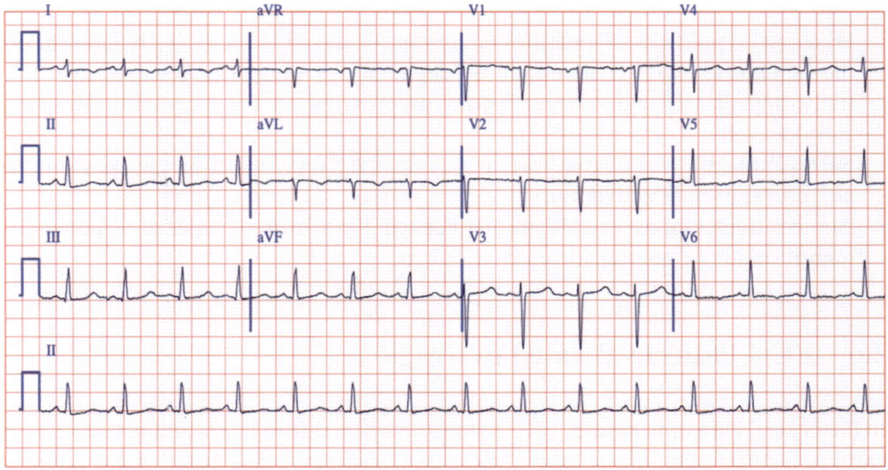

Fig. 2.22 Hypocalcemia. Nathanson LA, McClennen S, Safran C, Goldberger AL. ECG Wave-Maven: Self-Assessment Program for Students and Clinicians. http://ecg.bidmc.harvard.edu

2.5.9.3 Peaked T Wave

- Hyperkalemia (Fig. 2.23): Peaked T waves may be observed on the ECG, typically with a narrow base and tall amplitude. Associated findings may include widened QRS complexes, prolonged PR intervals, and flattened P waves.
- Early repolarization: Peaked T waves with a characteristic "tombstone" appearance may be present on the ECG, particularly in precordial leads (V2–V5).
- Acute myocardial ischemia/infarction: Peaked T waves may be observed in leads facing the ischemic region, typically in the early stages of myocardial ischemia. Associated findings may include ST-segment elevation and chest pain.

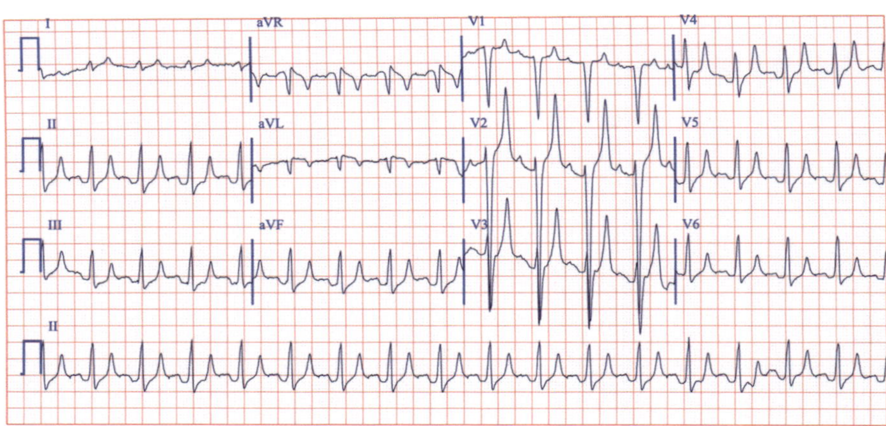

Fig. 2.23 Hyperkalemia, peaked T waves. Nathanson LA, McClennen S, Safran C, Goldberger AL. ECG Wave-Maven: Self-Assessment Program for Students and Clinicians. http://ecg.bidmc.harvard.edu

- Hyperacute phase of myocardial infarction: Peaked T waves may be present on the ECG, often with concomitant ST-segment elevation. The T waves may initially appear tall and narrow before progressing to broader and symmetrically peaked.
- BBB: Peaked T waves may occur as secondary repolarization changes due to altered ventricular activation.
- Acute intracranial events: diagnosis: Peaked T waves may occur as a secondary manifestation of neurogenic cardiac effects.

2.6 ECG Patterns Related to Drugs

In the critical care unit, certain ECG patterns may be due to drugs and influenced by various factors including comorbidities, critical illness, pharmacological interactions, and drug toxicity [22]. Pharmacists play a crucial role in understanding potential drug effects, thereby contributing to improving clinical outcomes and mitigating adverse events [23–25].

The most important ECG patterns with clinical relevance for pharmacists are discussed below.

2.6.1 *Patterns Associated with Specific Drugs or Toxics*

- **Tricyclic antidepressants:** These drugs can block fast sodium channels, prolonging QRS duration and delaying conduction. They can produce sinus tachycardia due to anticholinergic and alpha-1 antagonism and interfere with ventricular repolarization, leading to QT prolongation. A characteristic ECG finding is an R wave in aVR.

- **Antipsychotics:** These medications may induce bradycardia, sinus tachycardia, ventricular arrhythmias, or prolongation of QRS and QTc intervals.
- **Digoxin:** Arrhythmogenic effects of digoxin include triggered activity, automatism enhancement, and vagal tone augmentation, manifesting as PR interval prolongation, "reverse tick" or "Salvador Dali sagging" ST-segment depression, and shortened T-wave amplitude. Toxicity may be suspected with ventricular automatism, junctional tachycardia, atrial fibrillation, atrial tachycardia, AV block, ventricular fibrillation, and other arrhythmias.
- **Ethanol:** Ethanol toxicity increases sympathetic tone, impairs repolarization, and affects QTc duration, leading to sinus tachycardia, atrial tachycardia, atrial fibrillation, ventricular tachycardia, and prolongation of PR, QRS, and QTc intervals [22].
- **Cocaine:** Cocaine affects sodium, calcium, and potassium channels and exerts adrenergic agonism [22]. This can potentially cause sinus tachycardia, ventricular tachycardia, QTc prolongation, TdP, idioventricular rhythms, and asystole.
- **Organophosphates:** Toxicity is associated with sinus tachycardia/bradycardia, intraventricular conduction delays, variable AV blocks, and prolongation of PR, QRS, and QTc intervals.

2.6.2 *Specific Wave or Interval Impairments*

- **P wave:** Prolongation may result from sodium and potassium channel blockade.
- **PR interval:** Prolongation may occur due to vagal stimulation, beta-blockers, calcium channel antagonists, adenosine, and acetylcholinesterase inhibitors.
- **QRS complex:** Prolongation can be induced by sodium channel blockers.
- **QT interval:** Digoxin may shorten QT duration, while acetylcholinesterase inhibitors and several other drugs can prolong it.

References

1. Jackevicius C. Pharmacist participation in CPR needs resuscitation. Can J Hosp Pharm. 2015;68(4):275–6.
2. Kronick SL, Kurz MC, Lin S, et al. Part 4: Systems of care and continuous quality improvement: 2015 American Heart Association Guidelines Update for Cardiopulmonary Resuscitation and Emergency Cardiovascular Care. Circulation. 2015;132(18 Suppl 2):S397–413.
3. Bayés de Luna A, Fiol-Sala M, Bayés-Genís A, Baranchuk A. Clinical electrocardiography: a textbook. 5th ed. Wiley-Blackwell; 2021. ISBN: 1119536456.
4. Bayés de Luna A, Baranchuk A. Clinical arrhythmology. 2nd ed. Wiley-Blackwell; 2017. ISBN: 1119212758.
5. Baranchuk A. Atlas of advanced electrocardiogram interpretation. London: REMEDICA; 2013. www.ECGAtlas.com.

6. Kotsialou Z, Makris N, Gall S. Fundamentals of the electrocardiogram and common cardiac arrhythmias. Anaesth. Intensive Care Med. 2024;25:219–22.
7. Rautaharju PM, Surawicz B, Gettes LS, et al. AHA/ACCF/HRS recommendations for the standardization and interpretation of the electrocardiogram: part IV: the ST segment, T and U waves, and the QT interval: a scientific statement from the American Heart Association Electrocardiography and Arrhythmias Committee, Council on Clinical Cardiology; the American College of Cardiology Foundation; and the Heart Rhythm Society: endorsed by the International Society for Computerized Electrocardiology. Circulation. 2009;119(10):e241–50.
8. El-Sherif N, Turitto G, Boutjdir M. Acquired long QT syndrome and torsade de pointes. Pacing Clin Electrophysiol. 2018;41(4):414–21.
9. Xing LY, et al. Electrocardiographic markers of subclinical atrial fibrillation detected by implantable loop recorder: insights from the LOOP Study. Europace. 2023;25(5):euad014.
10. Kaakeh Y, Overholser BR, Lopshire JC, et al. Drug-induced atrial fibrillation. Drugs. 2012;72(12):1617–30.
11. Johner N, Namdar M, Shah DC. Typical Atrial Flutter: A Practical Review. J Cardiovasc Electrophysiol. 2025.
12. Liwanag M, Willoughby C. Atrial Tachycardia. 2023 Jun 26. In: StatPearls [Internet]. Treasure Island (FL): StatPearls Publishing; 2025.
13. Power DA, et al. Cardiovascular complications of interatrial conduction block: JACC state-of-the-art review. J Am Coll Cardiol. 2022;79(12):1199–211.
14. Escalante Perez S, et al. Bloqueo interauricular avanzado atípico: una presentación poco común del síndrome de Bayés. Arch Cardiol Mex. 2022;92(4):553–5.
15. Nedios S, et al. P-wave duration and interatrial block as predictors of ischemic stroke: a systematic review and meta-analysis. Europace. 2024;26(Supplement_1):euae102.656.
16. De Luna AB, Massó-Van Roessel A, Robledo LAE. The diagnosis and clinical implications of interatrial block. Eur Cardiol. 2015;10(1):54.
17. Pavone C, Pelargonio G. Reversible causes of atrioventricular block. Cardiol Clin. 2023;41(3):411–8.
18. Chen LY, et al. P wave parameters and indices: a critical appraisal of clinical utility, challenges, and future research—a consensus document endorsed by the International Society of Electrocardiology and the International Society for Holter and Noninvasive Electrocardiology. Circ Arrhythm Electrophysiol. 2022;15(4):e010435.
19. Gupta S, Khakh P, Miranda-Arboleda AF, et al. Pattern recognition and inductive-deductive reasoning: two cornerstones of electrocardiogram teaching. Can J Cardiol. 2024. S0828-282X(24)00300-3.
20. Nadeau-Routhier C, Baranchuk A. Electrocardiography in practice: what to do? Queens University Apple Books; 2016.
21. Surawicz B, Knilans T. Chou's electrocardiography in clinical practice: adult and pediatric. 6th ed. Saunders Elsevier; 2008. ISBN: 1416037748
22. Tisdale JE, Chung MK, Campbell KB, et al. Drug-induced arrhythmias: a scientific statement from the American Heart Association. Circulation. 2020;142(15):e214–33.
23. Institute for Safe Medication Practices. Preventing medication errors during codes. [Internet]. Available from: https://www.ismp.org/resources/preventing-medication-errors-during-codes.
24. Lipshutz AK, Morloc LL, Shore AD, et al. Medication errors associated with code situations in U.S. hospitals: direct and collateral damage. Jt Comm J Qual Patient Saf. 2008;34(1):46–56.
25. Pozzolini A, Rio T, Padeletti M, et al. Complex arrhythmias due to reversible causes. Card Electrophysiol Clin. 2019;11(2):375–90.

Further Reading

Zipes DP, Calkins H, Daubert JP, et al. ACC/AHA/HRS advanced training statement on clinical cardiac electrophysiology (a revision of the ACC/AHA 2006 update of the clinical competence statement on invasive electrophysiology studies, catheter ablation, and cardioversion) Heart Rhythm. 2015;2016;13(1):e3–e37.

Chapter 3
The Role of Chest Radiography in the Critical Care Unit

Fabio Macori

3.1 Introduction

Physical examination of patients can be challenging in the intensive care unit (ICU) due to the complexity of medical conditions and the devices often used to support life, and this is even more difficult when the patient is intubated. Portable chest X-rays are often used as an adjunct to the physical examination (Fig. 3.1a). Although it has some limitations in technical diagnostic capabilities, CXR is readily available and inexpensive and plays an important role in the daily evaluation of critically ill patients. Effective communication between radiologists and clinicians is essential to improve interpretation and ensure that quality care is provided to these patients.

It is recommended by the American College of Radiology (ACR) guidelines that portable chest radiography should be used for patients who have cardiopulmonary symptoms following cardiac or thoracic surgery, those who suffer from trauma, patients on monitoring and life support devices, and critically ill patients [1]. There are no strict guidelines dictating the frequency of chest radiography for ICU patients. However, several studies assessing the benefit of daily chest radiography in the ICU have been performed with varied findings. Patients who have acute cardiopulmonary problems are recommended to undergo daily chest radiography by the ACR. Chest radiographs should also be obtained immediately after the placement of endotracheal tubes, nasogastric tubes, vascular catheters, and chest tubes. Follow-up is necessary when the tube or catheter position is suspected to have changed or when otherwise clinically indicated. In the ICU, there are inherent challenges in chest radiography, which limit diagnostic accuracy. Many patients are unable to

F. Macori (✉)
Ospedale Santo Spirito Rome, Rome, RM, Italy
e-mail: fabio@macori.eu

Y. Alzaidi, M. A. Gebily (eds.), *The Pharmacist's Expanded Role in Critical Care Medicine*, https://doi.org/10.1007/978-3-031-77335-8_3

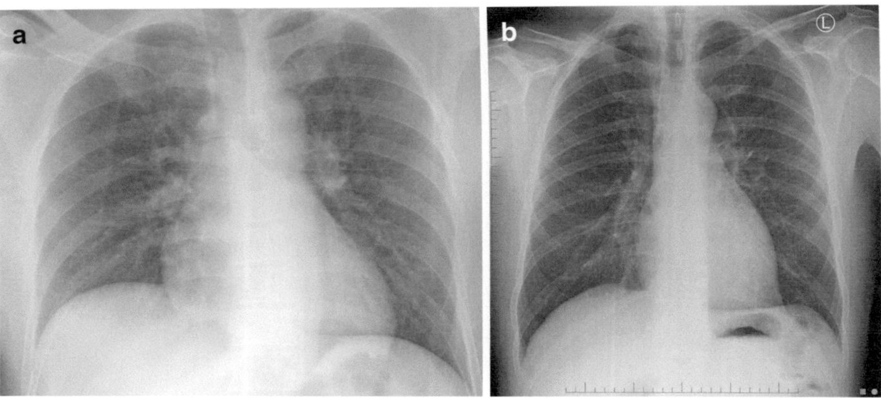

Fig. 3.1 Normal AP chest (**a**) and PA (**b**) for comparison

cooperate with the examination, which makes it difficult to obtain optimal upright (posterior–anterior) positioning (Fig. 3.1b). Radiographs are usually obtained in a semi-upright or supine anteroposterior (AP) position, and a lateral radiograph is often impractical. External monitoring devices, overlying tubes, and electrocardiographic leads may obscure underlying disease, mimic radiographic pathology, and create ambiguity regarding the positioning of other support equipment.

It is important to understand that the chest examination can vary depending on whether the patient is lying down or standing up. When a patient is lying down for an AP film, the cardiovascular structures may appear larger than they are, leading to a misdiagnosis of vascular cephalization. The vascular pedicle may also appear more prominent, which could be mistaken for congestive heart failure [2].

When interpreting chest radiographs of patients in intensive care units (ICUs), it is crucial to follow a systematic approach [3, 4]:

- Evaluate the position of all catheters and support devices.
- Check the patient's cardiovascular status.
- Search for abnormally increased lung opacification areas, which may indicate pneumonia or atelectasis.
- Assess the film for the amount and distribution of pleural fluid.
- Observe for any abnormal air collections, including pneumothorax, subcutaneous emphysema, pneumomediastinum, or pneumopericardium.

This systematic approach can help ensure accurate interpretation of chest radiographs in ICU patients.

3.2   Lines and Tubes [5, 6]

The evaluation of equipment is critical when imaging patients in ICUs. Early detection of malpositioning minimizes the risk of complications.

3.2.1   Endotracheal and Tracheostomy Tubes

Endotracheal tubes (Fig. 3.2) are used to provide mechanical ventilation to the patients who require short-term respiratory support. The tip of the tube must be positioned 4–6 cm above the carina. However, neck flexion may cause the tube to descend by up to 2 cm, while neck extension may cause it to ascend by up to 2 cm. An improperly positioned endotracheal tube can cause subsegmental atelectasis, lung collapse, pneumothorax, unintended extubation, larynx damage, esophageal intubation, and aspiration. Right-sided important bronchus intubation is more common due to the top angle of the right bronchus. Tracheostomy tubes are used for long-term intubation. The tube must be placed at the T3 stage and maintained with neck flexion and extension. The tube diameter must be 2/3 of the trachea's length, and the cuff ought not to distend the tracheal wall. Mediastinal air may be visible after tube placement.

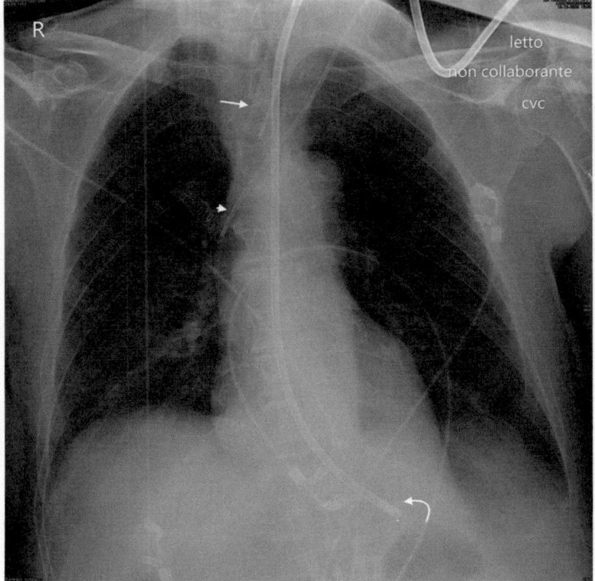

Fig. 3.2 Endotracheal tube (arrow), central venous catheter (arrowhead), and nasogastric tube (curved arrow)

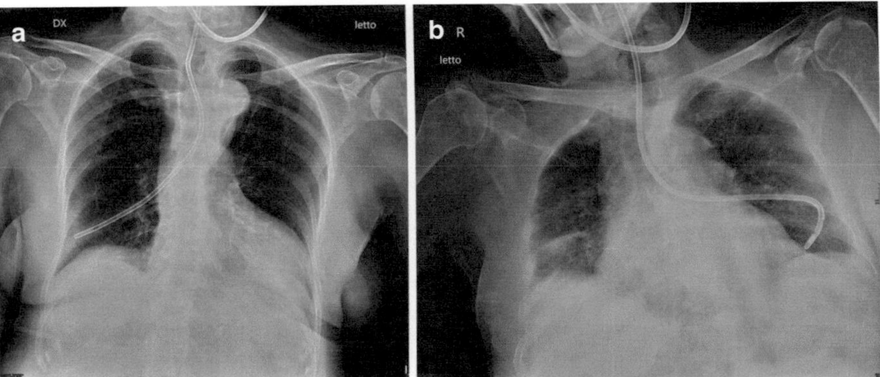

Fig. 3.3 Malposition of the nasogastric tube, inserted in the right bronchus, more frequent due to the angle of its origin (**a**), and left bronchus (**b**)

3.2.2 *Nasogastric Tube*

Gastroenteric tubes are used for feeding, drug administration, and suctioning. The best position of the tube tip is in the gastric antrum or the duodenum because it reduces the risk of aspiration (Fig. 3.2). Radiography is vital in detecting any odd vicinity of the tube, which could otherwise cause life-threatening headaches. Rare complications encompass pharyngeal and esophageal perforations. Tubes coiling within the pharynx or esophagus can create a high chance of aspiration. Enteric tubes terminating inside the trachea or bronchi (Fig. 3.3a, b) can cause bronchopulmonary damage and pneumonia. If the lung parenchyma is punctured, pneumothorax, pulmonary laceration, and pulmonary contusion should be considered. Therefore, an observe-up radiograph is vital if an enteric tube is placed within the airway.

3.2.2.1 Chest Tubes

Tube thoracostomy is often used for the removal of fluid or air from the pleural space (Fig. 3.4). The appropriate placement of a chest tube relies on whether the purpose is to remove air or fluid from the pleural space. For a pneumothorax evacuation, the tube's tip should face upwards, while it should face downwards for fluid drainage. In the case of loculated pleural fluid, the chest tube should be placed in the exact location of the loculation for effective drainage.

Improper placement of a chest tube can lead to ineffective pleural drainage. A radiopaque stripe on a radiograph can identify the tip and holes. The side hole should always be medial to the ribs' inner margin. Poor visualization of the non-opaque wall of the tube can indicate inadvertent placement in extrapleural soft tissues.

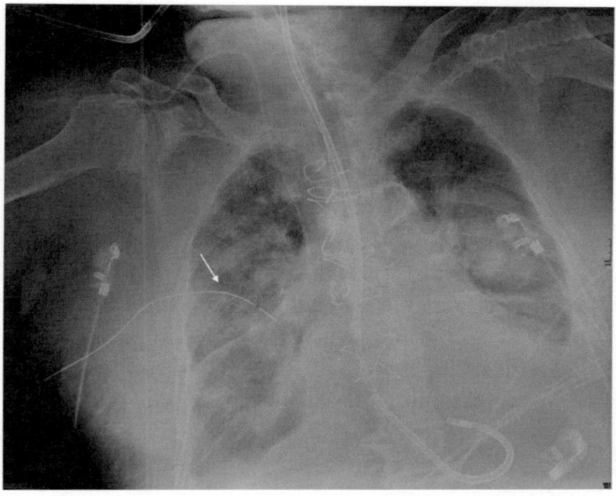

Fig. 3.4 Chest tube (arrow) of the right thorax. The study shows the findings of a bilateral pneumonia with pleural effusion and the history of sternotomy. The nasogastric tube is under the diaphragm, in the left quadrant

Ineffective drainage with chest tubes may be due to tube kinking, clotted blood or debris blockage, or tube tip blockage by the mediastinum. Chest tube advancement into the mediastinum can rarely cause heart or great vessel injury. Inserting the chest tube through the diaphragm into the abdomen may result in damage to the liver, spleen, and stomach.

After prolonged pulmonary atelectasis, re-expansion pulmonary edema occurs when air or fluid is rapidly removed from the pleural space. Symptoms can appear 2–48 h after lung re-expansion and may last up to 2 days. Radiographic findings include unilateral airspace opacity, and CT scans may show ground-glass opacities, consolidation, and septal thickening. The exact cause is not fully known, but it is believed to be linked to increased pulmonary vascular permeability and depletion of surfactant.

A residual pleural or parenchymal line may appear on a chest radiograph after removing a chest tube, outlining the previous tube tract. It is important not to mistake this line for a pneumothorax.

3.2.3   *Central Venous Catheters*

Central venous catheters (CVCs) are used for venous access and central venous pressure monitoring in critically ill patients (Fig. 3.2). They can be placed through the subclavian, internal jugular, or femoral veins. Smaller catheters can be inserted through antecubital veins and remain for months. The CVC tip should be in the superior vena cava, just below the first rib, and slightly above the right atrium. The right atrium should be avoided to prevent arrhythmia, myocardial rupture, and cardiac tamponade.

It is important to verify the correct positioning of a central venous catheter (CVC) through radiography, as malpositioning can occur in up to 40% of cases. Misplacement can affect central venous pressure measurement accuracy and cause adverse effects due to the infusion of potentially toxic substances. Misplaced CVCs can terminate in the right heart or central systemic veins. Inadvertent catheterization of the subclavian artery will present with a pulsatile flow in the catheter and an abnormal catheter position on a radiograph.

Pneumothorax is a common complication after CVC insertion, occurring in up to 5% of cases. Always get a chest radiograph after CVC placement. In the ICU, an upright or contralateral decubitus radiograph detects small pneumothoraxes, which can become larger in positively ventilated patients.

Vascular perforation during catheterization is life-threatening. Radiographic findings indicating vascular injury include unusual catheter placement, apical cap, new pleural effusion, and mediastinal widening. The catheter's gently curved tip and its position against the lateral wall of the SVC may indicate a venous perforation. Extravascular positioning can cause fluid buildup in the mediastinum or pleural space. A contrast medium can confirm proper catheter placement.

The catheter may knot, loop, or kink during placement. Prolonged placement can cause venous thrombosis, leading to pulmonary embolism. In 1% of cases, the catheter may fragment, causing "pinch-off syndrome." Fragmentation can result in arrhythmia, pulmonary embolism, or death. Minimally invasive endovascular retrieval techniques can recover catheter fragments.

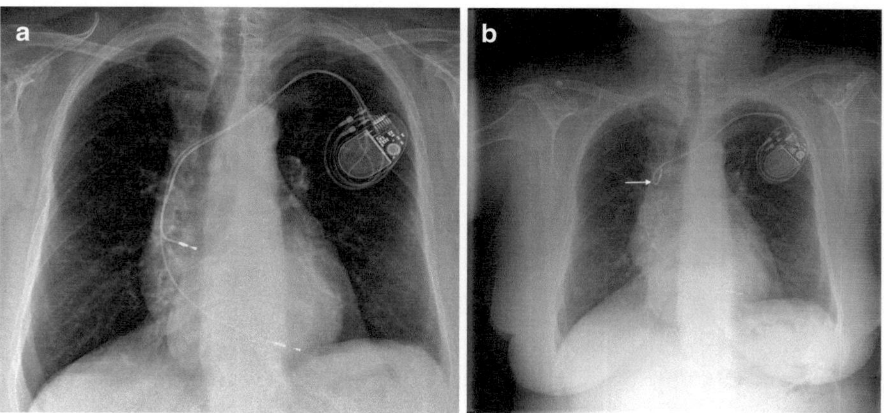

Fig. 3.5 Dual-lead pacemaker correctly positioned (**a**) and with a displaced lead (**b**) (arrow)

3.2.4 Cardiac Devices

Temporary and permanent cardiac pacemakers are used to treat conduction abnormalities (Fig. 3.5). Transvenous pacing is the preferred method for temporary pacing in the ICU; permanent pacemakers consist of a pulse generator implanted in the chest wall and lead wires with electrodes. They range from single lead to complex devices. Biventricular pacing or cardiac resynchronization therapy is a treatment option for severe congestive heart failure. The left ventricular pacing electrode can be inserted through the coronary sinus to stimulate the left ventricular myocardium. Combining an automatic implantable cardioverter-defibrillator (AICD) with a pacemaker can provide an additional benefit for these patients. AICD devices may have a single high-voltage shock coil or an additional coil in the SVC or brachiocephalic vein. External pacemaker-defibrillators are also commonly used in the ICU.

Electrode insertion can cause pneumothorax, vascular injury, and myocardial perforation (usually in the right ventricle). When the electrode tip extends beyond the heart's border, it is important to recognize and monitor for pericardial effusion and cardiac tamponade.

Lead fractures in pacemakers occur for various reasons, such as compression of the lead between the clavicle and the first rib or manipulation of the implanted pulse generator by the patient. Technological advancements have decreased the incidence of such fractures to 1–4%.

3.2.5 Arterial Catheters

The Swan-Ganz catheter measures pulmonary capillary wedge pressure to differentiate between cardiogenic and noncardiogenic pulmonary edema in critically ill patients.

A catheter is inserted into the main pulmonary arteries through the subclavian or internal jugular vein. The catheter tip should not extend beyond 2 cm of the hilum. Inflating the balloon should only happen during measurements. Pulmonary infarction can occur if the catheter is too distal, if the balloon is persistently inflated, or if a clot forms. A chest radiograph can determine the infarction as a wedge-shaped opacity.

CVC insertion complications such as misplacement, looping, coiling, knotting, pneumothorax, and vascular injury may occur in pulmonary artery catheter placement. Rare but serious complications include pulmonary artery rupture, dissection, and pseudoaneurysm. Pseudoaneurysm may cause new pulmonary nodules months after catheter removal. Balloon rupture and pulmonary artery-bronchial tree fistula are other rare complications.

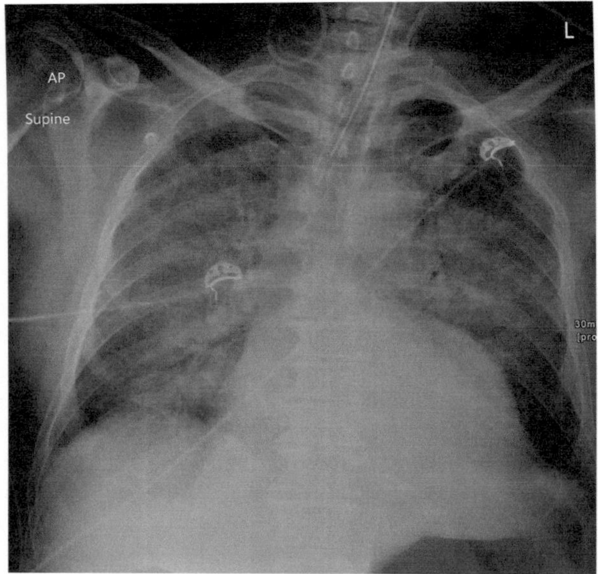

Fig. 3.6 Bilateral perihilar, mid, and lower zone predominant consolidation, most consistent with pulmonary edema. Moderate bilateral pleural effusions

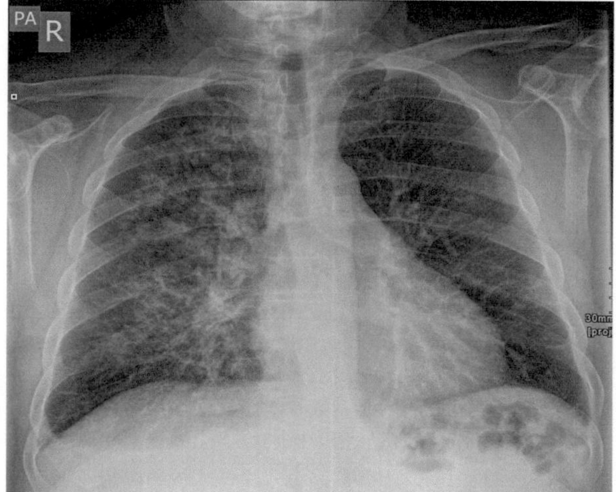

Fig. 3.7 Right perihilar, mid, and lower zone predominant consolidation in keeping with pulmonary edema

3.3 Cardiopulmonary Abnormalities

Several potential causes of increased lung opacification exist, but only a few are commonly seen in the ICU setting. These include pulmonary edema, pneumonia, atelectasis, and aspiration. The imaging characteristics of these entities are outlined below.

3.3.1 Pulmonary Edema

Pulmonary edema [7] is a frequent cause of diffuse parenchymal opacification in ICU patients (Figs. 3.6 and 3.7). It is important to differentiate between hydrostatic pulmonary edema (cardiogenic edema) and increased capillary permeability edema (noncardiogenic edema). While certain features can help distinguish between the two, it is only sometimes possible to differentiate them based solely on radiographic findings. Additionally, a patient may have both types of edema simultaneously.

Hydrostatic pulmonary edema, which is typically caused by congestive heart failure or volume overload, follows a predictable course. Increased pulmonary vascularity is followed by the sequential development of fluid in the interstitial compartments of the lungs and, subsequently, in the airspaces.

The interstitial compartment of the lungs has two major components: the peribronchovascular sheath and the interlobular septa. Fluid in the peribronchovascular sheath results in indistinct pulmonary vessels ("hilar haze") (Fig. 3.9) and peribronchial cuffing. This occurs when pulmonary venous pressures exceed the normal range of 8–12 mmHg. Fluid in the interlobular septa creates Kerley B (Fig. 3.10) or septal lines, which are linear opacities visible in the lung periphery. As interstitial edema becomes more severe, fluid can also accumulate in the subpleural space of the interlobar fissures, causing subpleural stripe or edema, which appears as a thickening of the interlobar fissures on chest radiographs.

As pulmonary venous pressure rises, fluid enters the alveolar spaces of the lungs. Airspace involvement can be detected by poorly defined lung opacities that coalesce to produce airspace consolidation, which may show air bronchograms. The presence of confluent, cloud-like lung opacities characterizes airspace consolidation. Airspace consolidation from hydrostatic pulmonary edema is usually bilateral and symmetric and often has a central or perihilar predominance. However, in some patients, alveolar pulmonary edema may be asymmetric or atypical in distribution. Although the appearance of pulmonary edema can vary among different patients, there is often a similar pattern in an individual patient from episode to episode. Thus, it is helpful to compare the current radiograph to the one obtained during a prior episode of pulmonary edema, particularly for patients with an asymmetric or atypical distribution.

Patients with hydrostatic pulmonary edema often have an enlarged heart, an increased vascular pedicle width, and pleural effusions. Patients with congestive heart failure typically have right-sided pleural effusions.

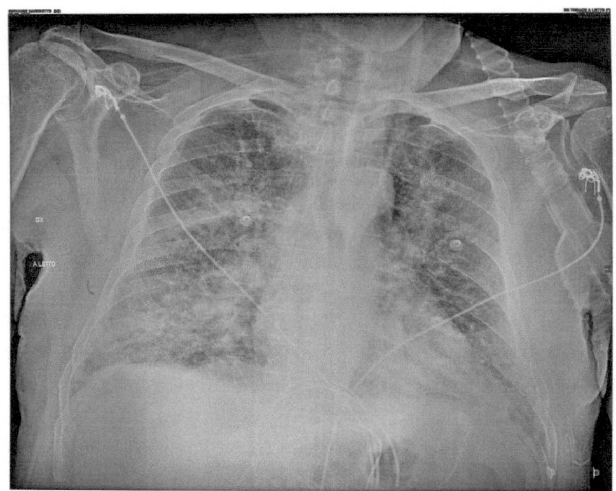

Fig. 3.8 Bilateral diffuse airspace opacification more likely in keeping with ARDS

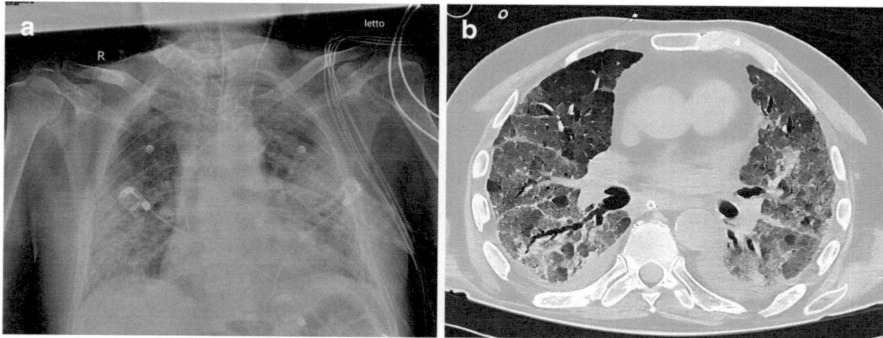

Fig. 3.9 Airspace opacification seen at the chest X-ray (**a**) confirmed at the CT (**b**) where a crazy paving is demonstrated. Bibasal pleural effusion

3.3.2 Acute Respiratory Distress Syndrome

Acute respiratory distress syndrome (ARDS) (Fig. 3.8) is a clinical syndrome characterized by hypoxemia resistant to oxygen therapy, absence of clinically apparent left atrial hypertension, and bilateral pulmonary opacification on the chest radiograph.

Pulmonary opacities on CT are often more heterogeneous than on the chest radiograph. A relatively symmetric ground-glass distribution predominates when ARDS is due to extrapulmonary causes. CT patterns in ARDS may be described as typical or atypical. Dense consolidation involves the posterior lungs in a dependent distribution in a typical pattern. Ground-glass opacities are seen in a nondependent distribution. In the atypical pattern, dense consolidation is seen in nondependent locations. The atypical distribution of consolidation is more likely to be found

Fig. 3.10 Complete collapse of the left lung

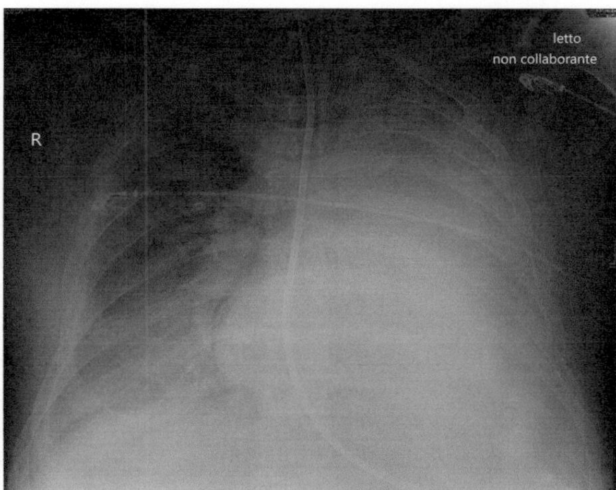

Fig. 3.11 Right basal linear atelectasis. The nasogastric tube is mispositioned, inserted in the left bronchus

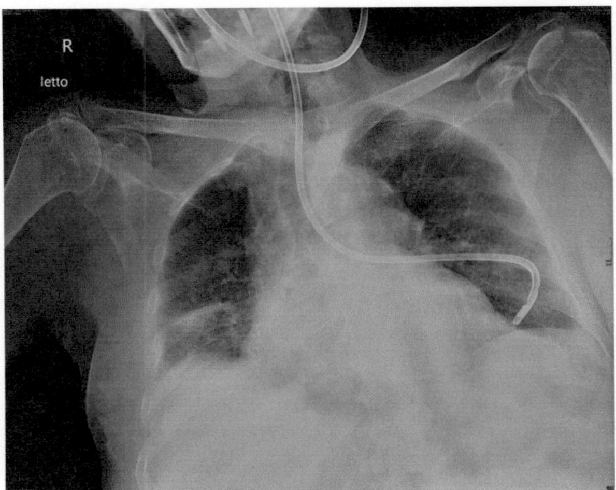

when ARDS is incited by pulmonary disease. Air bronchograms are frequently seen in both forms. "Crazy paving," a nonspecific CT appearance of interlobular septal thickening in a background of ground-glass attenuation, may also be seen (Fig. 3.9).

3.3.3 Atelectasis

Atelectasis, a decrease in lung volume, is the most common cause of pulmonary opacities in the ICU population. It is frequently found after general anesthesia and thoracic or upper abdominal surgery, occurring in up to 64% of patients in one surgical investigation. Atelectasis is usually subsegmental and can mimic pneumonia, particularly when signs of volume loss such as crowding of air bronchograms, fissural deviation, mediastinal shift, and diaphragmatic elevation are absent. Flat, platelike opacities are characteristic of discoid atelectasis. Complete lung collapse, lobar collapse, or segmental collapse can also be seen (Figs. 3.10 and 3.11). Atelectasis is categorized (according to mechanism) as obstructive, compressive, cicatricial, or adhesive. Adhesive atelectasis, common in premature neonates secondary to insufficient surfactant production, is not discussed further.

Obstructive atelectasis is the most common type of atelectasis. Impaired mucociliary function, increased secretions, and altered consciousness are predisposing factors. When only the distal, small airways are obstructed, crowded air bronchograms are seen. Air bronchograms are absent when the obstruction is more proximal in larger airways. Mucus plugging is a common cause of acute segmental, lobar, and complete lung collapse. The absence of air bronchograms in patients who have acute lobar collapse favors mucoid impaction as the etiology and predicts a higher rate of therapeutic success with bronchoscopy (79–89% in favorable patients).

Compressive atelectasis is the volume loss secondary to mass effect exerted on the lung. In the ICU population, pleural fluid is usually the cause. Other potential causes are thoracic tumor, pulmonary abscess, and severe cardiomegaly. Cicatricial

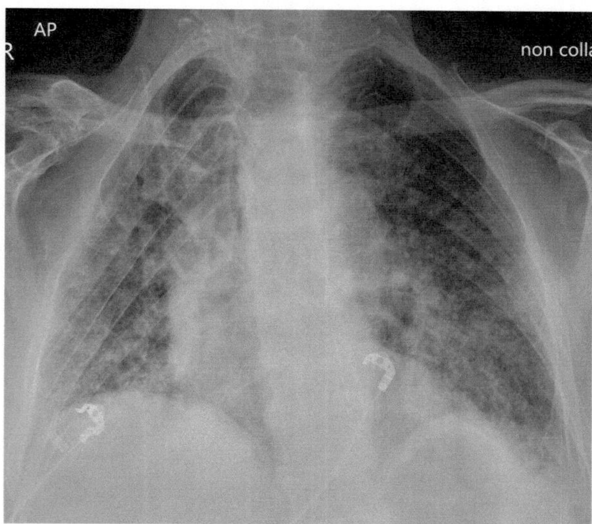

Fig. 3.12 Patchy, ill-defined ground glass, mostly on the dependent zone

atelectasis is the volume loss secondary to pulmonary fibrosis and can be seen in patients with underlying pulmonary disease or as a complication of ARDS.

On CT, atelectasis can often be identified by signs of volume loss. On contrast-enhanced CT, atelectasis results in relatively high attenuation of lung parenchyma, a useful feature distinguishing it from relatively lower attenuating consolidative processes such as pneumonia.

3.3.4 *Aspiration*

Intubation, diminished cough reflex, sedation, and enteric tube feeds increase aspiration risk. Aspiration can occur in mechanically ventilated patients despite adequate inflation of the endotracheal tube cuff. Clinically, aspiration events may go unnoticed or may be severe, causing respiratory distress. Aspiration can result in airway obstruction, chemical pneumonitis, or infectious pneumonia, depending on the volume and type of aspirate. Small amounts of aspirated saliva may result in no radiographic abnormality, whereas aspiration of large amounts of food substance increases the likelihood of aspiration pneumonia.

Patchy, ill-defined ground-glass, consolidative, and nodular opacities are the most frequently encountered radiographic manifestations of aspiration (Fig. 3.12). Opacities typically appear rapidly and are mostly located in the dependent regions of the lungs: the posterior segment of the upper lobes and the superior and posterior basal segments of the lower lobes. Opacities may increase in conspicuity over the first 1–2 days in aspiration pneumonitis but should resolve rapidly afterward. Aspiration pneumonia is likely present when opacities persist or increase over several days.

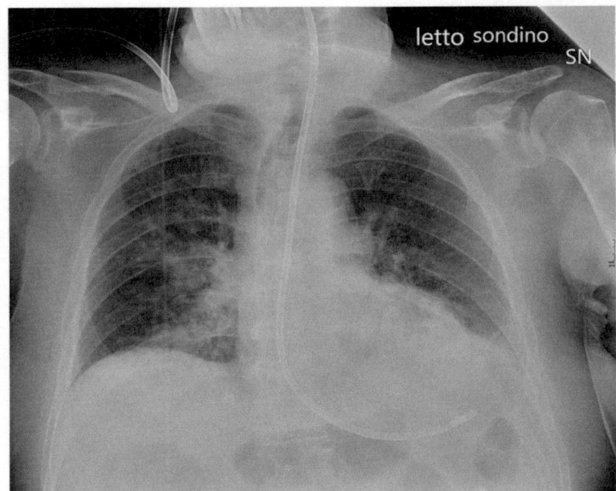

Fig. 3.13 Right basal lung inhomogeneous consolidation in keeping with pneumonia (*Acinetobacter*)

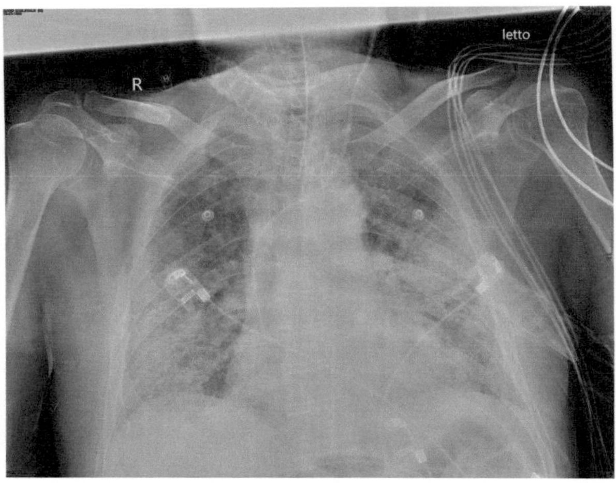

Fig. 3.14 Bilateral airspace consolidations

Patchy, dependent ground-glass and consolidative opacities are also seen on CT "tree-in-bud" opacities that result from inflammation of the distal airways. Although tree-in-bud opacities are nonspecific, when present in a dependent distribution, they are highly suggestive of aspiration.

3.3.5 Pneumonia

Pneumonia is another cause of pulmonary opacities in ICU patients. Aspiration and mechanical ventilation are two important risk factors for pneumonia in the ICU population. Ventilator-associated pneumonia occurs in 9–24% of patients ventilated for more than 48 h. Most pneumonias are caused by mixed anaerobic or, more frequently in the ventilated patient, aerobic gram-negative bacteria such as *Pseudomonas aeruginosa*.

Pneumonia may present as a focal consolidation on the chest radiograph (Fig. 3.13); however, it is often multifocal (Fig. 3.14). Pneumonia can be difficult to differentiate from other causes of pulmonary opacities such as atelectasis, aspiration, and pulmonary edema. Typically, pneumonia changes more slowly than these other entities. In addition, air bronchograms may be seen and differentiated from those seen in atelectasis by noting the absence of volume loss and crowding of bronchi.

When ARDS is present, the diagnostic accuracy of CT and chest radiography is diminished [3, 4]. The presence of underlying consolidation in ARDS limits the ability to exclude the presence of pneumonia. The incidence of pneumonia in patients who have diffuse lung injury at autopsy has been reported to be 58%.

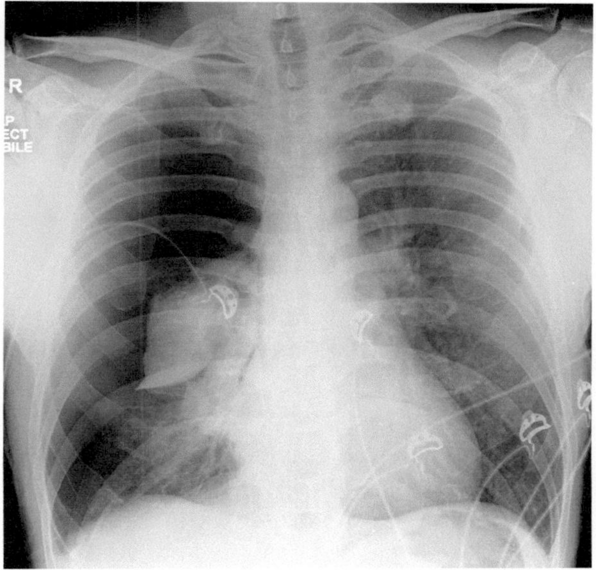

Fig. 3.15 Large right-sided pneumothorax with collapsed lung. No mediastinal shift. Case courtesy Prof. Frank Gaillard—Radiopaedia rID: 33269

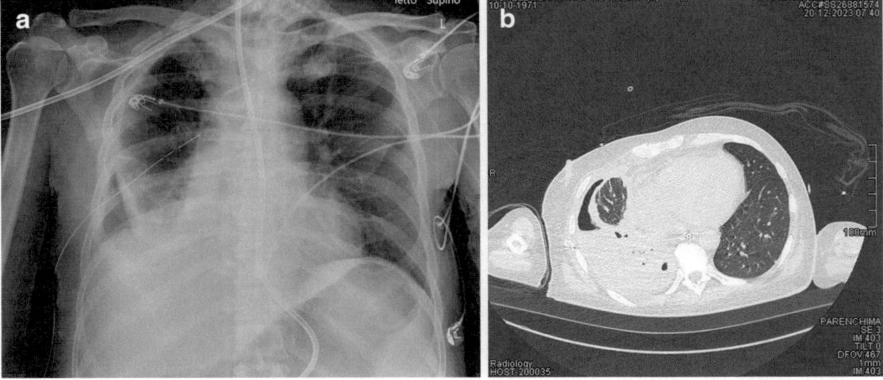

Fig. 3.16 Right basal hydropneumothorax (**a**) confirmed by the CT (**b**)

3.3.6 Pneumothorax, Pneumomediastinum, and Pleural Fluid

Pleural space abnormalities are common in the ICU and can include pneumothorax and pleural fluid. Pneumomediastinum is less common but important to recognize as it can indicate underlying tracheobronchial injury or alveolar rupture in a mechanically ventilated patient.

Pneumothorax can be caused by underlying pulmonary disease, trauma, or iatrogenesis. The classic sign of a thin, dense curvilinear pleural line, bordered by lung on one side and pleural air on the other, may be absent in supine ICU patients.

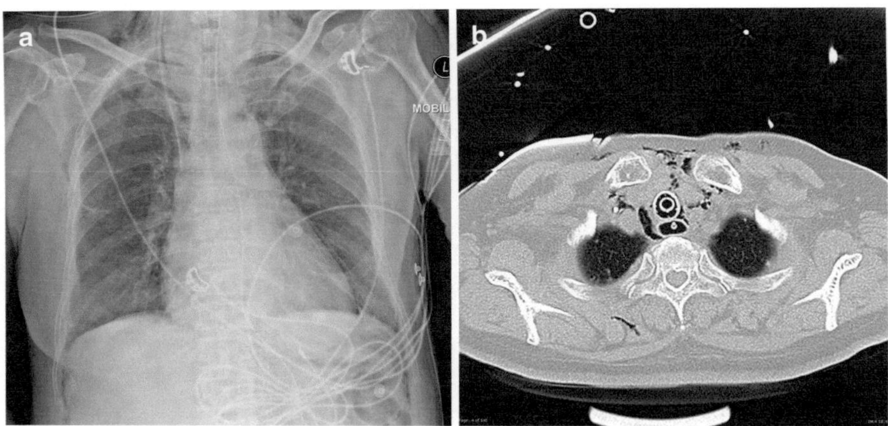

Fig. 3.17 Extensive pneumomediastinum extending into the neck and outlining the pericardium (**a**) confirmed by the CT (**b**). Right internal jugular central venous catheter and a nasogastric tube in situ

Detection requires a high degree of suspicion. A small pneumothorax can rapidly progress to tension in a ventilated patient, making recognition critical.

In the supine patient, pleural air initially accumulates in the anteromedial recess, which is the least dependent location in the hemithorax. Abnormal lucency at the lung base or projecting over the upper abdomen suggests pneumothorax. A lucent deep sulcus may be visualized in the medial or lateral hemithorax. In addition, mediastinum may be unusually well outlined. The lateral decubitus position is the most sensitive for detecting pleural air but is often impractical. When pneumothorax is suspected, an upright radiograph should be obtained for confirmation (Fig. 3.15).

Tension pneumothorax occurs when intrathoracic pressure is greater than atmospheric pressure. Radiographically, tension pneumothorax is most reliably diagnosed by inversion or flattening of the hemidiaphragm. Mediastinal shift may also be seen but is less reliable and frequently less pronounced in patients with acute respiratory distress syndrome (ARDS) due to reduced lung compliance.

Skin folds can mimic pneumothoraces, so important distinguishing features should be recognized. A skin fold is seen as a soft tissue-air interface, with radio-opacity on one side and normal lung on the other. In pneumothorax, a pleural line is often bordered by air on both sides: normal lung and pleural air. The diagnosis may be more complex when the lung is abnormally opaque, creating the illusion of a soft tissue-air interface. The opacity is a skin fold if pulmonary vessels extend peripheral to the interface. If no pulmonary vessels are seen peripherally, then a pneumothorax is present (Fig. 3.16).

Pneumomediastinum is extraluminal air within the mediastinum (Fig. 3.17). It can be seen in tracheobronchial injury, tracheostomy tube placement, mechanically ventilated patients, asthmatics, and esophageal rupture (although this is a rare cause). Pulmonary interstitial emphysema in the mechanically ventilated patient is a sign of alveolar rupture. Air may dissect the cephalad to the subcutaneous tissues of the neck and the caudad to the retroperitoneum.

Pleural fluid is common in ICU patients and is most frequently transudative. The supine radiograph is relatively insensitive in detecting pleural fluid and often underestimates the amount of pleural fluid. On the upright lateral radiograph, blunting of the costophrenic angle usually occurs when 200 mL of fluid is present but may be absent with as much as 500 mL. Layering pleural fluid is more difficult to detect on the supine radiograph. The costophrenic angle is often not blunted, and the supine radiograph may only demonstrate hazy "veil-like" opacification due to layering pleural fluid. The apex is the most dependent location in the supine patient, and pleural effusion may manifest as an apical cap.

Consolidation, atelectasis, and pleural fluid cause opacities on the chest radiograph and frequently coexist, particularly at the thoracic base. CT is useful in differentiating pleural fluid from pulmonary parenchymal disease and better characterizing loculated pleural fluid collections. Empyema is suggested when pleural fluid is bordered by enhancing, thick pleura. Hemothorax is suggested by relatively high-attenuation pleural fluid, commonly 35–70 Hounsfield units.

References

1. https://www.acr.org/-/media/ACR/Files/Practice-Parameters/Port-Chest-Rad.pdf.
2. Henry TS, Mellnick VM. Multisystem imaging of the critically ill patient. Radiol Clin North Am. 2020;58(1):xiii. https://doi.org/10.1016/j.rcl.2019.10.001.
3. Henschke CI, Yankelevitz DF, Wand A, Davis SD, Shiau M. Chest radiography in the ICU. Clin Imaging. 1997;21(2):90–103. https://doi.org/10.1016/0899-7071(95)00097-6.
4. Hill JR, Horner PE, Primack SL. ICU imaging. Clin Chest Med. 2008;29(1):59–76. https://doi.org/10.1016/j.ccm.2007.11.005.
5. Godoy MC, Leitman BS, de Groot PM, Vlahos I, Naidich DP. Chest radiography in the ICU: part 1, evaluation of airway, enteric, and pleural tubes. Am J Roentgenol. 2012;198(3):563–71. https://doi.org/10.2214/ajr.10.7226.
6. Godoy MC, Leitman BS, de Groot PM, Vlahos I, Naidich DP. Chest radiography in the ICU: part 2, evaluation of cardiovascular lines and other devices. Am J Roentgenol. 2012;198(3):572–81. https://doi.org/10.2214/ajr.11.8124.
7. Gluecker T, Capasso P, Schnyder P, Gudinchet F, Schaller MD, Revelly JP, et al. Clinical and radiologic features of pulmonary edema. Radiographics. 1999;19(6):1507–31.

Part II
Pulmonary Critical Care

Chapter 4
The Basics of Mechanical Ventilation

Tyler Peck and Richard M. Schwartzstein

4.1 Introduction

One of the most frequently used lifesaving interventions for critically ill patients is mechanical ventilation—the use of a machine that pumps gas, using positive pressure, into the lungs to ensure adequate exchange of oxygen and carbon dioxide to sustain life. Scenarios necessitating the use of mechanical ventilation include severe life-threatening respiratory failure due to respiratory system disease (e.g., pulmonary pathologies like pneumonia and acute asthma exacerbation, or neuromuscular diseases like Guillain-Barré syndrome and myasthenic crisis), protection of the airway from aspiration and adequate ventilation in patients with impaired consciousness, and maintenance of respiratory function during and after sedation–anesthesia used for surgery. The safe and effective use of mechanical ventilation requires collaboration of the entire intensive care unit (ICU) team, including critical care pharmacists.

While initial forms of mechanical ventilation included negative-pressure ventilation with devices such as the iron lung used widely during the polio epidemic of the 1950s, positive-pressure ventilation is the primary method of mechanical ventilation today. Positive-pressure ventilation can be delivered noninvasively via mask, nasal prongs, or helmet into the patient's upper airway (commonly referred to as noninvasive positive-pressure ventilation [NIPPV]) or invasively via laryngeal mask airway, endotracheal tube, or tracheostomy into the patient's lower airway. While NIPPV is an important critical care modality, this chapter focuses on invasive mechanical ventilation. Modern ventilators are complex computers that allow users to set a wide array of variables related to ventilation and provide advanced monitoring of patient physiology and patient-ventilator interactions.

T. Peck · R. M. Schwartzstein (✉)
Beth Israel Deaconess Medical Center, Harvard Medical School, Boston, MA, USA
e-mail: rschwart@bidmc.harvard.edu

Y. Alzaidi, M. A. Gebily (eds.), *The Pharmacist's Expanded Role in Critical Care Medicine*, https://doi.org/10.1007/978-3-031-77335-8_4

During the use of mechanical ventilation, pharmacists ensure appropriate support by recommending effective pharmacotherapy, particularly sedation and analgesia, reviewing medication regimens for efficacy and safety, and identifying potential medication adverse effects and interactions. This chapter serves to provide an overview of mechanical ventilation relevant to the critical care pharmacist, encompassing indications for its use, basic terminology and physiology, role of pharmacotherapy, common ventilator modes and settings, pathways forward after initiation of mechanical ventilation, and examples of common disease states in which mechanical ventilation is used.

4.2 Physiology of Respiration and Mechanical Ventilation

The physiology of respiration in mechanically ventilated patients is decidedly different from that of spontaneously breathing patients. Spontaneous breathing relies on the coordinated contraction and relaxation of respiratory muscles, primarily the diaphragm. During inhalation, the diaphragm contracts and lowers, expanding the chest cavity and lowering intrathoracic pressure. This pressure change creates a gradient, drawing air into the lungs. Conversely, exhalation is a passive process driven by the natural recoil of the lungs and chest wall. Gas exchange occurs by diffusion across the alveolar-capillary membrane in the lungs, where oxygen crosses from alveoli into the bloodstream, while carbon dioxide moves in the opposite direction.

Mechanical ventilation disrupts this natural physiology. In mechanically ventilated patients, an external device (ventilator) takes over the work of breathing. The ventilator delivers pressurized gas directly into the airways, bypassing the upper airway and relying on an endotracheal tube or tracheostomy for gas delivery into the lower airways. Positive pressure is maintained throughout the respiratory cycle (although may return to zero during expiration in some patients) and is the hallmark of mechanical ventilation. This positive pressure inflates the lungs, replacing the role of the diaphragm during inhalation. While gas exchange continues to occur passively across the alveolar-capillary membrane, the entire respiratory process becomes dependent on the ventilator settings and proper functioning of the ventilator circuit.

This shift from spontaneous to mechanical ventilation necessitates close monitoring and careful adjustments to ensure adequate gas exchange and prevent complications.

4.3 Indications for Mechanical Ventilation

The initiation of mechanical ventilation is warranted for critically ill patients who are unable to maintain adequate ventilation and gas exchange on their own. This inability to maintain respiratory function can be due to various reasons, each of which is an indication for the use of mechanical ventilation.

- *Acute hypoxemic respiratory failure*—Hypoxemia is a state of abnormally low blood oxygen levels which, in severe cases, can threaten life because of inadequate oxygen supply to tissues to allow cellular respiration and function. The causes of hypoxemia are impaired diffusion capacity (difficulty in oxygen moving from the alveolar compartment into the bloodstream; of note, because of the rapid equilibrium of oxygen between the alveolus and the blood, this mechanism only causes hypoxemia if there is an increase in the flow of blood through the pulmonary capillaries—i.e., a high cardiac output state as in exercise), hypoventilation (inadequate refreshment of gas in the alveoli as oxygen is removed by red blood cells, such that there is low oxygen availability for absorption into the pulmonary capillaries), ventilation-perfusion mismatch (poor matching of blood flow to the areas of the lung with the best supply of oxygen), shunt (blood flow through an abnormal pathway that bypasses the blood-alveolar interface), and low inhaled partial pressure of oxygen (uncommon at sea level). When blood oxygen levels are low due to diseases like pneumonia or acute respiratory distress syndrome (ARDS), mechanical ventilation provides the maximum possible delivery of oxygen to the alveoli, allowing for improved blood oxygen levels.
- *Acute hypercarbic respiratory failure*—Hypercarbia, or elevated carbon dioxide level in the blood, represents the inability of the respiratory system to remove enough of this waste product of cellular respiration to maintain a safe tissue environment. A common cause of this type of respiratory failure is an acute exacerbation of chronic obstructive pulmonary disease (COPD), in which obstructive airway disease causes severe impairment of alveolar ventilation and an accumulation of alveolar carbon dioxide ensues. Acute elevation of CO_2 levels in the blood is associated with respiratory acidosis and can cause worsening encephalopathy and eventually coma.
- *Altered consciousness*—Adequate respiration requires a patent airway through which alveolar gas can be exchanged with ambient air in the environment. States of altered consciousness can lead to airway obstruction due to aspiration of oropharyngeal contents (saliva, ingested food/liquid, etc.) and collapse of airway soft tissues (tongue occlusion of the airway). Any cause of severe encephalopathy can contribute to this process, including both primary neurologic pathology (e.g., stroke and seizure) and secondary causes (e.g., intoxication, sedating medications, and uremia).
- *Inability to maintain adequate ventilation without primary pulmonary disease*—Some patients are unable to ventilate adequately due to impaired activation of respiratory muscles without an underlying lung disease. This includes patients with neuromuscular weakness: for example, patients with spinal cord or phrenic nerve injury can be left unable to contract the diaphragm and thus have impaired ability to generate air movement. Alternatively, decreased respiratory muscle function can be caused by impaired respiratory drive due to a more central neurologic problem—this is the case with opioid overdose in which activation of opioid receptors in the brainstem causes inhibition of neurons that typically stimulate breathing.

4.4 Terminology Used in Mechanical Ventilation

Healthcare providers share a common language to describe the many parameters relevant to the use of mechanical ventilation. Familiarity with a few basic terms used to describe the settings and measurements in mechanical ventilation will allow pharmacists to understand this aspect of critical care management and communicate effectively with ICU team members.

Fraction of inspired oxygen (FiO₂) refers to the fraction or percentage of oxygen in the gas delivered to the patient from the ventilator. Ambient air (also called room air) in the environment typically contains 21% oxygen ($FiO_2 = 0.21$); ventilators can deliver up to 100% oxygen (or $FiO_2 = 1.0$) as selected by the clinician.

Airway pressure is the measured pressure in the patient's airway and can be measured at various stages of the respiratory cycle. A few examples of airway pressure are as follows:

- *Positive end-expiratory pressure (PEEP)* is the constant positive pressure applied to the airways at the end of exhalation before the next breath is initiated. Clinicians set the PEEP delivered by the ventilator. PEEP helps keep alveoli open (or "recruited") during expiration, which improves gas exchange and prevents lung injury from repeated closure–reopening of alveoli. High PEEP can cause overdistension of the lung tissue, which can impair gas exchange and cause decreased cardiac output (and hypotension) due to increased intrathoracic pressure and decreased venous return of blood to the heart.
- *Peak pressure (P_{peak})* is the highest pressure reached in the airway during inspiration and is generated by the movement of air through the respiratory system (Fig. 4.1).

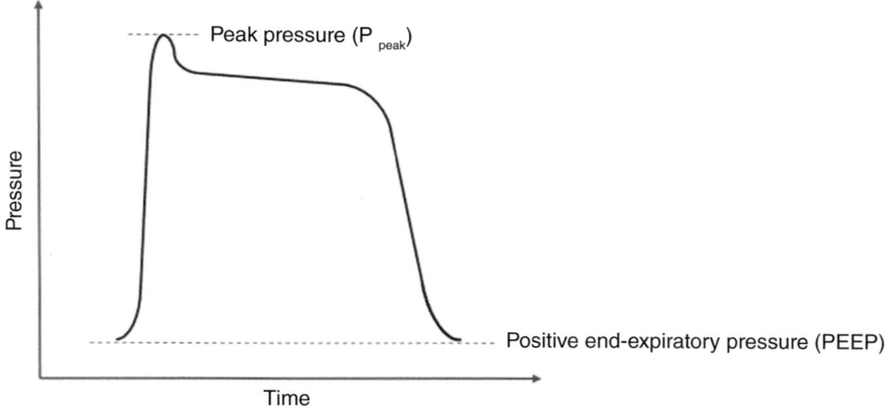

Fig. 4.1 Peak pressure and positive end-expiratory pressure (PEEP). During inspiration on positive-pressure ventilation, the airway pressure rises from the PEEP to the highest pressure of the respiratory cycle, known as the P_{peak}

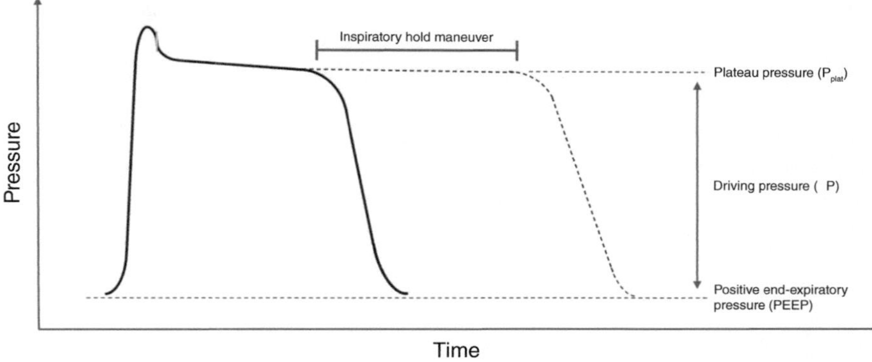

Fig. 4.2 Plateau pressure and driving pressure—the airway pressure when inspiratory flow has stopped and static equilibrium is reached is called the plateau pressure (P_{plat}), which can be measured using an inspiratory hold maneuver. The driving pressure (ΔP) is the difference between the plateau pressure and the positive end-expiratory pressure

- *Plateau pressure, or P_{plat}*, is the pressure remaining in the airway at the end of inspiration when flow has stopped (has reached equilibrium) (Fig. 4.2). This pressure can be measured on a ventilator by performing an end-inspiratory breath hold.
- *Driving pressure, or ΔP*, is the difference between the P_{plat} and PEEP and reflects the pressure that is distending the lungs during inspiration (Fig. 4.2). Excessive driving pressure contributes to ventilator-induced lung injury and is associated with increased mortality for patients on mechanical ventilation.

Tidal volume, or V_t, is the volume of gas delivered with each breath by the ventilator. Lower tidal volumes on the order of 6–8 mL/kg of ideal body weight are typically preferred, especially in lung injury and ARDS as higher tidal volumes in this population are associated with higher mortality.

Respiratory rate (RR) is the number of breaths delivered by the ventilator per minute. A respiratory rate is set on the ventilator by the clinician and represents the minimum number of breaths per minute the patient will receive; however, if the patient triggers additional breaths per minute, the observed respiratory rate will be higher than the set respiratory rate. Modern ventilators provide support or assistance for every breath triggered by the patient beyond the set respiratory rate.

Minute ventilation is the total volume of gas entering (or exiting) the lung per minute, which is equivalent to the tidal volume multiplied by the respiratory rate. The minute ventilation, sometimes referred to as the "minute volume," is a helpful metric of overall ventilation and can serve as a target for adequate ventilation especially when inadequate gas exchange or increased ventilatory demand is contributing to respiratory failure.

Compliance reflects the ease with which lungs expand when a given pressure is delivered, calculated as the tidal volume divided by the driving pressure. Low compliance indicates stiffness of the respiratory system and can be caused by stiff lungs or decreased coordination/stretch of the chest wall.

Airway resistance refers to the opposition to airflow within the airway, including both the patient's anatomic airway and the artificial tubing used to deliver breaths into the patient (e.g., the endotracheal tube). Increased airway resistance can be caused by airflow obstruction in the patient's airways as in bronchospasm and inflammation associated with asthma exacerbations or in the artificial airway as in kinking or mucus plugging of the endotracheal tube.

4.5 Modes of Mechanical Ventilation

In delivering breaths to patients receiving mechanical ventilation, the ventilator can be set to different modes that provide different methods of respiratory support, each with unique features, benefits, and cautions (Table 4.1). The ventilator mode should be selected based on the phase of respiratory failure for a given patient (active vs. resolving), specific aspects of the patient's respiratory physiology, and effort to minimize ventilator-induced lung injury. This section delves into three basic modes of mechanical ventilation that are widely used in ICU environments, acknowledging that this section is not exhaustive and there are many other modes used in patient care for various purposes [4].

Table 4.1 Modes of mechanical ventilation

Modes of Mechanical Ventilation	Parameters Set	Dependent Variables	Advantages and Disadvantages
Volume Control Ventilation (VCV)	• Tidal volume • Respiratory rate • PEEP • FiO2 • Inspiratory time • Inspiratory flow pattern	• Inspiratory airway pressures	• Tidal volume is constant and can ensure adequate ventilation without excessive breath volume • Flow pattern is fixed which can trigger patient discomfort
Pressure Control Ventilation (PCV)	• Inspiratory pressure • Respiratory rate • PEEP • FiO$_2$ • Inspiratory time	• Tidal volume	• Inspiratory pressure is set, which help avoid excessive airway pressure • Flow pattern is variable and determined by patient which can promote patient comfort • Tidal volume can vary, leading to inadequate ventilation or excessive tidal volumes
Pressure Support Ventilation (PSV)	• Inspiratory pressure • PEEP • FiO2 • Apnea ventilation trigger	• Tidal volume • Respiratory rate	• Because the patient completely sets the pattern of ventilation, this mode is considered most comfortable • PSV is helpful to use as a final step toward liberation from mechanical ventilation because ventilator support can be minimized • Ventilation can be highly variable and potentially inadequate

4.5.1 Volume Control Ventilation

Volume control ventilation (VCV) delivers a set tidal volume to the patient for a specified minimum number of breaths per minute. The volume delivered is regulated by the ventilator by providing a predetermined flow of inspired gas during the inspiratory time, after which flow ceases (volume = flow × time). The flow pattern and inspiratory time can be set on the ventilator to alter the inspiratory:expiratory (I:E) ratio which can be helpful in patients with obstructive lung disease in whom a prolonged expiratory time can allow more gas to be exhaled. VCV is an "assist-control mode," a method of ventilating a patient in which every breath triggered by the patient is fully supported with the set inspiratory settings, even if a given breath is beyond the set respiratory rate.

A major benefit of volume control ventilation is that tidal volume is fixed, thereby allowing for good control of delivered volumes to avoid potentially injurious larger tidal volumes. However, in this mode, inspiratory pressure is a dependent variable (based on the delivered tidal volume and the respiratory system compliance) and can cause a rise in transpulmonary pressure to excessive levels, contributing to ventilator-induced lung injury due to barotrauma. Also, because the rate and pattern of flow are both set on the ventilator, this can limit the patient's ability to alter flow breath to breath as is natural in spontaneous breathing and, consequently, can be more uncomfortable for patients ventilated in this mode, contributing to discomfort and patient-ventilator dyssynchrony.

4.5.2 Pressure Control Ventilation

Pressure control ventilation (PCV) delivers breaths with a set inspiratory pressure for a predetermined inspiratory time, during which there is less control of flow by the ventilator; the patient determines the flow based on how much effort they exert during inspiration. With no fixed amount of flow during the inspiratory time, there is no specific tidal volume delivered, and tidal volume can vary breath to breath based on patient effort, airway resistance, and respiratory system compliance—this is a potential hazard in patients who would benefit from low tidal volume ventilation with set tidal volumes. Because the patient is better able to regulate the inspiratory flow, this mode is considered more comfortable than volume control ventilation. Like volume control ventilation, the inspiratory:expiratory (I:E) ratio can be predetermined in pressure control ventilation because the inspiratory time is set by the clinician.

4.5.3 Pressure Support Ventilation

Pressure support ventilation (PSV) is used for patients who can initiate breaths on their own, with each of these breaths being supported with a set level of pressure delivered by the ventilator. Clinicians commonly use this mode for patients with resolving respiratory failure as a step toward liberation from mechanical ventilation. In PSV, patients have more control over their breathing pattern than with other ventilator modes; they can vary their respiratory rate, tidal volume, inspiratory time, and inspiratory flow. There is no minimum respiratory rate setting below which the ventilator would provide a control breath as in other modes; however, the ventilator monitors patients for episodes of apnea and will transition to a backup control mode of ventilation if the patient has an episode of apnea lasting a set duration of time (e.g., 20 seconds).

Major benefits of pressure support ventilation are that it allows for minimization of the amount of respiratory support the patient receives from the ventilator and is typically the most comfortable ventilator mode due to the patient's ability to alter their breath-to-breath respiratory pattern. There are potential downsides, however. Because the tidal volume is determined by the patient and is not limited to any specific volume, the patient can easily receive large tidal volumes that are potentially injurious. Additionally, patients may experience increased work of breathing to achieve their physiologically necessary minute ventilation if PSV settings are providing inadequate support; the ventilator does not assess patient effort, so clinical oversight to ensure adequate ventilator support is important.

4.6 Patient-Ventilator Interactions

Mechanical ventilation, while lifesaving, can become detrimental if the patient and ventilator are not in sync [5]. This mismatch, termed patient-ventilator dyssynchrony (PVD), arises when the ventilator's delivered breaths do not coincide with the patient's breathing efforts or demands. PVD can lead to a vicious cycle: increased patient work of breathing, discomfort, and potential ventilator-induced lung injury (VILI). Some forms of PVD reflect almost reflex-type interactions between the patient and machine, while others may be the consequence of patient breathing discomfort associated with the breathing parameters prescribed by the ventilator settings. By understanding the different types of PVD, healthcare providers can contribute to optimizing ventilator settings and ensuring non-harmful patient-ventilator interaction. In some cases, adjustments in sedation and analgesia may also be indicated, and pharmacologic neuromuscular blockade may even be required in cases of severe and clearly harmful dyssynchrony until other changes are made to promote safe ventilation. The various types of PVD can be broadly categorized based on the phase of the respiratory cycle where the mismatch occurs: trigger, flow, and cycle dyssynchrony [6].

4.6.1 Trigger Dyssynchrony

Trigger dyssynchrony involves issues with initiating a breath. An ineffective trigger occurs when the patient's effort fails to initiate a ventilator breath. Conversely, double triggering happens when a single patient effort triggers two ventilator breaths in quick succession. Auto-triggering arises when the ventilator misinterprets intrinsic airway fluctuations or ventilator circuit artifacts as patient effort, delivering unintended breaths. Finally, reverse triggering occurs when a ventilator breath delivered before the patient's expiration is complete, interrupting ongoing exhalation.

4.6.2 Flow Dyssynchrony

Flow dyssynchrony disrupts the inspiratory flow pattern. When the ventilator's delivered flow rate does not meet the patient's inspiratory demand, it can lead to patient effort to achieve a sufficient breath volume, increasing work of breathing and causing harmful swings in transpulmonary pressure. This can also cause patient discomfort, leading to increased need for sedation.

4.6.3 Cycle Dyssynchrony

Cycle dyssynchrony pertains to issues with breath termination. Premature cycling occurs when the ventilator ends inspiration before the patient completes inhalation, causing discomfort and potentially leading to a breath stacking, in which a second breath is delivered before the preceding exhalation is completed, which can cause volume accumulation and volutrauma. Conversely, delayed cycling happens when the ventilator fails to terminate inspiration despite the patient attempting to exhale, potentially leading to high airway pressure and barotrauma.

4.7 Complications of Mechanical Ventilation

While a lifesaving intervention, mechanical ventilation is not without its risks. Complications can arise from various factors, including ventilator settings, duration of ventilation, patient-ventilator interactions, and underlying patient condition. Here is a closer look at some of the potential complications associated with mechanical ventilation:

- *Ventilator-Induced Lung Injury (VILI)*: This umbrella term encompasses several lung injuries that can occur due to mechanical ventilation [7]. Two key contributors are volutrauma and barotrauma. Volutrauma refers to injury caused by delivering excessive tidal volumes, overstretching lung tissue and causing alveolar injury. Barotrauma, on the other hand, arises from high airway pressures during ventilation, potentially leading to alveolar rupture and air leaks (including pneumothorax and pneumomediastinum). Of note, barotrauma occurs due to excessive transpulmonary pressure (or distending pressure, the pressure exerted outward on the lung tissue relative to the pressure in the pleural space); high airway pressure itself is not necessarily injurious if balanced against an opposing pressure exerting an inward force on the lung, as in obesity or scuba diving. Additionally, atelectrauma, damage to the lung tissue due to mechanical shearing forces with repeated opening and closing (recruitment and derecruitment) of alveoli, can also occur during mechanical ventilation, due to insufficient use of PEEP to maintain lung recruitment.

- *Infections*: The presence of an endotracheal tube or tracheostomy disrupts the natural airway defenses, increasing the risk of ventilator-associated pneumonia (VAP). Pharmacists can play a crucial role in optimizing antibiotic selection and minimizing the emergence of antibiotic resistance in mechanically ventilated patients.
- *Airway Complications*: Mechanical ventilation can also lead to complications directly affecting the airway. Airway stenosis, a narrowing of the airway due to inflammation or scarring, can develop after prolonged endotracheal tube placement or as a result of tracheostomy placement. Airway bleeding can occur during–after tube placement (e.g., tracheoinnominate fistula) or as a consequence of airway suctioning through artificial airways.
- *Respiratory Muscle Atrophy*: When the ventilator takes over the work of breathing, respiratory muscles can weaken over time. This deconditioning, termed respiratory muscle atrophy, can make it challenging for patients to breathe independently upon attempts at liberation from the ventilator.

By understanding these potential complications, healthcare professionals, including critical care pharmacists, can strive to minimize their occurrence. Careful selection of ventilator settings, implementation of lung-protective ventilation strategies, judicious use of analgesics and sedation, meticulous infection control practices, and early initiation of weaning protocols are all crucial aspects of mitigating the risks associated with mechanical ventilation.

4.8 Pathways Forward Once Initiated on Mechanical Ventilation

While initiating mechanical ventilation provides vital support to critically ill patients, the ultimate goal is to transition them back to spontaneous breathing whenever possible. This section explores key pathways forward once mechanical ventilation has been initiated:

- *Spontaneous Awakening Trials (SATs) and Spontaneous Breathing Trials (SBTs)*: As the patient's condition improves, healthcare professionals can assess their readiness to breathe independently. A spontaneous awakening trial (SAT) evaluates the patient's level of consciousness and ability to follow simple commands after minimizing or discontinuing pharmacologic sedation. SBT can be performed in parallel with or separate from an SAT. During an SBT, the ventilator support is reduced or withdrawn for a predetermined period, typically to minimal ventilator support on pressure support ventilation, allowing the patient to breathe spontaneously. Pharmacists can play a role by ensuring that appropriate medication adjustments are made before and during the SBT to optimize respiratory drive and minimize the risk of complications. Successful completion of an SAT and SBT paves the way for extubation, the removal of the endotracheal tube.

- *Extubation*: Extubation signifies a major milestone in the recovery process. However, careful planning and meticulous attention to detail are crucial to ensure a smooth transition. Once a patient passes an SAT and SBT, healthcare providers should consider whether the patient has had adequate resolution of the initial cause of their respiratory failure leading to intubation, whether the patient may require additional procedures or diagnostic tests for which the patient should remain intubated (usually to be able to tolerate deep sedation), and whether the patient will be able to maintain adequate ventilation and gas exchange once removed from mechanical ventilation (e.g., will respiratory secretions or neuromuscular weakness prevent the patient from maintaining adequate respiratory function without mechanical ventilation). In some cases, patients may be extubated but subsequently placed on other respiratory support devices like NIPPV or high-flow nasal cannula (HFNC) to support respiratory function post-extubation and reduce the risk of post-extubation respiratory failure. Pharmacists contribute to the extubation process by reviewing medications that might affect airway reactivity or coughing, potentially causing difficulties after extubation. Additionally, they can recommend medications to manage pain and secretions, maximizing the likelihood of successful liberation from mechanical ventilation.
- *Tracheostomy Placement and Chronic Mechanical Ventilation*: In some cases, prolonged mechanical ventilation may be necessary. When long-term ventilation support is anticipated, placement of a tracheostomy, a surgical opening in the trachea, might be preferred over an endotracheal tube. This allows for improved patient comfort (and minimization of sedation) and can facilitate liberation from the ventilator (it is easier with a tracheostomy for the patient to attempt trials without ventilatory support). Pharmacists can play a role in managing medications specific to tracheostomy care, such as medications to promote secretion clearance. However, chronic mechanical ventilation requires ongoing monitoring and management by a specialized team to ensure optimal patient outcomes.

4.9 Mechanical Ventilation Management in Examples of Respiratory Failure

Although mechanical ventilation is used in a wide range of challenging situations and for many different lung diseases, two specific conditions can serve as models for its safe and effective application in critical care—acute respiratory distress syndrome (ARDS) and severe asthma exacerbation.

4.9.1 Acute Respiratory Distress Syndrome

ARDS is defined as acute onset of hypoxemia within a week of an insult known to cause ARDS with the presence of bilateral lung opacities on imaging (not explained by cardiogenic pulmonary edema, lung nodules, pleural effusions, or atelectasis as the primary cause of hypoxemia), necessitating the use of mechanical ventilation with PEEP of at least 5 cm H_2O (or NIPPV with expiratory pressure of at least 5 cm H_2O) or high-flow O_2 nasal cannula with a flow of at least 30 L/minute [8, 9]. Hypoxemia with a ratio of partial pressure of oxygen (PaO_2) to FiO_2 less than or equal to 300 mmHg qualifies as ARDS. The pathological hallmark of ARDS is the presence of alveolar injury and dysfunction, initially with significant interstitial and alveolar edema associated with marked inflammation, progressing later to proliferative and fibrotic phases of disease with resolution and recovery highly variable between patients.

The mainstay of mechanical ventilation strategy in ARDS is to support adequate oxygenation in the face of significant lung injury while safely ventilating the patient to avoid further lung injury. The term "lung-protective ventilation" encompasses this strategy and includes the important concept of low tidal volume ventilation, which calls for targeting tidal volume to 6–8 mL/kg corrected for ideal body weight (IBW) (and in some cases, even lower tidal volumes are used, down to 4 mL/kg IBW) to avoid volutrauma and limit driving pressure [10]. Additionally, plateau pressure of 30 cm H_2O or less is a common goal, as well as driving pressure of 15 cm H_2O or less, with the goal of limiting excessive inspiratory pressures to avoid the risk of barotrauma and excessive mechanical stress on the lung [11]. The team also strives to reduce the FiO_2 to 0.6 or less to avoid oxygen toxicity to the lung.

These targets, however, are balanced against PEEP to promote effective lung recruitment and prevent atelectasis, enhancing oxygenation and permitting reduced FiO_2. Applied PEEP should be carefully adjusted to achieve this goal while avoiding excessive PEEP that can cause overdistension of alveoli, thereby impairing gas exchange, impacting hemodynamics, and causing lung injury. There are various methods of titrating PEEP to the clinical scenario including increasing the PEEP systematically in response to increasing FiO_2 requirement, performing a decremental PEEP trial to assess for optimal PEEP using measurements of lung compliance and oxygenation, and employing esophageal manometry to estimate the transpulmonary pressure at end expiration [12].

Other advanced strategies used in parallel with mechanical ventilation are employed for more severe ARDS including prone positioning, pharmacologic neuromuscular blockade, use of inhaled pulmonary vasodilators, and use of extracorporeal membrane oxygenation. Prone positioning can remove the weight of the heart from compressing the lungs; this allows for better lung recruitment, which facilitates redistribution of pulmonary edema and tidal volume, and improved ventilation-perfusion matching [13]. Neuromuscular blockade can be used in patients with refractory hypoxemia and respiratory effort/patient-ventilator dyssynchrony that may be worsening their hypoxemia [14, 15].

4.9.2 Severe Asthma Exacerbation

Mechanical ventilation can also be difficult to manage in severe obstructive lung disease. A particularly striking example of this difficulty occurs in severe acute exacerbation of asthma requiring mechanical ventilation. Because of the remarkable ability of patients with asthma to compensate for impaired respiratory physiology, the reversible nature of asthma exacerbations with medical therapy, and the potential difficulty of mechanically ventilating them, healthcare providers typically make every effort to maximize the treatment of asthma to attempt rescue before proceeding with intubation and mechanical ventilation only if deemed necessary.

In an acute flare of asthma, airway inflammation, bronchospasm, and mucus plugging can lead to increasing airflow limitation. The muscle work associated with breathing increases as increased airway resistance causes both inhalation and exhalation to be effortful and difficult, with patients experiencing significant air hunger. Additionally, as expiratory flow is limited, full exhalation requires a longer time and can be truncated by the next inspiratory effort, leading to gas trapping, a phenomenon in which the lung becomes hyperinflated because an extra volume of air remains in the lungs at the end of exhalation beyond the normal relaxed volume or functional residual capacity. This process can occur cyclically such that the trapped volume of air at end exhalation continues to increase, leading to an increasing degree of hyperinflation, which shortens inspiratory muscles, further increasing the effort associated with breathing. Eventually, this can cause increased intrathoracic pressure, which impairs venous return, decreasing cardiac filling and causing hypotension or even cardiac arrest.

Once mechanical ventilation is initiated, it is imperative to monitor asthma patients for evidence of gas trapping and dynamic hyperinflation [16]. If increasing amounts of trapped air accumulate within the chest, there is additional pressure at end expiration above the applied PEEP; this observed PEEP in gas trapping is called "intrinsic PEEP" or "autoPEEP" [17]. On the ventilator, this phenomenon can be observed by performing an end-expiratory breath hold to assess for end-expiratory airway pressure and comparing this to the applied PEEP. Lung-protective ventilation with low tidal volumes targeted at 6–8 cc/kg of ideal body weight helps minimize the risk of volutrauma and limits the volume of inhaled gas that must be exhaled, decreasing the risk of dynamic hyperinflation. Inspiratory time can be shortened to allow for a longer expiratory phase, though a shorter inspiratory time with a fixed volume (as in volume control ventilation) means that inspiratory flow will be increased, which can lead to increased peak airway pressure.

Managing mechanically ventilated patients with severe asthma exacerbation also requires various pharmacologic measures. Standard therapies for acute asthma exacerbation include systemic steroids and inhaled bronchodilators (inhaled beta-agonists and muscarinic antagonists) with the goals of reducing airway inflammation and reducing airway resistance. Intravenous magnesium can be used as an adjunct therapy for bronchodilation, though the evidence for this is less clear. For patients requiring sedation, ketamine is an adjunctive sedating agent that provides both sedating/

analgesic and bronchodilating properties. Another supplementary treatment is the use of neuromuscular blockade for patients in whom safe mechanical ventilation is challenging due to significant respiratory effort by the patient; the use of neuromuscular blockade allows clinicians to take full control of a patient's ventilation temporarily, providing interventions by mechanical ventilation to address the patient's impaired ventilation, which may be poorly tolerated without sedation and neuromuscular blockade. Heliox (a gas mixture of helium and oxygen) can be used instead of a standard mixture of ambient air and supplemental oxygen, as the addition of low-density helium gas allows for decreased overall gas density and decreased airway resistance.

4.10 The Role of the Pharmacist in Mechanical Ventilation

Pharmacists play a pivotal role in ensuring safe and effective medication management for patients on mechanical ventilation. These patients often have complex medication regimens treating the pathologies underlying their critical illness and facilitating care through sedation, and even minor drug interactions or adverse effects can have significant consequences.

Mechanically ventilated patients often require sedation to tolerate the ventilator and prevent patient-ventilator dyssynchrony. Recent data suggest that up to 25% of patients who survive acute respiratory failure and a period of mechanical ventilation will suffer mental health issues post-extubation [1–3]. This is thought to be due to unrecognized dyspnea due to the underlying disease and/or the manner in which the ventilation is being provided and may occur despite relieving the work of breathing with mechanical ventilation. Thus, appropriate analgesia must be provided along with sedation. Pharmacists play a crucial role in selecting appropriate sedatives and analgesia, monitoring their effects on respiratory drive, and ensuring adequate pain/dyspnea control to minimize the need for excessive sedation. They can also recommend alternative routes of administration for medications, such as enteral or intravenous, if the usual routes are inaccessible.

Pharmacists actively collaborate with the interdisciplinary team, including intensivists, nurses, and respiratory therapists. They advocate for medication adjustments based on monitoring data and patient response, ensuring optimal synergy between medication therapy and ventilator management. Additionally, pharmacists can contribute to the development and implementation of evidence-based institutional protocols for sedation management and medication administration in mechanically ventilated patients.

4.11 Summary

Mechanical ventilation with positive-pressure support of ventilation is a mainstay of treatment in the ICU for patients with acute respiratory failure. Optimal management of these patients requires a solid understanding of the basic principles of the respiratory system and the interactions between the patient and the mechanical ventilator. Careful attention to pharmacological treatment, particularly the use of analgesics and sedative agents, is key to avoiding ventilator-induced lung injury and post-respiratory failure mental health issues as well as our efforts to minimize the duration of ventilatory support. The pharmacist is a vital member of the intensive care team whose contributions to the management of these patients are vital to ensuring a positive outcome.

References

1. Schwartzstein RM, Campbell ML. Dyspnea and mechanical ventilation: the emperor has no clothes. Am J Respir Crit Care Med. 2022;205:864–5. https://doi.org/10.1164/rccm.202201-0078ED.
2. Demoule A, Hajage D, Messika J, Jaber S, Diallo H, Coutrot M, Kouatchet A, Azoulay E, Fartoukh M, Hraiech S, Beuret P, Darmon M, Decavèle M, Ricard J-D, Chanques G, Mercat A, Schmidt M, Similowski T, Faure M, Demiri S, Ordan M-A, Mallet M, Berquier G, La Combe B, Emery M, Thiagarajah A, Belafia F, Capdevila M, Aarab Y, Combes A, Hekimian G, Le Gunnec L, Gouanne C, Taconet C, Papazian L, Forel J-M, Guervilly C, Adda M, Fabre X, Chakarian J-C, Philippon-Jouve B, Michelin F. Prevalence, intensity, and clinical impact of dyspnea in critically ill patients receiving invasive ventilation. Am J Respir Crit Care Med. 2022;205:917–26. https://doi.org/10.1164/rccm.202108-1857OC.
3. Demoule A, Decavele M, Antonelli M, Camporota L, Abroug F, Adler D, Azoulay E, Basoglu M, Campbell M, Grasselli G, Herridge M, Johnson MJ, Naccache L, Navalesi P, Pelosi P, Schwartzstein R, Williams C, Windisch W, Heunks L, Similowski T. Dyspnoea in acutely ill mechanically ventilated adult patients: an ERS/ESICM statement. Intensive Care Med. 2024;50:159–80. https://doi.org/10.1007/s00134-023-07246-x.
4. Chatburn RL. Classification of ventilator modes: update and proposal for implementation. Respir Care. 2007;52:301–23.
5. Blanch L, Villagra A, Sales B, Montanya J, Lucangelo U, Luján M, García-Esquirol O, Chacón E, Estruga A, Oliva JC, Hernández-Abadia A, Albaiceta GM, Fernández-Mondejar E, Fernández R, Lopez-Aguilar J, Villar J, Murias G, Kacmarek RM. Asynchronies during mechanical ventilation are associated with mortality. Intensive Care Med. 2015;41:633–41. https://doi.org/10.1007/s00134-015-3692-6.
6. Sottile PD. Albers D, Smith BJ, Moss MM. Ventilator dyssynchrony—detection, pathophysiology, and clinical relevance: a narrative review. Ann Thorac Med. 2020;15:190–8. https://doi.org/10.4103/atm.ATM_63_20.
7. Slutsky AS, Marco RV. Ventilator-induced lung injury. N Engl J Med. 2013;369:2126–36. https://doi.org/10.1056/NEJMra1208707.
8. The ARDS Definition Task Force*. Acute respiratory distress syndrome: the Berlin Definition. JAMA. 2012;307:2526–33. https://doi.org/10.1001/jama.2012.5669.
9. Matthay MA, Arabi Y, Arroliga AC, Bernard G, Bersten AD, Brochard LJ, Calfee CS, Combes A, Daniel BM, Ferguson ND, Gong MN, Gotts JE, Herridge MS, Laffey JG, Liu KD, Machado FR, Martin TR, McAuley DF, Mercat A, Moss M, Mularski RA, Pesenti A, Qiu H, Ramakrishnan N, Ranieri VM, Riviello ED, Rubin E, Slutsky AS, Thompson BT, Twagirumugabe T, Ware LB, Wick KD. A new global Definition of acute respiratory distress syndrome. Am J Respir Crit Care Med. 2024;209:37–47. https://doi.org/10.1164/rccm.202303-0558WS.
10. The Acute Respiratory Distress Syndrome Network. Ventilation with lower tidal volumes as compared with traditional tidal volumes for acute lung injury and the acute respiratory distress syndrome. N Engl J Med. 2000;342:1301–8. https://doi.org/10.1056/NEJM200005043421801.

11. Amato Marcelo BP, Meade MO, Slutsky AS, Laurent B, Costa Eduardo LV, Schoenfeld DA, Stewart TE, Matthias B, Daniel T, Alain M, Richard J-CM, Carvalho Carlos RR, Brower RG. Driving pressure and survival in the acute respiratory distress syndrome. N Engl J Med. 2015;372:747–55. https://doi.org/10.1056/NEJMsa1410639.

12. Heunks L, Piquilloud L, Demoule A. How we approach titrating PEEP in patients with acute hypoxemic failure. Crit Care. 2023;27:415. https://doi.org/10.1186/s13054-023-04694-1.

13. Claude G, Jean R, Jean-Christophe R, Pascal B, Arnaud G, Thierry B, Emmanuelle M, Michel B, Alain M, Olivier B, Marc C, Delphine C, Samir J, Sylvène R, Jordi M, Michel S, Gilles H, Christian B, Jack R, Marc G, Frédérique B, Gael B, Véronique L, Raphaele G, Loredana B, Louis A. Prone positioning in severe acute respiratory distress syndrome. N Engl J Med. 2013;368:2159–68. https://doi.org/10.1056/NEJMoa1214103.

14. Laurent P, Jean-Marie F, Arnaud G, Christine P-R, Gilles P, Anderson L, Samir J, Jean-Michel A, Didier P, Jean-Marie S, Jean-Michel C, Pierre C, Jean-Yves L, Claude G, Gwenaël P, Sophie M, Antoine R. Neuromuscular blockers in early acute respiratory distress syndrome. N Engl J Med. 2010;363:1107–16. https://doi.org/10.1056/NEJMoa1005372.

15. The National Heart, Lung, and Blood Institute PETAL Clinical Trials Network. Early neuromuscular blockade in the acute respiratory distress syndrome. N Engl J Med. 2019;380:1997–2008. https://doi.org/10.1056/NEJMoa1901686.

16. Stather DR, Stewart TE. Clinical review: mechanical ventilation in severe asthma. Crit Care. 2005;9:581–7. https://doi.org/10.1186/cc3733.

17. Junhasavasdikul D, Telias I, Grieco DL, Chen L, Gutierrez CM, Piraino T, Brochard L. Expiratory flow limitation during mechanical ventilation. Chest. 2018;154:948–62. https://doi.org/10.1016/j.chest.2018.01.046.

Chapter 5
Acute Respiratory Distress Syndrome

Lingye Chen and Bryan D. Kraft

5.1 Introduction

Acute respiratory distress syndrome (ARDS) is a common cause of acute respiratory failure in the intensive care unit (ICU) and is also highly lethal, with a mortality rate as high as 46% [8]. ARDS was first described as a clinical syndrome in 1967 by Ashbaugh et al. [7], who reported a case series of 12 patients with respiratory failure due to an acute-onset illness such as infection or trauma that was characterized by bilateral alveolar opacities on chest imaging, low lung compliance, and severe hypoxemia. Seven of the patients were intubated. Amazingly, Ashbaugh et al. proposed two potential therapies, positive end-expiratory pressure (PEEP) and corticosteroids, which are used, discussed, and studied to this day. Since the original description in 1967, the clinical definition of ARDS has been refined over time. In 1994, the American-European Consensus Conference defined ARDS by four criteria: acute-onset hypoxemia, arterial oxygen tension (PaO_2) to inspired oxygen fraction (FiO_2) (P/F) ratio $\leq$ 200, bilateral infiltrates on chest radiograph, and absence of left atrial hypertension or pulmonary artery wedge pressure $\leq$ 18 mmHg [9]. In 2012, the definition was updated by the ARDS Berlin Conference to include patients with an acute-onset illness ($\leq$7 days) due to a known etiology (i.e., infection);

L. Chen
Division of Pulmonary, Allergy, and Critical Care Medicine, Duke University School of Medicine, Durham, NC, USA
e-mail: Lingye.chen@duke.edu

B. D. Kraft (✉)
Division of Pulmonary, Allergy, and Critical Care Medicine, Duke University School of Medicine, Durham, NC, USA

Division of Pulmonary and Critical Care Medicine, Washington University School of Medicine, Saint Louis, MO, USA
e-mail: kraft@wustl.edu

Y. Alzaidi, M. A. Gebily (eds.), *The Pharmacist's Expanded Role in Critical Care Medicine*, https://doi.org/10.1007/978-3-031-77335-8_5

bilateral opacities on chest radiograph or computed tomogram not due to atelectasis, mass, or pleural effusion (Fig. 5.1) and not primarily due to congestive heart failure; and P/F ratio ≤ 300 on at least 5 cm H_2O of PEEP (if intubated) or continuous positive airway pressure (CPAP) if using noninvasive ventilation [36]. This definition further categorized patients as mild, moderate, and severe ARDS based on the degree of hypoxemia as measured by the P/F ratio (201–300, 101–200, and ≤ 100, respectively). The Berlin definition specified for the first time that patients can only meet ARDS criteria when they are treated with invasive or noninvasive positive-pressure ventilation. In 2024, the definition was updated again to be inclusive of resource-limited healthcare settings that may lack access to positive-pressure ventilation or the capability to measure arterial blood gases or perform chest radiographs. This new "Global Definition of ARDS" [55] was also derived in the post-COVID-19 era, where millions of patients developed ARDS and were treated noninvasively with heated, humidified high-flow nasal oxygen (HFNO). The 2024 Global Definition (Table 5.1) incorporates the use of HFNO as a support modality, the use of lung ultrasound to diagnose alveolar opacities, and the use of oxygen saturation by pulse oximetry (SpO_2) to FiO_2 (S/F) ratio to noninvasively grade the severity of hypoxemia.

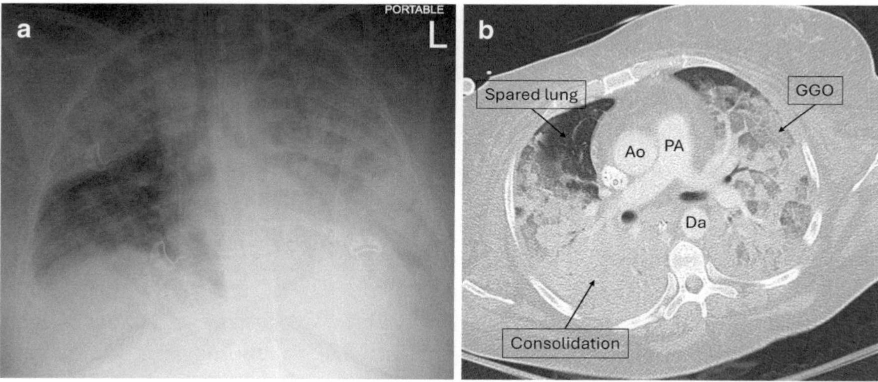

Fig. 5.1 Chest imaging in a patient with ARDS due to rhinovirus–enterovirus respiratory infection and *Streptococcus pneumoniae* bacterial pneumonia. (**a**) Portable anterior–posterior chest radiograph (L = left side) that shows consolidative opacities in the right upper lobe, left upper lobe, lingula, and left lower lobe. Also shown are an endotracheal tube overlying the trachea, a central venous catheter in the right internal jugular vein, and a dialysis catheter in the left internal jugular vein that terminates in the brachiocephalic vein. (**b**) Contrast-enhanced computed tomogram (CT) of the chest in the same patient on the same day showing right lower lobe consolidation, left upper lobe ground-glass opacities (GGO), and spared lung units in the right middle lobe. Also shown are the ascending aorta (Ao), main pulmonary artery (PA), and descending aorta (Da)

Table 5.1 2024 global definition of ARDS

Criteria for ARDS	Description
Characteristic cause or risk factor	A known predisposing risk factor or etiology is identifiable. Opacities are not *fully* explained by fluid overload, atelectasis, pleural effusion, or mass
Acute onset	Onset or acute worsening within 1 week
Bilateral lung opacities	Bilateral opacities are evident on chest radiography or computed tomography, or B-lines or consolidation is evident on lung ultrasound by a skilled ultrasound operator
Hypoxemia	
Non-intubated patients[a]	P/F ≤ 300 or S/F[b] ≤315 on HFNO[c] or NIPPV[d]
Intubated patients	Mild ARDS: P/F 201–300 or S/F[1] 236–315 Moderate ARDS: P/F 101–200 or S/F[b] 149–235 Severe ARDS: P/F ≤ 100 or S/F[b] ≤148
Resource-limited setting	S/F[b] ≤315

ARDS acute respiratory distress syndrome, *HFNO* heated, humidified, high-flow nasal oxygen, *NIPPV* noninvasive positive-pressure ventilation, *P/F* ratio of the partial pressure of arterial oxygen in mmHg to the fraction of inhaled oxygen, *S/F* ratio of the oxygen saturation measured by pulse oximetry to the fraction of inhaled oxygen. Adapted from Ref. [55]

[a]Fraction of inhaled oxygen is estimated by adding 0.03 for every liter per minute oxygen flow to 0.21

[b]Oxygen saturation by pulse oximetry cannot be higher than 97%

[c]At least 30 L per minute flow

[d]At least 5 cm H_2O end-expiratory pressure

5.2 Etiologies and Differential Diagnosis

Since 2020, ARDS has been a leading cause of death, with approximately 7 million deaths globally due to the COVID-19 pandemic. However, COVID-19 has not been the only ARDS pandemic (or near-pandemic) in recent memory. In 2003, the original Severe Acute Respiratory Syndrome Coronavirus 1 (SARS or SARS-CoV-1) caused over 1000 deaths in China [71]. During 2009–2010, the H1N1 swine influenza virus [63] caused over 100,000 deaths worldwide. In 2012, the Middle Eastern Respiratory Syndrome Coronavirus (MERS-CoV) [6] emerged and has caused nearly 1000 deaths (36% mortality rate) to date in Saudi Arabia and other Persian Gulf countries. Given the emergence of these four respiratory viruses that cause ARDS in only the last 25 years, it seems highly likely we will experience new respiratory virus pandemics, such as due to avian influenza or other preemergent coronaviruses, in the future. Additionally, not all ARDS spikes are due to infections: In 2019, there was a notable increase in ARDS cases due to electronic vaping-induced acute lung injury (EVALI) [51], later determined to be due to vitamin E acetate in vaping liquid [12]. Outside of pandemics, ARDS is still quite prevalent, with some estimates as high as 10% of all ICU patients, although clinician recognition of ARDS is poor [8]. Additional efforts are needed to improve clinical recognition of this syndrome so that appropriate treatments can be provided promptly to reduce the risk of ventilator-induced lung injury [42].

Many acute infectious or inflammatory conditions are known to predispose to the development of ARDS. These include primary causes of acute lung injury, such as pneumonia of any cause (e.g., bacterial, viral, fungal, mycobacterial), aspiration, inhalational lung injury (e.g., vaping), and near-drowning, and secondary (systemic) causes of acute lung injury, such as trauma, burns, acute pancreatitis, sepsis, and transfusion of blood products [91].

Additionally, several notable mimics of ARDS exist, including decompensated left ventricular failure, diffuse alveolar hemorrhage, acute interstitial pneumonia, pulmonary alveolar proteinosis, drug-induced pneumonitis, cryptogenic organizing pneumonia, and acute eosinophilic pneumonia. These mimics can be difficult to rule out at times, but common workups include echocardiography (to rule out left ventricular failure), bronchoalveolar lavage (to rule out diffuse alveolar hemorrhage, pulmonary alveolar proteinosis, and acute eosinophilic pneumonia), and obtaining additional clinical history such as the absence of inciting etiology (as can be seen in acute interstitial pneumonia) or a history of vaping, although other mimics such as cryptogenic organizing pneumonia and drug-induced pneumonitis can be hard to definitively exclude short of an open lung biopsy, which is not generally recommended in the acute setting.

5.3 Pathobiology

The pathobiology of ARDS has been elegantly elucidated over the last several decades using animal models of acute lung injury [17, 50]. The principal lesion is the breakdown of the lung's alveolar-capillary barrier due to toxins and acute inflammation (i.e., neutrophils), causing protein-rich exudative fluid to flood the alveolar space. This is accompanied by further inflammation and oxidative stress (i.e., reactive oxygen species) that cause mitochondrial, cellular, and tissue injury [49, 91]. The histopathologic hallmark of ARDS is diffuse alveolar damage (DAD) characterized by the formation of hyaline (fibrin) membranes, although some lung pathologists believe that hyaline membrane formation is exclusively a sign of oxygen toxicity. Pulmonary oxygen toxicity due to prolonged exposure to high FiO_2 (>0.6) can worsen existing lung injury and is indistinguishable from ARDS itself. Despite DAD being the characteristic histopathologic pattern seen, other histologic diagnoses have been identified in open lung biopsies of patients thought to have ARDS, such as bacterial pneumonia, organizing pneumonia, pulmonary embolism, diffuse alveolar hemorrhage, and lymphangitic tumor, though the DAD pattern is associated with the highest mortality [16]. After approximately 7 days, the lung begins to form a scar in the form of organizing pneumonia ("organization"), where the intra-alveolar fibrin serves as a scaffold for fibroblasts and myofibroblasts to lay down collagen. By day 14, the acute phase of ARDS has fully transitioned to the late fibroproliferative phase. ARDS will slowly resolve over days to weeks in many patients, but up to 40% or more of patients ultimately fail to display lung injury resolution and will not recover.

5.4 ARDS Phenotypes

Why some patients experience lung recovery and others do not is currently a matter of research. Recently, investigators have identified two distinct ARDS phenotypes that display different clinical outcomes [15, 54, 82]. These two phenotypes—a hypoinflammatory phenotype and a hyperinflammatory phenotype—display different mortality rates (~20% vs. ~50%, respectively) and different responses to treatments (more on this later) and likely represent two different pathobiologies. However, the hypoinflammatory phenotype may be a misnomer and more likely represents a poorly characterized or undifferentiated group. But what drives one phenotype over the other for a given patient is not yet known. However, in patients with pneumonia-induced ARDS (and probably sepsis-induced ARDS as well), one additional clear driver of severity is the size of the inoculum that leads to infection. Compared with lower inoculums, higher inoculums more readily overwhelm the lung's innate immune responses and lead to more severe lung injury [17, 18, 48].

5.5 Lung-Protective Ventilation

The cornerstone of ARDS management is lung-protective mechanical ventilation. In the landmark ARDS Network ARMA study published in 2000, patients treated with low tidal volume ventilation (6 ml/kg predicted body weight [PBW]) had significantly lower mortality and significantly more ventilator-free days, defined as days alive and free from mechanical ventilation, compared with patients treated with higher volumes (12 ml/kg PBW) [2]. For patients that were acidotic, tidal volumes of up to 8 ml/kg PBW (adjusted for pH >7.30) and respiratory rates up to 35 (adjusted for pH >7.15) were allowable. Oxygenation targets were PaO_2 of 55–80 mmHg or an SpO_2 of 88–95%. Plateau pressure targets were ≤30 cm H_2O. While not outlined in the study, peak airway pressure targets of ≤40 cm H_2O are also generally followed to reduce the risk of barotrauma.

Since the ARMA study, a number of subsequent studies have examined other aspects of lung-protective ventilation, including optimizing PEEP and targeting lower driving pressure (equal to the tidal volume divided by the compliance, or plateau pressure minus PEEP). In a landmark study in 2015, Amato et al. [4] showed that driving pressure was the strongest ventilator variable associated with survival, irrespective of tidal volume and plateau pressure. The risk of death was higher in patients with a driving pressure above 15–17 cm H_2O. In the observational LUNG-SAFE study, an international, multicenter study of 29,144 subjects, a driving pressure above 14 cm H_2O was associated with higher mortality [8]. These data suggest that a driving pressure of less than approximately 15 cm H_2O is ideal for lung protection; however, prospective evaluation of driving pressure is only just beginning [74], and a driving pressure-targeted strategy for ARDS has not yet been validated.

Other modalities of mechanical ventilation that offer theoretical lung protection have been explored, such as high-frequency oscillatory ventilation (HFOV). HFOV delivers a constant mean airway pressure to maintain alveolar recruitment and a respiratory rate of 3–15 Hz, the equivalent of hundreds of small tidal breaths per minute. Unlike conventional mechanical ventilation, HFOV avoids low end-expiratory pressures and high peak pressures, reducing the risk of ventilator-induced lung injury and improving PaO_2 [22]. However, in 2013, two landmark randomized, controlled trials demonstrated no mortality benefit or even harm associated with HFOV compared with conventional low tidal volume ventilation [34, 93]. Routine use of HFOV for the treatment of moderate-to-severe ARDS is, therefore, not recommended [32].

5.6 Positive End-Expiratory Pressure

Positive end-expiratory pressure (PEEP) is the airway pressure in mechanically ventilated patients applied during exhalation. PEEP has the effect of opening collapsed alveolar units and keeping them open throughout the respiratory cycle. This reduces atelectasis and improves oxygenation; however, too much PEEP can cause alveolar overdistention and worsen lung compliance. Providers must, therefore, determine the "best" PEEP for the individual patient, drawing from a number of available methods, such as clinician judgment, bedside PEEP titration (targeting best compliance or stress index), or more advanced techniques such as electrical impedance tomography and esophageal balloon manometry [42]. No method is better or worse than the other and should be chosen based on provider familiarity and availability of necessary equipment.

The ARDS Network published two PEEP/FiO_2 tables (a lower table and a higher table), which can serve as a guide for selecting PEEP levels (http://www.ardsnet. org/files/ventilator_protocol_2008-07.pdf). There is no definite benefit from a lower PEEP strategy compared with a higher PEEP strategy [14, 90], although in a subgroup of patients with moderate-to-severe ARDS (i.e., P/F $\leq$ 200), a higher PEEP strategy may be associated with lower mortality [23].

5.7 Conservative Fluid Management

Patients with ARDS frequently also have sepsis, hypovolemia, and/or shock and require intravenous fluid boluses; however, fluids can also worsen pulmonary edema due to the disrupted alveolar-capillary barriers (see Pathobiology). In a landmark ARDS Network study published in 2006, subjects randomized to a conservative fluid management strategy (defined as having a central venous pressure <4 mmHg and pulmonary artery wedge pressure <8 mm Hg) experienced significantly more ventilator-free days compared with a liberal fluid management strategy (defined as a central venous pressure of 10–14 mm Hg and a wedge pressure of 14–18 mm Hg) [60]. While it is rare in the present day to measure central venous pressure (and even rarer to measure pulmonary capillary wedge pressure) in patients with ARDS, the general concept of avoiding fluid overload in patients with ARDS has held. However, using latent class analysis, investigators have found that different ARDS phenotypes respond differently to fluids. For instance, the hyperinflammatory phenotype had significantly lower mortality in the liberal fluid group compared with the conservative fluid group (40% vs. 50%, respectively) [31]. Taken together, these data overall support an individualized approach to fluid management for each patient to balance the competing factors of supporting plasma volume for adequate perfusion while avoiding fluid overload and worsening pulmonary edema.

5.8   Moderate-to-Severe ARDS

In cases where the P/F ratio remains ≤150 despite optimizing lung-protective ventilation, PEEP, and fluid status, additional therapies may be necessary, such as prone positioning, neuromuscular blockade, corticosteroids, inhaled pulmonary vasodilators, and/or extracorporeal membrane oxygenation. The following sections discuss these salvage therapies and are most applicable to patients with moderate-to-severe ARDS.

5.9   Prone Positioning

Prone positioning is the placement of the patient on the stomach rather than the back (supine). Mechanical ventilation is still delivered in the usual low-volume, low-pressure mode. While turning critically ill patients from supine to prone involves skilled nursing and respiratory therapy support, there are several physiologic effects of prone positioning that mitigate hypoxemia in moderate-to-severe ARDS: In the supine position, atelectasis preferentially develops in the dependent posterior and basilar portions of the lungs [38, 75]. In addition, the transpulmonary pressure, or distention pressure, is higher in the anterior region and lower in the posterior region, leading to overdistention of the anterior alveoli and exacerbating collapse of the posterior alveoli, even in the presence of PEEP [38, 73]. At the same time, blood preferentially flows to these dependent and poorly ventilated regions, creating a shunt. In the prone position, however, the posterior atelectasis is reduced, as pressure is instead placed on the sternum and heart, and circulation now favors the better aerated anterior regions. This diversion of blood into ventilated alveoli alleviates shunt and ventilation-perfusion mismatch [73]. In addition, the difference in transpulmonary pressures between anterior and posterior regions is reduced, mitigating over and underdistention, respectively. These effects are particularly evident in obese patients [72].

Years of case series described short-term improvement in oxygenation with the use of prone positioning [25, 66, 73], but its use gained traction following the PROSEVA trial which demonstrated a remarkable mortality benefit (number needed to treat = 6) [43] in moderate-to-severe ARDS (P/F < 150). Later systematic reviews and meta-analyses confirmed that early prone positioning used in conjunction with lung-protective ventilation offers the greatest mortality reduction in severe ARDS [46, 57, 67, 85]. The current consensus is that patients with severe ARDS should undergo prone positioning for ≥12 hours per day (strong recommendation, moderate certainty of evidence) [76]. Due to discomfort associated with prone positioning, patients are generally expected to need increased sedation or even neuromuscular blockade (see next section), although neuromuscular blockade is not mandatory.

5.10 Neuromuscular Blockade

Neuromuscular blocking agents (NMBAs) paralyze respiratory muscles and can be employed when excess respiratory effort is thought to contribute to refractory hypoxemia or ventilator-induced lung injury. Spontaneous respiratory effort can occur even in patients receiving sedatives and can exacerbate lung injury. Excess skeletal muscle use and elevated heart rate can increase both oxygen demand and use. The respiratory pattern may become dyssynchronous with the ventilator, increase transpulmonary pressure, and result in self-induced lung injury. By relaxing respiratory muscles and eliminating spontaneous respirations, NMBAs reduce oxygen consumption [11], regional alveolar overdistention [92], and inflammatory cytokine levels [37].

In the landmark ACURASYS trial, early use of NMBA (cisatracurium 15 mg i.v. bolus followed by 37.5 mg/hour infusion × 48 hours) resulted in a statistically significant mortality benefit, a reduction in the number of days on the ventilator, and a reduction in multiorgan dysfunction [65]. As a result, NMBAs became the recommended salvage therapy in patients with moderate-to-severe ARDS [20]. However, since ACURASYS, early prone positioning also became the standard of care that improved ARDS survival, and the benefit of NMBAs was called into question. One such study evaluating the use of NMBAs was the ROSE trial, which used the same dosing strategy but found no mortality benefit and perhaps an increase in adverse cardiovascular events in the intervention group [61]. The discordant results between ACURASYS and ROSE are thought to be due to improved care practices that evolved since ACURASYS, such as optimization of PEEP, greater use of prone positioning, and less use of sedation. Additionally, both studies excluded subjects that were already receiving NMBA due to clinician judgment, which was more common in ROSE (13.5%) than in ACURASYS (4.3%). Therefore, NMBAs may be still indicated in patients with ventilator dyssynchrony or based on clinician judgment and should not be automatically discounted because of ROSE.

The current recommendation is to use NMBAs within 48 hours of severe ARDS (conditional recommendation, low certainty) if oxygenation or ventilation cannot be achieved using light sedation [3, 76]. The preferred NMBA is cisatracurium [40, 69], as it undergoes Hofmann elimination in the plasma and, therefore, does not depend on hepatic or renal metabolism, making this ideal for ICU patients who already have or are at risk for multiorgan dysfunction. Furthermore, its half-life of less than 30 minutes allows paralysis to be rapidly reversed.

Because NMBAs work only on voluntary skeletal muscles and have no sedative or analgesic effects, it is imperative to concomitantly administer heavy sedation and analgesia; otherwise, patients will have partial or full awareness while paralyzed. To minimize such discomfort, the common practice is to sedate patients until they reach a Richmond Agitation Sedation Scale (RASS) of −5, defined as comatose, prior to initiation of the NMBA.

5.11 Corticosteroids

Glucocorticoids inhibit the production of pro-inflammatory cytokines responsible for driving ARDS. Their role in the treatment of ARDS has been extensively studied, and the recommendation for their use has fluctuated over time. Earlier recommendation against routine use of corticosteroids for ARDS was based on a landmark randomized, controlled trial demonstrating no mortality benefit of methylprednisolone (single dose of 2 mg/kg followed by 0.5 mg/kg q6 hours × 14 days, then 0.5 mg/kg q12 hours × 7 days, then tapering) in patients with ARDS of at least 7 days' duration [84]. As such, the use of corticosteroids in ARDS was limited to patients with concomitant steroid-responsive processes such as septic shock [5, 83, 87], *Pneumocystis jirovecii* infection [30], and adrenal insufficiency [52].

Recently, however, the landscape has shifted in favor of using steroids to treat ARDS. During the COVID-19 pandemic, dexamethasone (6 mg qday × 10 days) was shown to significantly improve outcomes in hospitalized patients with COVID-19 pneumonia requiring oxygen support, including those with moderate-to-severe ARDS [77, 86]. Around the same time, dexamethasone (20 mg daily × 5 days, then 10 mg daily × 5 days) was also shown to significantly improve mortality in moderate-to-severe non-COVID ARDS (P/F < 200) without a signal for adverse effects such as hyperglycemia or neuromuscular weakness [89]. Moreover, hydrocortisone (continuous infusion of 200 mg per day × 4 or 7 days, then tapered for a total of 8 or 14 days) has been shown to reduce mortality in severe community-acquired pneumonia [21]. Currently, the American Thoracic Society recommends the use of corticosteroids in patients within the first 14 days of ARDS [76] while acknowledging some limitations to this recommendation. Initiating steroid treatment more than 14 days after ARDS onset, however, may be associated with higher mortality [53, 84]. Given the variability of clinical trials, there is no real consensus on which corticosteroid, dose, or duration is optimal. Moreover, the use of corticosteroids in non-intubated patients with non-COVID ARDS has not been studied.

5.12 Inhaled Pulmonary Vasodilators

The lung is the only organ in the human body that vasoconstricts in response to hypoxia. This highly intentional physiologic response serves to maximize capillary perfusion of only those alveolar units that participate in gas exchange. In ARDS, however, alveolar-capillary injury is widespread leading to shunt and hypoxic pulmonary vasoconstriction. Inhaled pulmonary vasodilators, such as inhaled nitric oxide (iNO) and epoprostenol, can be delivered exogenously to severely hypoxemic patients and offer the theoretical benefit of selectively vasodilating preserved alveolar-capillary units to maximize gas exchange and reduce shunt fraction and hypoxemia [78]. However, despite the physiologic improvement associated with inhaled pulmonary vasodilators, there is no accompanying improvement in hard outcomes such as survival [39, 44, 47]. These inhaled drugs are also used to reduce right ventricular afterload in the setting of cor pulmonale, an unfortunate yet common complication in severe ARDS (~25% incidence) that is associated with a high mortality [42].

5.13 Veno-Venous Extracorporeal Membrane Oxygenation

In cases of severe ARDS where it is not possible to provide tidal volumes and airway pressures within safe limits, and hypoxemia and hypercapnia are refractory to proning and other adjunctive salvage therapies, extracorporeal life support (ECLS) may be a rescue strategy. Veno-venous extracorporeal membrane oxygenation (VV ECMO) diverts blood from the central venous circulation into an external device whereby O_2 and CO_2 exchange occurs and oxygenated blood is returned back to the right heart [59]. VV ECMO can be used to support patients for days to weeks (or longer) waiting for lung recovery. VV ECMO requires trained personnel across multiple disciplines and is performed only at select medical centers.

The CESAR trial published in 2009 provided some of the initial evidence supporting the use of VV ECMO in patients with severe ARDS, demonstrating a mortality benefit in the intervention group—those patients that were randomized to transfer to an ECMO center (not to VV ECMO, itself) [70]. The study had numerous limitations including the lack of a standardized mechanical ventilation strategy and its randomization to an ECMO-capable center rather than to ECMO itself (where only 76% of subjects randomized to the ECMO center actually received ECMO). The study was also performed prior to the widespread use of prone positioning. Nevertheless, CESAR led to significantly increased adoption of VV ECMO for refractory ARDS. In an effort to address some of these shortcomings, the EOLIA trial published in 2018 randomized subjects with very severe ARDS (P/F <50 for 3 hours or <80 for 6 hours, or pH <7.25 and $PaCO_2$ $\geq$60 mmHg for 6 hours) to continued mechanical ventilation (control) or immediate VV ECMO cannulation (intervention) [19]. While EOLIA demonstrated no mortality benefit of VV ECMO compared to continued mechanical ventilation, 28% of the control group crossed over to the VV ECMO group due to refractory hypoxemia (57% of whom died). Subsequent post hoc analysis of EOLIA found a probable reduction in mortality by VV ECMO [41], and a meta-analysis also concluded that VV ECMO is associated with a reduction in mortality [58]. As a result, VV ECMO is recommended in selected patients with severe ARDS (conditional recommendation, low evidence) [76].

Given its resource intensity and risk of life-threatening complications, patient selection for VV ECMO should be deliberate with a focus on those patients with the highest likelihood of lung recovery. Patients who benefit most from VV ECMO are those under 50 years of age, in early-phase ARDS ($\leq$7 days), with reversible lung injury, and with single-organ dysfunction [80, 88]. Triggers for initiation are based commonly on EOLIA criteria assuming that the patient has failed to respond to optimization of mechanical ventilation and other salvage therapies such as higher PEEP, proning, and steroids [19, 70, 76].

Anticoagulation is generally initiated at the time of cannula insertion and may be continued for the duration of VV ECMO support to prevent clot formation within the oxygenator and circuit. However, it is not mandatory, and some centers do not routinely anticoagulate VV ECMO circuits at all. When used, the most common anticoagulant is unfractionated heparin (UFH), targeting an anti-Xa level of 0.3–0.5 or an activated partial thromboplastin time (aPTT) of 50–70 seconds [45]; however, the exact target ranges may vary clinically and by institution. In the case of documented or suspected heparin-induced thrombocytopenia, the preferred alternatives are the direct thrombin inhibitors argatroban [35] or bivalirudin [82] which are non-inferior to UFH. The use of anticoagulation and the development of circuit-induced von Willebrand syndrome or thrombocytopenia make bleeding, including intracranial hemorrhage, an unfortunate but recognized complication [19, 45, 58, 59].

Unlike anticoagulation, there is no recommendation for the use of sedation or analgesia, and its dosages are titrated based on patient needs. In early severe ARDS, deep sedation and even paralysis of patients on VV ECMO may be required to maintain low tidal volumes and airway pressures (see above). In the recovery phase, however, VV ECMO can be well tolerated in a fully awake patient. In fact, early mobilization with physical therapy, including in patients with femoral ECMO cannulation sites, is both safe and feasible [1, 13] and may improve functional independence at the time of hospital discharge [27].

Important changes in pharmacokinetics can occur when peripheral blood is circulated through a VV ECMO circuit. The addition of an extracorporeal circuit in general increases the volume of distribution and decreases the plasma concentration of hydrophilic drugs [81]. In addition, increased volume dilutes plasma proteins and increases free plasma concentrations of drugs that are otherwise albumin bound [26]. Meanwhile, lipophilic and protein-bound drugs tend to be sequestered in the circuit [81]. The effects of these pharmacokinetic alterations can lead to higher dosage requirements of sedation and analgesic agents and subtherapeutic plasma concentrations of antimicrobials [26].

5.14 Survivorship

Mortality from ARDS in the current era is estimated between 35% and 46% depending on the severity [8]. As a result of advances in critical care (low tidal volume ventilation, spontaneous awakening trials, improved management of sepsis), ARDS survival has increased over time [29]. With improved survivorship comes the increasingly recognized phenomenon of post-intensive care syndrome (PICS), an acquired or worsened state of cognitive, psychiatric, and/or physical dysfunction that persists for months to years in survivors of critical illness [33].

Prevalence of cognitive impairment and psychiatric disorders following ARDS have been reported to be 55% and 62%, respectively [56], with up to 40% of patients scoring similarly to patients with moderate traumatic brain injury and 26% to those with mild dementia [64]. The most commonly reported psychiatric diagnoses following critical illness survival are depression, anxiety, and post-traumatic stress disorder [10, 56]. Cognitive impairment is significantly associated with comorbid psychiatric symptoms [56].

Prolonged impairment in both lung function and muscle weakness has been widely described in survivors of ARDS. Restrictive ventilatory defects and impaired gas exchange are reported up to a year following the index event [28, 62]. Six-minute walk distances are also shortened though improve over time [68]. Persistent muscle weakness is associated with increased mortality at 5 years [24]. The cumulative effects of these physiologic derangements are reduced independence in activities of daily living and reduced quality of life [10, 33, 56].

Risk factors for PICS include the presence of preexisting comorbidities, baseline disability, severity of acute illness, blood glucose <100 mg/dl, longer duration of mechanical ventilation or ICU length of stay, presence of delirium, and prolonged exposure to sedatives, among others [10, 33, 56, 79]. While preexisting conditions are not modifiable, potentially modifiable variables such as sedation holidays, early mobilization, and more liberal glycemic control may reduce the likelihood or severity of long-term neuropsychiatric and physical dysfunction.

References

1. Abrams D, Madahar P, Eckhardt CM, Short B, Yip NH, Parekh M, Serra A, Dubois RL, Saleem D, Agerstrand C, Scala P, Benvenuto L, Arcasoy SM, Sonett JR, Takeda K, Meier A, Beck J, Ryan P, Fan E, Hodgson CL, Bacchetta M, Brodie D, MORE-PT Investigators. Early mobi-

lization during extracorporeal membrane oxygenation for cardiopulmonary failure in adults: factors associated with intensity of treatment. Ann Am Thorac Soc. 2022;19:90–8.

2. Acute Respiratory Distress Syndrome Network, Brower RG, Matthay MA, Morris A, Schoenfeld D, Thompson BT, Wheeler A. Ventilation with lower tidal volumes as compared with traditional tidal volumes for acute lung injury and the acute respiratory distress syndrome. N Engl J Med. 2000;342:1301–8.

3. Alhazzani W, Belley-Cote E, Moller MH, Angus DC, Papazian L, Arabi YM, Citerio G, Connolly B, Denehy L, Fox-Robichaud A, Hough CL, Laake JH, Machado FR, Ostermann M, Piraino T, Sharif S, Szczeklik W, Young PJ, Gouskos A, Kiedrowski K, Burns KEA. Neuromuscular blockade in patients with Ards: a rapid practice guideline. Intensive Care Med. 2020;46:1977–86.

4. Amato MB, Meade MO, Slutsky AS, Brochard L, Costa EL, Schoenfeld DA, Stewart TE, Briel M, Talmor D, Mercat A, Richard JC, Carvalho CR, Brower RG. Driving pressure and survival in the acute respiratory distress syndrome. N Engl J Med. 2015;372:747–55.

5. Annane D, Sebille V, Bellissant E, Ger-Inf-05 Study Group. Effect of low doses of corticosteroids in septic shock patients with or without early acute respiratory distress syndrome. Crit Care Med. 2006;34:22–30.

6. Arabi YM, Balkhy HH, Hayden FG, Bouchama A, Luke T, Baillie JK, Al-Omari A, Hajeer AH, Senga M, Denison MR, Nguyen-Van-Tam JS, Shindo N, Bermingham A, Chappell JD, Van Kerkhove MD, Fowler RA. Middle East respiratory syndrome. N Engl J Med. 2017;376:584–94.

7. Ashbaugh DG, Bigelow DB, Petty TL, Levine BE. Acute respiratory distress in adults. Lancet. 1967;2:319–23.

8. Bellani G, Laffey JG, Pham T, Fan E, Brochard L, Esteban A, Gattinoni L, Van Haren F, Larsson A, Mcauley DF, Ranieri M, Rubenfeld G, Thompson BT, Wrigge H, Slutsky AS, Pesenti A, LUNG SAFE Investigators, ESICM Trials Group. Epidemiology, patterns of care, and mortality for patients with acute respiratory distress syndrome in intensive care units in 50 countries. Jama. 2016;315:788–800.

9. Bernard GR, Artigas A, Brigham KL, Carlet J, Falke K, Hudson L, Lamy M, Legall JR, Morris A, Spragg R. The American-European consensus conference on Ards. Definitions, mechanisms, relevant outcomes, and clinical trial coordination. Am J Respir Crit Care Med. 1994;149:818–24.

10. Bienvenu OJ, Colantuoni E, Mendez-Tellez PA, Dinglas VD, Shanholtz C, Husain N, Dennison CR, Herridge MS, Pronovost PJ, Needham DM. Depressive symptoms and impaired physical function after acute lung injury: a 2-year longitudinal study. Am J Respir Crit Care Med. 2012;185:517–24.

11. Bishop MJ. Hemodynamic and gas exchange effects of pancuronium bromide in sedated patients with respiratory failure. Anesthesiology. 1984;60:369–71.

12. Blount BC, Karwowski MP, Shields PG, Morel-Espinosa M, Valentin-Blasini L, Gardner M, Braselton M, Brosius CR, Caron KT, Chambers D, Corstvet J, Cowan E, De Jesus VR, Espinosa P, Fernandez C, Holder C, Kuklenyik Z, Kusovschi JD, Newman C, Reis GB, Rees J, Reese C, Silva L, Seyler T, Song MA, Sosnoff C, Spitzer CR, Tevis D, Wang L, Watson C, Wewers MD, Xia B, Heitkemper DT, Ghinai I, Layden J, Briss P, King BA, Delaney LJ, Jones CM, Baldwin GT, Patel A, Meaney-Delman D, Rose D, Krishnasamy V, Barr JR, Thomas J, Pirkle JL, Lung Injury Response Laboratory Working Group. Vitamin E acetate in Bronchoalveolar-lavage fluid associated with Evali. N Engl J Med. 2020;382:697–705.

13. Braune S, Bojes P, Mecklenburg A, Angriman F, Soeffker G, Warnke K, Westermann D, Blankenberg S, Kubik M, Reichenspurner H, Kluge S. Feasibility, safety, and resource utilisation of active mobilisation of patients on extracorporeal life support: a prospective observational study. Ann Intensive Care. 2020;10:161.

14. Brower RG, Lanken PN, Macintyre N, Matthay MA, Morris A, Ancukiewicz M, Schoenfeld D, Thompson BT, National Heart, Lung, Blood Institute ARDS Clinical Trials Network.

Higher versus lower positive end-expiratory pressures in patients with the acute respiratory distress syndrome. N Engl J Med. 2004;351:327–36.

15. Calfee CS, Delucchi K, Parsons PE, Thompson BT, Ware LB, Matthay MA, NHLBI ARDS Network. Subphenotypes in acute respiratory distress syndrome: latent class analysis of data from two randomised controlled trials. Lancet Respir Med. 2014;2:611–20.

16. Cardinal-Fernandez P, Bajwa EK, Dominguez-Calvo A, Menendez JM, Papazian L, Thompson BT. The presence of diffuse alveolar damage on open lung biopsy is associated with mortality in patients with acute respiratory distress syndrome: a systematic review and meta-analysis. Chest. 2016;149:1155–64.

17. Chen L, Welty-Wolf KE, Kraft BD. Nonhuman primate species as models of human bacterial sepsis. Lab Anim (NY). 2019;48:57–65.

18. Chen L, Kraft BD, Roggli VL, Healy ZR, Woods CW, Tsalik EL, Ginsburg GS, Murdoch DM, Suliman HB, Piantadosi CA, Welty-Wolf KE. Heparin-based blood purification attenuates organ injury in baboons with Streptococcus pneumoniae pneumonia. Am J Physiol Lung Cell Mol Physiol. 2021;321:L321–35.

19. Combes A, Hajage D, Capellier G, Demoule A, Lavoue S, Guervilly C, Da Silva D, Zafrani L, Tirot P, Veber B, Maury E, Levy B, Cohen Y, Richard C, Kalfon P, Bouadma L, Mehdaoui H, Beduneau G, Lebreton G, Brochard L, Ferguson ND, Fan E, Slutsky AS, Brodie D, Mercat A, EOLIA Trial Group, REVA, and ECMONet. Extracorporeal membrane oxygenation for severe acute respiratory distress syndrome. N Engl J Med. 2018;378:1965–75.

20. Debacker J, Hart N, Fan E. Neuromuscular blockade in the 21st century management of the critically ill patient. Chest. 2017;151:697–706.

21. Dequin PF, Meziani F, Quenot JP, Kamel T, Ricard JD, Badie J, Reignier J, Heming N, Plantefeve G, Souweine B, Voiriot G, Colin G, Frat JP, Mira JP, Barbarot N, Francois B, Louis G, Gibot S, Guitton C, Giacardi C, Hraiech S, Vimeux S, L'her E, Faure H, Herbrecht JE, Bouisse C, Joret A, Terzi N, Gacouin A, Quentin C, Jourdain M, Leclerc M, Coffre C, Bourgoin H, Lengelle C, Caille-Fenerol C, Giraudeau B, Le Gouge A, CRICS-TriGGERSep Network. Hydrocortisone in severe community-acquired pneumonia. N Engl J Med. 2023;388:1931–41.

22. Derdak S, Mehta S, Stewart TE, Smith T, Rogers M, Buchman TG, Carlin B, Lowson S, Granton J, Multicenter Oscillatory Ventilation For Acute Respiratory Distress Syndrome Trial (MOAT) Study Investigators. High-frequency oscillatory ventilation for acute respiratory distress syndrome in adults: a randomized, controlled trial. Am J Respir Crit Care Med. 2002;166:801–8.

23. Dianti J, Tisminetzky M, Ferreyro BL, Englesakis M, Del Sorbo L, Sud S, Talmor D, Ball L, Meade M, Hodgson C, Beitler JR, Sahetya S, Nichol A, Fan E, Rochwerg B, Brochard L, Slutsky AS, Ferguson ND, Serpa Neto A, Adhikari NKJ, Angriman F, Goligher EC. Association of positive end-expiratory pressure and lung recruitment selection strategies with mortality in acute respiratory distress syndrome: a systematic review and network meta-analysis. Am J Respir Crit Care Med. 2022;205:1300–10.

24. Dinglas VD, Aronson Friedman L, Colantuoni E, Mendez-Tellez PA, Shanholtz CB, Ciesla ND, Pronovost PJ, Needham DM. Muscle weakness and 5-year survival in acute respiratory distress syndrome survivors. Crit Care Med. 2017;45:446–53.

25. Douglas WW, Rehder K, Beynen FM, Sessler AD, Marsh HM. Improved oxygenation in patients with acute respiratory failure: the prone position. Am Rev Respir Dis. 1977;115:559–66.

26. Dzierba AL, Abrams D, Brodie D. Medicating patients during extracorporeal membrane oxygenation: the evidence is building. Crit Care. 2017;21:66.

27. ECMO-PT Study Investigators, International ECMO Network. Early mobilisation during extracorporeal membrane oxygenation was safe and feasible: a pilot randomised controlled trial. Intensive Care Med. 2020;46:1057–9.

28. Elliott CG, Morris AH, Cengiz M. Pulmonary function and exercise gas exchange in survivors of adult respiratory distress syndrome. Am Rev Respir Dis. 1981;123:492–5.

29. Erickson SE, Martin GS, Davis JL, Matthay MA, Eisner MD, NIH NHLBI ARDS Network. Recent trends in acute lung injury mortality: 1996–2005. Crit Care Med. 2009;37:1574–9.

30. Ewald H, Raatz H, Boscacci R, Furrer H, Bucher HC, Briel M. Adjunctive corticosteroids for pneumocystis jiroveci pneumonia in patients with Hiv infection. Cochrane Database Syst Rev. 2015;2015(4):Cd006150.
31. Famous KR, Delucchi K, Ware LB, Kangelaris KN, Liu KD, Thompson BT, Calfee CS, ARDS Network. Acute respiratory distress syndrome subphenotypes respond differently to randomized fluid management strategy. Am J Respir Crit Care Med. 2017;195:331–8.
32. Fan E, Del Sorbo L, Goligher EC, Hodgson CL, Munshi L, Walkey AJ, Adhikari NKJ, Amato MBP, Branson R, Brower RG, Ferguson ND, Gajic O, Gattinoni L, Hess D, Mancebo J, Meade MO, Mcauley DF, Pesenti A, Ranieri VM, Rubenfeld GD, Rubin E, Seckel M, Slutsky AS, Talmor D, Thompson BT, Wunsch H, Uleryk E, Brozek J, Brochard LJ, American Thoracic Society, European Society of Intensive Care Medicine, and Society of Critical Care Medicine. An Official American Thoracic Society/European Society of Intensive Care Medicine/Society of Critical Care Medicine clinical practice guideline: mechanical ventilation in adult patients with acute respiratory distress syndrome. Am J Respir Crit Care Med. 2017;195:1253–63.
33. Fazzini B, Battaglini D, Carenzo L, Pelosi P, Cecconi M, Puthucheary Z. Physical and psychological impairment in survivors of acute respiratory distress syndrome: a systematic review and meta-analysis. Br J Anaesth. 2022;129:801–14.
34. Ferguson ND, Cook DJ, Guyatt GH, Mehta S, Hand L, Austin P, Zhou Q, Matte A, Walter SD, Lamontagne F, Granton JT, Arabi YM, Arroliga AC, Stewart TE, Slutsky AS, Meade MO, OSCILLATE Trial Investigators, Canadian Critical Care Trials Group. High-frequency oscillation in early acute respiratory distress syndrome. N Engl J Med. 2013;368:795–805.
35. Fisser C, Winkler M, Malfertheiner MV, Philipp A, Foltan M, Lunz D, Zeman F, Maier LS, Lubnow M, Muller T. Argatroban versus heparin in patients without heparin-induced thrombocytopenia during venovenous extracorporeal membrane oxygenation: a propensity-score matched study. Crit Care. 2021;25:160.
36. Force ADT, Ranieri VM, Rubenfeld GD, Thompson BT, Ferguson ND, Caldwell E, Fan E, Camporota L, Slutsky AS. Acute respiratory distress syndrome: the Berlin definition. Jama. 2012;307:2526–33.
37. Forel JM, Roch A, Marin V, Michelet P, Demory D, Blache JL, Perrin G, Gainnier M, Bongrand P, Papazian L. Neuromuscular blocking agents decrease inflammatory response in patients presenting with acute respiratory distress syndrome. Crit Care Med. 2006;34:2749–57.
38. Gattinoni L, Mascheroni D, Torresin A, Marcolin R, Fumagalli R, Vesconi S, Rossi GP, Rossi F, Baglioni S, Bassi F, et al. Morphological response to positive end expiratory pressure in acute respiratory failure. Computerized tomography study. Intensive Care Med. 1986;12:137–42.
39. Gebistorf F, Karam O, Wetterslev J, Afshari A. Inhaled nitric oxide for acute respiratory distress syndrome (Ards) in children and adults. Cochrane Database Syst Rev. 2016;2016:Cd002787.
40. Gill KV, Voils SA, Chenault GA, Brophy GM. Perceived versus actual sedation practices in adult intensive care unit patients receiving mechanical ventilation. Ann Pharmacother. 2012;46:1331–9.
41. Goligher EC, Tomlinson G, Hajage D, Wijeysundera DN, Fan E, Juni P, Brodie D, Slutsky AS, Combes A. Extracorporeal membrane oxygenation for severe acute respiratory distress syndrome and posterior probability of mortality benefit in a post hoc Bayesian analysis of a randomized clinical trial. Jama. 2018;320:2251–9.
42. Grotberg JC, Reynolds D, Kraft BD. Management of severe acute respiratory distress syndrome: a primer. Crit Care. 2023;27:289.
43. Guerin C, Reignier J, Richard JC, Beuret P, Gacouin A, Boulain T, Mercier E, Badet M, Mercat A, Baudin O, Clavel M, Chatellier D, Jaber S, Rosselli S, Mancebo J, Sirodot M, Hilbert G, Bengler C, Richecoeur J, Gainnier M, Bayle F, Bourdin G, Leray V, Girard R, Baboi L, Ayzac L, PROSEVA Study Group. Prone positioning in severe acute respiratory distress syndrome. N Engl J Med. 2013;368:2159–68.
44. Haeberle HA, Calov S, Martus P, Serna-Higuita LM, Koeppen M, Goll A, Bernard A, Zarbock A, Meersch M, Weiss R, Mehrlander M, Marx G, Putensen C, Bakchoul T, Magunia H,

Nieswandt B, Mirakaj V, Rosenberger P. Inhaled prostacyclin therapy in the acute respiratory distress syndrome: a randomized controlled multicenter trial. Respir Res. 2023;24:58.

45. Helms J, Frere C, Thiele T, Tanaka KA, Neal MD, Steiner ME, Connors JM, Levy JH. Anticoagulation in adult patients supported with extracorporeal membrane oxygenation: guidance from the scientific and standardization committees on perioperative and critical care haemostasis and thrombosis of the international society on thrombosis and haemostasis. J Thromb Haemost. 2023;21:373–96.

46. Hu SL, He HL, Pan C, Liu AR, Liu SQ, Liu L, Huang YZ, Guo FM, Yang Y, Qiu HB. The effect of prone positioning on mortality in patients with acute respiratory distress syndrome: a meta-analysis of randomized controlled trials. Crit Care. 2014;18:R109.

47. Karam O, Gebistorf F, Wetterslev J, Afshari A. The effect of inhaled nitric oxide in acute respiratory distress syndrome in children and adults: a Cochrane systematic review with trial sequential analysis. Anaesthesia. 2017;72:106–17.

48. Kraft BD, Piantadosi CA, Benjamin AM, Lucas JE, Zaas AK, Betancourt-Quiroz M, Woods CW, Chang AL, Roggli VL, Marshall CD, Ginsburg GS, Welty-Wolf K. Development of a novel preclinical model of pneumococcal pneumonia in nonhuman primates. Am J Respir Cell Mol Biol. 2014;50:995–1004.

49. Kraft BD, Pavlisko EN, Roggli VL, Piantadosi CA, Suliman HB. Alveolar mitochondrial quality control during acute respiratory distress syndrome. Lab Investig. 2023;103:100197.

50. Kulkarni HS, Lee JS, Bastarache JA, Kuebler WM, Downey GP, Albaiceta GM, Altemeier WA, Artigas A, Bates JHT, Calfee CS, Dela Cruz CS, Dickson RP, Englert JA, Everitt JI, Fessler MB, Gelman AE, Gowdy KM, Groshong SD, Herold S, Homer RJ, Horowitz JC, Hsia CCW, Kurahashi K, Laubach VE, Looney MR, Lucas R, Mangalmurti NS, Manicone AM, Martin TR, Matalon S, Matthay MA, Mcauley DF, Mcgrath-Morrow SA, Mizgerd JP, Montgomery SA, Moore BB, Noel A, Perlman CE, Reilly JP, Schmidt EP, Skerrett SJ, Suber TL, Summers C, Suratt BT, Takata M, Tuder R, Uhlig S, Witzenrath M, Zemans RL, Matute-Bello G. Update on the features and measurements of experimental acute lung injury in animals: an official American Thoracic Society workshop report. Am J Respir Cell Mol Biol. 2022;66:e1–e14.

51. Layden JE, Ghinai I, Pray I, Kimball A, Layer M, Tenforde MW, Navon L, Hoots B, Salvatore PP, Elderbrook M, Haupt T, Kanne J, Patel MT, Saathoff-Huber L, King BA, Schier JG, Mikosz CA, Meiman J. Pulmonary illness related to E-cigarette use in Illinois and Wisconsin - final report. N Engl J Med. 2020;382:903–16.

52. Liu L, Li J, Huang YZ, Liu SQ, Yang CS, Guo FM, Qiu HB, Yang Y. The effect of stress dose glucocorticoid on patients with acute respiratory distress syndrome combined with critical illness-related corticosteroid insufficiency. Zhonghua Nei Ke Za Zhi. 2012;51:599–603.

53. Lopinto J, Arrestier R, Peiffer B, Gaillet A, Voiriot G, Urbina T, Luyt CE, Bellaiche R, Pham T, Ait-Hamou Z, Roux D, Clere-Jehl R, Azoulay E, Gaudry S, Mayaux J, Mekontso Dessap A, Canoui-Poitrine F, De Prost N. High-dose steroids for nonresolving acute respiratory distress syndrome in critically ill covid-19 patients treated with dexamethasone: a multicenter cohort study. Crit Care Med. 2023;51:1306–17.

54. Maddali MV, Churpek M, Pham T, Rezoagli E, Zhuo H, Zhao W, He J, Delucchi KL, Wang C, Wickersham N, Mcneil JB, Jauregui A, Ke S, Vessel K, Gomez A, Hendrickson CM, Kangelaris KN, Sarma A, Leligdowicz A, Liu KD, Matthay MA, Ware LB, Laffey JG, Bellani G, Calfee CS, Sinha P, LUNG SAFE Investigators and the ESICM Trials Group. Validation and utility of Ards subphenotypes identified by machine-learning models using clinical data: an observational, multicohort, retrospective analysis. Lancet Respir Med. 2022;10:367–77.

55. Matthay MA, Arabi Y, Arroliga AC, Bernard G, Bersten AD, Brochard LJ, Calfee CS, Combes A, Daniel BM, Ferguson ND, Gong MN, Gotts JE, Herridge MS, Laffey JG, Liu KD, Machado FR, Martin TR, Mcauley DF, Mercat A, Moss M, Mularski RA, Pesenti A, Qiu H, Ramakrishnan N, Ranieri VM, Riviello ED, Rubin E, Slutsky AS, Thompson BT, Twagirumugabe T, Ware LB, Wick KD. A new global definition of acute respiratory distress syndrome. Am J Respir Crit Care Med. 2024;209:37–47.

56. Mikkelsen ME, Christie JD, Lanken PN, Biester RC, Thompson BT, Bellamy SL, Localio AR, Demissie E, Hopkins RO, Angus DC. The adult respiratory distress syndrome cognitive outcomes study: long-term neuropsychological function in survivors of acute lung injury. Am J Respir Crit Care Med. 2012;185:1307–15.

57. Munshi L, Del Sorbo L, Adhikari NKJ, Hodgson CL, Wunsch H, Meade MO, Uleryk E, Mancebo J, Pesenti A, Ranieri VM, Fan E. Prone position for acute respiratory distress syndrome: a systematic review and meta-analysis. Ann Am Thorac Soc. 2017;14:S280–8.

58. Munshi L, Walkey A, Goligher E, Pham T, Uleryk EM, Fan E. Venovenous extracorporeal membrane oxygenation for acute respiratory distress syndrome: a systematic review and meta-analysis. Lancet Respir Med. 2019;7:163–72.

59. Munshi L, Brodie D, Fan E. Extracorporeal support for acute respiratory distress syndrome in adults. Nejm Evid. 2022;1:Evidra2200128.

60. National Heart Lung Blood Institute Acute Respiratory Distress Syndrome Clinical Trials Network, Wiedemann HP, Wheeler AP, Bernard GR, Thompson BT, Hayden D, Deboisblanc B, Connors AF Jr, Hite RD, Harabin AL. Comparison of two fluid-management strategies in acute lung injury. N Engl J Med. 2006;354:2564–75.

61. National Heart Lung Blood Institute Petal Clinical Trials Network, Moss M, Huang DT, Brower RG, Ferguson ND, Ginde AA, Gong MN, Grissom CK, Gundel S, Hayden D, Hite RD, Hou PC, Hough CL, Iwashyna TJ, Khan A, Liu KD, Talmor D, Thompson BT, Ulysse CA, Yealy DM, Angus DC. Early neuromuscular blockade in the acute respiratory distress syndrome. N Engl J Med. 2019;380:1997–2008.

62. Neff TA, Stocker R, Frey HR, Stein S, Russi EW. Long-term assessment of lung function in survivors of severe Ards. Chest. 2003;123:845–53.

63. Novel Swine-Origin Influenza A Virus Investigation Team, Dawood FS, Jain S, Finelli L, Shaw MW, Lindstrom S, Garten RJ, Gubareva LV, Xu X, Bridges CB, Uyeki TM. Emergence of a novel swine-origin influenza A (H1N1) virus in humans. N Engl J Med. 2009;360:2605–15.

64. Pandharipande PP, Girard TD, Jackson JC, Morandi A, Thompson JL, Pun BT, Brummel NE, Hughes CG, Vasilevskis EE, Shintani AK, Moons KG, Geevarghese SK, Canonico A, Hopkins RO, Bernard GR, Dittus RS, Ely EW, BRAIN-ICU Study Investigators. Long-term cognitive impairment after critical illness. N Engl J Med. 2013;369:1306–16.

65. Papazian L, Forel JM, Gacouin A, Penot-Ragon C, Perrin G, Loundou A, Jaber S, Arnal JM, Perez D, Seghboyan JM, Constantin JM, Courant P, Lefrant JY, Guerin C, Prat G, Morange S, Roch A, ACURASYS Study Investigators. Neuromuscular blockers in early acute respiratory distress syndrome. N Engl J Med. 2010;363:1107–16.

66. Pappert D, Rossaint R, Slama K, Gruning T, Falke KJ. Influence of positioning on ventilation-perfusion relationships in severe adult respiratory distress syndrome. Chest. 1994;106:1511–6.

67. Park SY, Kim HJ, Yoo KH, Park YB, Kim SW, Lee SJ, Kim EK, Kim JH, Kim YH, Moon JY, Min KH, Park SS, Lee J, Lee CH, Park J, Byun MK, Lee SW, Rlee C, Jung JY, Sim YS. The efficacy and safety of prone positioning in adults patients with acute respiratory distress syndrome: a meta-analysis of randomized controlled trials. J Thorac Dis. 2015;7:356–67.

68. Parry SM. Nalamalapu SR, Nunna K, Rabiee A, Friedman LA, Colantuoni E, Needham DM, Dinglas VD. Six-minute walk distance after critical illness: a systematic review and meta-analysis. J Intensive Care Med. 2021;36:343–51.

69. Payen JF, Chanques G, Mantz J, Hercule C, Auriant I, Leguillou JL, Binhas M, Genty C, Rolland C, Bosson JL. Current practices in sedation and analgesia for mechanically ventilated critically ill patients: a prospective multicenter patient-based study. Anesthesiology. 2007;106:687–95.

70. Peek GJ, Mugford M, Tiruvoipati R, Wilson A, Allen E, Thalanany MM, Hibbert CL, Truesdale A, Clemens F, Cooper N, Firmin RK, Elbourne D, CESAR trial collaboration. Efficacy and economic assessment of conventional ventilatory support versus extracorporeal membrane oxygenation for severe adult respiratory failure (Cesar): a multicentre randomised controlled trial. Lancet. 2009;374:1351–63.

71. Peiris JS, Yuen KY, Osterhaus AD, Stohr K. The severe acute respiratory syndrome. N Engl J Med. 2003;349:2431–41.
72. Pelosi P, Croci M, Calappi E, Mulazzi D, Cerisara M, Vercesi P, Vicardi P, Gattinoni L. Prone positioning improves pulmonary function in obese patients during general anesthesia. Anesth Analg. 1996;83:578–83.
73. Pelosi P, Brazzi L, Gattinoni L. Prone position in acute respiratory distress syndrome. Eur Respir J. 2002;20:1017–28.
74. Pereira Romano ML, Maia IS, Laranjeira LN, Damiani LP, Paisani DM, Borges MC, Dantas BG, Caser EB, Victorino JA, Filho WO, Amato MBP, Cavalcanti AB. Driving pressure-limited strategy for patients with acute respiratory Distress syndrome. A pilot randomized clinical trial. Ann Am Thorac Soc. 2020;17:596–604.
75. Puybasset L, Cluzel P, Chao N, Slutsky AS, Coriat P, Rouby JJ. A computed tomography scan assessment of regional lung volume in acute lung injury. The Ct Scan Ards Study Group. Am J Respir Crit Care Med. 1998;158:1644–55.
76. Qadir N, Sahetya S, Munshi L, Summers C, Abrams D, Beitler J, Bellani G, Brower RG, Burry L, Chen JT, Hodgson C, Hough CL, Lamontagne F, Law A, Papazian L, Pham T, Rubin E, Siuba M, Telias I, Patolia S, Chaudhuri D, Walkey A, Rochwerg B, Fan E. An update on management of adult patients with acute respiratory distress syndrome: an official American Thoracic Society clinical practice guideline. Am J Respir Crit Care Med. 2024;209:24–36.
77. Recovery Collaborative Group, Horby P, Lim WS, Emberson JR, Mafham M, Bell JL, Linsell L, Staplin N, Brightling C, Ustianowski A, Elmahi E, Prudon B, Green C, Felton T, Chadwick D, Rege K, Fegan C, Chappell LC, Faust SN, Jaki T, Jeffery K, Montgomery A, Rowan K, Juszczak E, Baillie JK, Haynes R, Landray MJ. Dexamethasone in hospitalized patients with Covid-19. N Engl J Med. 2021;384:693–704.
78. Rossaint R, Falke KJ, Lopez F, Slama K, Pison U, Zapol WM. Inhaled nitric oxide for the adult respiratory distress syndrome. N Engl J Med. 1993;328:399–405.
79. Sasannejad C, Ely EW, Lahiri S. Long-term cognitive impairment after acute respiratory distress syndrome: a review of clinical impact and pathophysiological mechanisms. Crit Care. 2019;23:352.
80. Schmidt M, Bailey M, Sheldrake J, Hodgson C, Aubron C, Rycus PT, Scheinkestel C, Cooper DJ, Brodie D, Pellegrino V, Combes A, Pilcher D. Predicting survival after extracorporeal membrane oxygenation for severe acute respiratory failure. The respiratory extracorporeal membrane oxygenation survival prediction (Resp) score. Am J Respir Crit Care Med. 2014;189:1374–82.
81. Shekar K, Fraser JF, Smith MT, Roberts JA. Pharmacokinetic changes in patients receiving extracorporeal membrane oxygenation. J Crit Care. 2012;27(741):e9–18.
82. Sinha P, Delucchi KL, Chen Y, Zhuo H, Abbott J, Wang C, Wickersham N, Mcneil JB, Jauregui A, Ke S, Vessel K, Gomez A, Hendrickson CM, Kangelaris KN, Sarma A, Leligdowicz A, Liu KD, Matthay MA, Ware LB, Calfee CS. Latent class analysis-derived subphenotypes are generalisable to observational cohorts of acute respiratory distress syndrome: a prospective study. Thorax. 2022;77:13–21.
83. Sprung CL, Annane D, Keh D, Moreno R, Singer M, Freivogel K, Weiss YG, Benbenishty J, Kalenka A, Forst H, Laterre PF, Reinhart K, Cuthbertson BH, Payen D, Briegel J, CORTICUS Study Group. Hydrocortisone therapy for patients with septic shock. N Engl J Med. 2008;358:111–24.
84. Steinberg KP, Hudson LD, Goodman RB, Hough CL, Lanken PN, Hyzy R, Thompson BT, Ancukiewicz M, National Heart, Lung, and Blood Institute Acute Respiratory Distress Syndrome (ARDS) Clinical Trials Network. Efficacy and safety of corticosteroids for persistent acute respiratory distress syndrome. N Engl J Med. 2006;354:1671–84.
85. Sud S, Friedrich JO, Adhikari NKJ, Fan E, Ferguson ND, Guyatt G, Meade MO. Comparative effectiveness of protective ventilation strategies for moderate and severe acute respiratory distress syndrome. A network meta-analysis. Am J Respir Crit Care Med. 2021;203:1366–77.

86. Tomazini BM, Maia IS, Cavalcanti AB, Berwanger O, Rosa RG, Veiga VC, Avezum A, Lopes RD, Bueno FR, Silva M, Baldassare FP, Costa ELV, Moura RAB, Honorato MO, Costa AN, Damiani LP, Lisboa T, Kawano-Dourado L, Zampieri FG, Olivato GB, Righy C, Amendola CP, Roepke RML, Freitas DHM, Forte DN, Freitas FGR, Fernandes CCF, Melro LMG, Junior GFS, Morais DC, Zung S, Machado FR, Azevedo LCP, COALITION COVID-19 Brazil III Investigators. Effect of dexamethasone on days alive and ventilator-free in patients with moderate or severe acute respiratory distress syndrome and Covid-19: the codex randomized clinical trial. Jama. 2020;324:1307–16.
87. Tongyoo S, Permpikul C, Mongkolpun W, Vattanavanit V, Udompanturak S, Kocak M, Meduri GU. Hydrocortisone treatment in early sepsis-associated acute respiratory distress syndrome: results of a randomized controlled trial. Crit Care. 2016;20:329.
88. Tonna JE, Abrams D, Brodie D, Greenwood JC, Rubio Mateo-Sidron JA, Usman A, Fan E. Management of adult patients supported with venovenous extracorporeal membrane oxygenation (Vv Ecmo): guideline from the extracorporeal life support organization (Elso). Asaio J. 2021;67:601–10.
89. Villar J, Ferrando C, Martinez D, Ambros A, Munoz T, Soler JA, Aguilar G, Alba F, Gonzalez-Higueras E, Conesa LA, Martin-Rodriguez C, Diaz-Dominguez FJ, Serna-Grande P, Rivas R, Ferreres J, Belda J, Capilla L, Tallet A, Anon JM, Fernandez RL, Gonzalez-Martin JM, dexamethasone in ARDS network. Dexamethasone treatment for the acute respiratory distress syndrome: a multicentre, randomised controlled trial. Lancet Respir Med. 2020;8:267–76.
90. Walkey AJ, Del Sorbo L, Hodgson CL, Adhikari NKJ, Wunsch H, Meade MO, Uleryk E, Hess D, Talmor DS, Thompson BT, Brower RG, Fan E. Higher peep versus lower peep strategies for patients with acute respiratory distress syndrome: a systematic review and meta-analysis. Ann Am Thorac Soc. 2017;14:S297–303.
91. Ware LB, Matthay MA. The acute respiratory distress syndrome. N Engl J Med. 2000;342:1334–49.
92. Yoshida T, Torsani V, Gomes S, De Santis RR, Beraldo MA, Costa EL, Tucci MR, Zin WA, Kavanagh BP, Amato MB. Spontaneous effort causes occult pendelluft during mechanical ventilation. Am J Respir Crit Care Med. 2013;188:1420–7.
93. Young D, Lamb SE, Shah S, MacKenzie I, Tunnicliffe W, Lall R, Rowan K, Cuthbertson BH, Oscar Study Group. High-frequency oscillation for acute respiratory distress syndrome. N Engl J Med. 2013;368:806–13.

Chapter 6
Acute Exacerbations of Chronic Obstructive Pulmonary Disease

Laura C. McNamara, Alyse Reichheld, and Camille R. Petri

6.1 Introduction/Epidemiology

Chronic obstructive pulmonary disease (COPD) is a common, progressive respiratory disease marked by classic symptoms of dyspnea and cough, with objective evidence of airflow limitation. Despite these nearly universal findings, patients with COPD have heterogeneous lung disease, and thus a wide spectrum of clinical phenotypes exist. Proposed risk factors for this condition include tobacco use, genetic predisposition (i.e., alpha-1 antitrypsin deficiency), long-standing asthma, environmental pollution, and various occupational exposures, such as burning biomass fuel and several types of mining [1]. In light of these risk factors, the prevalence, already estimated to be at least 9–12% of the global population, is expected to increase over time [2–5].

The natural history of COPD is marked by episodic worsening of patients' respiratory symptoms, also referred to as COPD exacerbations (ECOPD). The severity of these exacerbations can vary, ranging from mild cases that can be effectively managed in the outpatient setting to severe cases necessitating admission to the intensive care unit. Studies estimate that between 15 and 30% of patients admitted with severe COPD exacerbation do not survive the hospitalization [6, 7]. As a result, COPD and its sequelae require significant healthcare resources and pose a major threat to patients' longevity and quality of life [8–10].

Herein, we provide a wholistic overview of COPD exacerbations. We describe the pathophysiology of COPD exacerbations to offer the context for proposed

L. C. McNamara · A. Reichheld
Department of Medicine, Beth Israel Deaconess Medical Center, Boston, MA, USA

C. R. Petri (✉)
Division of Pulmonary and Critical Care, Department of Medicine, Beth Israel Deaconess Medical Center, Harvard Medical School, Boston, MA, USA
e-mail: cpetri@bidmc.harvard.edu

Y. Alzaidi, M. A. Gebily (eds.), *The Pharmacist's Expanded Role in Critical Care Medicine*, https://doi.org/10.1007/978-3-031-77335-8_6

treatments and potential complications. Caring for these patients in the ICU requires a multidisciplinary approach, one in which pharmacists play an essential role.

6.2 Physiology

6.2.1 Basic Pulmonary Physiology of COPD

The diagnosis of COPD requires a constellation of clinical signs and symptoms in concert with specific pulmonary function abnormalities. Common subjective findings include cough, shortness of breath, and phlegm production. In order to make a diagnosis of COPD, patients must have these symptoms as well as characteristic changes on pulmonary function testing. Based on current best practices for spirometry interpretation, patients meet the criteria for obstruction when the ratio of forced expiratory volume in 1 s (FEV_1) to forced vital capacity (FVC) (FEV_1/FVC ratio) is less than the predicted fifth percentile, which is considered the lower limit of normal. Bronchodilator testing must also be negative; that is, neither FEV_1 nor FVC improve meaningfully after bronchodilator administration, indicating that the obstruction is nonreversible.

The hallmarks of pulmonary physiology in patients with COPD include this nonreversible airway obstruction, increased lung compliance (i.e., ability of the lung to stretch and expand), and gas exchange limitations. Risk factors (such as cigarette smoking or environmental exposures) trigger chronic inflammation and subsequent airway remodeling. This pathophysiology develops insidiously over time and is often progressive [11, 12]. In COPD, there is also heterogeneous distal airway and alveolar destruction, which is termed emphysema. Proposed mechanisms for this destruction include an imbalance between protease and antiprotease activity in the lung parenchyma as well as apoptosis of pneumocytes [13].

The nonreversible obstruction often develops as a result of thickened, yet poorly supported, airway walls, as well as reduced numbers of small airways [14]. Although not universal for all patients with COPD, many also have goblet cell mucus hypersecretion, which predisposes to occlusion of terminal airways, and characteristics of chronic bronchitis [15]. Together, these features combine to increase airway resistance, such that on spirometry, patients have a reduced FEV_1, leading to reduced expiratory airflow and obstruction.

Emphysema also contributes to a reduction in the elastic recoil of the lungs. Thus, the lungs are more compliant, putting patients at risk of developing air trapping and hyperinflation [16]. This can be recognized clinically on chest imaging (i.e., loss of diaphragm convexity as demonstrated in Fig. 6.1) or on physical exam (i.e., barrel deformity of the chest wall) but is formally diagnosed with lung volume testing [17, 18].

With the destruction of terminal airways, alveoli, and their adjacent pulmonary capillaries, patients also develop gas exchange limitations and ventilation/perfusion (V/Q) mismatch, with resultant chronic hypoxemic and/or hypercapnic respiratory

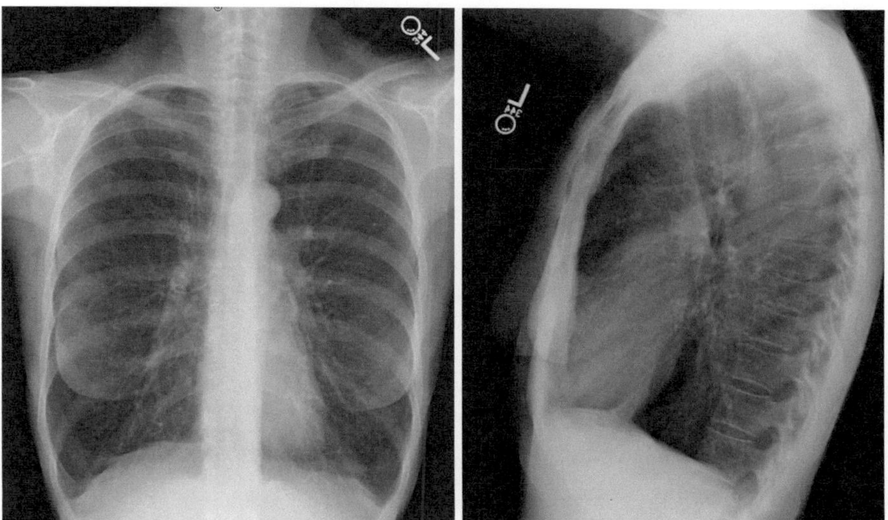

Fig. 6.1 Posterior–anterior and lateral chest radiographs demonstrating flattening of the diaphragm, suggestive of hyperinflation

failure. This multilevel destruction of the lung anatomy also predisposes patients to pulmonary hypertension.

6.2.2   *Physiology During COPD Exacerbation*

An acute worsening of underlying airway inflammation, often incited by some additional insult, is thought to precipitate exacerbations of COPD. The most common triggers include viral infections (of which rhinovirus is the most common), bacterial infections, and environmental exposures (i.e., increases in air pollution or tobacco use), though pulmonary emboli and cardiac conditions should also be considered (see Sect. 6.3.1) [19].

This acute on chronic airway inflammation results in increased airway edema, smooth muscle tone, and mucus production. Together, these aggravate the underlying pathophysiology of V/Q mismatch and increased airway resistance, leading to the common clinical findings of worsened hypoxemia, hypercapnia, tachypnea, increased sputum production, and dyspnea.

The dyspnea and increased ventilatory demand that patients experience during an exacerbation can also have harmful pathophysiologic consequences, particularly during a severe exacerbation. More specifically, as minute ventilation increases during an exacerbation, patients will have reduced expiratory time [16]. In the context of concurrent expiratory flow limitation, patients experience incomplete exhalation, which leads to serial increases in end-expiratory lung volume with each breath, a

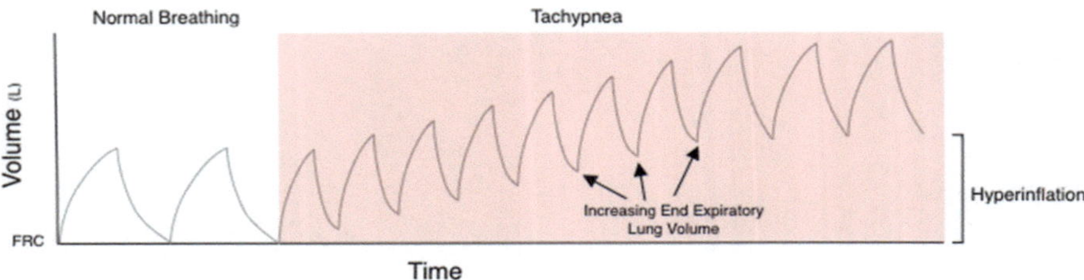

Fig. 6.2 Dynamic hyperinflation volume-time curve (showing increasing end-expiratory lung volumes during tachypnea, resulting in sequentially higher lung volumes). *FRC* functional residual capacity (lung volume achieved at rest, after passive exhalation)

phenomenon referred to as "dynamic hyperinflation" (Fig. 6.2). Dynamic hyperinflation may further impair respiratory function through the following mechanisms:

1. Increasing the patient's work of breathing (by virtue of initiating a breath at a higher resting lung volume).
2. Worsening mechanics of the respiratory system (due to reduced lung and chest wall compliance at higher lung volumes, which forces the patient to exert greater effort to successfully inspire).
3. Decreasing ventilatory efficiency (by changing the geometric configuration and length of the respiratory muscles, putting them in a disadvantaged position).
4. Increasing intrathoracic pressure (i.e., "intrinsic positive end-expiratory pressure [PEEP]"), thereby risking impaired right ventricular filling and cardiac output [20–22].

6.3 Diagnosis of COPD Exacerbation

6.3.1 Definition

While specific criteria defining a COPD exacerbation vary according to different sources, all agree that it is marked by an acute episode of worsened respiratory symptoms [23–25]. The hallmark features include increased dyspnea, cough, phlegm production, and/or sputum purulence. These symptoms often develop within 2 weeks prior to presentation and most commonly after an inciting trigger that leads to airway inflammation (see below in Sect. 6.2.2 for further details on this pathophysiology) [23, 24].

6.3.2 Differential Diagnoses and Evaluation

Essential to the diagnosis of ECOPD is a thorough workup to exonerate other potential causes of the patient's respiratory symptoms. In particular, other pulmonary conditions, such as pulmonary embolism, pneumonia, aspiration, and pneumothorax, and cardiac diseases, such as congestive heart failure, myocardial infarction, and arrhythmias, should be considered as alternative diagnoses. Patients with COPD are at increased risk for many of these conditions and are also susceptible to ECOPD triggered by them [26]. Nevertheless, it can be diagnostically challenging to determine the primary culprit of respiratory symptoms in patients with underlying COPD and associated comorbidities. The management of ECOPD should include a search for an inciting trigger, as patients often require treatment for this trigger in addition to COPD-directed treatments.

Close attention to the physical exam (e.g., looking for signs of volume overload) and thoughtful diagnostic workup can help identify confounding diagnoses and/or triggers. All patients should undergo chest imaging according to local resource availability. Chest radiograph and/or lung ultrasound can be useful in identifying pneumonia, pneumothoraces, pulmonary edema, and pleural effusions. We also recommend evaluating for infection with viral testing and sputum sample for gram stain and bacterial culture, as these results can be diagnostically relevant and can also help guide treatment (see below in Sect. 6.4.3 for further details on antimicrobials). The breadth of these tests should be guided by local resources and other epidemiologic considerations, such as seasonal variations of different respiratory pathogens. While C-reactive protein (CRP) and procalcitonin levels may help guide antibiotic usage, they have yet to be incorporated into COPD guidelines, and there is still significant debate regarding how they should best be used in this population (see below in Sect. 6.4.3 for further details on these acute-phase reactants). Because patients with COPD are at increased risk for pulmonary emboli, all patients should undergo a probability assessment to determine further workup with a d-dimer or CT pulmonary angiogram as clinically indicated, particularly when no other trigger has been identified [27]. Cardiac workup should include electrocardiogram, cardiac biomarkers with troponin and NT-pro BNP, and consideration of an echocardiogram.

6.3.3 Classification of Exacerbation Severity

Recent work aims to better characterize the severity of an individual's COPD exacerbation, both for guiding clinical care and advancing research. For example, the Rome Proposal integrates several objective clinical variables, specifically measures of dyspnea (using the validated visual analog score [VAS] for dyspnea), respiratory rate, heart rate, hypoxemia, hypercapnia, and inflammation (using the serum CRP), to classify patients as having either a mild, moderate, or severe exacerbation (Fig. 6.3) [24]. Other studies have looked at the relationship between eosinophilia, both in the sputum and peripheral blood, and COPD exacerbations. While results are limited and sometimes conflicting, there is a suggestion that peripheral eosinophilia is associated with an increased risk of moderate-to-severe exacerbations, but also improved short-term outcomes during an exacerbation [28, 29].

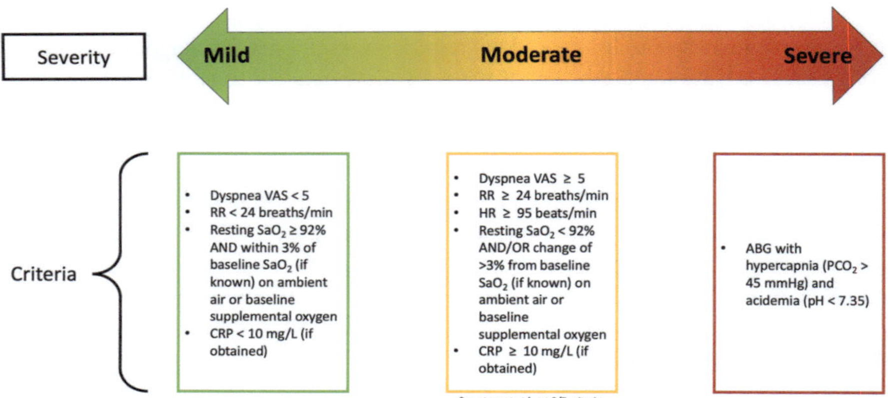

Fig. 6.3 Severity grading for ECOPD [24]. *SaO₂* oxygen saturation of arterial blood, *RR* respiratory rate, *HR* heart rate, *ABG* arterial blood gas, *PCO₂* partial pressure of carbon dioxide. Reprinted with permission of the American Thoracic Society. Copyright © 2024 American Thoracic Society. All rights reserved [24]. The American Journal of Respiratory and Critical Care Medicine is an official journal of the American Thoracic Society

6.3.4 Indications for ICU Admission

The treatment setting for patients with ECOPD should be determined by the severity of their presentation as well as local resources and practice patterns. In general, patients with features of severe exacerbation, such as those described in Fig. 6.3, should be considered for ICU admission. Other features that suggest life-threatening respiratory failure and warrant ICU admission include altered mental status, refractory hypoxemia (i.e., requiring fraction of inspired oxygen [FiO₂] ≥0.4) or hypercarbia (i.e., PaCO₂ > 60 mmHg or above the patient's baseline), severe acidemia (i.e., pH ≤7.25), refractory increased work of breathing (i.e., accessory muscle use and tachypnea), hemodynamic instability, and/or need for noninvasive or invasive mechanical ventilation [23].

6.4 Pharmacologic Treatment

6.4.1 Bronchodilators

6.4.1.1 Mechanism

The recommended initial bronchodilators for COPD exacerbations are short-acting beta-agonists (SABAs), either alone or in combination with short-acting muscarinic antagonists (SAMAs) [23]. SABAs stimulate beta₂ receptors, causing relaxation of airway smooth muscle and subsequent improvement in expiratory airflow. SAMAs block muscarinic cholinergic receptors, leading to decreased contraction of these smooth muscles as well as reducing the airway mucus hypersecretion that accompanies ECOPD [23, 30].

6.4.1.2 Evidence-Based Regimen and Dosing

The SABA-SAMA combination of albuterol and ipratropium results in greater spirometric improvements compared to albuterol alone in stable COPD, but evidence for acute exacerbations is scarce, with no additional benefit in pulmonary function observed after 90 min [31, 32]. Nevertheless, the combination is frequently utilized to treat COPD exacerbations [31, 33, 34]. It is further recommended that all patients either continue long-acting bronchodilators (LABAs, LAMAs, or a combination) during an acute exacerbation or start long-acting agents before hospital discharge [35].

Systematic reviews have demonstrated no difference in FEV_1 between short-acting bronchodilators delivered via metered-dose inhaler (MDI) and nebulizer [36]. Acutely symptomatic patients may be unable to adequately perform proper MDI technique, such that nebulized delivery of bronchodilators is preferred. Nebulizers are also a convenient and more effective medication delivery method for patients requiring noninvasive positive-pressure ventilation (NPPV) or high-flow nasal cannula (HFNC), as the medications can be delivered through these circuits without interruption of respiratory support [37, 38]. Conversely, in patients receiving invasive mechanical ventilation, if the appropriate technique is used by those administering the medication, MDIs are a safe and effective option [39].

For severe exacerbations, patients should typically receive a dose of short-acting bronchodilator, according to local pharmacy formulary, every hour for 2–3 hours. Examples of this include, but are not limited to, 1–2 puffs of albuterol MDI or a 3 cc nebulized solution of ipratropium 0.5 mg/albuterol 2.5 mg. Depending on the clinical response, time between treatments may be extended to every 2–3 hours [23]. If the patient is not responding to treatment, some clinicians will start continuous nebulized treatments, commonly albuterol monotherapy, although this practice is not recommended by the Global Initiative for Chronic Obstructive Lung Disease (GOLD) guidelines, likely given logistical challenges and a lack of robust data to support this practice [40, 41].

Methylxanthines, such as aminophylline and theophylline, provide bronchodilatory effects via nonselective phosphodiesterase inhibition. These agents should be avoided in exacerbations, however, as they disproportionately increase the risk of adverse effects, such as nausea, vomiting, tremors, and palpitations/arrhythmias, while providing only modest and inconsistent benefit in lung function [23, 42].

6.4.1.3 Adverse Effects

While practitioners should be aware of potential adverse effects, they rarely preclude the use of SABA and SAMA bronchodilators during a COPD exacerbation, given the clear benefits of bronchodilators in this setting. Due to the activation of beta$_2$ adrenergic receptors, SABAs may cause tremors, sinus tachycardia, and even arrhythmias in certain patients [43]. Physiologically, albuterol can also decrease serum potassium levels and produce lactic acidosis, particularly when administered at high doses or continuously [44–47]. These metabolic effects are transient and are rarely of clinical significance. The main adverse effect of SAMAs is dry mouth; some patients report a bitter metallic taste. Prior studies have reported a small increase in cardiovascular events in COPD patients treated with ipratropium, but larger clinical trials did not find an effect on cardiovascular event risk [48–53].

6.4.2 Glucocorticoid Therapy

6.4.2.1 Mechanism

The anti-inflammatory effects of glucocorticoids, which complement bronchodilators to improve airway resistance, are a key component in the treatment of moderate-to-severe ECOPD [54].

6.4.2.2 Evidence for Use

Prior studies have demonstrated that systemic glucocorticoids reduce recovery time, enhance lung function (FEV$_1$ specifically), improve oxygenation, lower the risk of treatment failure, and shorten hospital stays during COPD exacerbations [23, 55–57]. These studies, however, have primarily explored systemic glucocorticoids in ambulatory or hospital settings, while often excluding ICU patients. Two randomized controlled trials (RCTs) have explored the use of systemic glucocorticoids in critically ill patients with conflicting results. Alía and colleagues compared systemic glucocorticoids versus placebo and demonstrated that glucocorticoids decrease the duration of mechanical ventilation, reduce failure rates of noninvasive mechanical ventilation, and shorten ICU length of stay (LOS) [58]. Abroug and colleagues, however, did not find a significant difference in these outcomes but saw higher rates of clinically relevant hyperglycemia with glucocorticoid use [59]. Of note, these studies used different formulations of glucocorticoids, which will be addressed in further detail below, and neither study met their enrollment targets due to difficulty identifying patients not already started on glucocorticoids. A meta-analysis found that systemic glucocorticoids seem to have greater treatment success for non-critically ill patients compared to critically ill patients [60]. Nevertheless, considering this efficacy in less severe ECOPD, systemic glucocorticoids remain essential in managing COPD exacerbations in critically ill patients. As an aside, although it is widely accepted that the use of glucocorticoids in patients with influenza pneumonia results in higher mortality, use in patients with ECOPD triggered by influenza is still recommended [61, 62].

6.4.2.3   Dose and Formulation

In non-critically ill patients with ECOPD, there is evidence to support the use of oral prednisone 40 mg daily or its equivalent [23, 63]. Limited data exist regarding the optimal medication, dose, and route for systemic glucocorticoids in patients with COPD exacerbations requiring ICU admission. Alía and colleagues, who conducted the previously mentioned trial that showed a benefit of systemic glucocorticoids in critically ill patients with COPD exacerbations, used high doses of methylprednisolone (0.5 mg/kg every 6 hours for 72 hours, 0.5 mg/kg every 12 hours on days four through six, and 0.5 mg/kg/day on days seven through day ten) [58].

Limited data exists regarding which glucocorticoid should be used in ECOPD in critically ill patients, though, as discussed above, Alía and colleagues did show benefit with methylprednisolone compared to placebo [64]. In non-ICU patients, studies have shown similar efficacy with methylprednisolone, prednisone, and prednisolone [55, 65]. There have not been head-to-head trials between different glucocorticoids in critically ill patients, but for non-ICU patients, methylprednisolone is equivalent to hydrocortisone in terms of treatment failure rate, length of emergency department stays, and dyspnea, but patients treated with hydrocortisone experience lower FEV_1, lower peak expiratory flow rates, and increased hyperglycemia [66]. Another study, also in non-ICU patients, comparing methylprednisolone to dexamethasone, found that those treated with dexamethasone had less improvement in FEV_1 and a longer duration of symptoms [67]. As such, when available, methylprednisolone, prednisolone, or prednisone should be the preferred systemic glucocorticoids in the treatment of ECOPD.

In terms of route of administration, the bioavailability of oral versus intravenous glucocorticoids is nearly equivalent, and thus efficacy is equivalent in non-critically ill patients [68, 69]. In critically ill patients, data is limited, but it is important to note that the previously mentioned positive clinical trial, by Alía et al., used intravenous methylprednisolone, while the negative trial, by Abroug et al., used oral prednisone [58, 59]. In our practice, it is common to use intravenous formulations for more severe exacerbations, for patients who are failing to respond to oral glucocorticoids, for patients with impaired gastrointestinal absorption, or for patients with inadequate oral access, such as those who are receiving noninvasive positive-pressure ventilation (NPPV). Prior studies have shown that in outpatients and hospitalized patients, high-dose nebulized budesonide seems to be non-inferior to oral or intravenous glucocorticoids, though its use in lieu of systemic glucocorticoids has not been studied in ICU patients and therefore is not recommended for this population presently [57, 70–72].

There is data to support a personalized approach to glucocorticoid dosing. One study utilized patient characteristics, symptoms, and laboratory analysis to create a personalized, severity-dependent dose for study participants and found that this approach led to higher initial doses of glucocorticoids and reduced in-hospital treatment failure compared to a fixed-dose approach, without an impact on hospital length of stay. As such, it is common for clinicians to use higher dosing for more severe exacerbations. There are limits to this approach, however. For example, in critically ill patients, one observational study found that treatment with lower dose glucocorticoids (<240 mg/day of methylprednisolone equivalent) compared to higher dose (>240 mg/day) in the first 2 days of treatment did not influence mortality but was associated with shorter days mechanically ventilated, ICU LOS, and overall hospital LOS [69, 73, 74]. Increasing evidence supports using personalized and more moderate doses of glucocorticoids rather than fixed or high doses during severe COPD exacerbations. As such, a thorough review of an individual's past response to glucocorticoids can inform future decisions about treatment regimens. When this information is unknown or not available, we recommend a dose equivalent of prednisone 40 mg daily for the vast majority of exacerbations; however, if patients are on chronic glucocorticoids, clinically deteriorating, or failing to improve, higher doses such as methylprednisolone 60 mg up to every 6 hours should be considered. Ongoing work is exploring the role of possible biomarkers, such as peripheral eosinophilia, to inform methods to decrease patient exposure to systemic glucocorticoids given their potential for significant side effects, which are addressed in greater detail below [75–78].

6.4.2.4 Duration

Data on the preferred duration of glucocorticoid treatment in critically ill patients with ECOPD is limited. The REDUCE trial (Reduction in the Use of Corticosteroids in Exacerbated COPD) showed that among non-ICU patients, a 5-day regimen is not inferior to a 14-day regimen, which is supported by subsequent systematic reviews [63, 79]. Based on this literature, several societies have adopted these shorter courses into their treatment guidelines for non-critically ill patients with ECOPD [23, 63, 80]. For critically ill patients, we again favor a personalized approach, relying on patients' past responses to not only glucocorticoid dosing but also duration. In our practice, courses of 5–14 days are generally considered standard, with longer courses being reserved for sicker patients [58].

Once the decided course is completed, the glucocorticoids can typically stop altogether. However, in severe cases when patients have not fully recovered, tapers can be considered to prevent abrupt worsening of respiratory symptoms; tapers are not generally indicated to prevent acute adrenal insufficiency.

6.4.2.5 Adverse Effects

Even brief courses of glucocorticoids are linked to heightened risks of pneumonia, sepsis, and mortality [81]. Corticosteroids cause hyperglycemia, hypernatremia, and fluid retention (due to their mineralocorticoid effects). Further, they are associated with delirium, development of ICU-acquired weakness, gastrointestinal bleeding, uncontrolled hypertension, and hospital-acquired infections [82]. Many of these effects are dose and duration dependent, highlighting the importance of ongoing efforts to reduce patients' overall exposure to systemic glucocorticoids. In the interim, it is important to proactively mitigate as well as monitor for these potential side effects. Examples of this include administering the medication earlier in the day to avoid sleep–wake cycle disruption. To prevent gastrointestinal bleeding, patients with a history of peptic ulcer disease, concurrent use of nonsteroidal anti-inflammatory drugs (NSAIDs), or therapeutic anticoagulation, or those who otherwise meet ICU stress ulcer prophylaxis recommendations, should receive a proton pump inhibitor for the duration of systemic glucocorticoid therapy [83].

6.4.3 Antimicrobials

6.4.3.1 Antibiotic Patient Selection

It is recommended that antibiotics only be given to patients who are most likely to have a bacterial infection or those who are the most ill [23]. About half of patients presenting with a COPD exacerbation have sputum cultures that grow bacteria; however, it can be challenging to distinguish infection from bacterial colonization, as up to 30% of patients with stable COPD also have bacterial colonization of their airways [84, 85]. In order to identify the patients most likely to benefit from antibiotics, the GOLD guidelines recommend providing empiric antibiotics to patients with increased sputum purulence if the patient also has associated dyspnea and/or increased sputum volume. Guidelines also recommend providing empiric antibiotics to any patient who requires invasive or noninvasive mechanical ventilation [23, 26, 86]. In critically ill patients who require mechanical ventilation, antibiotic therapy is associated with decreased mortality, duration of mechanical ventilation, and length of hospital stay [87, 88].

Studies have investigated whether acute-phase reactants (such as CRP and procalcitonin) can help identify patients who should receive antibiotics, but results are inconclusive to date. One study found that when CRP was low (<20 mg/L), there was a reduction in antibiotic use without an increase in treatment failure [89, 90]. Conversely, in ICU patients with a COPD exacerbation, the use of a procalcitonin-based algorithm (with a procalcitonin cutoff of 0.1 µg/L) to decide whether to initiate or stop antibiotics was associated with higher 3-month mortality [91]. A systematic review further elaborated that measuring procalcitonin in patients hospitalized with a COPD exacerbation did not significantly reduce antibiotic exposure [92]. Overall, more studies are needed to define the role of acute-phase reactants in informing antibiotic use in ECOPD.

6.4.3.2 Antibiotic Selection and Duration

Empiric antibiotic choice should be informed by any available historical patient microbiologic data and patient risk factors for *Pseudomonas* infection and based on local antibiograms. The most common bacterial pathogens triggering COPD exacerbations in hospitalized patients include *Haemophilus influenzae, Moraxella catarrhalis, Streptococcus pneumoniae,* and *Staphylococcus aureus.* While less common, atypical pathogens, such as *Chlamydophila pneumoniae* and *Mycoplasma pneumoniae,* can also lead to exacerbations. As such, standard therapy should target these pathogens specifically. Potential options include but are not limited to amoxicillin-clavulanate, a third-generation cephalosporin, or a macrolide, tetracycline, or respiratory quinolone [23]. Whenever possible, antibiotic selection should be further tailored based on updated results from the patient's current hospitalization.

In severe exacerbations, and thus for patients requiring ICU admission, *Pseudomonas* or other gram-negative bacilli should be considered [93–95]. The greatest predictor for *Pseudomonas* infection is the isolation of *Pseudomonas* on prior cultures [96]. Other risk factors include FEV_1 <30% predicted, active tobacco use, bronchiectasis on chest imaging, antibiotic use in the last 3 months, and chronic systemic glucocorticoid use [97–99]. For these patients, anti-pseudomonal agents, such as ciprofloxacin, levofloxacin, piperacillin-tazobactam, ceftazidime, or cefepime, should be initiated depending on local susceptibility patterns [94]. At any point in the presentation, if the patient has clinical signs and/or symptoms suggestive of pneumonia, antibiotics should be tailored to those specific treatment guidelines [100, 101].

Prior studies have shown that initiating antibiotics within the first 2 days of hospitalization is associated with decreased risks of treatment failure, in-hospital mortality, and 30-day readmission [102, 103]. It is recommended to evaluate clinical response at 48–72 hours, and the total duration of antibiotics should be 5–7 days [104, 105]. There are preliminary data to support shortening antibiotic duration further, though it is likely too early to implement this broadly, particularly in critically ill patients, and thus further prospective trials are warranted [106].

The decision regarding the route of antibiotic administration should be based on the patient's ability to tolerate oral medications and the pharmacokinetic properties of the antibiotic, though generally speaking there is no difference in efficacy [23].

6.4.3.3 Antivirals

Just as rates of bacterial infection approach 50% in patients with ECOPD, viral infections are just as prevalent, with some patients even experiencing bacterial and viral co-infection. The majority of viral infections are caused by rhinovirus, though human metapneumovirus, influenza, coronavirus, parainfluenza, and respiratory syncytial virus have also been implicated [84, 93]. Early treatment with oseltamivir (within 48 hours of symptom onset) in all critically ill patients infected with influenza is associated with improved survival and may be associated with shorter ICU LOS and duration of mechanical ventilation [107]. In patients presenting later, the clinical trajectory should guide treatment. Oral agents, such as oseltamivir, are recommended, but inhaled zanamivir can increase airway reactivity and subsequently worsen exacerbations [108]. Regarding other respiratory viruses, current guidelines suggest that patients with COPD exacerbations triggered by SARS-CoV-2 infections should be treated with the same standard of care as other COVID-19 patients, including consideration of antivirals (i.e., remdesivir), glucocorticoids (i.e., dexamethasone), IL-6 receptor blockers (i.e., tocilizumab), and/or JAK inhibitors (i.e., baricitinib) according to current evidence and recommendations [23]. In general, treatment of respiratory syncytial virus (RSV) with antivirals is not universally recommended for adults, as opposed to for children, and should only be considered on a case-by-case basis in severely immunocompromised patients [109].

6.4.4 *Symptomatic Treatment of Dyspnea + Anxiolysis*

6.4.4.1 Nonpharmacologic Interventions

The American Thoracic Society recommends that symptomatic treatment of COPD exacerbations should focus on both the psychological and physical components of dyspnea. Dyspnea may be improved with supplemental oxygen, if the patient is hypoxemic, or blowing cool air on the patient's face with a fan [110].

6.4.4.2 Opioids

If nonpharmacologic interventions are insufficient or if sedation is required in the context of invasive mechanical ventilation, opioids can be given to improve dyspnea. Although nebulized opioids have been anecdotally reported as a treatment for dyspnea, systemic reviews have shown no difference between nebulized opioids and placebo, so oral or intravenous administration is preferred [109, 111]. Further, for dyspnea relief, studies have not shown that any certain opioid is superior [112–114]. Opioids should be titrated to the effect of relieving dyspnea with frequent reassessment given that higher doses of opioids may lead to respiratory depression, a significant consequence amidst significant ECOPD. As such, opioid use should be of limited duration, provided at the lowest effective dose and weaned as able. Chronic opioid use for dyspnea palliation can be considered in patients otherwise optimized after acknowledging the risks and shared decision-making between patient and provider [115].

6.4.4.3 Benzodiazepines

Benzodiazepines can be considered in cases of distressing breathlessness, when opioids are not sufficiently effective, when they are contraindicated, or when the patients are in the last days of life. Overall, the evidence does not suggest significant benefits for these symptoms, so caution is advised due to potential side effects such as delirium and drowsiness as well as respiratory depression [116–118].

6.4.4.4 Dexmedetomidine

Dexmedetomidine, a continuous intravenous infusion often limited to the ICU setting, may improve dyspnea as it offers analgesic and anxiolytic properties without causing significant respiratory depression. It can be used as a potential alternative to respiratory depressing anxiolytics (i.e., benzodiazepines) for the management of dyspnea [119]. In patients with refractory dyspnea due to end-stage cancer, one retrospective study found that dexmedetomidine safely relieves symptoms [120]. Though its use in the ECOPD setting is not yet established in clinical guidelines, dexmedetomidine is an appealing option for the management of anxiolysis to help patients better tolerate noninvasive or invasive ventilation support.

6.4.4.5 Ketamine

By inhibiting catecholamine reuptake and decreasing production of inflammatory cytokines, ketamine can cause airway relaxation and alleviate bronchospasms [121–123]. Prior studies have reported that continuous ketamine infusion in patients with asthma improved gas exchange and chest compliance [124]. One prospective study, in patients with underlying COPD undergoing thoracic surgery with single-lung ventilation, demonstrated improved oxygenation and decreased shunt fraction [125]. However, a different RCT found that ketamine did not improve respiratory mechanics in mechanically ventilated patients with COPD exacerbation or status asthmaticus when compared to fentanyl infusion [126]. In light of these variable results, we consider ketamine as an alternative sedative when typical analgesia and sedation regimens are not effective for ECOPD patients requiring invasive mechanical ventilation. Nevertheless, more studies are needed to further explore the potential role of ketamine in the management of COPD exacerbations in critically ill patients.

6.4.5 Adjunctive Therapies

6.4.5.1 Magnesium

For patients with severe exacerbations, we recommend intravenous magnesium sulfate. It is thought that magnesium causes bronchodilation by inhibiting calcium influx into airway smooth muscle cells [127]. A systematic review showed that magnesium sulfate reduced hospital admissions for patients with acute COPD exacerbation [128]. Two milligrams dosed once intravenously is likely sufficient to achieve these desired effects.

6.4.5.2 Diuretics

Diuretics are commonly used in the management of heart failure, which often can coexist with COPD. When clinically indicated, one can consider using diuretics to further optimize a patient's respiratory status by decreasing cardiac preload and subsequently reducing pulmonary edema. When prescribing diuretics, it is important to monitor for potential adverse effects, including electrolyte imbalances and impaired renal function.

6.4.5.3 Vitamin D

Vitamin D has immune modulator effects and may attenuate inflammatory responses to viral and bacterial infections [129, 130]. A meta-analysis showed that vitamin D supplementation can reduce the rate of moderate or severe COPD exacerbations in deficient patients (<25 nmol/L) without an effect in those with higher levels, but more recent studies did not demonstrate this benefit [131, 132]. GOLD guidelines recommend screening all hospitalized patients with COPD exacerbation for vitamin D deficiency and supplementing when identified.

6.4.5.4 Venous Thromboembolism Prophylaxis

All patients who are hospitalized with acute COPD exacerbations, and with respiratory failure more generally, are at risk for the development of deep venous thrombosis and subsequent pulmonary embolism [27]. We recommend pharmacologic thromboprophylaxis for patients who do not have other contraindications [23, 133].

6.4.5.5 Smoking Cessation

For patients who use tobacco, hospitalizations provide an opportunity to promote smoking cessation, which, in addition to other systemic benefits, can improve COPD prognosis and risk of future exacerbations [134]. All patients who currently smoke should be offered nicotine replacement therapy (such as nicotine patches or nicotine lozenges) to decrease the risk of nicotine withdrawal, which can affect even patients receiving sedation with mechanical ventilation [23, 135–137].

6.4.5.6 Bowel Regimen

Although data is limited, constipation and abdominal bloating may interfere with diaphragmatic excursion and worsen feelings of breathlessness in COPD exacerbations [138]. We recommend monitoring for constipation and starting a gentle bowel regimen for patients admitted with COPD exacerbation.

6.4.5.7 Mucolytics

We do not recommend a standardized approach to the use of mucolytic agents (i.e., thiol or thiol-based derivatives such as nebulized N-acetylcysteine), which may help address the mucus hypersecretion seen in ECOPD. Given limited prospective data on these medications, we favor an individualized approach based on the patient's presenting symptoms and clinical findings [139].

6.4.5.8 Nutrition

Low body mass index in patients with COPD has been associated with worse outcomes, including mortality, exacerbations, and quality of life. For patients presenting with ECOPD, a thorough nutritional assessment and as-needed supplementation are essential not only to their immediate recovery but also to potentially reducing their risk for future exacerbations [140–142].

6.4.5.9 Post-Discharge Adjuncts

Efforts should be made to ensure that patients receive appropriate post-discharge follow-up for discussion of further measures to reduce the risk of subsequent exacerbation. This includes but is not limited to immunizations, smoking cessation as discussed above, and evaluation of candidacy for nocturnal NPPV, pulmonary rehabilitation, chronic suppressive antibiotics (i.e., azithromycin), and phosphodiesterase-4 inhibitors (i.e., roflumilast) [23].

6.5 ICU-Level Interventions

Respiratory support is a key pillar in the treatment of patients presenting with severe ECOPD who require admission to an ICU. Here, we describe an evidence-based approach to these types of support and their indications and contraindications. The first step is to determine if the patient's respiratory failure is driven by hypoxemia, hypercapnia, or a combination of both, as this will guide which type of support or device should be utilized. The second step is to titrate the device settings to objective markers of oxygenation and ventilation. Given the inaccuracies reported with pulse oximetry, particularly in individuals with darker skin tones, we recommend the additional use of arterial blood gas sampling to assist with clinical decisions regarding oxygen titration [143, 144]. Alternatively, venous blood gas sampling, which is less painful for the patient, logistically easier to obtain, and a reasonably accurate measure of pH, $PaCO_2$, and HCO_3-, can and should be utilized for titration of ventilatory support [145, 146]. In addition to blood gas analysis, close monitoring of patient's mental status, work of breathing, and device measurements (e.g., minute ventilation) should inform NPPV adjustments.

In patients with stable COPD, there are different oxygen saturation goals depending on the presence or absence of hypercapnia. In all patients with ECOPD though, supplemental oxygen should be titrated to achieve oxygen saturations of 88–92% (or PaO_2 60–70 mmHg). This has been associated with improved respiratory acidosis and mortality compared to higher oxygen saturation targets in this population [147–149]. Compared to oxygen targets, the decisions about $PaCO_2$ targets are more nuanced. They are dictated by the patient's baseline $PaCO_2$, as well as the patient's lung mechanics and other factors contributing to overall acid-base status.

6.5.1 Noninvasive Positive-Pressure Ventilation

Noninvasive positive-pressure ventilation (NPPV) is the delivery of ventilatory support with air or a combination of air and oxygen to a patient without an endotracheal tube. Ventilatory support is provided via a face mask that is tightly fitted with straps over the patient's head to ensure an adequate seal around the patient's mouth and nose. Colloquially, both bilevel positive airway pressure (BPAP) and continuous positive airway pressure (CPAP) fall under the umbrella of NPPV, though there are other forms of NPPV that are outside of the scope of this and are best managed by providers and respiratory therapists trained in acute and chronic respiratory failure. BPAP, which can treat both hypercapnia and hypoxemia, is considered the mode of choice for patients with ECOPD; therefore, the majority of our discussion will center there [150]. CPAP in general can be helpful in hypoxemic respiratory failure, but has limited benefit in hypercapnic respiratory failure, and therefore is not considered first line for ventilatory support in patients with ECOPD [151].

As opposed to continuous airway pressure that is delivered in CPAP, bilevel NPPV delivers both a higher inspiratory positive airway pressure (IPAP) and a lower expiratory positive airway pressure (EPAP). By providing pressure during inspiration, the IPAP is able to reduce the patient's work of breathing required to achieve a particular tidal volume. With pressure provided during exhalation, the EPAP stents open the airways and alveoli and over time counteract the high work of breathing that occurs during ECOPD (see Sect. 6.2.2). The difference between IPAP and EPAP values, referred to as the delta PAP, influences the resultant tidal volume (V_t). As such, a larger delta PAP should lead to a greater V_t and greater minute ventilation, and thus more ventilatory support [152]. In addition to these parameters, providers can set the delivered FiO_2 and a backup mandatory respiratory rate.

The indications for bilevel NPPV in ECOPD include the following:

1. Hypercapnic Respiratory Failure ($PaCO_2$ > 45 mmHg and pH <7.35).

Evidence: A Cochrane review of 17 studies showed improved mortality and risk of endotracheal intubation when NPPV with usual care was compared to usual care alone in patients presenting with ECOPD and respiratory acidosis (defined by the above laboratory values) [150]. In light of these benefits, many guidelines suggest usage of bilevel NPPV in patients with acute or acute on chronic hypercapnic respiratory failure due to ECOPD in an effort to prevent endotracheal intubation. It can also be considered as an alternative to endotracheal intubation if the patient is not acutely deteriorating, though this is a nuanced decision and requires a wholistic view of the patient and subsequent close monitoring [153]. We recommend reassessing no more than 2 hours after initiation of BPAP. Data suggests that if the pH remains <7.25 after 2 hours of BPAP, then the need for intubation is likely [154].

Comments: In ECOPD with hypercapnia but a normal pH, NPPV has not been shown to be beneficial. Given potential harms, many agree that it should not be offered in this clinical setting; instead, medical management and as-needed oxygen support should be prioritized [153]. Conversely, if intubation is not within a patient's care preferences, BPAP should be discussed and offered as an alternative treatment for ECOPD if the need arises.

2. Respiratory Distress or Hypoxemic Respiratory Failure.

Evidence: Brochard and colleagues looked at NPPV plus usual care compared to usual care alone in patients with ECOPD. To be included, patients had to have hypercapnic respiratory failure or meet at least two of the following criteria: tachypnea (respiratory rate >30 breaths per minute), hypoxemia ($PaO_2 < 45$ mmHg), or acidemia (pH <7.35) on room air. This study found improvement in respiratory rate, need for endotracheal intubation, as well as hospital LOS and in-hospital mortality in the NPPV arm [155].

Comments: For patients with respiratory distress or hypoxemia refractory to supplemental oxygen, bronchodilators, steroids, and IV magnesium, NPPV is a helpful form of respiratory support. NPPV use, though, should not delay intubation if invasive mechanical ventilation is ultimately required and best for the patient.

3. Post-extubation Support.

Evidence: Prospective randomized controlled trials have shown decreased risk of post-extubation failure when patients with chronic lung conditions or hypercapnia, and even more specifically with COPD, are extubated to bilevel NPPV as opposed to oxygen mask alone [156–158].

Comments: In patients with COPD exacerbations who are approaching extubation, BPAP should be utilized in the immediate post-extubation period to reduce the risk of post-extubation respiratory failure [153]. Given the differences in study protocols utilized, the optimum duration of BPAP post-extubation is not clear; however, likely a minimum of 6–8 hours per day for 1–2 days is required to achieve benefit [153, 156–159].

Contraindications to NPPV include need for emergent intubation, conditions that would place patients at risk of aspiration (e.g., copious secretions or emesis, inability to protect airway), recent facial trauma or surgery, and recent upper gastrointestinal surgery [160]. Altered mental status is a relative contraindication; if this is attributable to hypercapnia, it often improves with the ventilatory support BPAP offers [161]. If a patient is unable to tolerate wearing the NPPV mask, anxiolytic medications (as discussed further in Sect. 6.4.4) can be trialed, though generally this is an indication to pursue another form of respiratory support.

6.5.2 High-Flow Nasal Canula

After BPAP, high-flow nasal canula (HFNC) is the second-line respiratory support device for patients with a COPD exacerbation [162]. HFNC is a noninvasive device that delivers a gas with titratable FiO_2 at high flow rates (e.g., up to 70 L per minute). Physiologically, there are several benefits of this type of delivery system, which we have summarized here:

1. Decreases air entrainment: Air entrainment occurs when the patient inhales ambient air, in conjunction with the gas provided by a given respiratory support device. This mixing of gases, proportional to the flow rate of the device and minute ventilation of the patient, has the effect of reducing the true FiO_2 of inspired gas. This phenomenon is therefore common with lower flow oxygen devices, like nasal cannula or simple face mask, such that there is a limit to the amount of inspired oxygen that can be achieved. Because the airflow provided by HFNC matches or even exceeds the ventilatory demands of patients with respiratory failure, the FiO_2 of the gas delivered is not appreciably diluted by ambient air, and thus the set FiO_2 is delivered in full to the alveoli. Studies have shown that HFNC improves oxygenation without up-titration of the set FiO_2, suggesting that the flow rate has a greater role [163].
2. Decreased dead-space ventilation: The adult respiratory tract has about 150 cc of anatomic dead space, where gas exchange does not occur due to the structure of the nasal and oropharynx, larynx, and trachea [164]. The high airflow delivered by HFNC is able to wash out residual carbon dioxide from the respiratory tract and thereby improve ventilation [165]. It is proposed that this improves patient work of breathing as they no longer need to maintain as high of a minute ventilation [163].
3. Mild positive end-expiratory pressure (PEEP): At sufficient airflow velocity, HFNC is able to provide modest levels of PEEP. As the flow rate increases, so too does the pressure in the alveoli at the end of expiration. However, this effect likely does not exceed 5 cm H_2O [166].

Given these physiologic effects, the most robust evidence for HFNC use is in patients with acute hypoxemic respiratory failure. In this broad population, not specific to ECOPD, HFNC has been shown to reduce risk of intubation and perhaps even improve 90-day mortality [162, 167]. While these same benefits have not been reproduced in patients with hypercapnic respiratory failure, many of whom had ECOPD, there still may be a role for its use [162]. In these patients, HFNC appears to be non-inferior to NPPV in terms of gas exchange and work of breathing, and actually superior with regard to patient comfort [167, 168].

In light of this evidence, in patients with ECOPD, we recommend the use of HFNC under the following circumstances:

1. Intolerance of or failure of NPPV prior to consideration of endotracheal intubation and invasive mechanical ventilation.

2. Respiratory support for patients during short breaks from NPPV.
3. Post-extubation respiratory support if patients are unable to tolerate BPAP, which should otherwise be the device of choice [162].

Similar to NPPV, the major contraindication to HFNC is if the patient otherwise requires intubation and invasive mechanical ventilation. Other contraindications include altered mental status and intolerance of the device [169].

6.5.3 *Invasive Mechanical Ventilation*

Invasive mechanical ventilation (IMV) is a way to provide oxygenation and mandatory ventilation to patients, most often via an endotracheal tube or at times via a tracheostomy, for patients who have already undergone this procedure or who require prolonged IMV. These connections allow for a completely closed system by which critical care clinicians can provide high levels of respiratory support. When patients receive IMV via an endotracheal tube, analgosedation should be optimized to ensure patient comfort.

In patients with ECOPD, IMV is indicated for severe respiratory distress or life-threatening respiratory failure, failure of noninvasive options like BPAP or HFNC, or airway protection. We define failure of noninvasive options as worsened work of breathing or gas exchange. More specifically, pH <7.25 after 2 hours of BPAP has been associated with a >90% need for intubation [154]. Furthermore, if patients are unable to be liberated from BPAP within 48 hours, we recommend consideration of IMV. Beyond bedside observation, scoring tools such as the BAP-65 (which includes BUN, mental status, HR, and age) can help predict which patients with ECOPD will require IMV [170, 171]. Although many patients treated with NPPV initially will ultimately require endotracheal intubation, studies suggest that attempting NPPV does not cause harm and importantly identifies patients who do not require intubation; as such, this can lead to improved patient outcomes, specifically lower mortality and ICU LOS [172, 173].

After intubation, attention should focus on optimizing ventilator settings to enhance ventilation, oxygenation, resistance, and compliance, along with ensuring proper analgesia and sedation. These conversations should occur at the bedside with input from multiple members of the care team, including but not limited to the clinicians, respiratory therapists, and nurses. Many ventilator settings are dependent on the brand and model of the ventilator as well as the selected mode of support. Strategies for patients undergoing IMV are aimed at supporting the patient's oxygen and ventilation needs, while also preventing dynamic hyperinflation and its deleterious sequela (described in more detail in Sect. 6.2.2). In order to achieve these goals, we recommend:

1. Adhering to the general principles of lung-protective ventilation described elsewhere in order to minimize ventilator-associated lung injury [174]. There should be a particular emphasis on low tidal volumes (4–8 cc/kg of ideal body weight),

which reduces the risk of dynamic hyperinflation by providing smaller volumes that are easier to expire.

2. Prolonging the expiratory time to ensure complete exhalation and avoidance of dynamic hyperinflation. This can be achieved by slowing the respiratory rate and adjusting the inspiratory to expiratory ratio (I:E ratio) so that it is at least 1:3.
3. Permitting hypercapnia, as long as the pH is within a hemodynamically and metabolically safe range (i.e., >7.2), to allow for the lower tidal volumes and longer expiratory time discussed above.
4. Promoting ventilator-patient synchrony and reducing patient work of breathing, acknowledging that sedation and even paralysis may be required to achieve this [175].
5. Utilizing best PEEP titration strategies (i.e., pressure-volume loop, decremental PEEP, esophageal manometry) to help reduce patient's work of breathing and to stent open distal airways, thus improving total airway resistance [176]. The amount of applied PEEP should never exceed the amount of intrinsic PEEP [177].

Further titration of ventilator settings should take into account the patient's oxygen saturation, acid-base status, measurements of intrinsic PEEP, airway resistance, and compliance [178]. Patients should be assessed daily for spontaneous awakening and breathing trials and should be weaned from the ventilator safely but expeditiously, using NPPV and/or HFNC as post-extubation support (as discussed in detail in Sects. 6.5.1 and 6.5.2) [179].

6.6 Conclusion

COPD exacerbations result in significant utilization of healthcare resources, including ICU admissions, and high patient morbidity and mortality [180]. Optimization of pulmonary physiology during an acute exacerbation requires a multidisciplinary approach to address potential triggers, decrease airway inflammation, reduce airway resistance, and support adequate oxygenation and ventilation.

References

1. Eisner MD, Anthonisen N, Coultas D, et al. An official American Thoracic Society public policy statement: novel risk factors and the global burden of chronic obstructive pulmonary disease. Am J Respir Crit Care Med. 2010;182(5):693–718. https://doi.org/10.1164/rccm.200811-1757ST.
2. Boers E, Barrett M, Su JG, et al. Global burden of chronic obstructive pulmonary disease through 2050. JAMA Netw Open. 2023;6(12):e2346598. https://doi.org/10.1001/jamanetworkopen.2023.46598.
3. Varmaghani M, Dehghani M, Heidari E, Sharifi F, Saeedi Moghaddam S, Farzadfar F. Global prevalence of chronic obstructive pulmonary disease: systematic review and meta-analysis. East Mediterr Health J. 2019;25(1):47–57. https://doi.org/10.26719/emhj.18.014.

4. Ntritsos G, Franek J, Belbasis L, et al. Gender-specific estimates of COPD prevalence: a systematic review and meta-analysis. Int J Chron Obstruct Pulmon Dis. 2018;13:1507–14. https://doi.org/10.2147/COPD.S146390.

5. Safiri S, Carson-Chahhoud K, Noori M, et al. Burden of chronic obstructive pulmonary disease and its attributable risk factors in 204 countries and territories, 1990-2019: results from the global burden of disease study 2019. BMJ. 2022;378:e069679. https://doi.org/10.1136/bmj-2021-069679.

6. Seneff MG, Wagner DP, Wagner RP, Zimmerman JE, Knaus WA. Hospital and 1-year survival of patients admitted to intensive care units with acute exacerbation of chronic obstructive pulmonary disease. JAMA. 1995;274(23):1852–7.

7. Hoogendoorn M, Hoogenveen RT, van Mölken MPR, Vestbo J, Feenstra TL. Case fatality of COPD exacerbations: a meta-analysis and statistical modelling approach. Eur Respir J. 2011;37(3):508–15. https://doi.org/10.1183/09031936.00043710.

8. Chen S, Kuhn M, Prettner K, et al. The global economic burden of chronic obstructive pulmonary disease for 204 countries and territories in 2020–50: a health-augmented macroeconomic modelling study. Lancet Glob Health. 2023;11(8):e1183–93. https://doi.org/10.1016/S2214-109X(23)00217-6.

9. Srivastava K, Thakur D, Sharma S, Punekar YS. Systematic review of humanistic and economic burden of symptomatic chronic obstructive pulmonary disease. PharmacoEconomics. 2015;33(5):467–88. https://doi.org/10.1007/s40273-015-0252-4.

10. Sin DD, Anthonisen NR, Soriano JB, Agusti AG. Mortality in COPD: role of comorbidities. Eur Respir J. 2006;28(6):1245–57. https://doi.org/10.1183/09031936.00133805.

11. Baraldo S, Turato G, Badin C, et al. Neutrophilic infiltration within the airway smooth muscle in patients with COPD. Thorax. 2004;59(4):308–12. https://doi.org/10.1136/thx.2003.012146.

12. Turato G, Zuin R, Miniati M, et al. Airway inflammation in severe chronic obstructive pulmonary disease: relationship with lung function and radiologic emphysema. Am J Respir Crit Care Med. 2002;166(1):105–10. https://doi.org/10.1164/rccm.2111084.

13. Sharafkhaneh A, Hanania NA, Kim V. Pathogenesis of emphysema. Proc Am Thorac Soc. 2008;5(4):475–7. https://doi.org/10.1513/pats.200708-126ET.

14. McDonough JE, Yuan R, Suzuki M, et al. Small-airway obstruction and emphysema in chronic obstructive pulmonary disease. N Engl J Med. 2011;365(17):1567–75. https://doi.org/10.1056/NEJMoa1106955.

15. Kim V, Criner GJ. Chronic bronchitis and chronic obstructive pulmonary disease. Am J Respir Crit Care Med. 2013;187(3):228. https://doi.org/10.1164/rccm.201210-1843CI.

16. O'Donnell DE, Laveneziana P. Physiology and consequences of lung hyperinflation in COPD. Eur Respir Rev. 2006;15(100):61–7. https://doi.org/10.1183/09059180.00010002.

17. Shaker SB, Dirksen A, Bach KS, Mortensen J. Imaging in chronic obstructive pulmonary disease. COPD J Chronic Obstr Pulm Dis. 2007;4(2):143–61. https://doi.org/10.1080/15412550701341277.

18. Pierce JA, Ebert RV. The barrel deformity of the chest, the senile lung and obstructive pulmonary emphysema. Am J Med. 1958;25(1):13–22. https://doi.org/10.1016/0002-9343(58)90193-1.

19. Papi A, Luppi F, Franco F, Fabbri LM. Pathophysiology of exacerbations of chronic obstructive pulmonary disease. Proc Am Thorac Soc. 2006;3(3):245–51. https://doi.org/10.1513/pats.200512-125SF.

20. Macklem PT. Hyperinflation. Am Rev Respir Dis. 1984;129(1):1–2. https://doi.org/10.1164/arrd.1984.129.1.1.

21. Soffler MI, Hayes MM, Schwartzstein RM. Respiratory sensations in dynamic hyperinflation: physiological and clinical applications. Respir Care. 2017;62(9):1212–23. https://doi.org/10.4187/respcare.05198.

22. Jörgensen K, Müller MF, Nel J, Upton RN, Houltz E, Ricksten SE. Reduced intrathoracic blood volume and left and right ventricular dimensions in patients with severe emphysema: an MRI study. Chest. 2007;131(4):1050–7. https://doi.org/10.1378/chest.06-2245.

23. Agustí A, Celli BR, Criner GJ, et al. Global initiative for chronic obstructive lung disease 2023 report: GOLD executive summary. Eur Respir J. 2023;61(4):2300239. https://doi.org/10.1183/13993003.00239-2023.

24. Celli BR, Fabbri LM, Aaron SD, et al. An updated definition and severity classification of chronic obstructive pulmonary disease exacerbations: the Rome proposal. Am J Respir Crit Care Med. 2021;204(11):1251–8. https://doi.org/10.1164/rccm.202108-1819PP.

25. Kim V, Aaron SD. What is a COPD exacerbation? Current definitions, pitfalls, challenges and opportunities for improvement. Eur Respir J. 2018;52(5):1801261. https://doi.org/10.1183/13993003.01261-2018.

26. Beghé B, Verduri A, Roca M, Fabbri LM. Exacerbation of respiratory symptoms in COPD patients may not be exacerbations of COPD. Eur Respir J. 2013;41(4):993–5. https://doi.org/10.1183/09031936.00180812.

27. Anderson FA, Spencer FA. Risk factors for venous thromboembolism. Circulation. 2003;107(23_suppl_1):I-9–I-16. https://doi.org/10.1161/01.CIR.0000078469.07362.E6.

28. Vedel-Krogh S, Nielsen SF, Lange P, Vestbo J, Nordestgaard BG. Blood eosinophils and exacerbations in chronic obstructive pulmonary disease. The Copenhagen general population study. Am J Respir Crit Care Med. 2016;193(9):965–74. https://doi.org/10.1164/rccm.201509-1869OC.

29. Jabarkhil A, Moberg M, Janner J, et al. Elevated blood eosinophils in acute COPD exacerbations: better short- and long-term prognosis. Eur Clin Respir J. 2020;7(1):1757274. https://doi.org/10.1080/20018525.2020.1757274.

30. Calzetta L, Ritondo BL, Zappa MC, et al. The impact of long-acting muscarinic antagonists on mucus hypersecretion and cough in chronic obstructive pulmonary disease: a systematic review. Eur Respir Rev. 2022;31(164):210196. https://doi.org/10.1183/16000617.0196-2021.

31. McCrory DC, Brown CD. Anti-cholinergic bronchodilators versus beta2-sympathomimetic agents for acute exacerbations of chronic obstructive pulmonary disease. Cochrane Database Syst Rev. 2002;2003(4):CD003900. https://doi.org/10.1002/14651858.CD003900.

32. Campbell S. For COPD a combination of ipratropium bromide and albuterol sulfate is more effective than Albuterol Base. Arch Intern Med. 1999;159(2):156. https://doi.org/10.1001/archinte.159.2.156.

33. Moayyedi P, Congleton J, Page RL, Pearson SB, Muers MF. Comparison of nebulised salbutamol and ipratropium bromide with salbutamol alone in the treatment of chronic obstructive pulmonary disease. Thorax. 1995;50(8):834–7. https://doi.org/10.1136/thx.50.8.834.

34. COMBIVENT Inhalation Aerosol Study Group. In chronic obstructive pulmonary disease, a combination of ipratropium and albuterol is more effective than either agent alone. Chest. 1994;105(5):1411–9. https://doi.org/10.1378/chest.105.5.1411.

35. Kew KM, Mavergames C, Walters JAE. Long-acting beta2-agonists for chronic obstructive pulmonary disease. Cochrane Database Syst Rev. 2013;2013(10):CD010177. https://doi.org/10.1002/14651858.CD010177.pub2.

36. Van Geffen WH, Douma WR, Slebos DJ, Kerstjens HA. Bronchodilators delivered by nebuliser versus pMDI with spacer or DPI for exacerbations of COPD. Cochrane Database Syst Rev. 2016;2016(8):CD011826. https://doi.org/10.1002/14651858.CD011826.pub2.

37. Branconnier MP, Hess DR. Albuterol delivery during noninvasive ventilation. Respir Care. 2005;50(12):1649–53.

38. Colaianni-Alfonso N, MacLoughlin R, Espada A, et al. Delivery of aerosolized bronchodilators by high-flow nasal cannula during COPD exacerbation. Respir Care. 2023;68(6):721–6. https://doi.org/10.4187/respcare.10614.

39. Dhand R, Tobin MJ. Bronchodilator delivery with metered-dose inhalers in mechanically-ventilated patients. Eur Respir J. 1996;9(3):585–95. https://doi.org/10.1183/09031936.09.09030585.

40. McPeck M, Tandon R, Hughes K, Smaldone GC. Aerosol delivery during continuous nebulization. Chest. 1997;111(5):1200–5. https://doi.org/10.1378/chest.111.5.1200.

41. Reisner C, Lee J, Kotch A, Dworkin G. Comparison of volume output from two different continuous nebulizer systems. Ann Allergy Asthma Immunol. 1996;76(2):209–13. https://doi.org/10.1016/S1081-1206(10)63424-2.

42. Barr RG, Rowe BH, Camargo CA. Methylxanthines for exacerbations of chronic obstructive pulmonary disease. Cochrane Database Syst Rev. 2003;2003(2):CD002168. https://doi.org/10.1002/14651858.CD002168.

43. Page RL, O'Bryant CL, Cheng D, et al. Drugs that may cause or exacerbate heart failure: a scientific statement from the American Heart Association. Circulation. 2016;134(6):e32–69. https://doi.org/10.1161/CIR.0000000000000426.

44. Rodrigo GJ, Rodrigo C. Elevated plasma lactate level associated with high dose inhaled albuterol therapy in acute severe asthma. Emerg Med J EMJ. 2005;22(6):404–8. https://doi.org/10.1136/emj.2003.012039.

45. Zitek T, Cleveland N, Rahbar A, et al. Effect of nebulized albuterol on serum lactate and potassium in healthy subjects. Heard K, ed. Acad Emerg Med. 2016;23(6):718–21. https://doi.org/10.1111/acem.12937.

46. Montoliu J. Potassium-lowering effect of albuterol for hyperkalemia in renal failure. Arch Intern Med. 1987;147(4):713. https://doi.org/10.1001/archinte.1987.00370040095017.

47. Windom HH, Burgess CD, Siebers RWL, et al. The pulmonary and extrapulmonary effects of inhaled β-agonists in patients with asthma. Clin Pharmacol Ther. 1990;48(3):296–301. https://doi.org/10.1038/clpt.1990.152.

48. Tashkin DP, Celli B, Senn S, et al. A 4-year trial of tiotropium in chronic obstructive pulmonary disease. N Engl J Med. 2008;359(15):1543–54. https://doi.org/10.1056/NEJMoa0805800.

49. Singh S, Loke YK, Furberg CD. Inhaled anticholinergics and risk of major adverse cardiovascular events in patients with chronic obstructive pulmonary disease: a systematic review and meta-analysis. JAMA. 2008;300(12):1439–50. https://doi.org/10.1001/jama.300.12.1439.

50. Kesten S, Jara M, Wentworth C, Lanes S. Pooled clinical trial analysis of tiotropium safety. Chest. 2006;130(6):1695–703. https://doi.org/10.1378/chest.130.6.1695.

51. Anthonisen NR, Connett JE, Enright PL, Manfreda J, Lung Health Study Research Group. Hospitalizations and mortality in the lung health study. Am J Respir Crit Care Med. 2002;166(3):333–9. https://doi.org/10.1164/rccm.2110093.

52. Rodrigo GJ, Castro-Rodriguez JA, Nannini LJ, Plaza Moral V, Schiavi EA. Tiotropium and risk for fatal and nonfatal cardiovascular events in patients with chronic obstructive pulmonary disease: systematic review with meta-analysis. Respir Med. 2009;103(10):1421–9. https://doi.org/10.1016/j.rmed.2009.05.020.

53. Celli B, Decramer M, Leimer I, Vogel U, Kesten S, Tashkin DP. Cardiovascular safety of tiotropium in patients with COPD. Chest. 2010;137(1):20–30. https://doi.org/10.1378/chest.09-0011.

54. Williams DM. Clinical pharmacology of corticosteroids. Respir Care. 2018;63(6):655–70. https://doi.org/10.4187/respcare.06314.

55. Davies L, Angus RM, Calverley PM. Oral corticosteroids in patients admitted to hospital with exacerbations of chronic obstructive pulmonary disease: a prospective randomised controlled trial. Lancet Lond Engl. 1999;354(9177):456–60. https://doi.org/10.1016/s0140-6736(98)11326-0.

56. Thompson WH, Nielson CP, Carvalho P, Charan NB, Crowley JJ. Controlled trial of oral prednisone in outpatients with acute COPD exacerbation. Am J Respir Crit Care Med. 1996;154(2 Pt 1):407–12. https://doi.org/10.1164/ajrccm.154.2.8756814.

57. Maltais F, Ostinelli J, Bourbeau J, et al. Comparison of nebulized budesonide and oral prednisolone with placebo in the treatment of acute exacerbations of chronic obstructive pulmonary disease: a randomized controlled trial. Am J Respir Crit Care Med. 2002;165(5):698–703. https://doi.org/10.1164/ajrccm.165.5.2109093.

58. Alía I, de la Cal MA, Esteban A, et al. Efficacy of corticosteroid therapy in patients with an acute exacerbation of chronic obstructive pulmonary disease receiving ventilatory support. Arch Intern Med. 2011;171(21):1939–46. https://doi.org/10.1001/archinternmed.2011.530.

59. Abroug F, Ouanes-Besbes L, Fkih-Hassen M, et al. Prednisone in COPD exacerbation requiring ventilatory support: an open-label randomised evaluation. Eur Respir J. 2014;43(3):717–24. https://doi.org/10.1183/09031936.00002913.

60. Abroug F, Ouanes I, Abroug S, et al. Systemic corticosteroids in acute exacerbation of COPD: a meta-analysis of controlled studies with emphasis on ICU patients. Ann Intensive Care. 2014;4:32. https://doi.org/10.1186/s13613-014-0032-x.

61. Ni YN, Chen G, Sun J, Liang BM, Liang ZA. The effect of corticosteroids on mortality of patients with influenza pneumonia: a systematic review and meta-analysis. Crit Care Lond Engl. 2019;23(1):99. https://doi.org/10.1186/s13054-019-2395-8.

62. Studer S, Rassouli F, Waldeck F, Brutsche MH, Baty F, Albrich WC. No evidence of harmful effects of steroids in severe exacerbations of COPD associated with influenza. Infection. 2022;50(3):699–707. https://doi.org/10.1007/s15010-021-01743-1.

63. Leuppi JD, Schuetz P, Bingisser R, et al. Short-term vs conventional glucocorticoid therapy in acute exacerbations of chronic obstructive pulmonary disease: the REDUCE randomized clinical trial. JAMA. 2013;309(21):2223. https://doi.org/10.1001/jama.2013.5023.

64. Arcos DB, Krishnan JA, Vandivier RW, et al. High-dose versus low-dose systemic steroids in the treatment of acute exacerbations of chronic obstructive pulmonary disease: systematic review. Chronic Obstr Pulm Dis J COPD Found. 2016;3(2):580–8. https://doi.org/10.15326/jcopdf.3.2.2015.0178.

65. Niewoehner DE, Erbland ML, Deupree RH, et al. Effect of systemic glucocorticoids on exacerbations of chronic obstructive pulmonary disease. Department of Veterans Affairs Cooperative Study Group. N Engl J Med. 1999;340(25):1941–7. https://doi.org/10.1056/NEJM199906243402502.

66. Aggarwal P, Wig N, Bhoi S. Efficacy of two corticosteroid regimens in acute exacerbation of chronic obstructive pulmonary disease. Int J Tuberc Lung Dis. 2011;15(5):687–92. https://doi.org/10.5588/ijtld.10.0540.

67. Li H, He G, Chu H, Zhao L, Yu H. A step-wise application of methylprednisolone versus dexamethasone in the treatment of acute exacerbations of COPD. Respirology. 2003;8(2):199–204. https://doi.org/10.1046/j.1440-1843.2003.00468.x.

68. de Jong YP, Uil SM, Grotjohan HP, Postma DS, Kerstjens HAM, van den Berg JWK. Oral or IV prednisolone in the treatment of COPD exacerbations: a randomized, controlled, double-blind study. Chest. 2007;132(6):1741–7. https://doi.org/10.1378/chest.07-0208.

69. Lindenauer PK. Association of Corticosteroid Dose and Route of administration with risk of treatment failure in acute exacerbation of chronic obstructive pulmonary disease. JAMA. 2010;303(23):2359. https://doi.org/10.1001/jama.2010.796.

70. Ställberg B, Selroos O, Vogelmeier C, Andersson E, Ekström T, Larsson K. Budesonide/formoterol as effective as prednisolone plus formoterol in acute exacerbations of COPD. A double-blind, randomised, non-inferiority, parallel-group, multicentre study. Respir Res. 2009;10(1):11. https://doi.org/10.1186/1465-9921-10-11.

71. Ding Z, Li X, Lu Y, et al. A randomized, controlled multicentric study of inhaled budesonide and intravenous methylprednisolone in the treatment on acute exacerbation of chronic obstructive pulmonary disease. Respir Med. 2016;121:39–47. https://doi.org/10.1016/j.rmed.2016.10.013.

72. Gunen H, Hacievliyagil SS, Yetkin O, Gulbas G, Mutlu LC, In E. The role of nebulised budesonide in the treatment of exacerbations of COPD. Eur Respir J. 2007;29(4):660–7. https://doi.org/10.1183/09031936.00073506.

73. Kiser TH, Allen RR, Valuck RJ, Moss M, Vandivier RW. Outcomes associated with corticosteroid dosage in critically ill patients with acute exacerbations of chronic obstructive pulmonary disease. Am J Respir Crit Care Med. 2014;189(9):1052–64. https://doi.org/10.1164/rccm.201401-0058OC.

74. Vondracek SF, Hemstreet BA. Retrospective evaluation of systemic corticosteroids for the management of acute exacerbations of chronic obstructive pulmonary disease. Am J Health Syst Pharm. 2006;63(7):645–52. https://doi.org/10.2146/ajhp050316.

75. Hurst JR, Vestbo J, Anzueto A, et al. Susceptibility to exacerbation in chronic obstructive pulmonary disease. N Engl J Med. 2010;363(12):1128–38. https://doi.org/10.1056/NEJMoa0909883.
76. Buttery S, Lewis A, Oey I, et al. Patient experience of lung volume reduction procedures for emphysema: a qualitative service improvement project. ERJ Open Res. 2017;3(3):00031–2017. https://doi.org/10.1183/23120541.00031-2017.
77. Bafadhel M, McKenna S, Terry S, et al. Blood eosinophils to direct corticosteroid treatment of exacerbations of chronic obstructive pulmonary disease: a randomized placebo-controlled trial. Am J Respir Crit Care Med. 2012;186(1):48–55. https://doi.org/10.1164/rccm.201108-1553OC.
78. Sivapalan P, Lapperre TS, Janner J, et al. Eosinophil-guided corticosteroid therapy in patients admitted to hospital with COPD exacerbation (CORTICO-COP): a multicentre, randomised, controlled, open-label, non-inferiority trial. Lancet Respir Med. 2019;7(8):699–709. https://doi.org/10.1016/S2213-2600(19)30176-6.
79. Walters JAE, Tan DJ, White CJ, Gibson PG, Wood-Baker R, Walters EH. Systemic corticosteroids for acute exacerbations of chronic obstructive pulmonary disease. Cochrane Database Syst Rev. 2014;2014(9):CD001288. https://doi.org/10.1002/14651858.CD001288.pub4.
80. Wedzicha JA, Miravitlles M, Hurst JR, et al. Management of COPD exacerbations: a European Respiratory Society/American Thoracic Society guideline. Eur Respir J. 2017;49(3):1600791. https://doi.org/10.1183/13993003.00791-2016.
81. Waljee AK, Rogers MAM, Lin P, et al. Short term use of oral corticosteroids and related harms among adults in the United States: population based cohort study. BMJ. 2017;357:j1415. https://doi.org/10.1136/bmj.j1415.
82. Young A, Marsh S. Steroid use in critical care. BJA Educ. 2018;18(5):129–34. https://doi.org/10.1016/j.bjae.2018.01.005.
83. Targownik LE, Fisher DA, Saini SD. AGA clinical practice update on De-prescribing of proton pump inhibitors: expert review. Gastroenterology. 2022;162(4):1334–42. https://doi.org/10.1053/j.gastro.2021.12.247.
84. Papi A, Bellettato CM, Braccioni F, et al. Infections and airway inflammation in chronic obstructive pulmonary disease severe exacerbations. Am J Respir Crit Care Med. 2006;173(10):1114–21. https://doi.org/10.1164/rccm.200506-859OC.
85. Zalacain R, Sobradillo V, Amilibia J, et al. Predisposing factors to bacterial colonization in chronic obstructive pulmonary disease. Eur Respir J. 1999;13(2):343–8. https://doi.org/10.1034/j.1399-3003.1999.13b21.x.
86. Miravitlles M, Kruesmann F, Haverstock D, Perroncel R, Choudhri SH, Arvis P. Sputum colour and bacteria in chronic bronchitis exacerbations: a pooled analysis. Eur Respir J. 2012;39(6):1354–60. https://doi.org/10.1183/09031936.00042111.
87. Nouira S, Marghli S, Belghith M, Besbes L, Elatrous S, Abroug F. Once daily oral ofloxacin in chronic obstructive pulmonary disease exacerbation requiring mechanical ventilation: a randomised placebo-controlled trial. Lancet Lond Engl. 2001;358(9298):2020–5. https://doi.org/10.1016/S0140-6736(01)07097-0.
88. Deniel G, Cour M, Argaud L, Richard JC, Bitker L. Early antibiotic therapy is associated with a lower probability of successful liberation from mechanical ventilation in patients with severe acute exacerbation of chronic obstructive pulmonary disease. Ann Intensive Care. 2022;12(1):86. https://doi.org/10.1186/s13613-022-01060-2.
89. Prins HJ, Duijkers R, van der Valk P, et al. CRP-guided antibiotic treatment in acute exacerbations of COPD in hospital admissions. Eur Respir J. 2019;53(5):1802014. https://doi.org/10.1183/13993003.02014-2018.
90. Butler CC, Gillespie D, White P, et al. C-reactive protein testing to guide antibiotic prescribing for COPD exacerbations. N Engl J Med. 2019;381(2):111–20. https://doi.org/10.1056/NEJMoa1803185.

91. Daubin C, Valette X, Thiollière F, et al. Procalcitonin algorithm to guide initial antibiotic therapy in acute exacerbations of COPD admitted to the ICU: a randomized multicenter study. Intensive Care Med. 2018;44(4):428–37. https://doi.org/10.1007/s00134-018-5141-9.

92. Chen K, Pleasants KA, Pleasants RA, et al. Procalcitonin for antibiotic prescription in chronic obstructive pulmonary disease exacerbations: systematic review, meta-analysis, and clinical perspective. Pulm Ther. 2020;6(2):201–14. https://doi.org/10.1007/s41030-020-00123-8.

93. Sykes A, Mallia P, Johnston SL. Diagnosis of pathogens in exacerbations of chronic obstructive pulmonary disease. Proc Am Thorac Soc. 2007;4(8):642–6. https://doi.org/10.1513/pats.200707-101TH.

94. Dixit D, Bridgeman MB, Madduri RP, Kumar ST, Cawley MJ. Pharmacological management and prevention of exacerbations of chronic obstructive pulmonary disease in hospitalized patients. P T Peer-Rev J Formul Manag. 2016;41(11):703–12.

95. Soler N, Torres A, Ewig S, et al. Bronchial microbial patterns in severe exacerbations of chronic obstructive pulmonary disease (COPD) requiring mechanical ventilation. Am J Respir Crit Care Med. 1998;157(5):1498–505. https://doi.org/10.1164/ajrccm.157.5.9711044.

96. Garcia-Vidal C, Almagro P, Romaní V, et al. Pseudomonas aeruginosa in patients hospitalised for COPD exacerbation: a prospective study. Eur Respir J. 2009;34(5):1072–8. https://doi.org/10.1183/09031936.00003309.

97. Gallego M, Pomares X, Espasa M, et al. Pseudomonas aeruginosa isolates in severe chronic obstructive pulmonary disease: characterization and risk factors. BMC Pulm Med. 2014;14:103. https://doi.org/10.1186/1471-2466-14-103.

98. Parameswaran GI, Sethi S. Pseudomonas infection in chronic obstructive pulmonary disease. Future Microbiol. 2012;7(10):1129–32. https://doi.org/10.2217/fmb.12.88.

99. Monsó E, Garcia-Aymerich J, Soler N, et al. Bacterial infection in exacerbated COPD with changes in sputum characteristics. Epidemiol Infect. 2003;131(1):799–804.

100. Kalil AC, Metersky ML, Klompas M, et al. Management of Adults with Hospital-acquired and Ventilator-associated Pneumonia: 2016 clinical practice guidelines by the Infectious Diseases Society of America and the American Thoracic Society. Clin Infect Dis. 2016;63(5):e61–e111. https://doi.org/10.1093/cid/ciw353.

101. Metlay JP, Waterer GW, Long AC, et al. Diagnosis and treatment of adults with community-acquired pneumonia. An official clinical practice guideline of the American Thoracic Society and Infectious Diseases Society of America. Am J Respir Crit Care Med. 2019;200(7):e45–67. https://doi.org/10.1164/rccm.201908-1581ST.

102. Stefan MS, Rothberg MB, Shieh MS, Pekow PS, Lindenauer PK. Association between antibiotic treatment and outcomes in patients hospitalized with acute exacerbation of COPD treated with systemic steroids. Chest. 2013;143(1):82–90. https://doi.org/10.1378/chest.12-0649.

103. Rothberg MB, Pekow PS, Lahti M, Brody O, Skiest DJ, Lindenauer PK. Antibiotic therapy and treatment failure in patients hospitalized for acute exacerbations of chronic obstructive pulmonary disease. JAMA. 2010;303(20):2035–42. https://doi.org/10.1001/jama.2010.672.

104. Masterton RG, Burley CJ. Randomized, double-blind study comparing 5- and 7-day regimens of oral levofloxacin in patients with acute exacerbation of chronic bronchitis. Int J Antimicrob Agents. 2001;18(6):503–12. https://doi.org/10.1016/s0924-8579(01)00435-6.

105. Gupta N, Haley R, Gupta A, Sethi S. Chronic obstructive pulmonary disease in the intensive care unit: antibiotic treatment of severe chronic obstructive pulmonary disease exacerbations. Semin Respir Crit Care Med. 2020;41(6):830–41. https://doi.org/10.1055/s-0040-1708837.

106. Messous S, Trabelsi I, Bel Haj Ali K, et al. Two-day *versus* seven-day course of levofloxacin in acute COPD exacerbation: a randomized controlled trial. Ther Adv Respir Dis. 2022;16:175346662210997. https://doi.org/10.1177/17534666221099729.

107. Moreno G, Rodríguez A, Sole-Violán J, et al. Early oseltamivir treatment improves survival in critically ill patients with influenza pneumonia. ERJ Open Res. 2021;7(1):00888–2020. https://doi.org/10.1183/23120541.00888-2020.

108. Li M, Han GC, Chen Y, et al. Efficacy of oseltamivir compared with zanamivir in COPD patients with seasonal influenza virus infection: a randomized controlled trial. Braz J Med Biol Res. 2020;54(2):e9542. https://doi.org/10.1590/1414-431X20209542.

109. Beaird OE, Freifeld A, Ison MG, et al. Current practices for treatment of respiratory syncytial virus and other non-influenza respiratory viruses in high-risk patient populations: a survey of institutions in the Midwestern respiratory virus collaborative. Transpl Infect Dis. 2016;18(2):210–5. https://doi.org/10.1111/tid.12510.

110. Schwartzstein RM, Lahive K, Pope A, Weinberger SE, Weiss JW. Cold facial stimulation reduces breathlessness induced in Normal subjects. Am Rev Respir Dis. 1987;136(1):58–61. https://doi.org/10.1164/ajrccm/136.1.58.

111. Farncombe M, Chater S, Gillin A. The use of nebulized opioids for breathlessness: a chart review. Palliat Med. 1994;8(4):306–12. https://doi.org/10.1177/026921639400800406.

112. Simon ST, Köskeroglu P, Gaertner J, Voltz R. Fentanyl for the relief of refractory breathlessness: a systematic review. J Pain Symptom Manag. 2013;46(6):874–86. https://doi.org/10.1016/j.jpainsymman.2013.02.019.

113. Clemens KE, Klaschik E. Effect of hydromorphone on ventilation in palliative care patients with dyspnea. Support Care Cancer. 2008;16(1):93–9. https://doi.org/10.1007/s00520-007-0310-3.

114. Pang GS, Qu LM, Tan YY, Yee ACP. Intravenous fentanyl for dyspnea at the end of life: lessons for future research in dyspnea. Am J Hosp Palliat Care. 2016;33(3):222–7. https://doi.org/10.1177/1049909114559769.

115. Nici L, Mammen MJ, Charbek E, et al. Pharmacologic Management of Chronic Obstructive Pulmonary Disease. An official American Thoracic Society clinical practice guideline. Am J Respir Crit Care Med. 2020;201(9):e56–69. https://doi.org/10.1164/rccm.202003-0625ST.

116. Janssen DJA, Ekström M, Currow DC, et al. COVID-19: guidance on palliative care from a European Respiratory Society international task force. Eur Respir J. 2020;56(3):2002583. https://doi.org/10.1183/13993003.02583-2020.

117. Simon ST, Higginson IJ, Booth S, Harding R, Weingärtner V, Bausewein C. Benzodiazepines for the relief of breathlessness in advanced malignant and non-malignant diseases in adults. Cochrane Database Syst Rev. 2016;10(10):CD007354. https://doi.org/10.1002/14651858.CD007354.pub3.

118. Jolly E, Aguirre L, Jorge E, Luna C. Acute effect of lorazepam on respiratory muscles in stable patients with chronic obstructive pulmonary disease. Medicina (Mex). 1996;56(5 Pt 1):472–8.

119. Mano A, Murata T, Date K, et al. Dexmedetomidine for dyspnoea. BMJ Support Palliat Care. 2023;13(e1):e84–5. https://doi.org/10.1136/bmjspcare-2020-002334.

120. Li N, Cui M, Wang Y. Effect of Dexmedetomidine for palliative sedation for refractory Dyspnoea in patients with terminal-stage cancer. Cancer Manag Res. 2023;15:291–9. https://doi.org/10.2147/CMAR.S404934.

121. Min ZM, Ning QY, Zhu W, et al. Protective effects of ketamine on allergen-induced airway inflammatory injure and high airway reactivity in asthma: experiment with rats. Zhonghua Yi Xue Za Zhi. 2007;87(19):1308–13.

122. Goyal S, Agrawal A. Ketamine in status asthmaticus: a review. Indian J Crit Care Med. 2013;17(3):154–61. https://doi.org/10.4103/0972-5229.117048.

123. Hirshman CA, Downes H, Farbood A, Bergman NA. Ketamine block of bronchospasm in experimental canine asthma. Br J Anaesth. 1979;51(8):713–8. https://doi.org/10.1093/bja/51.8.713.

124. Huber FC, Gutierrez J, Corssen G. Ketamine: its effect on airway resistance in man. South Med J. 1972;65(10):1176–80. https://doi.org/10.1097/00007611-197210000-00003.

125. Karacaer F, Biricik E, Ilgınel M, et al. Effects of ketamine infusion on oxygenation in patients with chronic obstructive pulmonary disease undergoing lung cancer surgery. Turk J Anaesthesiol Reanim. 2023;51(1):16–23. https://doi.org/10.5152/TJAR.

126. Nedel W, Costa R, Mendez G, Marin L, Vargas T, Marques L. Negative results for ketamine use in severe acute bronchospasm: a randomised controlled trial. Anaesthesiol Intensive Ther. 2020;52(3):215–8. https://doi.org/10.5114/ait.2020.97765.
127. Gourgoulianis KI, Chatziparasidis G, Chatziefthimiou A, Molyvdas PA. Magnesium as a relaxing factor of airway smooth muscles. J Aerosol Med. 2001;14(3):301–7. https://doi.org/10.1089/089426801316970259.
128. Ni H, Aye SZ, Naing C. Magnesium sulfate for acute exacerbations of chronic obstructive pulmonary disease. Cochrane Database Syst Rev. 2022;5(5):CD013506. https://doi.org/10.1002/14651858.CD013506.pub2.
129. Greiller CL, Martineau AR. Modulation of the immune response to respiratory viruses by vitamin D. Nutrients. 2015;7(6):4240–70. https://doi.org/10.3390/nu7064240.
130. Greiller CL, Suri R, Jolliffe DA, et al. Vitamin D attenuates rhinovirus-induced expression of intercellular adhesion molecule-1 (ICAM-1) and platelet-activating factor receptor (PAFR) in respiratory epithelial cells. J Steroid Biochem Mol Biol. 2019;187:152–9. https://doi.org/10.1016/j.jsbmb.2018.11.013.
131. Jolliffe DA, Greenberg L, Hooper RL, et al. Vitamin D to prevent exacerbations of COPD: systematic review and meta-analysis of individual participant data from randomised controlled trials. Thorax. 2019;74(4):337–45. https://doi.org/10.1136/thoraxjnl-2018-212092.
132. Rafiq R, Aleva FE, Schrumpf JA, et al. Vitamin D supplementation in chronic obstructive pulmonary disease patients with low serum vitamin D: a randomized controlled trial. Am J Clin Nutr. 2022;116(2):491–9. https://doi.org/10.1093/ajcn/nqac083.
133. Bertoletti L, Quenet S, Laporte S, et al. Pulmonary embolism and 3-month outcomes in 4036 patients with venous thromboembolism and chronic obstructive pulmonary disease: data from the RIETE registry. Respir Res. 2013;14(1):75. https://doi.org/10.1186/1465-9921-14-75.
134. Godtfredsen NS, Vestbo J, Osler M, Prescott E. Risk of hospital admission for COPD following smoking cessation and reduction: a Danish population study. Thorax. 2002;57(11):967–72. https://doi.org/10.1136/thorax.57.11.967.
135. van Eerd EAM, van der Meer RM, van Schayck OCP, Kotz D. Smoking cessation for people with chronic obstructive pulmonary disease. Cochrane Database Syst Rev. 2016;2016(8):CD010744. https://doi.org/10.1002/14651858.CD010744.pub2.
136. Lucidarme O, Seguin A, Daubin C, et al. Nicotine withdrawal and agitation in ventilated critically ill patients. Crit Care Lond Engl. 2010;14(2):R58. https://doi.org/10.1186/cc8954.
137. Rigotti NA, Arnsten JH, McKool KM, Wood-Reid KM, Singer DE, Pasternak RC. The use of nicotine-replacement therapy by hospitalized smokers. Am J Prev Med. 1999;17(4):255–9. https://doi.org/10.1016/s0749-3797(99)00095-1.
138. Delmastro M, Santoro C, Nava S. Respiratory changes during defecation in patients with chronic respiratory failure. Eur Respir J. 2004;23(4):617–9. https://doi.org/10.1183/0903193 6.04.00084504.
139. Papadopoulou E, Hansel J, Lazar Z, et al. Mucolytics for acute exacerbations of chronic obstructive pulmonary disease: a meta-analysis. Eur Respir Rev. 2023;32(167):220141. https://doi.org/10.1183/16000617.0141-2022.
140. Beijers RJHCG, Steiner MC, Schols AMWJ. The role of diet and nutrition in the management of COPD. Eur Respir Rev. 2023;32(168):230003. https://doi.org/10.1183/1600061 7.0003-2023.
141. Zhang R, Lu H, Chang Y, Zhang X, Zhao J, Li X. Prediction of 30-day risk of acute exacerbation of readmission in elderly patients with COPD based on support vector machine model. BMC Pulm Med. 2022;22(1):292. https://doi.org/10.1186/s12890-022-02085-w.
142. Gattermann Pereira T, Lima J, Silva FM. Undernutrition is associated with mortality, exacerbation, and poorer quality of life in patients with chronic obstructive pulmonary disease: a systematic review with meta-analysis of observational studies. J Parenter Enter Nutr. 2022;46(5):977–96. https://doi.org/10.1002/jpen.2350.
143. Sjoding MW, Dickson RP, Iwashyna TJ, Gay SE, Valley TS. Racial bias in pulse oximetry measurement. N Engl J Med. 2020;383(25):2477–8. https://doi.org/10.1056/NEJMc2029240.

144. Fawzy A, Wu TD, Wang K, et al. Racial and ethnic discrepancy in pulse oximetry and delayed identification of treatment eligibility among patients with COVID-19. JAMA Intern Med. 2022;182(7):730–8. https://doi.org/10.1001/jamainternmed.2022.1906.

145. McKeever TM, Hearson G, Housley G, et al. Using venous blood gas analysis in the assessment of COPD exacerbations: a prospective cohort study. Thorax. 2016;71(3):210–5. https://doi.org/10.1136/thoraxjnl-2015-207573.

146. McCanny P, Bennett K, Staunton P, McMahon G. Venous vs arterial blood gases in the assessment of patients presenting with an exacerbation of chronic obstructive pulmonary disease. Am J Emerg Med. 2012;30(6):896–900. https://doi.org/10.1016/j.ajem.2011.06.011.

147. Echevarria C, Steer J, Wason J, Bourke S. Oxygen therapy and inpatient mortality in COPD exacerbation. Emerg Med J. 2021;38(3):170–7. https://doi.org/10.1136/emermed-2019-209257.

148. O'Driscoll BR, Howard LS, Earis J, Mak V. British Thoracic Society guideline for oxygen use in adults in healthcare and emergency settings. BMJ Open Respir Res. 2017;4(1):e000170. https://doi.org/10.1136/bmjresp-2016-000170.

149. Austin MA, Wills KE, Blizzard L, Walters EH, Wood-Baker R. Effect of high flow oxygen on mortality in chronic obstructive pulmonary disease patients in prehospital setting: randomised controlled trial. BMJ. 2010;341:c5462. https://doi.org/10.1136/bmj.c5462.

150. Osadnik CR, Tee VS, Carson-Chahhoud KV, Picot J, Wedzicha JA, Smith BJ. Non-invasive ventilation for the management of acute hypercapnic respiratory failure due to exacerbation of chronic obstructive pulmonary disease. Cochrane Database Syst Rev. 2017;2017:7. https://doi.org/10.1002/14651858.CD004104.pub4.

151. Ameen A, Zedan M, El Shamly M. Comparison between continuous positive airway pressure and bilevel positive pressure ventilation in treatment of acute exacerbation of chronic obstructive pulmonary disease. Egypt J Chest Dis Tuberc. 2012;61(3):95–101. https://doi.org/10.1016/j.ejcdt.2012.10.018.

152. MacIntyre NR. Physiologic effects of noninvasive ventilation. Respir Care. 2019;64(6):617–28. https://doi.org/10.4187/respcare.06635.

153. Rochwerg B, Brochard L, Elliott MW, et al. Official ERS/ATS clinical practice guidelines: noninvasive ventilation for acute respiratory failure. Eur Respir J. 2017;50(2):1602426. https://doi.org/10.1183/13993003.02426-2016.

154. Confalonieri M, Garuti G, Cattaruzza MS, et al. A chart of failure risk for noninvasive ventilation in patients with COPD exacerbation. Eur Respir J. 2005;25(2):348–55. https://doi.org/10.1183/09031936.05.00085304.

155. Brochard L, Mancebo J, Wysocki M, et al. Noninvasive ventilation for acute exacerbations of chronic obstructive pulmonary disease. N Engl J Med. 1995;333(13):817–22. https://doi.org/10.1056/NEJM199509283331301.

156. Ornico SR, Lobo SM, Sanches HS, et al. Noninvasive ventilation immediately after extubation improves weaning outcome after acute respiratory failure: a randomized controlled trial. Crit Care. 2013;17(2):R39. https://doi.org/10.1186/cc12549.

157. Ferrer M, Sellarés J, Valencia M, et al. Non-invasive ventilation after extubation in hypercapnic patients with chronic respiratory disorders: randomised controlled trial. Lancet Lond Engl. 2009;374(9695):1082–8. https://doi.org/10.1016/S0140-6736(09)61038-2.

158. Nava S, Gregoretti C, Fanfulla F, et al. Noninvasive ventilation to prevent respiratory failure after extubation in high-risk patients. Crit Care Med. 2005;33(11):2465–70. https://doi.org/10.1097/01.ccm.0000186416.44752.72.

159. Girault C, Bubenheim M, Abroug F, et al. Noninvasive ventilation and weaning in patients with chronic Hypercapnic respiratory failure. Am J Respir Crit Care Med. 2011;184(6):672–9. https://doi.org/10.1164/rccm.201101-0035OC.

160. Society BPGL and BT. Non-invasive ventilation in acute respiratory failure. Thorax. 2002;57(3):192–211. https://doi.org/10.1136/thorax.57.3.192.

161. Díaz GG, Alcaraz AC, Talavera JCP, et al. Noninvasive positive-pressure ventilation to treat Hypercapnic coma secondary to respiratory failure. Chest. 2005;127(3):952–60. https://doi.org/10.1378/chest.127.3.952.
162. Oczkowski S, Ergan B, Bos L, et al. ERS clinical practice guidelines: high-flow nasal cannula in acute respiratory failure. Eur Respir J. 2022;59(4):2101574. https://doi.org/10.1183/13993003.01574-2021.
163. Mauri T, Turrini C, Eronia N, et al. Physiologic effects of high-flow nasal cannula in acute hypoxemic respiratory failure. Am J Respir Crit Care Med. 2017;195(9):1207–15. https://doi.org/10.1164/rccm.201605-0916OC.
164. Fowler WS. Lung function studies; the respiratory dead space. Am J Physiol. 1948;154(3):405–16. https://doi.org/10.1152/ajplegacy.1948.154.3.405.
165. Möller W, Celik G, Feng S, et al. Nasal high flow clears anatomical dead space in upper airway models. J Appl Physiol Bethesda Md 1985. 2015;118(12):1525–32. https://doi.org/10.1152/japplphysiol.00934.2014.
166. Parke RL, Eccleston ML, McGuinness SP. The effects of flow on airway pressure during nasal high-flow oxygen therapy. Respir Care. 2011;56(8):1151–5. https://doi.org/10.4187/respcare.01106.
167. Frat JP, Thille AW, Mercat A, et al. High-flow oxygen through nasal cannula in acute hypoxemic respiratory failure. N Engl J Med. 2015;372(23):2185–96. https://doi.org/10.1056/NEJMoa1503326.
168. Papachatzakis I, Velentza L, Kontogiannis S, Trakada G. High flow nasal cannula with warm humidified air versus non-invasive mechanical ventilation in respiratory failure type II. Eur Respir J. 2017;50(suppl 61):PA2182. https://doi.org/10.1183/1393003.congress-2017.PA2182.
169. Nishimura M. High-flow nasal cannula oxygen therapy in adults. J Intensive Care. 2015;3(1):15. https://doi.org/10.1186/s40560-015-0084-5.
170. Shorr AF, Sun X, Johannes RS, Yaitanes A, Tabak YP. Validation of a novel risk score for severity of illness in acute exacerbations of COPD. Chest. 2011;140(5):1177–83. https://doi.org/10.1378/chest.10-3035.
171. Tabak YP, Sun X, Johannes RS, Gupta V, Shorr AF. Mortality and need for mechanical ventilation in acute exacerbations of chronic obstructive pulmonary disease: development and validation of a simple risk score. Arch Intern Med. 2009;169(17):1595–602. https://doi.org/10.1001/archinternmed.2009.270.
172. Squadrone E, Frigerio P, Fogliati C, et al. Noninvasive vs invasive ventilation in COPD patients with severe acute respiratory failure deemed to require ventilatory assistance. Intensive Care Med. 2004;30(7):1303–10. https://doi.org/10.1007/s00134-004-2320-7.
173. Antón A, Güell R, Gómez J, et al. Predicting the result of noninvasive ventilation in severe acute exacerbations of patients with chronic airflow limitation. Chest. 2000;117(3):828–33. https://doi.org/10.1378/chest.117.3.828.
174. Neto SCGB, Torres-Castro R, Lima Í, Resqueti VR, Fregonezi GAF. Weaning from mechanical ventilation in people with neuromuscular disease: a systematic review. BMJ Open. 2021;11(9):e047449. https://doi.org/10.1136/bmjopen-2020-047449.
175. Davidson AC, Banham S, Elliott M, et al. BTS/ICS guideline for the ventilatory management of acute hypercapnic respiratory failure in adults. Thorax. 2016;71(Suppl 2):ii1–ii35. https://doi.org/10.1136/thoraxjnl-2015-208209.
176. Smith TC, Marini JJ. Impact of PEEP on lung mechanics and work of breathing in severe airflow obstruction. J Appl Physiol Bethesda Md 1985. 1988;65(4):1488–99. https://doi.org/10.1152/jappl.1988.65.4.1488.
177. MacIntyre NR, McConnell R, Cheng KCG. Applied PEEP during pressure support reduces the inspiratory threshold load of intrinsic PEEP. Chest. 1997;111(1):188–93. https://doi.org/10.1378/chest.111.1.188.

178. Reddy RM, Guntupalli KK. Review of ventilatory techniques to optimize mechanical ventilation in acute exacerbation of chronic obstructive pulmonary disease. Int J Chron Obstruct Pulmon Dis. 2007;2(4):441–52.
179. MacIntyre N, Huang YC. Acute exacerbations and respiratory failure in chronic obstructive pulmonary disease. Proc Am Thorac Soc. 2008;5(4):530–5. https://doi.org/10.1513/pats.200707-088ET.
180. Prediletto I, Giancotti G, Nava S. COPD exacerbation: why it is important to avoid ICU admission. J Clin Med. 2023;12(10):3369. https://doi.org/10.3390/jcm12103369.

Chapter 7
Acute Asthma Exacerbation in the Intensive Care Unit

Kevin G. Correa and Lauren E. Eggert

7.1 Introduction

7.1.1 What Is Asthma?

Asthma is a heterogeneous, chronic respiratory disease that is characterized by variable airway obstruction through hyperresponsive bronchoconstriction and bronchial inflammation [1]. The diagnosis of asthma is made based on a combination of clinical symptoms such as cough, wheezing, shortness of breath, and chest tightness and a demonstration of variable airflow obstruction [1, 2]. Asthma on spirometry typically presents as a reversible, obstructive ventilatory defect notable for a reduced peak expiratory flow (PEF), forced exhalatory volume in 1 second (FEV-1), and forced vital capacity (FEV-1/FVC) ratio, and sometimes there is also evidence of air trapping or hyperinflation [1, 2]. The severity of asthma symptoms may correlate to the severity of a decrease in PEF and FEV-1 at home or in clinic and can be used to trend response to therapeutic agents [1, 2]. The cornerstone management of asthma revolves around controlling airway inflammation to reduce obstructive symptoms by targeting the several molecular pathways that lead to inflammation and bronchoconstriction [1]. As a result of chronic inflammation, the airway, or bronchioles, may undergo remodeling, leading to increased bronchoconstriction, thickened bronchioles, and mucus production [3] (Fig. 7.1).

Asthma is one of the most common inflammatory diseases and is known to affect more than 300 million individuals worldwide [1]. The prevalence of asthma varies from country to country, with estimates ranging from 1% to 29% of the population. It is one of the few diseases that can develop in people of all ages, from young

K. G. Correa (✉) · L. E. Eggert
Division of Pulmonary, Allergy, and Critical Care Medicine, Stanford University, Palo Alto, CA, USA
e-mail: correak@stanford.edu; leggert1@stanford.edu

Y. Alzaidi, M. A. Gebily (eds.), *The Pharmacist's Expanded Role in Critical Care Medicine*, https://doi.org/10.1007/978-3-031-77335-8_7

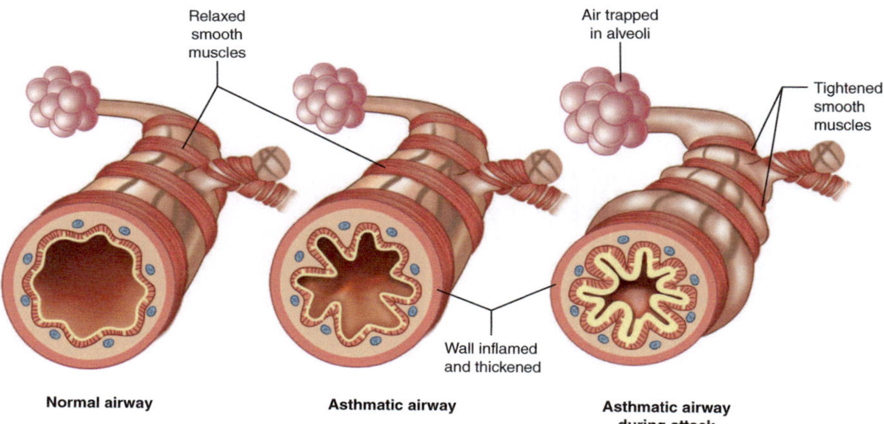

Fig. 7.1 Diagram depicting the bronchioles, or airways, in normal, asthma, and exacerbation state. Note the decreased lumen size and increased bronchoconstriction in the asthmatic and exacerbation airways

children to late adulthood, with onset and severity closely linked to genetics and environmental factors [1]. Social factors have also been shown to play a significant role in the severity and control of asthma with worse outcomes in populations identified as minorities and from lower socioeconomic backgrounds [1]. Asthma is heterogeneous, and several distinct phenotypes have been described, including but not limited to the following: allergic, exercise-induced, obesity-associated, and nonallergic [1]. To address asthma's large global health impact, the Global Initiative for Asthma (GINA) was created which provides guidance to clinicians regarding asthma management in an evidence-based manner [2].

7.1.2 What Is an Asthma Exacerbation?

The key goal of asthma management is to target minimal to no day-to-day symptoms and minimize the risk for exacerbations. The range of medications required to keep an individual's asthma under control varies widely, which owes to the disease's heterogeneity. Several disease-specific questionnaires have been developed to assess one's asthma symptoms and can be used as an objective measurement of a medication's impact on their asthma control. Given asthma's close interplay with environmental factors, control can vary throughout the year and medication changes may be necessary in one's disease course.

An exacerbation is defined as asthma with rapidly worsening symptoms and clinical deterioration [1]. The hyperresponsive and inflamed bronchioles of the airway lead to overt bronchoconstriction and airflow obstruction, which can be demonstrated by worsening obstruction on spirometry and/or a decreased PEF [4]. In addition, the remodeled bronchioles are subjected to mucus hypersecretion, which additionally leads to further airway occlusion and subsequent hyperinflation [4]. Prompt recognition of exacerbation symptoms is crucial as early assessment and intervention are necessary to prevent significant morbidity and mortality. The range of severity of an asthma exacerbation can be from mild which can be managed as an outpatient to severe and life-threatening, requiring admission to the intensive care unit (ICU). Asthma exacerbations are a frequent cause of emergency room visits and hospital admissions [5]. The presence and rate of exacerbations have become a standard benchmark for assessing a patient's asthma control. Preventing exacerbations is a key therapeutic target for medical treatment of asthma.

7.1.3 *Exacerbation Triggers and Risk Factors for More Severe Exacerbations*

In many exacerbations, there is a clear culprit responsible for causing the acute asthma symptoms. These triggers can be infectious or noninfectious, such as smoke, pollution, cold weather, or allergen exposure [1]. As individuals understand their asthma symptoms in relation to their environment, they will become more familiar with their triggers and can work to purposefully avoid such exposures. Asthmatics will have their own threshold on how much exposure of a trigger they need to provoke an exacerbation. Additionally, repeated exposures may provoke further immune system sensitization leading to more pronounced symptoms with decreased trigger exposure [1]. Unfortunately, many asthma triggers are variable and unpredictable, hence the importance of obtaining baseline asthma control. Table 7.1 highlights some of the most common triggers for asthma exacerbations.

Table 7.1 Review of common triggers of asthma exacerbations

Category	Trigger
Infectious	Bacterial infections (bronchitis, tracheitis, pneumonia) Viral infections (rhinovirus, SARS-CoV-2, RSV, etc.) Fungal spores, *aspergillus* colonization
Allergens	Pollen Grasses Trees Dust mites, cockroaches Pet dander
Irritants	Cleaning agents and solutions Preservatives Cold air or weather changes Wildfires or pollution Strong odors
Miscellaneous	Aspirin (aspirin exacerbated respiratory disease ie. AERD) Gastric reflux Exercise

The major challenge that presents to clinicians is gauging the severity and trajectory of an asthmatic presenting to seek care with an exacerbation. Not all exacerbations that present for medical evaluation require hospitalization, and many can be safely treated as an outpatient with oral corticosteroids, inhaled bronchodilators, and close outpatient follow-up. If present, there are several risk factors that raise concern for increased risk of a severe exacerbation requiring hospital admission including escalation to the ICU. Risk factors include prior asthma exacerbation requiring ICU level of care, need for invasive or noninvasive ventilation, history of recent exacerbation with known difficult-to-control asthma, steroid-dependent asthma, elderly patients with significant comorbidities, and pregnant individuals presenting with exacerbation [4, 5]. Upon arrival to the emergency department, patients experiencing an asthma exacerbation should be assessed in a timely manner as early identification and management of ICU-bound patients are vital.

7.2 Diagnosis

Evaluation of the asthmatic presenting in an exacerbation requires a comprehensive review of the patient's clinical presentation and available objective data. Triage and initial management in the first hour within emergency department arrival are crucial as clinical deterioration can occur rapidly. Early interventions performed in the emergency department can shape the hospital course for a patient. The main indications for an asthmatic to require ICU level of care include worsening clinical status refractory to initial therapies, increased work of breathing with concern for impending respiratory failure, carbon dioxide retention with respiratory acidosis or respiratory failure requiring invasive or noninvasive ventilation, significant comorbidities that may complicate hospital course, and a history of a prior exacerbation requiring ICU-level care [4, 5].

7.2.1 Physical Examination

The initial physical examination is fundamental to correctly identifying the level of care a patient needs upon presentation to the emergency department. In addition to the initial exam, serial examinations are necessary to assess a patient's response to initial interventions, especially because clinical status can quickly change during the course of severe exacerbations [5]. When in doubt about the level of care, it is always better to monitor an exacerbation in the ICU, as delays or transfers of care can lead to increased morbidity. Therefore, clinicians should pay particular attention to specific findings on the exam which can signal patients at higher risk for needing ICU level of care. Table 7.2 highlights the main physical exam findings that are indicative of a severe or life-threatening exacerbation.

Table 7.2 Common physical exam findings in asthma exacerbations

Organ system	Exam finding
Neurologic	Altered mental status (CO_2 narcosis), fatigue, lethargy
Head, eyes, ears, nose, and throat (HEENT)	Nasal flaring, stridor (can be if in the setting of anaphylaxis), sternocleidomastoid (SCM) retractions, pursed-lip breathing
Cardiovascular	Tachycardia, hypotension (can be if in the setting of anaphylaxis)
Pulmonary	Tachypnea, use of accessory breathing muscles (tripod breathing), wheezing, decreased breath sounds ("silent chest" due to hyperinflation)
Abdominal	Paradoxical abdominal breathing, emesis, and diarrhea (can be in the setting of anaphylaxis)
Extremities/ musculoskeletal	Cyanosis, skin rash, or flushing (can be in the setting of anaphylaxis)

7.2.2 *Laboratory Data*

As highlighted previously, the underlying etiology of an asthma exacerbation can be infectious or noninfectious. Therefore, initial workup sent in an exacerbation should include labs to rule out common triggers. Initial labs should include a complete blood cell count with differential to assess for leukocytosis and eosinophilia and basic metabolic panel to evaluate for any electrolyte abnormalities and renal function for medication dosing. In noninfectious triggers of exacerbations, laboratory studies may be completely normal [5]. Initial infectious workup may include laboratory tests such as a nasal swab testing for common respiratory viruses and serum procalcitonin to help assess the likelihood of bacterial infection. If supported by further clinical symptoms or data, additional studies could be considered such as respiratory gram stain and culture, blood cultures, inflammatory markers, and a troponin and NT-proBNP to rule out comorbid cardiac disease [5]. Certain infectious triggers of exacerbations may have treatment options to either shorten the duration of exacerbation or prevent progression to severe disease such as influenza and SARS-CoV-2 infections.

Patients in exacerbation are tachypneic and have a degree of hyperventilation that can be expected. Since asthma is a disease of the airways and not the lung parenchyma, oxygen saturation can be expected to be normal in a mild-moderate exacerbation. If an arterial blood gas is obtained in exacerbation, then the expected findings range from normal to a mild respiratory alkalosis occurring from hyperventilation. If serial blood gases demonstrate retention of CO_2 (hypercapnia), a patient may become hypoxic due to hypercapnia, which is a key concern for impending respiratory failure because of respiratory fatigue or "tiring out," and the patient may require urgent ventilatory support [4].

Given that corticosteroids are the cornerstone of asthma exacerbation management, close attention should be paid to blood glucose in patients with a known history of diabetes or insulin resistance as uncontrolled hyperglycemia can lead to further adverse events. In the ICU, patients can have their hyperglycemia readily addressed with either subcutaneous insulin or a continuous insulin infusion.

Fig. 7.2 Chest X-rays in the majority of asthma exacerbations are low yield. One of the more common findings as demonstrated below is hyperinflation

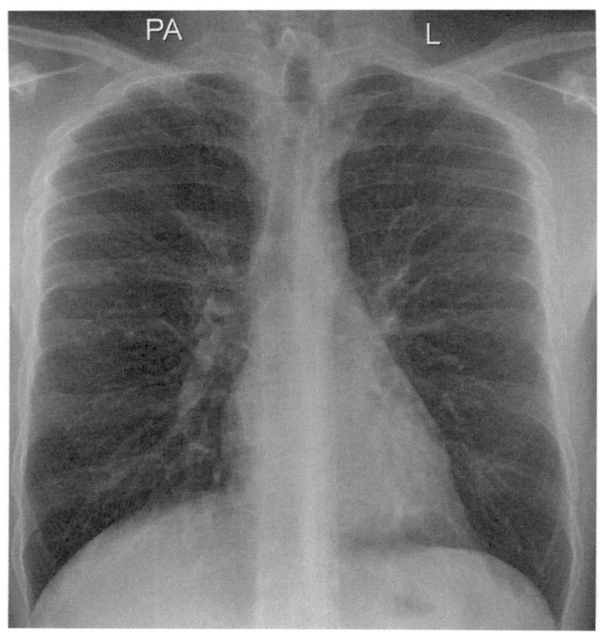

7.2.3 Radiographic Findings

The role of radiologic studies in asthma exacerbations is limited. Unless the exacerbation was triggered by pneumonia which can be seen on a chest X-ray or high-resolution computed tomography (CT) scan of the chest, most asthma exacerbations have an unremarkable chest X-ray [5]. Chest X-ray may demonstrate hyperinflation and flattened diaphragms due to air trapping from airway obstruction. A CT of the chest may demonstrate findings that are consistent with chronic airway inflammation such as bronchial wall thickening, and mucus plugging. Normal imaging findings do not exclude the diagnosis of an asthma exacerbation. Even in the ICU setting, there is limited utility to obtaining serial imaging unless there were prior findings requiring follow-up. In many instances, imaging is used to rule out an alternative diagnosis such as pulmonary embolism, pneumothorax, or pneumonia (Fig. 7.2).

7.3 Medical Management of Exacerbations

The management of an acute asthma exacerbation centers around reversing the underlying pathophysiology. As described previously, an exacerbation is represented by uncontrolled hyperresponsiveness of the airway as a result of inflammation and bronchoconstriction. The backbone of exacerbation management is thus through corticosteroids to temper airway inflammation and inhaled bronchodilators to relieve bronchoconstriction [5]. In severe exacerbations requiring the medical ICU, there may be limited initial response to treatment due to the degree of airway inflammation and bronchoconstriction. This poses a clinical challenge as continued patient deterioration may occur despite initiating the correct therapies. In these difficult cases, several other therapies have been proposed with varying degrees of potential clinical benefit and data to support their use.

7.3.1 Standard-of-Care Therapy

Corticosteroids are the mainstay of therapy for acute asthma exacerbations by acting to decrease airway inflammation [1, 5]. These are given in addition to bronchodilators which act to relieve bronchial wall smooth muscle constriction. Together, these therapies act to alleviate airflow obstruction, reduce air trapping and hyperinflation, and, thus, relieve patient symptoms and improve clinical status.

Ideal dosing of systemic corticosteroids in asthma exacerbations remains unclear. A previously published meta-analysis and systematic review comparing low-dose versus high-dose systemic corticosteroids for asthma exacerbations found no additional benefit with higher doses of systemic corticosteroids compared to lower doses [7]. Low-dose corticosteroids were defined as $\leq$80 mg of methylprednisolone or $\leq$400 mg of hydrocortisone per day. However, patients who were in the ICU or receiving mechanical ventilation were excluded from these trials. There are no randomized controlled trials to dictate the dosing of systemic corticosteroids for patients requiring systemic corticosteroids in the intensive care unit, and thus, it is often left to clinician discretion. In general, higher dosages of systemic steroids and IV formulations tend to be used more frequently for patients admitted to the ICU, especially if requiring invasive ventilation.

While dosing remains nebulous, what is known is that earlier time to corticosteroid administration is associated with improved outcomes. Studies have demonstrated that patients who receive corticosteroids within 1 hour of emergency department arrival have fewer admissions for asthma [8]. While these studies did not evaluate ICU patients, it does suggest that early control of inflammation is key for optimal outcomes. In adult subjects in this study, the dosage of corticosteroid ranged from 500 mg of IV hydrocortisone (equivalent to 100 mg of methylprednisolone) to 125 mg of IV methylprednisolone, which is the most frequently used dosage in emergency departments in the United States [5].

There are two major types of inhaled bronchodilators that are used in acute asthma management: short-acting beta$_2$ adrenergic receptor agonists (SABAs), and short-acting anticholinergics (SAAC). The most encountered type of SABA is salbutamol, better known as albuterol, and for SAAC, it is ipratropium. Albuterol and ipratropium can be given as either a nebulizer or a metered-dose inhaler (MDI).

Studies have not shown a benefit of using nebulizers over MDIs; however, MDIs are more cost effective [9]. More doses of an MDI are required to reach an equivalent dosage of medication in a nebulized solution [9]. A meta-analysis and systematic review evaluated the benefit of addition of SAAC to SABA monotherapy in acute asthma. The results consistently demonstrated that combination usage of SABA/SAAC, at single or multiple doses, was more effective at reducing the risk for hospitalization and improving lung function than either medication alone [10, 11]. Dosages and frequencies for inhaled medications varied in the studies; however, ranges included albuterol 2.5–5 mg from hourly to several times per hour, and ipratropium 0.5 mg with similar frequency. In the ICU, inhaled bronchodilators are usually started as a continuous nebulization and then are spaced out as the patient improves clinically.

7.3.2 *Indications for Antibiotics*

Bacterial infections as triggers for asthma exacerbations only make up as small number of total exacerbations [12]. However, starting empiric antibiotics remains a common practice among providers [12]. Several studies have been published investigating whether the addition of antibiotics to the standard of care improves outcomes in asthma exacerbations. These studies excluded patients with confirmed bacterial infections warranting antibiotics. In a meta-analysis and systematic review of these studies, there was limited evidence to suggest that the addition of empiric antibiotics improved symptoms or airflow obstruction [12, 13]. The antibiotic classes that were studied included macrolides and penicillins, and there was no difference in outcomes by antibiotic class. However, like prior studies, patients admitted to the ICU were excluded from these studies. In cases of severe asthma requiring ICU admission, antibiotic coverage is usually initiated empirically, and then the decision to continue is readdressed after reviewing preliminary data to better rule in or rule out infection.

In addition to white blood cell count and culture data, serum procalcitonin measurements have been explored in asthma to guide the initiation and discontinuation of antibiotics. Procalcitonin, a pre-hormone to calcitonin, rises with bacterial infections but not with viral infections and has been studied extensively in relation to airway infections [5]. In one randomized, controlled trial, the procalcitonin level was used to decide whether to initiate and when to discontinue antibiotics versus clinician discretion. The group where procalcitonin levels were used to guide decisions on antibiotics had reduced the use of antibiotics without differences in clinical outcomes [14]. While it is not available in all health systems, serum procalcitonin may be of assistance when making decisions regarding antibiotic initiation and/or discontinuation.

7.3.3 Potential Adjunctive Therapies

7.3.3.1 Inhaled Corticosteroids (ICSs)

ICSs are the mainstay of the management of outpatient asthma; however, they play a limited role in the management of acute asthma exacerbations [2, 15]. This is largely due to the use of enteral or intravenous corticosteroids that are at doses much higher than the inhaled form can deliver. However, one argument that is made for the use of ICS is immediate delivery to the affected region [15]. Previous studies evaluating the use of ICS in acute asthma exacerbations have primarily looked at the use of adjunctive ICS to prevent hospitalization, and in most studies, the need for ICU admission or status asthmaticus was an exclusion criterion. In a pooled meta-analysis and systematic review, ICS use in acute asthma, either versus placebo or in addition to systemic corticosteroids, resulted in decreased hospital admissions [15]. Further studies analyzing the benefit of ICS on other important outcomes and in more severe exacerbations are needed. Adjunctive ICS use combined with systemic corticosteroids should be considered for use in patients with severe asthma exacerbations in the ICU in addition to standard-of-care therapy, especially since they are generally well tolerated with minimal potential for adverse effects.

7.3.3.2 Intravenous (IV) Magnesium Sulfate (MgSO$_4$)

The use of IV magnesium sulfate has been well described as an adjunctive treatment for severe asthma when there is clinical deterioration despite the initiation of standard-of-care medications [5, 16]. Its mechanism of action is still unclear, but it is believed that magnesium sulfate promotes bronchial wall smooth muscle relaxation and may also mitigate airway inflammation [16]. In a meta-analysis of placebo-controlled trials evaluating the efficacy of a one-time bolus of IV magnesium sulfate, its use resulted in a reduced need for hospital admission and improved lung function [16]. Of the studies available, only one study evaluated the effect of IV magnesium sulfate on the need for admission to the ICU, which did not show any significant difference compared to placebo [16]. Nonetheless, a one-time bolus of IV magnesium sulfate should be considered in all patients being admitted to the ICU for severe asthma given potential benefits and lack of significant adverse effects.

7.3.3.3 Inhaled Magnesium Sulfate (MgSO$_4$)

While the use of IV magnesium sulfate is well described and frequently used in clinical practice, the use of inhaled magnesium sulfate is less common. The nebulized solution is prepared by diluting the IV formulation or dissolving MgSO4 into sterile water; however, there are no FDA-approved formulations of nebulized magnesium sulfate currently available [17]. The use of inhaled magnesium sulfate has been investigated in asthma refractory to the initial standard of care. In a review of trials investigating the benefit of inhaled magnesium sulfate in addition to SABA/SAAC, doses of inhaled magnesium sulfate ranged from one to three (spaced out by 30-min intervals) [17]. Another meta-analysis of seven studies showed varying results, and the authors concluded that there may be a small benefit to the addition of inhaled magnesium sulfate, with a low confidence level [17]. Given the relative safety of the medication, its use could be considered in life-threatening circumstances in areas where it is available for use.

7.3.3.4 Intravenous (IV) Aminophylline

Aminophylline belongs to the drug class of methylxanthines, which includes theophylline. Both medications have historically been used for the treatment of chronic asthma for their weak bronchodilator effects. They have since been mostly replaced by stronger bronchodilators such as inhaled beta$_2$-agonists [18]. IV aminophylline has been proposed as an adjunct to inhaled beta$_2$-agonists in the treatment of acute asthma. A meta-analysis of 17 studies did not show any significant improvement in airflow or need for systemic corticosteroids with the use of IV aminophylline [18]. Additionally, patients treated with aminophylline experienced a higher incidence of nausea, vomiting, palpitations, and/or arrhythmias [18]. Because of these potential side effects and minimal evidence for benefit, IV aminophylline should be avoided in patients experiencing severe asthma requiring ICU admission. Nausea and vomiting may increase the risk for aspiration in patients and may also predispose them to dangerous arrhythmias when used in combination with SABAs.

7.3.3.5 Intravenous (IV) Beta$_2$-Agonists

The use of inhaled beta$_2$-agonists is the standard of care in acute asthma; however, the IV formulations of these drugs, such as bedoradrine and terbutaline, are rarely used. These drugs have mostly been studied in pediatric patients, in which there was no difference in the rates of ICU admissions with or without the drug [19]. Only one study has looked at the addition of IV beta$_2$-agonists to the standard of care in adult patients, and it did not lead to a reduction in hospital admissions [19].

7.3.3.6 Leukotriene Antagonists (LTRAs)

LTRAs such as montelukast are commonly used in the outpatient setting for the management of allergic asthma [2]. Production of leukotrienes by the immune system as a response to allergic triggers leads to bronchoconstriction and subsequent asthma symptoms [20]. Several studies have evaluated the impact of LTRAs in acute asthma as adjuncts to standard-of-care therapy. A meta-analysis showed a small improvement in airflow but no significant difference in hospital admission rates with IV or oral LTRAs. There was a slight, although nonsignificant, trend towards a reduction in hospital admissions in the IV group [20]. However, there are currently no FDA-approved IV LTRAs available commercially.

7.3.3.7 Intramuscular (IM) or IV Epinephrine

As highlighted in the earlier sections, anaphylaxis may mimic a severe asthma exacerbation. Untreated, both have a high mortality rate, and early recognition and appropriate treatment are paramount. IM epinephrine is the standard-of-care treatment for anaphylaxis. Epinephrine activates both alpha- and beta-adrenergic receptors and therefore could potentially be used in acute asthma exacerbations. A previous meta-analysis included studies in which epinephrine was administered in any formulation to patients with acute asthma exacerbations [21]. Epinephrine was found to be similarly efficacious to selective beta$_2$-agonists, but epinephrine had more side effects, and there was no clinical benefit when any form of epinephrine was added to inhaled beta$_2$-agonists in acute asthma [21]. Therefore, there is no data to support the use of epinephrine for severe asthma in the ICU aside from in patients with concomitant confirmed or suspected anaphylaxis.

7.3.3.8 Inhaled Anesthetics

Inhalational anesthetics such as isoflurane have been studied in patients with severe asthma requiring invasive mechanical ventilation [22]. Inhalational isoflurane stimulates the beta-adrenergic receptor leading to bronchial wall smooth muscle relaxation and bronchodilation [22]. In the limited number of cases in which isoflurane has been used, patients had generally already received many of the adjunctive therapies previously discussed. Clinical improvement was reported in all patients receiving isoflurane therapy, with a duration of therapy ranging from 16 to 34 hours [22]. Pursuant to local hospital policy, the presence of an anesthesiologist may be required when using inhaled isoflurane.

7.3.3.9 Inhaled Helium-Oxygen (Heliox)

The combination of oxygen-helium mixtures has long been used for patients with severe asthma exacerbations given that it reduces airway resistance [23, 24]. It has been studied in both mechanically ventilated patients and non-ventilated patients. For patients with acute asthma exacerbations not requiring mechanical ventilation, placebo-controlled trials have not demonstrated improved outcomes with heliox [23]. However, the primary outcomes in many of these studies were limited to rates of hospital admission and did not assess more seriously ill patients. One prospective observational study evaluated heliox in patients requiring mechanical ventilation for asthma or COPD exacerbations (high airway resistance states), without demonstrable improvement in measures of airway resistance [24].

7.3.3.10 Intravenous Ketamine

Ketamine has been used as an adjunct for severe asthma when there is clinical deterioration despite standard-of-care therapy [25]. Ketamine has many properties with potential benefit in severe asthma. It acts as a direct bronchodilator, stimulating beta$_2$-adrenergic receptors, and has indirect bronchodilator effects through the inhibition of vagal stimulation that leads to bronchoconstriction [25]. Data supporting the use of IV ketamine as an adjunctive therapy for severe asthma in the ICU come primarily from case reports. There is some data that ketamine, when given as an infusion, reduced the risk for requiring mechanical ventilation. In mechanically ventilated patients who received ketamine, improvement in clinical status and decreased airway resistance have been reported [25]. The limited data available suggests that IV ketamine is one of the few adjunctive therapies which may be particularly beneficial in patients with severe asthma requiring ICU admissions. High-quality studies are needed to validate these benefits. Also, this is another medication which may require the presence of an anesthesiologist for administration.

7.3.4 Emerging and Investigational Therapies

7.3.4.1 Subcutaneous (SC) Biologics

Biologics in asthma are a relatively new therapy. These monoclonal antibodies target cytokines in the Th2 inflammatory pathway and are used in the outpatient setting to treat patients with uncontrolled asthma symptoms or frequent exacerbations despite maximal inhaler therapy [26]. The role of these therapies in acute asthma is unknown. In one patient case, the biologic dupilumab was used as an adjunct for an asthma exacerbation that did not respond to the standard of care. Following SC administration of dupilumab, there was notable patient improvement [26]. Given the low side effect profile and potential benefits of these medications in acute asthma exacerbations, further studies are needed evaluating these therapies in the acute setting.

7.4 Airway Management of Exacerbations

ICU admission and the need for mechanical ventilation are associated with increased morbidity and mortality in patients with severe asthma exacerbations [27]. Therefore, it is crucial to promptly identify patients at risk for progressive respiratory failure. Asthma is a disease of the airways, and hypoxemia is not typically present in most asthma exacerbations [5]. In many cases, patients do not require high amounts of supplemental oxygen, and providers should aim to keep oxygen saturation >92% [5]. Impending respiratory failure is often signaled by respiratory muscle fatigue, mental status changes, lethargy, or hypercapnia and should be promptly treated with noninvasive or invasive ventilatory support [5].

7.4.1 Noninvasive Ventilation (NIV)

The use of NIV in severe asthma may help to provide enough respiratory support to stave off the need for intubation and mechanical ventilation. NIV can assist with alleviating the patient's work of breathing and correcting hypercapnia that may lead to CO_2 narcosis—a common cause of intubation in delayed presentations of severe asthma exacerbations [4]. Modalities of NIV include continuous positive-pressure ventilation (CPAP) and bilevel positive pressure ventilation (BiLevel). For severe asthma exacerbations, bilevel pressure support ventilation is preferred and titrated at the discretion of the intensivist to augment ventilation [4, 27]. Support for the use of NIV in severe asthma exacerbations is mostly coopted from the literature supporting the use of NIV in COPD exacerbations, which are similar physiologically to asthma exacerbations [27]. A large, multicenter, cohort study evaluating outcomes of NIV use in severe asthma exacerbations found that its use was associated with a reduction in the need for invasive mechanical ventilation and also a small mortality benefit [27]. NIV should be considered for appropriately selected patients with severe asthma exacerbations in the ICU.

7.4.2 Invasive Mechanical Ventilation (IMV)

Progression of an asthma exacerbation to IMV is concerning and indicates severe disease. This severe state is notable for high airway resistance (P_{peak}) and hyperinflation [28, 29]. Intensivists and respiratory therapists should closely monitor the airway resistance and auto-PEEP, a marker for hyperinflation [29, 30]. Medication adjuncts can be considered if there is limited response to standard of care while patients receive IMV. Downstream complications of uncontrolled hyperinflation and high airway resistance include barotrauma, pneumothorax, and hypotension [29, 30]. Deep sedation may be required to address ventilator dyssynchrony until improvement in respiratory dynamics. If unable to obtain ventilator synchrony despite sedation, paralytics may be considered [29]. Once improved from a respiratory status, mechanical support and sedation should be weaned as tolerated by the patient. Extubation should be considered once there has been significant improvement in disease state (Fig. 7.3).

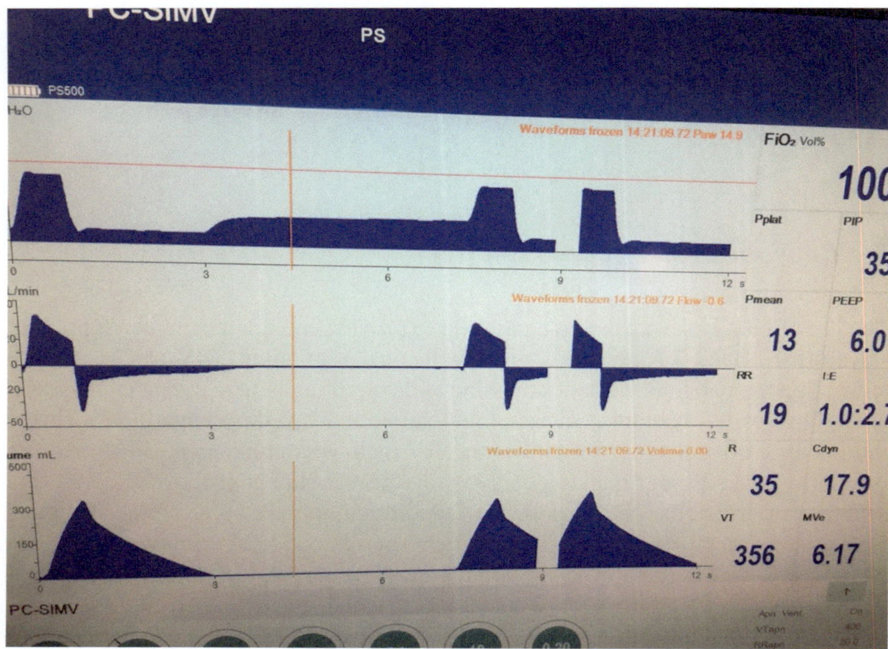

Fig. 7.3 Ventilator screen demonstrating obstruction and auto-PEEPing in an asthmatic patient

7.5 Extracorporeal Membrane Oxygenation (ECMO) in Exacerbations

ECMO is a form of mechanical circulatory support that can be used to support patients with profound hypoxemic respiratory failure and/or cardiovascular failure. It functions by removing blood via a drainage cannula inserted either in a central vein or in an artery, passing it through an oxygenator and pump and then delivered back into the body via a return cannula [31]. The configuration of ECMO is determined by the disease state and the amount of support required by the patient [31]. The use of ECMO for refractory severe asthma is rare; however, it has been described in the literature as salvage therapy when invasive mechanical ventilation was insufficient. There is limited evidence to support the use of ECMO as salvage therapy. A retrospective, cohort study evaluating 127 asthma exacerbations requiring ECMO support demonstrated an association with lower mortality in the ECMO group versus propensity-matched models [31]. While further studies are required to explore this subject, ECMO as a rescue modality can be considered if there is further clinical deterioration despite maximal patient optimization following the initiation of invasive mechanical ventilation.

7.6 De-escalation of Care

As an asthma exacerbation improves, the patient will note improved work of breathing, reduced cough, resolution of wheezing, and improved air movement on auscultation. Corticosteroids should be transitioned to oral when tolerated and continued until at least discharge, if not continued as a slow taper through outpatient follow-up. Use of SABAs and SAACs should be spaced out from continuous to every few hours and then used on an as-needed basis. Near discharge, patients should be restarted on their home ICS if not continued during hospitalization. If a patient was not previously on an ICS, this should be started prior to discharge and continued until outpatient follow-up. The GINA guidelines are a helpful resource for identifying an ideal inhaler regimen for a patient. Inhaler teaching should occur with a respiratory therapist before discharge, and patients should be given a spacer if appropriate and instructed on its use.

7.6.1 Outpatient Follow-Up

Patients who require admission for an asthma exacerbation should be referred to a pulmonologist as an outpatient [5]. Inhalers and medications should be reconciled based on symptoms, and triggers should be reviewed to prevent future exacerbations. In certain cases, patients with severe asthma exacerbations are discharged on a tapered oral corticosteroid regimen that should be carefully discontinued. Symptoms may return if corticosteroids are weaned too quickly. If asthma symptoms remain persistent and severe despite maximal inhaler therapy requiring oral steroids, addition of biologics should be considered.

7.7 Summary

Asthma is an inflammatory disease of the respiratory airways that results in symptoms of shortness of breath, wheezing, and cough. Mainstay therapy of outpatient asthma is through inhaled corticosteroids and bronchodilators. An asthma exacerbation is defined by acute worsening of asthma symptoms, and it requires escalation of care to properly manage. Exacerbations can be triggered by infectious and non-infectious etiologies. The standard of care in an asthma exacerbation is centered around corticosteroids and frequent administration of bronchodilators. Exacerbations can be severe and progress to profound respiratory failure requiring the ICU. Several adjunct therapies have been studied in severe asthma that does not initially respond to the standard of care, each with varying levels of efficacy. Respiratory status should be closely monitored with the goal to avoid invasive mechanical ventilation as it carries an increased risk for mortality. Studies show some mortality benefits with using noninvasive ventilation to prevent the need for invasive mechanical ventilation. Once improved and discharged, patients with a history of an asthma exacerbation requiring ICU admission are considered high risk and should have close outpatient pulmonology follow-up.

References

1. Holgate ST, Wenzel S, Postma DS, Weiss ST, Renz H, Sly PD. Asthma. Nat Rev Dis Primers. 2015;1(1):1–22. https://doi.org/10.1038/nrdp.2015.25.
2. 2023 GINA Main Report. Global Initiative for Asthma—GINA. Accessed March 14, 2024. https://ginasthma.org/2023-gina-main-report/.
3. What is Asthma? Welcome to the NAEP©. Accessed May 11, 2024. https://www.asthmasa. org/what-is-asthma/.
4. Phipps P. The pulmonary physician in critical care * 12: acute severe asthma in the intensive care unit. Thorax. 2003;58(1):81–8. https://doi.org/10.1136/thorax.58.1.81.
5. Hasegawa K, Craig SS, Teach SJ, Camargo CA. Management of asthma exacerbations in the emergency department. J Allergy Clin Immunol Pract. 2021;9(7):2599–610. https://doi. org/10.1016/j.jaip.2020.12.037.
6. Manser R, Reid D, Abramson MJ. Corticosteroids for acute severe asthma in hospitalised patients. Cochrane Database Syst Rev. 2001;2001:CD001740. https://doi. org/10.1002/14651858.CD001740.
7. Rowe BH, Spooner C, Ducharme F, Bretzlaff J, Bota G. Early emergency department treatment of acute asthma with systemic corticosteroids. Cochrane Database Syst Rev. 2001;2001:CD002178. https://doi.org/10.1002/14651858.CD002178.
8. Cates CJ, Welsh EJ, Rowe BH. Holding chambers (spacers) versus nebulisers for beta-agonist treatment of acute asthma. Cochrane Database Syst Rev. 2013;2014:CD000052. https://doi. org/10.1002/14651858.CD000052.pub3.
9. Kirkland SW, Vandenberghe C, Voaklander B, Nikel T, Campbell S, Rowe BH. Combined inhaled beta-agonist and anticholinergic agents for emergency management in adults with asthma. Cochrane Database Syst Rev. 2017;2017:CD001284. https://doi. org/10.1002/14651858.CD001284.pub2.
10. Rodrigo GJ, Castro-Rodriguez JA. Anticholinergics in the treatment of children and adults with acute asthma: a systematic review with meta-analysis. Thorax. 2005;60(9):740–6. https:// doi.org/10.1136/thx.2005.047803.
11. Normansell R, Sayer B, Waterson S, Dennett EJ, Forno MD, Dunleavy A. Antibiotics for exacerbations of asthma. Cochrane Database Syst Rev. 2018;2018:CD002741. https://doi. org/10.1002/14651858.CD002741.pub2.
12. Johnston SL, Szigeti M, Cross M, et al. Azithromycin for acute exacerbations of asthma: the AZALEA randomized clinical trial. JAMA Intern Med. 2016;176(11):1630–7. https://doi. org/10.1001/jamainternmed.2016.5664.
13. Tang J, Long W, Yan L, et al. Procalcitonin guided antibiotic therapy of acute exacerbations of asthma: a randomized controlled trial. BMC Infect Dis. 2013;13(1):596. https://doi.org/10.118 6/1471-2334-13-596.
14. Edmonds ML, Milan SJ Jr, CAC, Pollack CV, Rowe BH. Early use of inhaled corticosteroids in the emergency department treatment of acute asthma. Cochrane Database Syst Rev. 2012;12:CD002308. https://doi.org/10.1002/14651858.CD002308.pub2.
15. Kew KM, Kirtchuk L, Michell CI, Griffiths B. Intravenous magnesium sulfate for treating adults with acute asthma in the emergency department. Cochrane Database Syst Rev. 2014;2014(5):CD010909. https://doi.org/10.1002/14651858.CD010909.pub2.

16. Knightly R, Milan SJ, Hughes R, et al. Inhaled magnesium sulfate in the treatment of acute asthma. Cochrane Database Syst Rev. 2017;11:CD003898. https://doi.org/10.1002/14651858. CD003898.pub6.
17. Nair P, Milan SJ, Rowe BH. Addition of intravenous aminophylline to inhaled beta$_2$-agonists in adults with acute asthma. Cochrane Database Syst Rev. 2012;2012:12. https://doi. org/10.1002/14651858.CD002742.pub2.
18. Travers AH, Milan SJ, Jones AP Jr, CAC, Rowe BH. Addition of intravenous beta$_2$-agonists to inhaled beta$_2$-agonists for acute asthma. Cochrane Database Syst Rev. 2012;12(12):CD010179. https://doi.org/10.1002/14651858.CD010179.
19. Watts K, Chavasse RJ. Leukotriene receptor antagonists in addition to usual care for acute asthma in adults and children. Cochrane Database Syst Rev. 2012;2012(5):CD006100. https:// doi.org/10.1002/14651858.CD006100.pub2.
20. Baggott C, Hardy JK, Sparks J, et al. Epinephrine (adrenaline) compared to selective beta-2-agonist in adults or children with acute asthma: a systematic review and meta-analysis. Thorax. 2022;77(6):563–72. https://doi.org/10.1136/thoraxjnl-2021-217124.
21. Johnston RG, Noseworthy TW, Friesen EG, Yule HA, Shustack A. Isoflurane therapy for status asthmaticus in children and adults. Chest. 1990;97(3):698–701. https://doi.org/10.1378/ chest.97.3.698.
22. Rodrigo GJJ, Pollack CV, Rodrigo C, Rowe BH. Heliox for nonintubated acute asthma patients. Cochrane Database Syst Rev. 2006;2006(4):CD002884. https://doi.org/10.1002/14651858. CD002884.
23. Leatherman JW, Romero RS, Shapiro RS. Lack of benefit of heliox during mechanical ventilation of subjects with severe air-flow obstruction. Respir Care. 2018;63(4):375–9. https://doi. org/10.4187/respcare.05893.
24. Goyal S, Agrawal A. Ketamine in status asthmaticus: a review. Indian J Crit Care Med. 2013;17(3):154–61. https://doi.org/10.4103/0972-5229.117048.
25. Kim BG, Park DW, Park TS, et al. A case of biologic use in acute asthma exacerbation refractory to conventional management. J Allergy Clin Immunol Pract. 2023;11(9):2922–5. https:// doi.org/10.1016/j.jaip.2023.06.064.
26. Althoff MD, Holguin F, Yang F, et al. Noninvasive ventilation use in critically ill patients with acute asthma exacerbations. Am J Respir Crit Care Med. 2020;202(11):1520–30. https://doi. org/10.1164/rccm.201910-2021OC.
27. Yartsev A. Ventilation strategies for Status Asthmaticus | Deranged Physiology. Accessed May 11, 2024. https://derangedphysiology.com/main/required-reading/ respiratory-medicine-and-ventilation/Chapter611/ventilation-strategies-status-asthmaticus-0.
28. Laher AE, Buchanan SK. Mechanically ventilating the severe asthmatic. J Intensive Care Med. 2018;33(9):491–501. https://doi.org/10.1177/0885066617740079.
29. Leatherman J. Mechanical ventilation for severe asthma. Chest. 2015;147(6):1671–80. https:// doi.org/10.1378/chest.14-1733.
30. Zakrajsek JK, Min SJ, Ho PM, et al. Extracorporeal membrane oxygenation for refractory asthma exacerbations with respiratory failure. Chest. 2023;163(1):38–51. https://doi. org/10.1016/j.chest.2022.09.029.

Chapter 8
Acute Pulmonary Embolism

Soyoung Kristi Kim and Lauren A. Igneri

8.1 Introduction

Pulmonary embolism (PE) is a common yet serious clinical presentation of venous thromboembolism (VTE). VTE, including deep vein thrombosis (DVT) and PE, is the third most common acute cardiovascular syndrome globally, behind myocardial infarction and stroke [59]. Globally, the incidence of PE is reported to be between 39 (in Hong Kong) and 115 (in the United States) per 100,000 population [113].

Acute PE may present with varying degrees of critical illness, ranging from incidental findings of asymptomatic PE to hemodynamic instability or cardiac arrest in high-risk patients with PE. Despite numerous advancements in the management of PE, the mortality rate for PE continues to be high. In high-risk patients, the 30-day mortality can be as high as 22% [73]. An analysis of epidemiologic databases reported the overall age-adjusted mortality per 100,000 populations as 2.84 in 2006 compared to 2.81 in 2019 [118].

Given the incidence and severity of illness associated with PE, pharmacist clinicians should have an expanded understanding of the diagnostic process for the detection and management of PE. Pharmacists should be aware of the high rates of VTE that are associated with critical illness and develop during hospitalization. Hospital-acquired VTE accounts for more than half of all VTE reported in the United States [38]. The incidence of PE in critically ill patients in the intensive care unit (ICU) ranges from 1.4% to 2.9%, although the true incidence including undetected or asymptomatic PE may be higher [73].

S. K. Kim · L. A. Igneri (✉)
Clinical Pharmacy Specialist, Critical Care, Department of Pharmacy,
Cooper University Health Care, Camden, NJ, USA
e-mail: Igneri-Lauren@CooperHealth.edu

Y. Alzaidi, M. A. Gebily (eds.), *The Pharmacist's Expanded Role in Critical Care Medicine*, https://doi.org/10.1007/978-3-031-77335-8_8

8.1.1 Risk Factors for VTE

Risk factors for the development of VTE are characterized as either acquired or inherited. Acquired risk factors include comorbidities such as hypertension, recent surgery, immobility, cancer, and obesity [101]. Patients may also have inherited risk factors for hypercoagulable states. The concept of antithrombin deficiency leading to the loss of thrombin activity was proposed as early as 1905, forming the basis for there being genetic risk factors for VTE [22, 101]. Additional risk factors for inherited thrombophilia include factor V Leiden mutation, prothrombin gene mutation, and deficiencies in protein S or C [22]. The identification of reversible or irreversible acquired risk factors will play an important role in delineating provoked and unprovoked VTE, which determines the duration of anticoagulation therapy [59]. Table 8.1 describes the weak, moderate, and strong predisposing factors for VTE.

8.1.2 Pathophysiology of VTE

VTE often results from the presence of optimal conditions for thrombus formation as described by Virchow's triad. This includes alterations in blood flow (e.g., venous stasis), endothelial damage, and hypercoagulable state as described above [101].

Table 8.1 Predisposing factors for VTE

Weak risk factors	Moderate risk factors	Strong risk factors
Diabetes mellitus	Arthroscopic knee surgery	Fracture of lower limb
Hypertension	Autoimmune diseases	Recent hospitalization for heart failure or atrial fibrillation/flutter
Immobility/bed rest	Blood transfusion	Hip or knee replacement
Increasing age	Central venous lines	Major trauma
Laparoscopic surgery	Intravenous catheters and leads	Myocardial infarction
Obesity	Chemotherapy	Previous VTE
Pregnancy	Congestive heart failure or respiratory failure	Spinal cord injury
Varicose veins	Erythropoiesis-stimulating agents	
	Hormone replacement therapy (depends on formulation)	
	In vitro fertilization	
	Oral contraceptive therapy	
	Post-partum period	
	Infection (specifically pneumonia, urinary tract infection, and HIV)	
	Inflammatory bowel disease	
	Cancer (highest risk in metastatic disease)	
	Paralytic stroke	
	Superficial vein thrombosis	
	Thrombophilia	

Thrombi typically form in the deep veins of the lower extremities, usually at sites of decreased flow such as valve cusps. Once microthrombi are formed due to venous stasis or endothelial injury, blood flow is further impeded. This progresses to further vascular injury and clot formation, perpetually activating the coagulation cascade [71]. Thrombus that originates from a venous bed may resolve completely or partially via recanalization, organization, and/or lysis or continue to expand and embolize to the pulmonary circulation [71, 101].

8.1.3 PE Definitions and Classifications

8.1.3.1 Pathogenesis of PE

PE often results from a thrombus originating in the lower extremity proximal veins (e.g., iliac, femoral, or popliteal) that travels to the pulmonary vasculature. Emboli follow normal venous circulation, from the vena cava to the right atrium and ventricle, and then ultimately to the pulmonary artery and its branches. The presence of specific patient factors such as the use of pacemakers, implantable defibrillators, and indwelling central venous catheters may increase the risk of an upper extremity DVT that embolizes the pulmonary arteries [71, 101]. In the Registro Informatizado de la Enfermedad Tromboembolica (RIETE) registry of patients with documented VTE, the rates of PE at 90 days were similar regardless of the origin of the thrombus in the upper or lower extremity [74]. In rare instances, thrombus may originate directly from the pulmonary vasculature without evidence of DVT. Factors such as endothelial cell dysfunction, hypoxia, and inflammation may lead to this phenomenon of in situ PE. This can be observed in patients with trauma (such as chest contusions), sickle cell disease, pulmonary tuberculosis, and other systemic diseases. Seldom, pulmonary embolism develops from non-thrombotic causes, such as air, fat, or tumor emboli that obstruct the pulmonary artery or its branches [71, 110]. The pathophysiology, diagnosis, and management of non-thrombotic PE are beyond the scope of this chapter. There are multiple ways to characterize PE, including its anatomic location, chronicity, and risk stratification, which are described in Table 8.2.

8.1.3.2 Anatomic Location

The anatomic location of thrombi further stratifies PE. A large clot that lodges at the bifurcation of the main pulmonary artery leads to a saddle PE. A saddle embolus obstructs the blood flow to both the right and left pulmonary arteries. Smaller emboli that travel beyond the pulmonary artery bifurcation can lodge distally in the lobar, segmental, or subsegmental branches. Occlusions of a distal pulmonary artery (segmental and subsegmental) can lead to pulmonary infarction, potentially causing ischemia, hemorrhage, and tissue necrosis. Due to the location of the emboli, saddle

Table 8.2 Characterization of PE

Characteristics	Categories	Definition
Anatomic	Saddle	Emboli at the bifurcation of the main pulmonary artery
	Lobar	Emboli at the lobar branches
	Segmental	Emboli at the segmental branches
	Subsegmental	Emboli at the subsegmental branches
Chronicity	Acute	Immediate or recent symptoms
	Subacute	Symptoms over weeks to months
	Chronic	Symptoms lasting months to years
Risk	Low	Refer to Table 8.5
	Intermediate-low	
	Intermediate-high	
	High	

PE was historically assumed to be associated with more hemodynamic compromise compared to PE caused by distal thrombi. However, no difference in mortality was observed between a saddle and non-saddle PE in a recent retrospective review, which highlights the importance of cautiously monitoring all patients for signs of decompensation regardless of the anatomic location of the emboli [41].

8.1.3.3 Chronicity

Patients can present with acute, subacute, or chronic PE. The duration of patient symptoms such as cough or shortness of breath differentiates patients into one of the three categories. Patients with acute PE present with immediate or recent symptoms, whereas those with subacute PE may report symptoms that are presented insidiously over weeks to months [26, 96]. In contrast, patients with chronic PE often present with symptoms lasting months to years. Although most patients recover fully after the resolution of acute embolism, approximately 30–50% of patients have perfusion defects and residual pulmonary obstruction at 6 months from diagnosis despite anticoagulation [115].

Patients with chronic PE may develop pulmonary hypertension from unresolved pulmonary occlusions in the pulmonary arteries, subsequent fibrosis, and remodeling of the pulmonary vessels leading to elevated pulmonary vascular resistance (PVR) [76]. This unique pathophysiology is known as chronic thromboembolic pulmonary hypertension (CTEPH), also designated as Group 4 pulmonary hypertension by the World Health Organization. Although the incidence of CTEPH is not clearly defined, it is identified in 0.5–9% of patients following acute PE [115].

Treatment for CTEPH can be highly variable and requires multidisciplinary team evaluation. All eligible patients without contraindications should receive indefinite anticoagulation. For patients that are operable candidates, pulmonary thromboendarterectomy (PTE) may be a curative therapy. In recent years, balloon pulmonary angioplasty emerged as an established treatment option for patients who are not surgical candidates [115]. Patients may also receive pulmonary hypertension-specific therapies, such as pulmonary vasodilators or remodeling agents that lower the pulmonary vascular resistance (PVR) and pulmonary artery pressure (PAP) [52]. Riociguat, a soluble guanylate cyclase stimulator approved for use in inoperable CTEPH or persistent CTEPH following PTE, was shown to improve 6-minute walking distance and PVR in the CHEST-1 study [33].

8.1.3.4   Risk Stratification

Patients are further categorized according to the risk of mortality and poor outcomes. Previously, PE was often stratified as massive, submassive, or nonmassive/low risk depending on the hemodynamic stability, although definitions of hemodynamic stability have varied. The 2011 scientific statement from the American Heart Association defined massive PE as an acute PE with sustained hypotension, pulselessness, or persistent profound bradycardia. The term submassive PE was utilized to describe acute PE without systemic hypotension but with either RV dysfunction or myocardial necrosis, and low-risk PE was defined as acute PE in the absence of the clinical markers of adverse prognosis that define massive or submassive PE [42]. These definitions are important to acknowledge since historical primary literature frequently utilized such terminology to stratify patients. Newer guidelines, including the one published by the European Society of Cardiology in 2020, transitioned to categorizing PE as high, intermediate-high, intermediate-low, and low risk [59]. The risk stratification ultimately guides diagnostic and treatment strategies in PE, which are discussed in forthcoming sections.

8.1.4   Clinical Presentation

8.1.4.1   Symptoms

Patients with acute PE may present with a multitude of nonspecific symptoms or with abnormal cardiopulmonary exams that mimic numerous other disease states including:

- Pleuritic chest pain
- Dyspnea
- Apprehension
- Angina chest pain
- Cough
- Diaphoresis
- Hemoptysis

- Lightheadedness
- Leg or thigh pain/swelling
- Orthopnea
- Palpitations
- Syncope
- Wheezing

PE should be included in the differential diagnosis when unexplained or rapid-onset dyspnea, pleuritic chest pain, or hemoptysis is present. Particularly, in patients with preexisting heart or pulmonary disease, dyspnea may be the most prominent symptom. However, dyspnea was experienced by 73% of patients with PE despite no preexisting cardiopulmonary conditions in the PIOPED II registry, at rest or with exertion [98]. Pleuritic chest pain is typically the result of pleural irritation from distal emboli that causes pulmonary infarction, whereas chest pain that mimics acute coronary syndrome or aortic dissection may be caused by RV ischemia from extensive central PE [101]. Symptoms suggestive of DVT (e.g., erythema, warmth, pain, swelling, tenderness) may also warrant further evaluation for PE, as PE often arises from a thrombus in the lower extremity. In the same registry, 44% of patients with PE experienced concomitant leg or thigh symptoms [98].

Patients with high-risk PE may present with hemodynamic instability such as systemic hypotension, RV dysfunction, presyncope or syncope, and even cardiopulmonary arrest [59, 101]. These features are more pronounced in patients with a greater magnitude of embolism or in patients with preexisting cardiac comorbidities [59, 101]. Finally, some patients with PE may be asymptomatic on presentation, making workup challenging.

8.1.4.2 Physician Examination

Similarly to presenting symptoms, patients with PE may have variable physical exam findings that mimic other disease states [101]:

- Anxiety
- Chest-wall tenderness
- Fever
- Heart failure
- Leg or thigh swelling/tenderness
- Neck vein distention
- Shock
- Tachycardia
- Tachypnea
- Wheezing

Patients with PE frequently present with tachypnea and tachycardia, which may confound the diagnoses by mimicking potential infectious etiologies. Particularly when patients have concomitant fever or shock, the treatment team may focus the management on antimicrobials for pneumonia or sepsis. The pharmacist's involvement in the appropriate evaluation of these nonspecific clinical findings can minimize unnecessary antimicrobial usage in patients with PE.

The severity of a patient's physical examination may depend on the patient's baseline cardiopulmonary reserve. Patients with a concomitant cardiac or pulmonary disease may not possess the adequate compensatory mechanism to overcome the clot burden in the pulmonary vasculature, leading to worsening hemodynamics [71, 101].

8.1.4.3 Cardiopulmonary Compromise

Pulmonary embolism may impair not only gas exchange, but also systemic circulation [59]. Whereas small emboli block the peripheral arteries and precipitate pulmonary infarction, large saddle embolus can obstruct the main pulmonary artery and have a grave impact on the cardiovascular system.

Hypoxemia from PE develops due to various mechanisms. The obstruction of the pulmonary vascular bed causes decreased capillary blood flow, leading to intrapulmonary shunting, increased alveolar dead space, ventilation-perfusion (V/Q) ratio mismatch, and decreased mixed venous oxygen saturation. V/Q mismatch occurs from zones of reduced flow in the obstructed vessels and zones of overflow in non-obstructed vessels. Atelectasis, alveolar hemorrhage, or bronchoconstriction can also lead to worsening shunt physiology [101, 110]. Low CO from RV failure also contributes to the reduced mixed venous oxygen saturation.

PE may cause hemodynamic alterations to varying degrees. When less than 20% of the pulmonary vascular bed is occluded by thromboemboli, patients without pre-existing cardiopulmonary disease are able to elicit compensatory mechanisms to support near-normal hemodynamics [101]. PE-induced hypoxemia causes neurohormonal activation of thromboxane A2 and serotonin, leading to initial vasoconstriction and increased PVR. When 30–40% of the pulmonary bed is occluded, PAP increases, and the RV adapts by increasing the stroke volume to maintain cardiac output (CO). This compensatory mechanism temporarily improves flow through the obstructed pulmonary vascular bed and stabilizes systemic blood pressure. However, the effect is short-lived as the thin-walled RV cannot generate a consistent mean PAP >40 mmHg. When pulmonary obstruction exceeds 50–60%, or when the compensatory mechanism is overwhelmed, drastic cardiovascular collapse can ensue. The increase in PVR leads to RV dilation, increased RV wall tension, and flattening of the interventricular septum, which alter the contractility of the myocardium. Ultimately, abrupt RV failure and desynchronization of the ventricles result in LV filling impedance, reduction in CO, and hemodynamic instability [101]. RV failure is attributed as the main cause of death in severe PE [59]. Patients with preexisting cardiopulmonary disease may have an exaggerated response to smaller degrees of pulmonary vascular occlusion, leading to severe pulmonary hypertension disproportionate to the degree of obstruction from acute PE [101].

8.2 Diagnosis and Risk Assessment

8.2.1 *Diagnostic Workup*

8.2.1.1 Clinical Pretest/Scores

Clinical pretest probability scoring is a cornerstone of diagnostic algorithms for PE as it guides selection of tests based on an assessment of the patient's signs and symptoms, risk factors for PE, presence of DVT, and whether PE is the most likely diagnosis, thereby allocating resources to patients most likely to derive benefit from testing (e.g., confirm or refute diagnosis of PE) [59]. Comparatively, pretest assessment using clinical gestalt lacks standardization, and preference should be to use clinical prediction rules for workup of PE.

The pharmacist clinician should be familiar with the most common pretest probability scores as they inform the need for further diagnostic testing and provide an opportunity to strategize potential initial anticoagulation selection while confirmatory tests are pending. The most widely used clinical pretest scores for PE include the Wells scores, Geneva Clinical Prediction, and PE Rule-Out Criteria and are compared in Table 8.3.

The Wells score incorporates seven criteria with the evaluation of D-dimer to estimate the clinical pretest probability of PE as either low, moderate, or high and is one of the most widely utilized and validated pretest probability scoring tools for PE [111, 112]. In the study validating the score in the emergency department (ED), PE was excluded in patients with a low pretest score and negative D-dimer and no imaging was performed. Comparatively, 40.6% of patients in the high-probability group and 16.2% in the moderate-probability group with positive D-dimer were diagnosed with PE. Only 1.3% of patients in the low-probability group re-presented back to the ED and were ultimately diagnosed with PE [112]. Subsequently, the score was simplified to "PE unlikely" or "PE likely" and validated in the Christopher Study [106]. In patients classified as unlikely, PE was excluded if the D-dimer was normal, and most patients did not receive anticoagulation. Only 0.5% were found to have subsequent PE at 3-month follow-up [106]. This score was also validated in conjunction with the use of an age-adjusted D-dimer cutoff in ADJUST-PE, a multicenter, multinational prospective management outcome study of outpatients with suspected PE [88]. Similarly, the Geneva clinical prediction rule, which originally incorporated seven variables, was revised to eight variables, simplified, and then validated in the ADJUST-PE [88].

To prevent unnecessary testing for PE in the emergency department (ED) setting, the Pulmonary Embolism Rule-Out Criteria (PERC) were developed to identify those with a low risk for PE who do not require further workup [59]. When there is low clinical suspicion for PE and the patient meets all eight criteria, a diagnosis of PE should not be pursued. Penaloza and colleagues found that when all PERC criteria were met in patients with a low gestalt assessment, PE prevalence was zero [80]. Subsequently, a prospective, observational study demonstrated that PERC had

Table 8.3 Comparison of Wells scores, Geneva Clinical Prediction, and PE Rule-Out Criteria [59, 88, 111, 112]

Wells Score		Geneva Clinical Prediction			PE Rule-out Criteria Rule
			Clinical Decision Rule Points		
Variables	**Points**	**Variables**	**Original**	**Simplified**	**Variables**
Clinically suspected DVT	3	Previous PE or DVT	3	1	Age <50 years
Alternative diagnosis is less likely than PE	3	Heart rate			Pulse <100 beats/ minute
		75–94 beats/minute	3	1	
		≥95 beats/minute	5	2	
Heart rate >100 beats/min	1.5	Surgery or fracture within past month	2	1	Pulse oximetry >94%
Immobilization or surgery in previous 4 weeks	1.5	Hemoptysis	2	1	No unilateral leg swelling
History of VTE	1.5	Active cancer	2	1	No hemoptysis
Hemoptysis	1	Unilateral lower-limb pain	3	1	No surgery or trauma within 4 weeks
Malignancy or treatment for it in previous 6 months	1	Pain on lower-limb deep venous palpation and unilateral edema	4	1	No prior DVT or PE
		Age > 65	1	1	No oral hormone use

Interpretation

Clinical Probability	Points	Clinical Probability	Points		Clinical Probability
Three-level prediction		*Three-level score*			If all variables met combined with low clinical suspicion for PE, diagnosis of PE should not be pursued
High probability	≥6.5	Low	0–3	0–1	
Moderate probability	4.5–6.0	Intermediate	4–10	2–4	
Low probability	≤4	High	≥11	≥5	
Two-level prediction		*Two-level score*			
High probability	>4	PE unlikely	0–5	0–2	
Low probability	≤4	PE likely	≥6	≥3	

a low rate of false-negatives for excluding PE in low-risk patients, and a crossover cluster-randomized trial found that PERC was noninferior to the gestalt method [30, 81].

8.2.1.2 D-Dimer-Level Interpretations

D-dimer levels become elevated in acute thrombosis due to activation of the coagulation cascade and plasmin-mediated enzymatic degradation of cross-linked fibrin clot [50]. While normal D-dimer levels (generally <500 ng/mL) have a high negative predictive value to rule out PE, high D-dimer levels have a low positive predictive value and are not useful as a confirmatory test [59].

Several D-dimer assays are available, but the quantitative enzyme-linked immunosorbent assay (ELISA) has >95% sensitivity to exclude PE in patients with low or intermediate pretest probability. Many studies have shown that a negative D-dimer in combination with low or intermediate clinical pretest probability scores excludes PE without the need for further testing [30, 80, 81, 88, 112]. When anticoagulation is withheld due to the negative result, the risk of developing PE at 3 months is <1% [14].

It is important for the pharmacist clinician to be aware of disease states that may cause false elevations in D-dimer to aid with the interpretation of result, especially when used in conjunction with pretest probability scoring. Other physiologic states or conditions that may result in elevated D-dimer in the absence of VTE include pregnancy, malignancy, cigarette smoking, trauma, infection, or sepsis. Additionally, patients who are older, immobilized, and with autoimmune disorders or have had recent surgery may have an elevated D-dimer without having VTE [12].

Recently, alternative D-dimer thresholds have been evaluated to optimize the proportion of patients who ultimately receive confirmatory imaging studies and are found to have PE.

Several studies have shown that D-dimer levels increase with age, limiting the utility of D-dimer thresholds <500 ng/mL to rule out PE in older individuals, especially those greater than age 80. The age-adjusted D-dimer threshold of patient age multiplied by 10 ng/mL in individuals over age 50 has been prospectively evaluated. In the ADJUST-PE study, clinical pretest probability scoring was evaluated with either the simplified Geneva score or the two-level Wells score. Patients with low/intermediate or unlikely probability had D-dimer testing performed, with a negative test defined as <500 ng/mL (patient age <50) or less than the age-adjusted level (patient age ≥50). In patients with D-dimer between 500 and their age-adjusted threshold, the rate of VTE at 3 months was 0.3%. Among patients >75 years, the use of age-adjusted D-dimer increased the proportion of patients in whom PE could be excluded from 6.4% with the standard threshold to 29.7% without any additional false-negative findings [88].

Due to the risks associated with radiation and contrast media, clinical probability-adapted D-dimer thresholds have been evaluated to reduce exposure to confirmatory testing in patients unlikely to have PE. The PEGeD study used the Wells clinical pretest probability scoring with D-dimer <1000 ng/mL in low-probability and <500 ng/mL in moderate-probability patients to exclude PE and further workup in the outpatient or emergency department setting. Of all patients determined not to have PE and did not receive treatment, only one patient developed VTE at 3 months. Importantly, the use of probability-adapted D-dimer thresholds resulted in 17.6% less patients receiving chest imaging for PE workup compared to the traditional threshold of <500 ng/mL for low- or moderate-probability patients [50].

In the YEARS study, clinical pretest probability scoring with three of the original Wells criteria (i.e., YEARS items)—(1) clinical signs of DVT, (2) hemoptysis, and (3) PE is the most likely diagnosis—was applied to inpatients and outpatients with suspected PE. PE was excluded if patients had zero YEARS criteria and D-dimer <1000 ng/mL or ≥ 1 YEARS criteria and D-dimer <500 ng/mL; otherwise, computed tomography pulmonary angiography (CTPA) was pursued. Use of YEARS criteria and clinical probability-adjusted D-dimer resulted in a <1% risk of VTE at 3 months and a 14% decrease in CTPA testing among patients of all ages compared to the use of standard Wells criteria and D-dimer <500 ng/mL [107].

Similarly, YEARS criteria and clinical probability-adapted D-dimer thresholds were evaluated in pregnant women in the Artemis study. Compression ultrasonography evaluating for DVT was pursued if patients had no YEARS criteria and D-dimer ≥1000 ng/mL or ≥1 YEARS criteria and D-dimer ≥500 ng/mL. If DVT was not identified on ultrasound, only then was CTPA pursued to minimize radiation exposure during pregnancy. This algorithm safely ruled out PE across all trimesters but was most efficient in avoiding CTPA in patients who began the study during their first trimester [108].

Based on recent literature, it is reasonable to use an age or clinical probability-adapted D-dimer threshold in conjunction with pretest probability scoring to guide further workup for PE.

8.2.2 Computed Tomography Pulmonary Angiography (CTPA)

CTPA is the gold standard for confirming the presence of PE. Intravenous radiopaque contrast allows for the visualization and detection of filling defects in the pulmonary arteries on computed tomography. For patients with a low or intermediate probability of PE, guidelines suggest that a negative CTPA is adequate to exclude PE. However, the negative predictive value is low for patients with high clinical probability [59]. Figure 8.1 shows filling defects (pulmonary thromboemboli) in bilateral pulmonary arteries, which are consistent with acute PE.

8.2.3 Mortality Risk Assessment

Risk factors for PE-associated morbidity and mortality were poorly understood until the publication of the International Cooperative Pulmonary Embolism Registry (ICOPER) data from 2110 patients with proven PE in 1999. Overall, 4.2% of

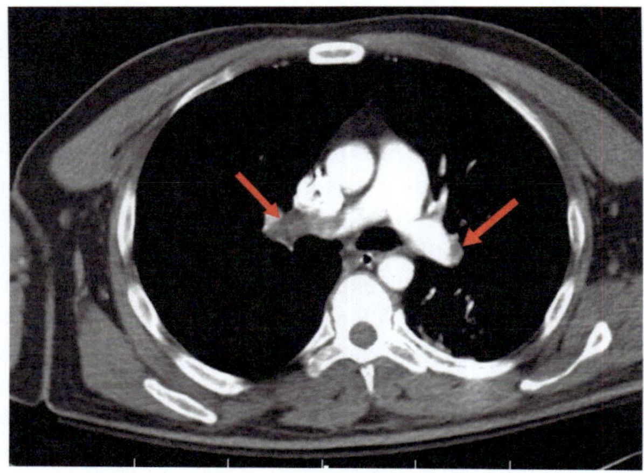

Fig. 8.1 CTPA demonstrating filling defects (pulmonary thromboemboli) in bilateral pulmonary arteries consistent with acute PE. *CTPA* computed tomography pulmonary angiography

patients presented with hemodynamic instability. However, the presence of hemodynamic instability (SBP <90 mmHg) at presentation was associated with a higher mortality at 3 months (58.3%) compared to those who were hemodynamically stable (15.1%). Multiple-regression modeling demonstrated that age over 70 years, cancer, congestive heart failure, chronic obstructive pulmonary disease, systolic arterial hypotension, tachypnea, and right ventricular hypokinesis on echocardiography were significant indicators of poor prognosis [35]. Findings from this registry shaped future studies seeking to identify risk factors for high-risk PE.

8.2.3.1 PE Severity Index Score

The pulmonary embolism severity index (PESI) score is the most validated clinical score for risk stratification of patients presenting with PE (Table 8.4). It was derived from a study of over 15,000 patients at 186 Pennsylvania hospitals to predict 30-day mortality in PE and then validated in a European study of 221 inpatients with PE. Patients who did not meet any PESI criteria were considered low-risk PE and found to have 30-day mortality rates of 1.5% or less [4]. Another study found 90-day mortality using the original score in low-risk patients (classes I–II) to be 1.1% compared with 11.1% in moderate- to very-high-risk patients (risk classes III–V). Ultimately, the score was simplified, and the RIETE validation cohort demonstrated a 1.1% 30-day mortality in the low-risk group versus 8.9% in the high-risk group [45]. Overall, the PESI score has a 99% negative predictive value and is a useful tool to identify patients at low risk of death who may be managed as an outpatient for PE [24].

8.2.3.2 Prognostic Indicators

While anticoagulation is the first-line treatment for hemodynamically stable patients with PE, patients demonstrating poor prognostic indicators may require thrombolytic therapy or surgical or mechanical thrombectomy. Review of prognostic

Table 8.4 Pulmonary Embolism Severity Index Score [10]

Pulmonary Embolism Severity Index Score		
Parameters	**Original**	**Simplified**
Age	Age in years	1 point (if age >80 years)
Altered mental status	+60 points	–
Arterial oxyhemoglobin saturation <90%	+20 points	1 point
Cancer	+30 points	1 point
Chronic heart failure	+10 points	1 point
Chronic pulmonary disease	+10 points	–
Male sex	+10 points	
Pulse rate ≥110 beats/minute	+20 points	1 point
Respiratory rate >30/min	+20 points	–
Systolic BP <100 mm Hg	+30 points	1 point
Temperature <35°C	+20 points	–
Interpretation		
Risk Stratification	**30-day mortality**	
Low risk	Class I: ≤65 points (0%–1.6%) Class II: 66–85 points (1.7%–3.5%)	0 points (1%)
Moderate risk High risk Very high risk	Class III: 86–105 points (3.2%–7.1%) Class IV:106–125 points (4%–11.4%) Class V: >125 points (10%–24.5%)	≥1 point (10.9%)

indicators is especially important for those with intermediate-risk PE since evidence of RV dysfunction or cardiac ischemia portends an increased risk of mortality and may necessitate a higher level of care or additional intervention. Pharmacists should be familiar with poor prognostic indicators.

Transthoracic echocardiography of the RV may detect changes in ventricular function caused by acute pressure overload from PE. Findings consistent with RV dysfunction include right ventricular hypokinesis and dilatation, interventricular septal flattening and paradoxical motion toward the left ventricle, tricuspid regurgitation, pulmonary hypertension, and loss of inspiratory collapse of the inferior vena cava [10]. These findings of acute PE without right ventricular dysfunction on CTPA are shown in Fig. 8.2.

Patients presenting with acute PE and RV/LV diameter ratio of 1 or greater and tricuspid annular plane systolic excursion (TAPSE) less than 16 mm are at increased risk of 30-day PE-related mortality or need for rescue thrombolysis, even if they are initially hemodynamically stable [59, 85]. Similarly, an RV/LV diameter ratio of 0.9 or greater on CTPA is associated with a fivefold increased risk for PE-related mortality or clinical deterioration [8, 70]. Figure 8.3 demonstrates these findings of acute PE causing right ventricular dysfunction on CTPA.

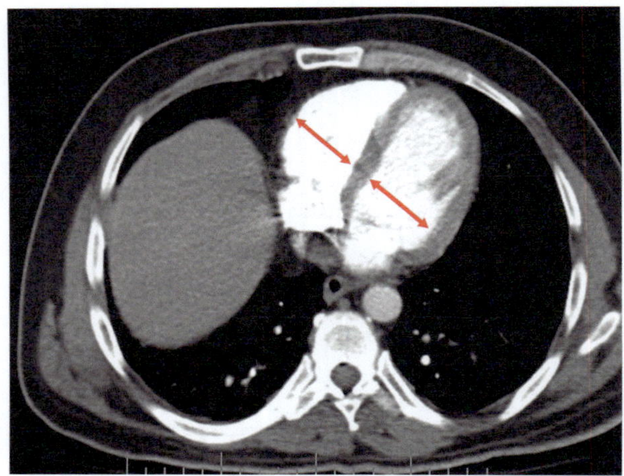

Fig. 8.2 CTPA of acute pulmonary embolism without right ventricular dysfunction. Note: RV/LV diameter ratio <1. *CTPA* computed tomography pulmonary angiography; *RV/LV* right ventricular to left ventricular ratio

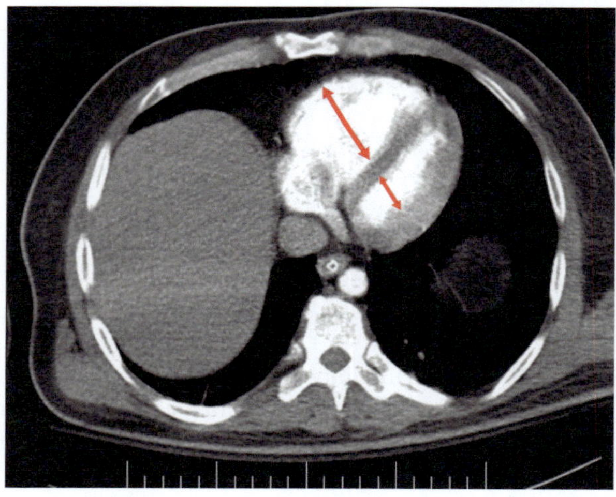

Fig. 8.3 CTPA of acute pulmonary embolism with right ventricular dysfunction. Note: RV/LV diameter ratio >1; Same patient from Fig. 8.2 after presenting with recurrent, high risk PE. *CTPA* computed tomography pulmonary angiography, *RV/LV* right ventricular to left ventricular ratio

Serum B-type natriuretic peptide (BNP) and N-terminal pro-B-type natriuretic peptide (NT-proBNP) are markers of RV dilatation in PE. A meta-analysis of 1132 patients with acute PE demonstrated that BNP or NT-proBNP elevations were associated with nearly sevenfold increases in complicated hospital course or 30-day mortality [55].

High-risk electrocardiographic (ECG) findings may represent RV dysfunction in PE [48]. While the most common ECG changes in acute PE include tachycardia, T-wave inversion in lead V1, and ST elevation in lead aVR, the following findings are predictors of hemodynamic collapse and 30-day mortality: heart rate above 100 beats/minute, $S_1Q_3T_3$ pattern, complete right bundle branch block, inverted T waves in V_1-V_4, ST elevation in aVR, and atrial fibrillation [93].

In the setting of PE, troponin elevations represent myocardial injury due to RV overload and are associated with increased risk for short-term, PE-related mortality, and serious adverse events even in hemodynamically stable patients [6, 10]. Since

Table 8.5 Pulmonary embolism classification based on prognostic indicators [10, 48, 59]

	Hemodynamic instability	**RV dysfunction**	**Myocardial injury**

	Cardiac arrest
	Obstructive shock
	  Systolic BP < 90 mm Hg
	  Vasopressors required to
	  achieve systolic
	  BP ≥ 90 mm Hg with
	  evidence of end-organ
	  hypoperfusion
	Persistent hypotension
	  Systolic BP < 90 mm Hg
	  or a systolic BP drop
	  ≥40 mm Hg for >15 min
	  not from another cause
		RV dilatation
		  Apical four-chamber
		  RV/LV diameter of ≥1
		  on CTPA or TTE.
		  Elevation of
		  BNP > 90 pg/mL or
		  N-terminal prohormone
		  BNP > 500 pg/mL
		ECG findings
		  HR > 100 beats/minute
		  $S_1Q_3T_3$ pattern
		  Complete right bundle
		  branch block
		  Inverted T waves in
		  V_1–V_4
		  ST elevation in aVR
		  Atrial fibrillation
			Troponin T
			  >0.1 ng/mL
			High sensitivity
			troponin T
			  <75 years old:
			  ≥ 14 pg/mL
			  ≥75 years old:
			  ≥ 45 pg/mL
			Tropnin I
			  >0.4 ng/mL

High risk	Present	Present	Present *Comment: Troponin measurement not required if hemo-dynamic instability or RV dysfunction*
Intermediate risk			
High risk features	–	Present	Present
Low risk features	–	≤1 indicator present	
Low risk	–	–	–

BNP brain naturietic peptide, *BP* blood pressure, *CTPA* computed tomography pulmonary angiography, *ECG* electrocardiogram, *HR* heart rate, *LV* left ventricle, *PESI* Pulmonary Embolism Severity Index, *RV* right ventricle, *sPESI* Simplified Pulmonary Embolism Severity Index, *TTE* transthoracic echocardiogram

Adapted with permission from: Konstantinides et al. [59]

[a]Cardiac arrest, obstructive shock (systolic BP <90 mm Hg or vasopressors required to achieve systolic BP ≥90 mm Hg, with end-organ hypoperfusion), or persistent hypotension (systolic BP <90 mm Hg or a systolic BP drop ≥40 mm Hg for >15 min) not from another cause

[b]If hemodynamic instability plus CTPA-confirmed PE and/or evidence of RV dysfunction on TTE are seen, neither PESI calculation nor troponin measurement are additionally required to classify high-risk PE

[c]Signs of RV dysfunction or elevated cardiac biomarker levels may be present, despite a calculated PESI I-II or sPESI of zero. Current guidelines recommend classification into the intermediate-risk category

age and renal function impact levels, age-adjusted cutoffs for high-sensitivity troponin T are useful to identify patients who may benefit from additional monitoring and/or early reperfusion therapy [46].

Evaluation of prognostic indicators in conjunction with PESI scoring forms the basis of PE classification, as outlined in Table 8.5.

8.3 Initial Management per Risk Stratification

8.3.1 Initial Management

Patients with a high or intermediate clinical probability of PE should be initiated on anticoagulation without delay while the workup is in progress [59]. The pharmacist clinician should work with the treatment team to guide initial management, including the choice of anticoagulant as well as supportive care based on the patient's risk stratification (Table 8.6).

8.3.1.1 Low-Risk PE

Patients presenting to the ED with low-risk PE have a lower rate of 30-day mortality, and appropriateness for early discharge should be assessed. Advanced interventions such as reperfusion therapy or surgery are not routinely performed for low-risk

Table 8.6 Treatment considerations based on the severity of PE

PE Classification	Care Site	Anticoagulation	Reperfusion Therapies	Considerations
Low risk	Early discharge for eligible patients	Rapid anticoagulation with an oral AC (e.g., apixaban or rivaroxaban) is preferred over parenteral AC; Certain OAC will require initial treatment with a parenteral AC	Not routinely recommended	Patients with adequate family/ social support and easy access to medication without other reason for hospitalization can be considered for early discharge
Intermediate-low risk	Hospitalize	Oral AC or parenteral AC (LMWH or fondaparinux preferred)	Not routinely recommended	Consider other patient/disease factors when determining oral vs parenteral AC
Intermediate-high risk	Hospitalize with close monitoring	Parenteral AC (consider UFH if concern for hemodynamic decompensation)	Not routinely recommended however may be beneficial in severe cases	Monitor closely for clinical deterioration refractory to standard anticoagulation
High risk	Hospitalize; admit to a critical care unit	Parenteral AC (e.g., UFH)	Consider immediate reperfusion therapies	Provide supportive care (oxygen, hemodynamic optimization, mechanical circulatory support) in addition to reperfusion therapy

AC anticoagulation, *LMWH* low molecular weight heparin, *OAC* oral anticoagulation, *UFH* unfractionated heparin

PE. Home treatment may be appropriate for patients with a low risk of PE-related death, no serious comorbidities or concomitant conditions requiring hospitalization, and no barriers to compliance with outpatient treatment. The pharmacist clinician is poised to provide anticoagulation counseling, address patient questions, and relay signs and symptoms that would warrant re-presentation back to the ED.

For patients appropriate to receive home treatment, rapid anticoagulation with a direct oral anticoagulant (DOAC) is preferred over inpatient treatment with 5 days of a parenteral anticoagulant [59, 99]. Notably, certain oral anticoagulants including dabigatran and edoxaban require initial treatment with a parenteral anticoagulation for a minimum of 5 days prior to transitioning to the oral agent. Vitamin K antagonists (VKAs) such as warfarin require an overlap with a parenteral anticoagulant upon initiation until a therapeutic INR between 2.0 and 3.0 is achieved, typically for a minimum of 5 days. In contrast, apixaban and rivaroxaban can be initiated immediately following the PE diagnosis as the sole agent. Apixaban and rivaroxaban require higher initial doses when initiating upon diagnosis of a PE according to the FDA-approved package insert, for 7 and 21 days, respectively [59, 77, 99]. The choice of oral anticoagulant depends on patient-specific factors such as renal function, affordability, drug-drug interactions, and other comorbidities such as antiphospholipid antibody syndrome. Frequency of dosing (e.g., once daily or twice daily) is an important factor for patients with concern for medication compliance. For a patient who otherwise has no contraindications, the use of a DOAC is preferred over vitamin K antagonists (VKA) [77]. Additional considerations for oral anticoagulants are listed in Table 8.7.

Table 8.8 outlines the initiation and maintenance phases of each oral anticoagulant. Patients not eligible for rapid anticoagulation with apixaban or rivaroxaban will require initial management with a parenteral anticoagulant. Subcutaneous injections of low-molecular-weight heparin (LMWH) or fondaparinux can be administered at home with appropriate patient education. The choice of anticoagulant for specific populations, such as those experiencing pregnancy or cancer, is discussed further in forthcoming sections.

Patient access to medical care and social support must be considered prior to discharge to ensure proper outpatient care and anticoagulant treatment [59]. Patients with a history of poor compliance or those who cannot afford medications are not ideal candidates for early discharge during the acute phase of PE [77].

8.3.1.2 Intermediate-Risk PE

PE is categorized as an intermediate risk if a patient presents with clinical signs of severe PE without evidence of hemodynamic instability such as cardiac arrest or hypotension. Patients are stratified as having intermediate-risk PE if meeting the criteria for PESI class III–V or sPESI ≥ 1 or if there is evidence of RV dysfunction and/or myocardial injury. Patients in the intermediate-risk category are not candidates for early discharge home treatment, and hospitalization for close monitoring is recommended. The initial management of intermediate-risk PE also includes

Table 8.7 Considerations and characteristics of oral AC

Medication	Requires initial parenteral AC	Can initiate immediately on diagnosis	Maintenance Dose Frequency per Day	Routine Dose Monitoring	Major Drug Interactions	Use in Renal Dysfunction (ESRD, CrCl <30 ml/min)
Factor Xa Inhibitors						
Apixaban		✓	Twice		CYP3A4	✓
Rivaroxaban		✓	Once		CYP3A4	
Edoxaban	✓		Once		P-glycoprotein	✓[*]
Direct Thrombin Inhibitor						
Dabigatran	✓		Twice		P-glycoprotein	
Vitamin K Antagonist						
Warfarin	✓	✓	Once	✓	Multiple CYP450 and dietary interactions	✓

[*]Edoxaban may not be ideal for VTE treatment in patients with CrCl >95 ml/min

Table 8.8 Initiation and maintenance dosing of oral anticoagulants for the treatment of PE

Medication	Initiation phase	Maintenance phase
Apixaban	10 mg twice daily for 7 days upon diagnosis of PE	5 mg twice daily
Rivaroxaban	15 mg twice daily for 21 days upon diagnosis of PE	20 mg once daily with meals
Edoxaban	Requires 5–10 days of parenteral anticoagulation prior to initiation	60 mg once daily
Dabigatran	Requires 5–10 days of parenteral anticoagulation prior to initiation	150 mg twice daily
Warfarin	Requires overlap with a parenteral anticoagulation upon initiation until therapeutic INR is achieved (typically for 5 days)	Patient-specific dose to maintain INR between 2 and 3

anticoagulation without delay while the workup is in progress. However, pharmacist clinicians should work with the care team to anticipate the risk for decompensation or need for intervention as this will impact the choice of initial anticoagulation.

Patients with intermediate-risk PE can be further categorized as intermediate-low risk if they do not have both RV dysfunction and myocardial injury. They may be treated with either a parenteral anticoagulant or a rapid-acting oral anticoagulant similar to the management of low-risk PE. If a parenteral agent is chosen, LMWH or fondaparinux is recommended over the use of unfractionated heparin (UFH). LMWH and fondaparinux can be given subcutaneously, whereas UFH is administered as a continuous intravenous infusion. UFH requires close monitoring of anti-Xa activity to ensure therapeutic levels and carry a higher risk of bleeding and heparin-induced thrombocytopenia [59, 77, 99]. However, individual patient factors and pharmacokinetics of each agent should be considered when choosing a parenteral anticoagulant. For example, UFH may be preferred in patients with renal dysfunction or in certain situations where a shorter acting, quickly reversible agent is optimal.

PE is classified as an intermediate-high risk if both RV dysfunction and myocardial injury are present. Patients with intermediate-high risk are at a higher risk of progressive hemodynamic decompensation. Even though routine thrombolytic use is not recommended to all patients in this category, reperfusion therapies may be beneficial, particularly in the setting of elevated lactate ≥ 2 mmol/L, elevated BNP, elevated shock index (HR/SBP) >1, or concomitant DVT [39]. In patients who are likely to receive systemic thrombolysis, it may be prudent to administer intravenous UFH infusion given its shorter half-life compared to subcutaneous injections. UFH should target factor Xa inhibition of 0.3–0.7 units/mL [72]. Additionally, subcutaneous anticoagulants such as LMWH or fondaparinux may not have reliable absorption in the setting of hypoperfusion [48, 59, 77]. The route, dose, and additional considerations for each parenteral anticoagulant are described in Table 8.9.

Table 8.9 Parenteral anticoagulants for the treatment of PE in adults [20, 32, 114]

Medication	Route	Dose	Dosing Weight Considerations	Dose Adjustment	Consideration
Unfractionated and low molecular weight heparins					
UFH	IV	80 units/kg IV bolus followed by 18 units/kg/h infusion	Use actual body weight; consider lower doses in patients with obesity	Titrate to therapeutic aPTT (1.5–2.5 times control) or anti-factor Xa (0.3–0.7 units/mL) according to institutional protocol	Preferred in patients with hemodynamic instability or renal dysfunction; monitor for heparin resistance or heparin-induced thrombocytopenia
Dalteparin	SC	200 units/kg every 24 h 100 units/kg twice daily	Use actual body weight to a maximum of 190 kg	Routine monitoring of anti-factor Xa is not performed however may be considered in patients with high risk of bleeding or ≥150 kg	Not recommended in patients on dialysis or CrCl <30 mL/min
Enoxaparin	SC	1 mg/kg twice daily 1.5 mg/kg every 24 h CrCl <30 mL/min: 1 mg/kg every 24 h	Use actual body weight; consider lower doses in patients with obesity*	Routine monitoring of anti-factor Xa is not performed however may be considered in patients with high risk of bleeding or ≥150 kg	Not recommended in patients on dialysis
Tinzaparin	SC	175 anti-Xa units/kg every 24 h	Use actual body weight; a fixed upper dose limit is not recommended	Routine monitoring of anti-factor Xa is not performed however may be considered in patients with high risk of bleeding, CrCl 20–<30 mL/min, or obesity	Not recommended in patients on dialysis or CrCl <20 mL/min
Factor Xa inhibitor (indirect thrombin inhibitor)					
Fondaparinux	SC	<50 kg: 5 mg every 24 h 50–100 kg: 7.5 mg every 24 h >100 kg: 10 mg every 24 h	Limited data available in patients with BMI >45 kg/m² or >150 kg	Routine monitoring of anti-factor Xa is not performed	Not recommended in patients on dialysis or CrCl <30 mL/min

(continued)

Table 8.9 (continued)

Medication	Route	Dose	Dosing Weight Considerations	Dose Adjustment	Consideration
Direct thrombin inhibitors					
Argatroban	IV	2 mcg/kg/min 0.25–1.5 mcg/kg/min if critically ill, hepatic dysfunction, or heart failure	Use actual body weight	Titrate to therapeutic aPTT (1.5–3 times control) according to institutional protocol	Commonly reserved for patients with heparin-induced thrombocytopenia or heparin resistance
Bivalirudin	IV	0.15–0.2 mg/kg/h or CrCl <60 mL/min: 0.04–0.08 mg/kg/h	Use actual body weight	Titrate to therapeutic aPTT (1.5–2.5 times control) according to institutional protocol	Commonly reserved for patients with heparin-induced thrombocytopenia or heparin resistance

*Additional dosing considerations are described in Table 8.10

aPTT activated partial thromboplastin time, *CrCl* creatinine clearance, *HIT* heparin-induced thrombocytopenia, *IV* intravenous, *PE* pulmonary embolism, *SC* subcutaneous, *UFH* unfractionated heparin

8.3.2 High-Risk PE

High-risk PE is classically defined with the presence of hemodynamic instability or cardiac arrest. Patients can present with persistent hypotension (systolic BP <90 mmHg or drop ≥40 mmHg lasting longer than 15 min) or obstructive shock requiring vasopressor support despite adequate filling status and end-organ hypoperfusion [59]. It is important to distinguish the cause of hemodynamic instability in PE since other critical illnesses can present similarly, such as new-onset arrhythmia, hypovolemia, or sepsis. Patients with high-risk PE will require immediate interventions, such as hemodynamic support or reperfusion therapy, in addition to anticoagulation. Given the patient's critical illness and the potential for additional interventions, a parenteral anticoagulant with a quick onset and offset of action is preferred. UFH is typically the agent of choice in patients without contraindications to heparinoids, with the same factor Xa inhibition targets regardless of whether thrombolysis is administered [72]. There are studies that have utilized LMWH safely in the setting of thrombolysis [54, 92]. However, it may be prudent to consider the patient's increased risk of bleeding as well as the need for quick reversal pending invasive procedures, especially with the advent of advanced endovascular therapies for PE.

The emergent use of thrombolytics and/or interventional procedures is described in the forthcoming sections.

Supportive care is crucial for patients with high-risk PE who present with hypoxemia, shock, or acute RV failure. Supplemental oxygen should be administered to patients with $SaO_2 < 90\%$. In patients who are refractory to conventional oxygen supplementation, high-flow oxygen or mechanical ventilation (invasive or noninvasive) may be considered. Intubation should be proceeded with caution, as RV dysfunction predisposes patients to severe decompensation with anesthesia and positive-pressure ventilation [59]. Optimal induction agents should minimize the incidence of hypotension. When providing mechanical ventilation, the 2019 ESC guidelines recommend 6 mL/kg of tidal volume and end-inspiratory plateau pressure <30 cm H_2O [59].

In patients with acute RV failure associated with PE, CO and volume status should be closely monitored. Cautious use of intravenous crystalloids administered at low volumes $\leq$500 mL can help identify patients with low CO that are preload dependent. Patients with a normal or low central venous pressure (CVP) may particularly benefit from volume optimization. However, aggressive volume administration may have a paradoxical effect of decreasing CO by over-distending the RV. Vasoactive medications such as norepinephrine or dobutamine are often utilized to support reduced perfusion. Norepinephrine, a mixed alpha/beta$_1$-adrenergic receptor agonist, increases systemic blood pressure but may lead to worsened tissue perfusion due to excessive vasoconstriction. An inotropic agent such as dobutamine can increase CO but may worsen hypotension requiring additional vasopressor support [59]. Vasodilator therapy may decrease PAP and PVR; however, it also decreases systemic blood pressure when given intravenously. The efficacy of inhaled vasodilators such as nitric oxide or prostacyclins is limited in the context of RV dysfunction from acute PE.

At centers that provide mechanical circulatory support (MCS), the temporary use of venoarterial extracorporeal membrane oxygenation (VA-ECMO) may be helpful in stabilizing a patient with high-risk PE. However, ECMO may predispose the patient to additional harm, including increased risk for bleeding or infection. Patient outcomes vary depending on the clinician expertise and experience. In patients with cardiac arrest associated with acute PE, advanced life support guidelines are followed, with an early consideration for thrombolytic therapy [59].

8.3.3 Definitive Anticoagulation Duration

The duration of anticoagulation post-PE depends on patient-specific factors, provoking events, and risk of recurrence (Table 8.10). All patients with PE should be treated with anticoagulation for a minimum of 3 months, with an option to extend to 6 months. In certain cases, indefinite anticoagulation may be warranted. The decision for anticoagulation duration will require a careful assessment of risk factors. Patients who have an identifiable, major transient risk factor that is reversible have a lower risk of VTE recurrence and can discontinue therapy after 3 months. On the other hand, patients without any identifiable risk factors, or patients with active cancer, recurrent VTE, or antiphospholipid antibody syndrome, may warrant lifelong anticoagulation [59]. In patients who are eligible for extended anticoagulation without cancer receiving DOACs, a reduced dose of apixaban or rivaroxaban can be considered after the first 6 months of therapy.

Table 8.10 Duration of definitive anticoagulation [25]

Persistent risk factor	Prior VTE	Presence of Transient/ Reversible Risk factor	Duration of anticoagulation
No identified persistent risk factor	First episode of PE	Major risk factor present	Discontinue after 3 months
		Minor risk factor present	Consider indefinite beyond 3 months
		No identifiable risk factor present	Consider indefinite beyond 3 months
	Recurrent PE	No major risk factor present	Recommend indefinite beyond 3 months
Cancer	–	–	Recommend indefinite or until cancer is cured
Antiphospholipid antibody syndrome	–	–	Recommend indefinite beyond 3 months
Other persistent risk factor	–	–	Consider indefinite beyond 3 months

8.4   Systemic Thrombolytic Therapy

Due to the risk of bleeding with systemic thrombolytic therapy, it should be reserved for use in patients with PE that present with high-risk features, including hypotension (e.g., SBP <90 mmHg or a drop of 40 mm Hg or more for more than 15 minutes), bradycardia, or pulselessness [59, 77, 99]. It may be considered for those with intermediate PE whose clinical course suggests imminent progression to hemodynamic decompensation after starting anticoagulation provided that the risk for bleeding remains low.

8.4.1   Evidence for Systemic Thrombolysis in PE

8.4.1.1   High-Risk PE

Thrombolysis in high-risk PE is based on low-level evidence evaluating the use of alteplase, streptokinase, urokinase, reteplase, and desmoteplase in this population [59, 77, 99].

The only prospective study of thrombolytics in high-risk PE randomized eight patients with PE-associated cardiogenic shock to receive 1,500,000 IU streptokinase IV over 1 hour and heparin 10,000 units IV bolus followed by infusion or heparin alone. The trial was stopped early after all four patients in the heparin-only group died within 3 hours of randomization compared to zero in the thrombolytic/heparin group, $p = 0.02$ [44]. Although there were significant limitations with this study, including small sample size and difference in time from PE onset to randomization (2.5 hours in the streptokinase plus heparin group versus 34.75 hours in the heparin-only group), time to onset of shock was similar between groups. Ultimately, right ventricular myocardial infarction and massive PE were identified on autopsy in the heparin-only group, suggesting that the prompt administration of thrombolytic therapy was responsible for improving outcomes in the thrombolytic/heparin group [44].

Thereafter, studies describing outcomes of patients who received thrombolysis in high-risk PE are largely registry based. In ICOPER, 4.2% of patients with confirmed PE presented with hemodynamic instability, and 13% were treated with thrombolysis. The adjusted mortality rate in hemodynamically unstable patients was 58.3%. Major bleeding occurred in 10.5% of the cohort and was noted to be more common in patients that received thrombolytic therapy [35]. RIETE was an international, multicenter, prospective registry study of 15,520 patients with acute VTE that found that patients with acute, symptomatic, high-risk PE had an OR 16.3 (95% CI, 8.50–31.4) of developing a fatal PE [63]. Out of the overall cohort, 1.2% received thrombolytic therapy, but no bleeding outcomes were described [63].

The EMPEROR study was a prospective, multicenter, observational registry describing the diagnosis, treatment, and outcomes of patients presenting to the ED with acute PE [84]. PE was confirmed in 1880 patients, with 33 receiving alteplase ($n = 29$) or tenecteplase ($n = 4$) in the ED and 12 receiving alteplase after hospital admission. Among the patients receiving thrombolytics in the ED, only 9.1% met the definition of high-risk PE (e.g., hypotension on presentation). Of the 20 patients with confirmed PE that died, 12 presented with at least one high-risk feature (e.g., SBP <90 mmHg, elevated troponin, or RV hypokinesis), but only 3 patients received thrombolytics. In patients that received thrombolysis, no deaths were attributable to bleeding complications [84].

Due to the increased risk of death seen when thrombolytics are withheld or delayed in high-risk PE, it would be unethical to perform a future randomized, controlled trial comparing modern thrombolytic therapies (e.g., alteplase or tenecteplase) with anticoagulation to anticoagulation alone. Therefore, outcomes following the administration of these thrombolytics in patients with high-risk PE are described in case reports and cohort studies only [13, 94].

Despite the low-quality evidence, guidelines recommend the use of fibrin-specific, second- and third-generation thrombolytics (alteplase and tenecteplase, respectively) over first-generation, non-fibrin-specific thrombolytics (streptokinase and urokinase) due to their more favorable administration and pharmacokinetic profiles [59, 77, 99]. Table 8.11 describes the dosing and pharmacokinetic considerations of thrombolytic therapy for PE.

8.4.1.2 Intermediate-Risk PE

Routine use of reperfusion therapy with systemic thrombolytics is not recommended in all intermediate-risk PE because of the high risk for bleeding complications. However, select patients with intermediate-risk PE may benefit provided that the risk for bleeding complications does not outweigh the potential benefits gained from thrombolysis.

Table 8.11 Dosing and pharmacokinetic considerations of thrombolytic therapy for PE

Thrombolytic	Dosing studied in PE			Half-life
	High risk	Intermediate risk	Cardiac arrest	
Alteplase	100 mg IV infusion over 2 h*	100 mg IV over 2 h* 50 mg IV over 2 h* 0.5 mg/kg (patients less than 50 kg) over 2 h 0.6 mg/kg over 2 h	50 mg IV push over 1 min (may repeat after 15 min of CPR) 50 mg IV infusion over 15 min (continue CPR for 15 min)	5 min

Tenecteplase	–	Weight-based IV push.
		  <60 kg: 30 mg
		  ≥60–<70 kg: 35 mg
		  ≥70–<80 kg: 40 mg
		  ≥80–<90 kg: 45 mg
		  ≥90 kg: 50 mg
			Weight-based IV push.
			  <60 kg: 30 mg
			  ≥60–<70 kg: 35 mg
			  ≥70–<80 kg: 40 mg
			  ≥80–<90 kg: 45 mg
			  ≥90 kg: 50 mg
				Initial: 20–24 min
				Terminal: 90–130 min

Streptokinase	250,000 units IV loading dose infused over 15–30 min then 100,000 units/h for 12–24 h	1.5 million units IV infusion over 2 h 250,000 units IV loading dose infused over 15–30 min then 100,000 units/h for 12–24 h	–	18 min

*May opt to administer alteplase 100 mg dose as 10 mg IV bolus followed by 90 mg over 2 h; 50 mg dose as 10 mg IV bolus followed by 40 mg over 2 h

The pharmacist clinician can assist in identifying patients with intermediate-high-risk PE who are at imminent risk of developing hemodynamic collapse, where systemic thrombolytic therapy may be considered:

- Presence of RV dysfunction
- Troponin elevations
- sPESI ≥1
- Lactate of ≥2 mmol/L
- Confirmed concomitant DVT
- BNP elevations
- Shock index (heart rate/systolic BP) >1 [39, 59, 77, 99]

Much controversy exists surrounding the choice of systemic thrombolytic therapy, dosing strategy, and timing of administration in intermediate-risk PE. Select, pivotal studies evaluating thrombolytic therapy in intermediate-risk PE are reviewed herein.

The largest prospective study evaluating alteplase for intermediate-risk PE randomized 256 patients with RVD on echocardiogram or RV strain on ECG to alteplase 100 mg versus placebo in addition to heparin [56]. Significantly more patients met the composite endpoint of in-hospital mortality or need for treatment escalation in the placebo versus alteplase groups (24.6% versus 11%, $p = 0.006$), which was driven by the need for treatment of hypotension, use of rescue thrombolysis, intubation, CPR, surgical embolectomy, or catheter-based intervention. Mortality was not statistically significant between the alteplase and placebo groups (3.4% versus 2.2%, $p = 0.71$), and there were no differences in major or fatal bleeding [56].

MOPETT was a prospective, open-label study evaluating a "safe dose" of alteplase in PE. One hundred twenty-one patients with symptomatic PE in ≥ 2 lobes were randomized to either alteplase 50 mg (patients <50 kg received 0.5 mg/kg) with anticoagulation or anticoagulation alone. Alteplase significantly reduced the incidence of pulmonary hypertension or recurrent PE at 28 months (16% versus 63%, $p < 0.001$), and no bleeding events occurred in either group [92]. Notably, the incidence of pulmonary hypertension was higher compared to prior literature, and nearly 80% of patients in the alteplase group received enoxaparin 1 mg/kg (maximum 80 mg) every 12 hours, which differs from other thrombolytic studies utilizing heparin as the main anticoagulant. Importantly, RVD was not a requirement for inclusion potentially indicating a less critically ill patient population than in the previous Konstantinides study [56].

Due to the lack of clear evidence to support one alteplase dosing strategy over another for PE, there is widespread use of either 50 mg ("half-dose") or 100 mg ("full-dose") depending on clinician assessment of an individual's risk for decompensation versus benefit. A retrospective cohort study including data from 3768 patients across 420 hospitals in the Premier Healthcare Database compared outcomes in patients receiving 50 mg versus 100 mg alteplase for PE. There was no difference in hospital mortality (13% versus 15%, $p = 0.3$), cerebral hemorrhage (0.5% versus 0.4%, $p = 0.67$), gastrointestinal bleeding (1.6% versus 1.6%, $p = 0.99$), acute blood loss anemia (6.9% versus 4.6%, $p = 0.11$), or documented fibrinolytic adverse events (2.6% versus 2.8%, $p = 0.82$) with half-dose versus full-dose alteplase [53]. However, patients receiving half-dose alteplase represented a less critically ill population as they were less likely to require vasopressor therapy (23.3% versus 39.4%, $p < 0.01$) and invasive ventilation (14.3% vs. 28.5%, $p < 0.01$) at baseline compared to patients receiving full-dose, which is likely a result of clinician selection bias. A propensity-matched analysis found that half-dose alteplase was associated with increased treatment escalation (53.8% versus 41.4%, $p < 0.01$) due to the need for secondary thrombolysis (25.9% versus 7.3%, $p < 0.01$) and catheter thrombus fragmentation (14.2% vs. 3.8%, $p < 0.01$), as well as a higher median cost of care ($103,843 versus $76,495 $p < 0.01$) [53].

PEITHO is the largest study of thrombolytic therapy in intermediate-risk PE. This international, multicenter, double-blinded trial randomized 1006 patients with PE complicated by RVD and elevated troponin (intermediate-high risk based on current PE classification) to either weight-based tenecteplase or placebo in combination with heparin. Tenecteplase was associated with a significant reduction in death or hemodynamic compromise at day 7 (OR 0.44; 95% CI, 0.23–0.87; $p = 0.02$). However, hemodynamics drove the difference in the primary outcome as there was no difference in death within 7 and 30 days. Unfortunately, compared to placebo, tenecteplase increased major extracranial bleeding at 7 days (OR 5.55; 95% CI, 2.3–13.39; $p < 0.001$) and stroke (OR 12.10; 95% CI, 1.57–93.39; $p = 0.003$), with ten hemorrhagic strokes occurring in the tenecteplase group compared to one in the placebo group [72]. Additionally, no difference in long-term survival, dyspnea, functional limitation, residual pulmonary hypertension, RVD, or CTEPH was seen in a 24-month outcome follow-up in 709 of the original patients in the PEITHO study [58]. These findings suggest that the benefit of systemic thrombolysis in patients with intermediate-high-risk PE may be countered by the increased risk of major bleeding. At this time, it is unknown whether alternative, lower dose tenecteplase strategies may have a more favorable risk-benefit ratio in intermediate-risk PE, similar to recent ischemic stroke literature.

Systemic thrombolytics should be reserved for patients with intermediate-high-risk PE at imminent risk for progression to hemodynamic collapse. The pharmacist clinician must be familiar with the nuances, strengths, and limitations of guideline recommendations and primary literature surrounding thrombolytic dosing in PE and be prepared to collaborate with the critical care team to develop individualized care plans.

8.4.1.3 Cardiac Arrest

It is estimated that 2–10% of cardiac arrests are attributable to suspected or confirmed PE [29]. Use of thrombolytic therapy in conjunction with standard ACLS resuscitation pathways has been proposed to resolve both coronary and pulmonary thromboses. Current cardiopulmonary resuscitation guidelines recommend adjunctive thrombolytic therapy, surgical embolectomy, and mechanical embolectomy as emergency treatment options when PE is the confirmed cause of cardiac arrest and suggest thrombolysis be considered when PE is the suspected cause of cardiac arrest [78].

A double-blind, prospective study randomized 233 patients to receive either alteplase 100 mg IV over 15 minutes or placebo if unresponsive to one minute of standard ACLS therapy for out-of-hospital cardiac arrest (OHCA) with pulseless electrical activity [1]. No significant difference was seen in survival to hospital discharge in the alteplase (0.9%) versus placebo (0%) groups ($p = 0.99$) or in any secondary endpoint including the return of spontaneous circulation (ROSC), hospital LOS, hemorrhage, or neurologic outcomes [1]. The low rate of survival in either group as well as the low number of patients with confirmed PE may have contributed to the inability to show a difference between interventions.

Another double-blind, multicenter trial done in Europe randomized 1050 patients with witnessed OHCA to either weight-based tenecteplase or placebo as an adjunct to prehospital CPR, but was ultimately terminated early due to interim analysis showing no difference in survival, ROSC, hospital admission, 24-hour survival, survival to hospital discharge, or neurologic outcome. The rate of intracranial hemorrhage was significantly higher in patients who received tenecteplase versus placebo (RR 6.95; 95% CI, 1.59–30.41; p = 0.006), highlighting safety concerns with the administration of thrombolytics to all-comers with cardiac arrest [11].

However, benefit from thrombolytics may be seen in patients with confirmed PE. A retrospective, observational, multicenter study of 14,253 adult patients with OHCA reported outcomes among a total of 246 patients with confirmed PE. Fifty-eight patients were given thrombolytics as part of the resuscitative effort, with the majority receiving tenecteplase (74%) followed by alteplase (24%). Thirty-day survival was higher in the thrombolysis group (16%) versus control (6%), p = 0.005, but no significant difference in good neurologic recovery was seen (adjusted RR 1.97; 95% CI, 0.70–5.56) [43]. A recent systematic review and meta-analysis of thrombolytic therapy in cardiac arrest from presumed or confirmed PE included 803 patients from 13 studies and found that IV thrombolysis was associated with higher rates of ROSC (OR 2.55, 95% CI, 1.50–4.34), but no significant difference in survival to hospital discharge (OR 1.41, 95% CI, 0.79–2.41) or bleeding complications (OR 2.21, 95% CI, 0.95–5.17) [29]. Notably, there was significant heterogeneity among thrombolytic agent choice and dosing.

Based on these findings, it is reasonable to attempt thrombolysis in conjunction with standard resuscitative measures for cardiac arrest if there is confirmation of or high suspicion of PE.

8.4.1.4 Contraindications to Thrombolytic Therapy

Most contraindications to thrombolytic therapy that are traditionally utilized in acute ischemic stroke should be considered relative in the setting of life-threatening, high-risk PE as early thrombolytic intervention has been shown to improve in-hospital mortality for hemodynamically unstable patients or those requiring mechanical ventilation [59, 97]. The pharmacist clinician should be familiar with the contraindication and relative contraindication stratification based on PE severity, which are described in Table 8.12.

8.4.2 Timing of Anticoagulation in Relation to Thrombolysis

In high-risk PE, it is important to initiate anticoagulation immediately while creating a plan for either systemic thrombolysis or alternative reperfusion therapies. Historically, there has been discordance among major guidelines as to whether heparin should be held during thrombolytic infusion administration. The 2008 CHEST guidelines suggest that it is acceptable to either continue or suspend UFH infusion during thrombolytic administration as these two practices have never been

Table 8.12 Contraindications to thrombolytic therapy

	Contraindications	Relative Contraindications
High-risk PE	Active internal bleeding. Recent intracranial hemorrhage.	Structural intracranial disease. Previous intracranial hemorrhage. Ischemic stroke within 3 months. Recent brain or spinal surgery. Recent head trauma with fracture or brain injury. Bleeding diathesis. Pregnancy.
Intermediate-risk PE	Structural intracranial disease. Previous intracranial hemorrhage. Ischemic stroke within 3 months. Active internal bleeding. Recent brain or spinal surgery. Recent head trauma with fracture or brain injury. Bleeding diathesis.	SBP >180 mm Hg. DBP >110 mm Hg. Recent bleeding (non-intracranial). Recent surgery. Recent invasive procedure. Ischemic stroke >3 months ago. Anticoagulated. Traumatic cardiopulmonary resuscitation. Pericarditis, pericardial fluid. Diabetic retinopathy. Pregnancy. Age >75 years or low body weight <65 kg. Female. Black race.

DBP diastolic blood pressure, *PE* pulmonary embolism, *SBP* systolic blood pressure
Reprinted from Ref. [39]

compared. They cite that US regulatory bodies recommend suspension of IV UFH during the 2-h alteplase 100 mg infusion, but other countries may continue with IV UFH while alteplase is infusing [47]. The 2014 ESC guidelines recommend that IV UFH should be stopped during administration of streptokinase or urokinase, but may be continued during alteplase infusion [57]. In cases when systemic thrombolysis is being administered, it is reasonable to continue IV UFH up until the initiation of alteplase infusion and discontinue while alteplase is infusing to reduce the risk of bleeding events. After the 2-h alteplase infusion is complete, an activated partial thromboplastin time (aPTT) should be assessed immediately, and UFH should only be resumed once the aPTT is less than two times the patient's baseline (or 80 seconds or less) [48]. A small study in healthy volunteers showed that aPTT may be prolonged following alteplase administration [103]. Clinical judgment should be used when determining the optimal time to restart IV UFH infusion, especially for patients who had short durations or no exposure to IV UFH prior to thrombolytic infusion. There is a paucity of evidence to guide an appropriate strategy for restarting heparin infusion based on anti-Xa monitoring, but it would be reasonable to wait for the anti-Xa level to drop to 0.7 units/mL or less before resuming heparin.

8.5 Alternative Reperfusion Therapies (Surgical Embolectomy, Endovascular Therapies)

8.5.1 Indications for Interventional Therapies

There are numerous interventional therapies performed for the management of PE, including catheter-directed clot fragmentation or aspiration, mechanical embolectomy, local thrombolysis, and a combination of pharmaco-mechanical approaches [86]. These techniques allow the restoration of pulmonary blood flow by relieving the obstruction which improves RV function. Even partial recanalization of the pulmonary arteries can improve hemodynamic stability, and complete removal of the thrombus is not always necessary.

There is a lack of high-quality controlled clinical trials that compare the efficacy and safety of these various techniques. Therefore, catheter-directed therapies are not currently considered first-line. According to the 2019 ESC guidelines, CDT can be considered for two categories of PE: high risk and intermediate-high risk. CDT can be considered for patients with high-risk PE if they have contraindications to or failure of systemic thrombolysis. Additionally, patients with intermediate-high-risk PE that experience treatment failure with anticoagulation or have contraindications to or failure of systemic thrombolysis should also be considered for CDT [59]. The 2021 CHEST guideline recommends the consideration of interventional therapies for high-risk PE patients with shock, high risk of bleeding, or failure of systemic thrombolysis [99].

Treatment failure in the setting of PE management is not clearly defined or agreed upon but generally describes a lack of improvement or further hemodynamic deterioration. Lack of hemodynamic improvement is assessed 2–4 hours after the completion of systemic thrombolysis, immediately after the completion of local thrombolytic infusion, or 24–48 hours after therapeutic anticoagulation. Patients with a lack of improvement or progressively worsening hemodynamics should be considered for rescue reperfusion therapy in discussion with members of the PE response team (PERT). Patients who develop life-threatening cardiorespiratory instability (requiring CPR, mechanical ventilation, catecholamine administration, or ECMO) should be evaluated emergently for treatment escalation [86].

8.5.2 Percutaneous Mechanical Interventions

Numerous techniques have been used for mechanical disruption or aspiration of thrombus to treat PE without the use of pharmacologic thrombolysis (Table 8.13). Despite the lack of comparative efficacy data, these devices offer an alternative treatment option for patients with contraindications to thrombolytic therapy [25]. Wire disruption, balloon fragmentation, and rotating pigtail catheters have been

Table 8.13 Available endovascular devices for percutaneous interventions for PE

Endovascular Devices	Catheter-directed thrombolysis	Aspiration Thrombectomy	Mechanical Fragmentation	Rheolytic Thrombectomy
AngioJet (Boston Scientific)	✓	✓		✓
Angiovac cannula (AngioDynamics)		✓		
Aspirex catheter (Straub Medical LLC)		✓	✓	
BASHIR endovascular catheter (Thrombolex)	✓	✓	✓	
Cragg-McNamara catheters (Medtronic)	✓			
EkoSonic endovascular system (EKOS Corp.)	✓ (USAT)			
FlowTriever (Inari Medical)		✓	✓	
Fountain infusion system (Merit Medical)	✓			
Indigo System (Penumbra)		✓	✓	
Uni-Fuse (AngioDynamics)	✓			

USAT ultrasound-assisted catheter-directed thrombolysis

used to fragment proximal PE into smaller pieces, which more readily undergo endogenous thrombolysis. However, clot fragmentation can increase the risk of distal embolization and vascular wall injury [86].

8.5.2.1 Mechanical, Aspiration, and Rheolytic Thrombectomy

Thrombus extraction can be performed by applying suction through large-bore catheters and aspirating. The Indigo mechanical thrombectomy system (Penumbra) is an example of an aspiration device with mechanical fragmentation and a continuous vacuum pump. In the prospective, single-arm, multicenter EXTRACT-PE study of patients with symptomatic acute PE with baseline RV/LV ratio greater than 0.9, the use of the Indigo system reduced the mean RV/LV ratio at 48 hours (mean reduction 0.43; $p < 0.0001$) [95]. The FlowTriever System (Inari) is another aspiration technology used with or without mechanical fragmentation. It uses self-expanding mesh disks that disrupt, entrap, and retract the clot for extraction. In the prospective FLARE study including patients with acute intermediate-risk PE, the FlowTriever System significantly also improved the RV/LV ratio at 48 hours (mean reduction

0.38; $p < 0.0001$) with minimal major bleeding [105]. Although other devices such as the Amplatz thrombectomy device (ev3 Inc) and the Greenfield device (Boston Scientific) have been used in the past, they are seldom used due to their bulkiness and rigidity [25].

Rheolytic thrombectomy is performed using a high-pressure saline jet which creates a pressure gradient and disrupts the thrombus, allowing for its aspiration. It can also spray a thrombolytic agent directly into the clot. The AngioJet PE (Boston Scientific) has a black box warning due to reports of asystole, bradycardia, and hemodynamic decompensation, possibly due to the releases of bradykinin, adenosine, or potassium during rheolytic thrombectomy [25].

8.5.2.2 Catheter-Directed Thrombolysis

Catheter-directed thrombolysis (CDT) delivers a low dose of a thrombolytic agent directly into the pulmonary artery or into the thrombus. Typically, alteplase is infused as a continuous infusion of 0.5–1.0 mg/h for up to 24 hours, resulting in the patient receiving about one-third of the systemic thrombolysis dose. Given the local delivery and the reduced dose, CDT may cause less life-threatening bleeds such as ICH or gastrointestinal bleeding, while increasing efficacy by achieving higher concentrations at the site of the thrombus [25]. Uni-Fuse (AngioDynamics), Cragg-McNamara (Medtronic), and Fountain infusion system (Merit Medical) are examples of CDT.

CDT can also be performed via ultrasound-accelerated catheters equipped with ultrasound transducers. The transducer emits pulsed high-frequency ultrasound waves which dissociate fibrin strands of the thrombus to enhance the penetration of fibrinolytic drugs. The use of EkoSonic Endovascular System (EKOS) was evaluated in numerous studies including ULTIMA, SEATTLE II, and OPTALYSE PE. All three studies demonstrated a reduction in the RV/LV ratio [60, 82, 102]. The variances in thrombolytic dosing and duration, as well as concomitant anticoagulation, are described in Table 8.14.

Despite the preference of many centers to utilize USAT over standard CDT, no high-quality study supports its superior efficacy. The SUNSET PE trial compared USAT using the EKOS catheter to standard non-ultrasound-assisted CDT. In this randomized, multicenter, single-blind study, there was no significant difference in the thrombus load reduction by the mean PA raw thrombus score reduction (9 ± 6 vs. 10 ± 6, respectively; $p = 0.76$) [5]. Although the use of CDT, particularly USAT, has been adopted widely, no controlled studies exist comparing CDT to systemic thrombolysis in PE.

During a catheter-directed therapy procedure, parenteral anticoagulation should be continued unless contraindicated, typically with UFH. There is no strong consensus on the dose or target anticoagulation intensity during these procedures, including during local thrombolysis. Patients may be switched to an oral anticoagulant or an alternative parenteral agent (such as LMWH) if they remain hemodynamically stable after the removal of the catheter [86].

Table 8.14 Summary of studies evaluating the use of EkoSonic Endovascular System [25]

Study, year	Study design	Study arm	rtPA dose	UFH dose	Conclusion
ULTIMA 2013	Multicenter RCT of patients with acute intermediate-risk PE and RV/LV ratio ≥1	Systemic UFH with USAT vs systemic UFH alone	10–20 mg over 15 h	Therapeutic target aPTT corresponding to anti-factor Xa 0.3–0.7 units/mL	Mean decrease in RV/LV ratio from baseline to 24 h: 0.3 with USAT vs 0.03 with systemic UFH alone ($p < 0.001$)
SEATTLE II 2015	Prospective, multicenter, single-arm study of patients with massive or submassive PE and RV/LV ratio ≥0.9	Systemic UFH with USAT	1 mg/h for 24 h with a unilateral catheter or 1 mg/h/catheter for 12 h with bilateral catheters	Therapeutic aPTT (60–80 s) before and after procedure; intermediate intensity during the procedure (aPTT 40–60 s) removal of the device (aPTT 60–80 s)	Mean RV/LV ratio from baseline to 48 h: 1.55 vs 1.13 ($p < 0.0001$)
OPTALYSE PE 2018	Multicenter RCT of patients with acute intermediate-risk PE and RV/LV ratio ≥0.9	Systemic UFH with USAT	Four dosing regimens: 2 mg/h per catheter for 2 h (range 4–8 mg) 1 mg/h per catheter for 4 h (range 4–8 mg) 1 mg/h per catheter for 6 h (range 6–12 mg) 2 mg/h per cathether for 6 h (range 12–24 mg)	Therapeutic aPTT before and after procedure; UFH dose reduced to 300–500 units/h during the thrombolytic infusion	All 4 dosing regimens improved RV/LV ratio from baseline (24%; $p = 0.0001$; 22.6%; $p = 0.0001$; 26.3%; $p = 0.0001$; 25.5%; $p = 0.0001$)

aPTT activated partial thromboplastin time, *RCT* randomized controlled clinical trial, *RV/LV* right ventricular to left ventricular ratio, *UFH* unfractionated heparin, *USAT* ultrasound-assisted catheter-directed thrombolysis

8.5.3 Surgical Embolectomy

Surgical embolectomy is also an alternative reperfusion therapy provided to some patients with intermediate- or high-risk PE when appropriate resources are available. Surgical embolectomy can be beneficial in patients with a contraindication for thrombolysis, extensive proximal thrombus burden, clot-in-transit, or paradoxical embolism [25]. After initiating cardiopulmonary bypass, incisions are made to the two main pulmonary arteries to remove or suction the thrombus.

8.5.4 Mechanical Circulatory Support

MCS devices such as VA-ECMO provide temporary alleviation for patients with RV dysfunction that develop cardiogenic shock or cardiac arrest. MCS is typically used in combination with other reperfusion therapies such as surgical embolectomy, as the efficacy of ECMO with anticoagulation alone is controversial [89].

8.6 Expanded Role of the Critical Care Pharmacist

8.6.1 PE Response Team (PERT)

PERTs are comprised of a multidisciplinary group of clinicians with expertise in the diagnosis and medical, surgical, and interventional management of PE. The concept of the PERT team was developed due to increasing patient complexity and the rise in therapeutic options for managing PE.

The PERT brings together multiple specialists including cardiology, pulmonology, hematology, vascular medicine, critical care, cardiothoracic surgery, interventional radiology, and critical care/emergency medicine pharmacy to rapidly evaluate patients with high- and intermediate-risk PE, formulate a treatment plan, and assemble necessary resources to provide the highest level of care [59, 89]. In addition to conventional treatment with anticoagulation and systemic thrombolytic therapy, emerging endovascular and surgical interventions may be more appropriate when clinical expertise and institutional resources are available, especially for patients with contraindications to systemic thrombolytic therapy.

The Cleveland Clinic found that patients treated by the PERT ($n = 426$) had lower rates of major or clinically relevant nonmajor bleeding (17.0% vs. 8.3%, $p = 0.002$), shorter time to initiation of therapeutic anticoagulation (16.3 vs. 12.6 hours, $p = 0.009$), decreased 30-day/inpatient mortality (8.5% vs. 4.7%, $p = 0.03$), and decreased use of inferior vena cava filters (22.2% vs. 16.4%, $p = 0.004$) than those treated prior to the implementation of the PERT ($n = 343$) [16]. Beth Israel Deaconess evaluated outcomes pre- and post-PERT implementation among 2042 patients hospitalized for acute PE. Out of 1158 patients presenting post-PERT implementation, the PERT team evaluated 14.2% of patients. While a reduction in PE-related mortality was not observed post-PERT implementation (2.9% versus 2.6%, $p = 0.89$), there was a significant decrease in the use of systemic thrombolysis (2.1% versus 3.8%, $p = 0.02$) and increased use of catheter-directed therapy (3.3% versus 1.3%, $p = 0.05$) compared to pre-PERT implementation [15].

While increased compliance with treatment algorithms, facilitation of medication ordering and administration, and access to drug information, including review of potential contraindications to therapy, have been seen with pharmacist involvement in other response teams (e.g., cardiopulmonary arrest, stroke, sepsis), there is a paucity of literature describing the pharmacist clinician's impact on outcomes as a member of the PERT.

The largest retrospective, observational study of 573 adult patients with massive or submassive PE sought to describe the role of the pharmacist on the PERT team ($n = 137$ pre-PERT and $n = 436$ post-PERT). The pharmacist participated in the care of 70% of patients in the post-PERT group and intervened in 73% of those cases, with the majority of interventions involving a pharmacist facilitating the ordering or administration of the anticoagulant or thrombolytic (58%). The post-PERT groups had significantly shorter median times from diagnosis to anticoagulation administration (post-PERT with a pharmacist, 63 minutes versus post-PERT without a pharmacist, 75.5 minutes) compared to the pre-PERT group (104 minutes), $p = 0.0001$. Additionally, significantly more patients in the post-PERT groups received LMWH compared to UFH when a pharmacist was involved (69.5%) versus without a pharmacist (53.3%), $p = 0.0019$. Post-PERT groups had significantly reduced major bleeding events (post-PERT with a pharmacist, 4.6% versus post-PERT without a pharmacist, 9.9%) compared to the pre-PERT group (14.6%), $p = 0.0013$ [37]. A small retrospective, observational study of 32 patients found that the median time to thrombolytic administration was significantly shorter after the introduction of a pharmacist as a member of the PERT (23 minutes versus 54 minutes, $p = 0.007$) [9]. Additionally, an exploratory analysis revealed that a higher percent of patients had an aPTT obtained before restarting the anticoagulant in the post-intervention group (84.6%) compared to the pre-intervention group (68.8%), which may account for the longer median time to resumption of anticoagulation after systemic thrombolysis seen in the post-intervention group (312 minutes versus 115.5 minutes) [9].

A retrospective study characterized anticoagulant prescribing patterns in patients evaluated by a PERT that included a pharmacist member [61]. Of the 209 patients prescribed anticoagulation at discharge, DOACs were the most common agent (47.4%) followed by warfarin (29.2%) and LMWH (23.4%). The most common intervention made was the initiation of a DOAC upon discharge; however, patients with a higher median BMI (35.4 kg/m^2) were more likely to be prescribed warfarin than DOACs (30 kg/m^2) or LMWH (29.6 kg/m^2), $p = 0.02$. Patients prescribed a DOAC versus warfarin had a shorter median LOS (6.1 versus 10.9 days, $p < 0.05$), and multivariable linear regression analysis found that selection of a DOAC at discharge was the only factor associated with reduced LOS (OR $-$ 0.6, 95% CI -1.01 to -0.18, $p < 0.01$) [61].

These studies demonstrate that pharmacist clinicians play a key role in the management of patients with PE, especially when serving as members of the PERT. Pharmacists can identify patients with moderate- or high-risk PE likely to derive benefit from thrombolytic therapy, screen for contraindications to therapy, and provide recommendations for anticoagulant therapy based on patient-specific factors. Additionally, pharmacists may improve throughput by facilitating the order, admixture, and administration process for thrombolytic and anticoagulant therapies for PE.

8.6.2 Enhancing the Safe Use of Thrombolytics

The thrombolytic therapy landscape has become increasingly complex as new clinical uses and dosing strategies have been evaluated for PE, acute ischemic stroke, and myocardial infarction [17]. Critical care pharmacists are poised to serve as an important resource for the healthcare team, whether it be by providing real-time drug information, selection, and preparation assistance at the bedside or engineering policies and order sets to guide appropriate thrombolytic selection, dosing, storage, and availability.

8.6.2.1 Medication Errors Associated with Thrombolytic Therapy

Errors with confusion between alteplase and tenecteplase have been reported to the FDA and the Institute for Safe Medication Practices (ISMP). From 2000 to 2014, the FDA received 21 reports of wrong drug errors associated with tenecteplase, many due to the use of abbreviations TPA and TNK or TNKase in the ordering process. Additionally, many institutions have both thrombolytics accessible on formulary for different indications.

At one hospital, alteplase was the formulary agent for stroke and PE, but tenecteplase was the formulary agent for ST-segment elevation myocardial infarction (STEMI) due to the lower cost compared to alteplase for this indication. A 72 kg patient presenting with stroke was ordered a weight-based dose of alteplase 65 mg (0.9 mg/kg). Unfortunately, the pharmacist was off service during this time. Both alteplase and tenecteplase were stored in the automatic dispensing cabinet (ADC) in the ED, and the nurse inadvertently retrieved tenecteplase, thinking that the "T" in TPA was for tenecteplase. A second nurse double-checked the dosing, but not the product selection. While tenecteplase is not FDA approved for stroke, 40 mg would be the dose for 72 kg if being treated for PE or STEMI. This patient received tenecteplase 65 mg, a 25 mg higher dose than appropriate for thrombolysis in other indications [18]. While no bleeding complications resulted from this error, this case underscores the potential for error and complications with having multiple thrombolytics on the formulary.

Administration of tenecteplase accidentally using the alteplase dosing regimen for stroke (0.9 mg/kg) would result in patients receiving higher dose than the recommended tenecteplase dose for PE in every patient weight category, and if a patient were to receive tenecteplase at the maximum recommended dose of alteplase (90 mg), they would receive nearly twofold the maximum recommended dose of tenecteplase (50 mg) [17].

8.6.2.2 Strategies to Mitigate Errors with Thrombolytics

Use of abbreviations for tenecteplase ("TNK"/"TNKase") and alteplase ("TPA") may lead to errors in prescribing and transcribing verbal, phone, and electronic orders, especially since these agents are used in similar settings (e.g., ED, critical care units) [17]. The FDA and ISMP recommend placing orders using either the full brand or the generic name for these agents [40, 104]. Abbreviations should be removed from all standardized order sets, treatment protocols, and ADCs to avoid confusion [17, 18, 40, 104]. Pharmacists can promote culture change by using full generic or brand name when discussing thrombolytics and providing instruction and feedback to prescribers to refrain from using these abbreviations. Some institutions have configured their electronic medical record (EMR) to automatically correct the full drug name if a thrombolytic abbreviation is entered [19].

Order sets should be clearly labeled for a given indication and guide clinicians to select the correct drug, dose, and administration time for that indication (SCCM Drug Shortage Alert 2023). Other safety measures that may be implemented within the EMR to reduce errors include adding weight-based dose limits, dual sign-offs of an independent double-check among healthcare providers prior to drug administration, and requiring nurses to document patient monitoring post-thrombolytic administration [19]. An extra safety layer exists for institutions that have implemented EMR interoperability with infusion pumps and barcode scanning, which provides a double-check of the right patient, drug, dose, and administration rate [19].

Having more than one thrombolytic in the hospital formulary and stocked in the same ADC increases the risk for medication errors. When multiple fibrinolytics are in the hospital formulary, the supply should be separated and clearly labeled. The Society of Critical Care Medicine recommends pharmacy personnel prepare each thrombolytic dose when possible to decrease the risk of error by clinicians who are not familiar with these drugs [79]. Many institutions have also opted to create indication-specific thrombolytic kits containing drugs and supplies (e.g., dosing cards, drug, diluent, syringes, infusion bag, tubing) to ensure correct drug selection, dosing, preparation, and administration.

Critical care pharmacists should leverage key stakeholders to ensure that appropriate, continuous education is given and competency assessed for all clinicians caring for patients with acute PE requiring thrombolytics including prescribers, technicians, and nurses. Training may include online modules, in-services, written memos, and hands-on simulations that focus on dosing, administering, monitoring, and locating the correct thrombolytic [19, 79].

8.6.3   *Anticoagulation in Special Populations*

During the acute phases of PE, the patient's risk stratification is the major determinant of the choice of anticoagulation. When determining the post-acute-phase management, additional patient-specific factors must be considered to select the appropriate anticoagulation strategy.

8.6.3.1   Renal Dysfunction

The degree of renal dysfunction is a crucial factor to consider when determining the patient's anticoagulation. DOACs are cleared renally in varying degrees, ranging from 80% renal clearance for dabigatran and 25% for apixaban [99]. Historically,

VKA has been recommended over DOACs for patients with renal dysfunction due to the lack of data in this population. However, there are additional disadvantages associated with chronic VKA therapy, including frequent blood draws for INR level as well as multiple food and drug interactions. VKA also increases the risk of calciphylaxis, which ESRD patients are already at a high risk of developing [75]. Considering the above concerns of VKA, recent studies have evaluated the use of DOACs, particularly apixaban, in renal impairment and dialysis-dependent patients. A meta-analysis of 10 atrial fibrillation or VTE studies reported the safety outcomes of 6693 and 19,836 ESRD patients receiving apixaban or warfarin, respectively. The risk ratio was 0.69 ($p = 0.0002$) for major bleeding and 0.74 ($p = 0.0002$) for clinically relevant bleeding, both in favor of apixaban. The risk of thrombosis was not statistically different [117]. Given that apixaban has the least renal clearance of the DOACs, it is a reasonable treatment option for patients with renal dysfunction without any dose adjustments. Dabigatran, rivaroxaban, and edoxaban should be avoided in patients with a severe degree of renal impairment or on hemodialysis.

For patients who are maintained on parenteral anticoagulants, renal dysfunction may also pose a concern for drug selection and dosing. Although UFH can be safely used for patients with CrCl <30 mL/min, it must be administered continuously via the intravenous route and is not a suitable option for long-term management post-discharge. In patients with CrCl 15–30 mL/min not on dialysis, reduced-dose LMWH (e.g., enoxaparin 1 mg/kg daily) can be used [59]. However, it is important to note that these recommendations may not apply to patients with acute kidney injury or patients with fluctuating renal function.

8.6.3.2   Extremes of Body Weight

Even though DOACs are generally preferred for the treatment of VTE, there is a paucity of data regarding the safety and efficacy of the available dosing regimens on patients with extremes of body weight. Given the lack of data, the 2016 International Society on Thrombosis and Haemostasis (ISTH) guideline recommended against using DOACs in patients with a BMI $\geq$40 kg/m^2 or weight $\geq$120 kg [66]. This recommendation was modified in the 2021 update with a focus on patients with obesity. For treatment of VTE, rivaroxaban or apixaban at standard doses is recommended regardless of BMI or weight [67]. Although several studies demonstrated changes in pharmacokinetics with rivaroxaban and apixaban in obese patients, most peaks and troughs were within the usual range [68]. In contrast, dabigatran and edoxaban are not recommended for use in this population [67]. The limited PK data for dabigatran revealed that 20% of patients >120 kg had peak plasma concentration below the usual treatment range [83]. However, the correlation between drug level and therapeutic efficacy has not been proven, which makes the application of drug levels difficult in clinical practice. Given the lack of specific therapeutic target levels for DOACs, drug-specific levels are not routinely recommended for any DOACs. The level alone should not alter clinical decision-making without a suspicion for treatment failure. Additionally, calibrated levels may not be readily available at all institutions.

A large observational study was published after the ISTH guideline update in 2021, demonstrating the efficacy of DOACs in higher body weight patients. In a retrospective cohort study of 5626 adult patients with BMI $\geq$35 kg/m^2 or weight $\geq$120 kg with a VTE, no difference in the 12-month recurrence rate was observed between DOAC and warfarin use. Patients receiving DOACs had lower rates of major bleeding compared to warfarin (0.5% vs. 2.4%; OR 4.25 (2.19, 8.22)). Notably, 10% of the study population had a BMI $\geq$50 kg/m^2, suggesting safety in even the morbidly obese population [69]. This is an area of rapidly evolving data, and pharmacist clinicians can play a major role in the decision-making process to determine the optimal oral anticoagulation strategy for patients with obesity.

LMWH is typically dosed based on total body weight (TBW); however, this may pose a concern in patients at extremes of body weight. Due to its hydrophilicity, high molecular weight, and plasma protein binding, enoxaparin does not distribute well into the adipose tissue. Therefore, previous trials frequently utilized a "dose cap" or maximum initial dose of 150 mg in patients with a body weight >150 kg to avoid over-anticoagulation. Additionally, patients with BMI $\geq$40 kg/m^2 tended to have more supratherapeutic peak anti-Xa levels on 1 mg/kg TBW regimen compared to 0.8 mg/kg [21]. In retrospective studies, patients with a higher body weight or BMI achieved therapeutic anti-Xa levels at doses equivalent to 0.7–1 mg/kg [21, 64, 109]. Given these findings, an initial dose cap of 150 mg per dose can be considered for patients weighing >150 kg or an initial weight-based dose of 0.7–0.8 mg/kg per dose for patients with BMI $\geq$40 kg/m^2. Although routine monitoring of LMWH via anti-Xa assay is not recommended due to the lack of efficacy data, it may be considered on a patient-specific basis to serve as a surrogate for the degree of anticoagulation [91]. In patients with low body weight receiving LMWH, the standard weight-based dose of 1 mg/kg per dose is suggested [91]. In a study that included patients treated for symptomatic acute VTE, there was no difference in recurrent VTE across various weight brackets. There was a higher overall bleeding complication rate in patients under 50 kg; however, the conclusion may be confounded by external factors such as the use of NSAIDs [7].

8.6.3.3 Pregnancy and Breastfeeding

Numerous oral anticoagulants such as VKA and DOACs carry teratogenicity concerns and thus are not recommended for pregnant patients. UFH and LMWH do not cross the placenta and are safe treatment options for patients while pregnant. LMWH is preferred over UFH given its more predictable pharmacokinetics and lower risk of heparin-induced thrombocytopenia [59]. Standard LMWH applies to pregnant patients; however, the question has been raised regarding the need for dose escalation with increasing body weight in pregnancy. A practice bulletin from the American College of Obstetricians and Gynecologists discusses the role of periodic anti-Xa level measurements to target a peak level between 0.6 and 1 units/mL in patients receiving twice-daily LMWH, although only a few patients required dose escalation [3]. The 2020 ESC guidelines recommend against routine anti-Xa level monitoring due to the lack of efficacy data [59]. In patients with heparin-induced thrombocytopenia, fondaparinux is a reasonable alternative despite solid data and potential for minor transplacental passage [3, 23, 59]. Systemic thrombolytics are considered a relative contraindication in pregnant patients. The risks and benefits should be weighed cautiously, and the standard recommendations for thrombolytic therapy should be followed for high-risk and intermediate-high-risk patients. In patients who are breastfeeding, LMWH and VKA can be used safely. DOACs should be avoided given the lack of fetal safety and efficacy profile [59]. Fondaparinux, danaparoid, and UFH are potential options.

8.6.3.4 Cancer

Previous guidelines such as the CHEST 2016 recommendations have given preference to LMWH as the anticoagulation of choice in patients with malignancy [49]. However, recent trials have demonstrated the efficacy and safety of select DOACs such as rivaroxaban, edoxaban, and apixaban in this population [2, 87, 116]. Multiple guidelines since then have incorporated rivaroxaban and edoxaban into their recommendations [27, 51, 100]. Although apixaban is an acceptable option for patients with malignancy, it was omitted from some of the current guidelines since the study was published after the guideline updates. The recently updated guidelines from CHEST and the International Initiative on Thrombosis and Cancer guideline include apixaban in addition to rivaroxaban and edoxaban as an initial DOAC option [28, 65, 99]. Due to the concern of increased gastrointestinal and genitourinary bleeding, rivaroxaban and edoxaban are generally avoided in patients with gastrointestinal tract malignancies [28]. Apixaban does not appear to carry the same risk and is thus the preferred option in this population. Dabigatran does not have adequate data for use as the first line in patients with cancer and does not have a role in most guidelines [99]. The NCCN has a conditional recommendation to use dabigatran as an acceptable alternative for patients who are not candidates for long-term LMWH [100].

8.6.3.5 Treatment Failure

There is a lack of data regarding the management of patients who are deemed anticoagulant treatment failures (e.g., recurrent or new VTE while on therapeutic anticoagulation). Prior to determining failure, pharmacists can perform a thorough patient interview to assess medication compliance. Although VKA adherence can be predicted by measuring the INR, DOAC levels are not readily available in many institutions [90]. However, anti-Xa measurements could detect the presence of factor Xa inhibitors and may be a useful tool, even if the calibrated levels are not available. In patients who are deemed noncompliant, any modifiable barriers to adherence should be addressed—mainly, insurance coverage or affordability, frequency of dosing, or incomplete understanding of administration instructions.

Even when patients are compliant with their anticoagulant regimen, treatment failure may still ensue from other factors that decrease drug levels. Rivaroxaban, for example, requires administration with the largest meal of the day to ensure adequate absorption. The site of absorption is also crucial to evaluate for patients requiring enteral administration of medication due to the inability to ingest orally. The distal tip of various feeding tubes may terminate in different sites (e.g., stomach, small intestine), which may drastically impact the absorption of DOACs. For example, rivaroxaban is mainly absorbed in the stomach and thus will have reduced absorption when it is released distal to the stomach. In contrast, apixaban is absorbed in the small intestine and the stomach, and potentially in the colon as well [67, 68].

Pharmacists may also consider drug interactions that may lead to DOAC failure by reviewing the patient's full medication history. Drug interactions mediated by CYP-450 or P-glycoprotein transport may decrease the concentration of DOACs. Specifically, reports of treatment failure are increasing with the concomitant use of antiseizure medications such as phenobarbital, phenytoin, and carbamazepine [36]. Uniquely, the use of DOACs with valproic acid or levetiracetam was also associated with high rates of thromboembolic events, despite no apparent drug interaction [31, 34].

If pharmacotherapy-related causes of treatment failure have been ruled out, patients may have other disease states that may contribute to treatment failure. For example, patients with antiphospholipid antibody syndrome should preferentially be treated with warfarin over DOACs, as DOACs were associated with an increased risk of recurrent thrombosis in this population [59]. If patients develop heparin-induced thrombocytopenia, the continued use of heparinoids may trigger new thromboses. Additionally, patients who underwent bariatric surgery may have questionable absorption of DOACS, which may lead to treatment failure. The 2021 ISTH guideline recommended against the use of DOACs in the immediate phase of post-bariatric surgery [67, 68]. However, strong data for this claim is not available. In a study involving 102 post-bariatric surgery patients, the recurrence rates of VTE were 0% and 1.7% while receiving apixaban and rivaroxaban, respectively [62]. If the above concerns were addressed and the patient does not have any modifiable or identified cause of treatment failure while on an anticoagulant, it may be reasonable to switch to an alternate agent.

8.7 Conclusion

While anticoagulation remains the cornerstone of PE management, assessment of patient-specific factors, risk for morbidity and mortality from PE, and risk for bleeding complications informs the decision to utilize systemic thrombolytic therapy, need for advanced interventional reperfusion procedures, as well as long-term anticoagulant choice and duration of therapy. The pharmacist clinician is a highly qualified member of the healthcare team to lead nuanced discussions on the risks and benefits of anticoagulant and thrombolytic therapies not only at the individual patient level, but also through the development of institutional PE treatment pathways and implementation of safety measures. Additionally, pharmacist clinicians have demonstrated to be a valuable member of the PERT by facilitating thrombolytic and anticoagulation administration and improving the safety and overall care of patients with PE.

References

1. Abu-Laban RB, Christenson JM, Innes GD, van Beek CA, Wanger KP, McKnight RD, MacPhail IA, Puskaric J, Sadowski RP, Singer J, Schechter MT, Wood VM. Tissue plasminogen activator in cardiac arrest with pulseless electrical activity. N Engl J Med. 2002;346(20):1522–8.
2. Agnelli G, Becattini C, Meyer G, et al. Apixaban for the treatment of venous thromboembolism associated with cancer. N Engl J Med. 2020;382(17):1599–607.
3. American College of Obstetricians and Gynecologists' Committee on Practice Bulletins—Obstetrics. ACOG practice bulletin no. 196: thromboembolism in pregnancy. Obstet Gynecol. 2018;132(1):e1–e17.
4. Aujesky D, Obrosky DS, Stone RA, et al. A prediction rule to identify low-risk patients with pulmonary embolism. Arch Intern Med. 2006;166:169–75.
5. Avgerinos ED, Jaber W, Lacomis J, Markel K, McDaniel M, Rivera-Lebron BN, Ross CB, Sechrist J, Toma C, Chaer R, SUNSET sPE Collaborators. Randomized trial comparing standard versus ultrasound-assisted thrombolysis for submassive pulmonary embolism: the SUNSET sPE trial. JACC Cardiovasc Interv. 2021;14:1364–73.
6. Bajaj A, Saleeb M, Rathor P, et al. Prognostic value of troponins in acute nonmassive pulmonary embolism: a meta-analysis. Heart Lung. 2015;44:327–34.
7. Barba R, Marco J, Martín-Alvarez H, et al. The influence of extreme body weight on clinical outcome of patients with venous thromboembolism: findings from a prospective registry (RIETE). J Thromb Haemost. 2005;3:856–62.
8. Becattini C, Agnelli G, Vedovati MC, et al. Multidetector computed tomography for acute pulmonary embolism: diagnosis and risk stratification in a single test. Eur Heart J. 2011;32:1657–63.
9. Berdahl GJ, Cascone AE, Ackerbauer KA, Feeney ME. Reduction in thrombolytic door-to-needle time with addition of pharmacist to pulmonary embolism response team. J Am Coll Clin Pharm. 2023;6:864–9.
10. Beri S, Pastores SM. Thrombolytic therapy for submassive pulmonary embolism. In: Oropello JM, Pastores SM, Kvetan V, editors. Critical care. McGraw Hill; 2017.
11. Böttiger BW, Arntz HR, Chamberlain DA, et al. Thrombolysis during resuscitation for out-of-hospital cardiac arrest. N Engl J Med. 2008;359:2651–62.
12. Bounds EJ, Kok SJ. D Dimer. [Updated 2023 Aug 31]. In: StatPearls [Internet]. Treasure Island, FL: StatPearls Publishing; 2023. Available from: https://www.ncbi.nlm.nih.gov/books/NBK431064/.
13. Caldicott D, Parasivam S, Harding J, Edwards N, Bochner F. Tenecteplase for massive pulmonary embolus. Resuscitation. 2002;55(2):211–3.
14. Carrier M, Righini M, Djurabi RK, et al. VIDAS D-dimer in combination with clinical pretest probability to rule out pulmonary embolism: a systematic review of management outcome studies. Thromb Haemost. 2009;101:886–92.
15. Carroll BJ, Beyer SE, Mehegan T, et al. Changes in care for acute pulmonary embolism through a multidisciplinary pulmonary embolism response team. Am J Med. 2020;133:1313–21.e6.
16. Chaudhury P, Gadre SK, Schneider E, et al. Impact of multidisciplinary pulmonary embolism response team availability on management and outcomes. Am J Cardiol. 2019;124:1465–9.

17. Chester KW, Corrigan M, Schoeffler JM, et al. Making a case for the right '-ase' in acute ischemic stroke: alteplase, tenecteplase, and reteplase. Expert Opin Drug Saf. 2019;18:87–96.

18. Cohen MR, Smetzer JL. Alteplase and tenecteplase confusion; lack of e-prescribing interoperability leads to double dosing; accidental overdoses involving fluorouracil infusions. Hosp Pharm. 2015;50:849–54.

19. Cox J, Hilton R. Patient safety network series highlight august 2023: transitions from alteplase to tenecteplase for acute ischemic stroke. Crit Care Med. 2023;23(3):14.

20. Cuker A, Arepally GM, Chong BH, et al. American Society of Hematology 2018 guidelines for management of venous thromboembolism: heparin-induced thrombocytopenia. Blood Adv. 2018;2:3360–92.

21. Curry MA, LaFollette JA, Alexander BR, Evans KS, Tran RH, Kempton CL. Evaluation of treatment-dose enoxaparin in acutely ill morbidly obese patients at an Academic Medical Center: a randomized clinical trial. Ann Pharmacother. 2019;53(6):567–73.

22. Dahlbäck B. Advances in understanding pathogenic mechanisms of thrombophilic disorders. Blood. 2008;112(1):19–27.

23. Dempfle CE. Minor transplacental passage of fondaparinux in vivo. N Engl J Med. 2004;350:1914–5.

24. Donzé J, Le Gal G, Fine MJ, et al. Prospective validation of the pulmonary embolism severity index: a clinical prognostic model for pulmonary embolism. Thromb Haemost. 2008;100:943–8.

25. Dudzinski DM, Giri J, Rosenfield K. Interventional treatment of pulmonary embolism. Circ Cardiovasc Interv. 2017;10:e004345.

26. Ellis DA, Neville E, Hall RJ. Subacute massive pulmonary embolism treated with plasminogen and streptokinase. Thorax. 1983;38(12):903–7.

27. Farge D, Frere C, Connors JM, et al. 2019 international clinical practice guidelines for the treatment and prophylaxis of venous thromboembolism in patients with cancer. Lancet Oncol. 2019;20(10):e566–81.

28. Farge D, Frere C, Connors JM, et al. 2022 international clinical practice guidelines for the treatment and prophylaxis of venous thromboembolism in patients with cancer, including patients with COVID-19. Lancet Oncol. 2022;23(7):e334–47.

29. Feltes J, Popova M, Hussein Y, Pierce A, Yamane D. Thrombolytics in cardiac arrest from pulmonary embolism: a systematic review and meta analysis. J Intensive Care Med. 2023;30:8850666231214754.

30. Freund Y, Cachanado M, Aubry A, et al. Effect of the pulmonary embolism rule-out criteria on subsequent thromboembolic events among low-risk emergency department patients: the PROPER randomized clinical trial. JAMA. 2018;319:559–66.

31. Galgani A, Palleria C, Iannone LF, De Sarro G, Giorgi FS, Maschio M, Russo E. Pharmacokinetic interactions of clinical interest between direct oral anticoagulants and antiepileptic drugs. Front Neurol. 2018;9:1067.

32. Garcia DA, Baglin TP, Weitz JI, et al. Parenteral anticoagulants: antithrombotic therapy and prevention of thrombosis, 9th ed: American College of Chest Physicians Evidence-Based Clinical Practice Guidelines. Chest. 2012;141(suppl 2):e24S–43S.

33. Ghofrani HA, D'Armini AM, Grimminger F, et al. Riociguat for the treatment of chronic thromboembolic pulmonary hypertension. N Engl J Med. 2013;369(4):319–29.

34. Giustozzi M, Mazzetti M, Paciaroni M, Agnelli G, Becattini C, Vedovati MC. Concomitant use of direct oral anticoagulants and antiepileptic drugs: a prospective cohort study in patients with atrial fibrillation. Clin Drug Investig. 2021;41(1):43–51.

35. Goldhaber SZ, Visani L, De Rosa M. Acute pulmonary embolism: clinical outcomes in the International Cooperative Pulmonary Embolism Registry (ICOPER). Lancet. 1999;353(9162):1386–9.

36. Gronich N, Stein N, Muszkat M. Association between use of pharmacokinetic-interacting drugs and effectiveness and safety of direct acting Oral anticoagulants: nested case-control study. Clin Pharmacol Ther. 2021;110(6):1526–36.

37. Groth CM, Acquisto NM, Wright C, Marinescu M, McNitt S, Goldenberg I, Cameron SJ. Pharmacists as members of an interdisciplinary pulmonary embolism response team. J Am Coll Clin Pharm. 2022;5(4):390–7.

38. Henke PK, Kahn SR, Pannucci CJ, et al. Call to action to prevent venous thromboembolism in hospitalized patients: a policy statement from the American Heart Association. Circulation. 2020;141:e914–31.

39. Igneri LA, Hammer JM. Systemic thrombolytic therapy for massive and submassive pulmonary embolism. J Pharm Pract. 2020;33:74–89.

40. Institute for Safe Medication Practices (ISMP). ISMP list of error-prone abbreviations, symbols, and dose designations. ISMP; 2021.

41. Isath A, Shah R, Bandyopadhyay D, et al. Dispelling the saddle pulmonary embolism myth (from a comparison of saddle versus non-saddle pulmonary embolism). Am J Cardiol. 2023;201:341–8.

42. Jaff MR, McMurtry MS, Archer SL, et al. Management of massive and submassive pulmonary embolism, iliofemoral deep vein thrombosis, and chronic thromboembolic pulmonary hypertension: a scientific statement from the American Heart Association. Circulation. 2011;123(16):1788–830.

43. Javaudin F, Lascarrou JB, Le Bastard Q, et al. Research Group of the French National Out-of-Hospital Cardiac Arrest Registry (GR-RéAC).Thrombolysis during resuscitation for out-of-hospital cardiac arrest caused by pulmonary embolism increases 30-day survival: findings from the French National Cardiac Arrest Registry. Chest. 2019;156:1167–75.

44. Jerjes-Sanchez C, Ramírez-Rivera A, de Lourdes García M, et al. Streptokinase and heparin versus heparin alone in massive pulmonary embolism: a randomized controlled trial. J Thromb Thrombolysis. 1995;2:227–9.

45. Jiménez D, Aujesky D, Moores L, et al. RIETE Investigators. Simplification of the pulmonary embolism severity index for prognostication in patients with acute symptomatic pulmonary embolism. Arch Intern Med. 2010;170:1383–9.

46. Kaeberich A, Seeber V, Jiménez D, et al. Age-adjusted high-sensitivity troponin T cut-off value for risk stratification of pulmonary embolism. Eur Respir J. 2015;45:1323–31.

47. Kearon C, Kahn SR, Agnelli G, et al. Antithrombotic therapy for venous thromboembolic disease: American College of Chest Physicians Evidence-Based Clinical Practice Guidelines (8th Edition). Chest. 2008;133(6 Suppl):454S–545S.

48. Kearon C, Akl EA, Comerota AJ, et al. Antithrombotic therapy for VTE disease: antithrombotic therapy and prevention of thrombosis, 9th ed: American College of Chest Physicians Evidence-Based Clinical Practice Guidelines. Chest. 2012;141(suppl 2):e419S–96S.

49. Kearon C, Akl EA, Ornelas J, et al. Antithrombotic therapy for VTE disease: CHEST guideline and expert panel report. Chest. 2016;149(2):315–52.

50. Kearon C, de Wit K, Parpia S, et al. Diagnosis of pulmonary embolism with d-Dimer adjusted to clinical probability. N Engl J Med. 2019;381:2125–34.

51. Key NS, Khorana AA, Kuderer NM, et al. Venous thromboembolism prophylaxis and treatment in patients with cancer: ASCO clinical practice guideline update. J Clin Oncol. 2020;38(5):496–520.

52. Kim NH, Delcroix M, Jais X, et al. Chronic thromboembolic pulmonary hypertension. Eur Respir J. 2019;53(1):1801915.

53. Kiser TH, Burnham EL, Clark B, et al. Half-dose versus full-dose alteplase for treatment of pulmonary embolism. Crit Care Med. 2018;46:1617–25.

54. Kline JA, Nordenholz KE, Courtney DM, Kabrhel C, Jones AE, Rondina MT, Diercks DB, Klinger JR, Hernandez J. Treatment of submassive pulmonary embolism with tenecteplase or placebo: cardiopulmonary outcomes at 3 months: multicenter double-blind, placebo-controlled randomized trial. J Thromb Haemost. 2014;12(4):459–68.

55. Klok FA, Mos IC, Huisman MV. Brain-type natriuretic peptide levels in the prediction of adverse outcome in patients with pulmonary embolism: a systematic review and meta-analysis. Am J Respir Crit Care Med. 2008;178:425–30.

56. Konstantinides S, Geibel A, Heusel G, Heinrich F, Kasper W. Heparin plus alteplase compared with heparin alone in patients with submassive pulmonary embolism. N Engl J Med. 2002;347(15):1143–50.

57. Konstantinides SV, Torbicki A, Agnelli G, et al. 2014 ESC guidelines on the diagnosis and management of acute pulmonary embolism. Eur Heart J. 2014;35(43):3033–69.

58. Konstantinides SV, Vicaut E, Danays T, Becattini C, Bertoletti L, Beyer-Westendorf J, Bouvaist H, Couturaud F, Dellas C, Duerschmied D, Empen K, Ferrari E, Galiè N, Jiménez D, Kostrubiec M, Kozak M, Kupatt C, Lang IM, Lankeit M, Meneveau N, Palazzini M, Pruszczyk P, Rugolotto M, Salvi A, Sanchez O, Schellong S, Sobkowicz B, Meyer G. Impact of thrombolytic therapy on the long-term outcome of intermediate-risk pulmonary embolism. J Am Coll Cardiol. 2017;69(12):1536–44.

59. Konstantinides SV, Meyer G, Becattini C, et al. 2019 ESC guidelines for the diagnosis and management of acute pulmonary embolism developed in collaboration with the European Respiratory Society (ERS). Eur Heart J. 2020;41:543–603.

60. Kucher N, Boekstegers P, Müller OJ, et al. Randomized, controlled trial of ultrasound-assisted catheter-directed thrombolysis for acute intermediate-risk pulmonary embolism. Circulation 2014;129(4):479–86.

61. Kuhrau S, Masic D, Mancl E, Brailovsky Y, Porcaro K, Morris S, Haines J, Charo K, Fareed J, Darki A. Impact of pulmonary embolism response team on anticoagulation prescribing patterns in patients with acute pulmonary embolism. J Pharm Pract. 2022;35(1):38–43.

62. Kushnir M, Gali R, Alexander M, Billett HH. Direct oral Xa inhibitors for the treatment of venous thromboembolism after bariatric surgery. Blood Adv. 2023;7(2):224–6.

63. Laporte S, Mismetti P, Décousus H, Uresandi F, Otero R, Lobo JL, Monreal M, RIETE Investigators. Clinical predictors for fatal pulmonary embolism in 15,520 patients with venous thromboembolism: findings from the Registro Informatizado de la Enfermedad TromboEmbolica venosa (RIETE) Registry. Circulation. 2008;117(13):1711–6.

64. Lee YR, Palmere PJ, Burton CE, Benavides TM. Stratifying therapeutic enoxaparin dose in morbidly obese patients by BMI class: a retrospective cohort study. Clin Drug Investig. 2020;40(1):33–40.

65. Lyman GH, Carrier M, Ay C, et al. American Society of Hematology 2021 guidelines for management of venous thromboembolism: prevention and treatment in patients with cancer. Blood Adv. 2021;5(4):927–74.

66. Martin K, Beyer-Westendorf J, Davidson BL, et al. Use of the direct oral anticoagulants in obese patients: guidance from the SSC of the ISTH. J Thromb Haemost. 2016;14:1308–13.

67. Martin KA, Beyer-Westendorf J, Davidson BL, et al. Use of direct oral anticoagulants in patients with obesity for treatment and prevention of venous thromboembolism: updated communication from the ISTH SSC Subcommittee on Control of Anticoagulation. J Thromb Haemost. 2021a;19:1874–82.

68. Martin AC, Thomas W, Mahir Z, et al. Direct oral anticoagulant concentrations in obese and high body weight patients: a cohort study. Thromb Haemost. 2021b;121(2):224–33.

69. Martin KA, Lancki N, Li C, et al. DOAC compared with warfarin for VTE in patients with obesity: a retrospective cohort study conducted through the VENUS network. J Thromb Thrombolysis. 2023;55(4):685–90.

70. Meinel FG, Nance JW Jr, Schoepf UJ, et al. Predictive value of computed tomography in acute pulmonary embolism: systematic review and meta-analysis. Am J Med. 2015;128:747–59.e2.

71. Meyer NJ, Schmidt GA. Pulmonary embolic disorders: thrombus, air, and fat. In: Hall JB, Schmidt GA, Kress JP, editors. Principles of critical care. 4th ed. McGraw Hill; 2014. Available at https://accessmedicine.mhmedical.com/content.aspx?bookid=1340§ionid=80031468.

72. Meyer G, Vicaut E, Danays T, et al. PEITHO Investigators. Fibrinolysis for patients with intermediate-risk pulmonary embolism. N Engl J Med. 2014;370:1402–11.

73. Millington SJ, Aissaoui N, Bowcock E, et al. High and intermediate risk pulmonary embolism in the ICU. Intensive Care Med. 2023;50(2):195–208. https://doi.org/10.1007/s00134-023-07275-6.

74. Muñoz FJ, Mismetti P, Poggio R, et al. Clinical outcome of patients with upper-extremity deep vein thrombosis: results from the RIETE Registry. Chest. 2008;133:143–8.
75. Nigwekar SU, Kroshinsky D, Nazarian RM, et al. Calciphylaxis: risk factors, diagnosis, and treatment. Am J Kidney Dis. 2015;66(1):133–46.
76. Nishiyama KH, Saboo SS, Tanabe Y, et al. Chronic pulmonary embolism: diagnosis. Cardiovasc Diagn Ther. 2018;8:253–71.
77. Ortel TL, Neumann I, Ageno W, et al. American Society of Hematology 2020 guidelines for management of venous thromboembolism: treatment of deep vein thrombosis and pulmonary embolism. Blood Adv. 2020;4:4693–738.
78. Panchal AR, Bartos JA, Cabañas JG, et al. Part 3: Adult basic and advanced life support: 2020 American Heart Association guidelines for cardiopulmonary resuscitation and emergency cardiovascular care. Circulation. 2020;142:S366–468.
79. Patel MK, Wang S, Wang WM. Society of Critical Care Medicine Drug Shortage Alert, Thrombolytics. June 2023. Available from: https://www.sccm.org/sccm/media/PDFs/Drug-Shortage-Alert-Thrombolytics.pdf.
80. Penaloza A, Roy PM, Kline J, et al. Performance of age-adjusted D-dimer cut-off to rule out pulmonary embolism. J Thromb Haemost. 2012;10:1291–6.
81. Penaloza A, Soulié C, Moumneh T, et al. Pulmonary embolism rule-out criteria (PERC) rule in European patients with low implicit clinical probability (PERCEPIC): a multicentre, prospective, observational study. Lancet Haematol. 2017;4:e615–21.
82. Piazza G, Hohlfelder B, Jaff M, et al. A prospective, single-arm, multicenter trial of ultrasound-facilitated, catheter-directed, low-dose fibrinolysis for acute massive and submassive pulmonary embolism: the SEATTLE II study. J Am Coll Cardiol Intv. 2015;8(10):1382–92.
83. Piran S, Traquair H, Chan N, Bhagirath V, Schulman S. Peak plasma concentration of direct oral anticoagulants in obese patients weighing over 120 kilograms: a retrospective study. Res Pract Thromb Haemost. 2018;2(4):684–8.
84. Pollack CV, Schreiber D, Goldhaber SZ, Slattery D, Fanikos J, O'Neil BJ, Thompson JR, Hiestand B, Briese BA, Pendleton RC, Miller CD, Kline JA. Clinical characteristics, management, and outcomes of patients diagnosed with acute pulmonary embolism in the emergency department: initial report of EMPEROR (Multicenter Emergency Medicine Pulmonary Embolism in the Real World Registry). J Am Coll Cardiol. 2011;57(6):700–6.
85. Pruszczyk P, Goliszek S, Lichodziejewska B, et al. Prognostic value of echocardiography in normotensive patients with acute pulmonary embolism. JACC Cardiovasc Imaging. 2014;7:553–60.
86. Pruszczyk P, Klok FA, Kucher N, et al. Percutaneous treatment options for acute pulmonary embolism: a clinical consensus statement by the ESC Working Group on Pulmonary Circulation and Right Ventricular Function and the European Association of Percutaneous Cardiovascular Interventions. EuroIntervention. 2022;18(8):e623–38.
87. Raskob GE, van Es N, Verhamme P, et al. Edoxaban for the treatment of cancer-associated venous thromboembolism. N Engl J Med. 2018;378(7):615–24.
88. Righini M, Van Es J, Den Exter PL, et al. Age-adjusted D-dimer cutoff levels to rule out pulmonary embolism: the ADJUST-PE study. JAMA. 2014;311:1117–24.
89. Rivera-Lebron B, McDaniel M, Ahrar K, et al. Diagnosis, treatment and follow up of acute pulmonary embolism: consensus practice from the PERT Consortium. Clin Appl Thromb Hemost. 2019;25:1076029619853037.
90. Rodger MA, Miranda S, Delluc A, et al. Management of suspected and confirmed recurrent venous thrombosis while on anticoagulant therapy. What next? Thromb Res. 2019;180:105–9.
91. Sebaaly J, Covert K. Enoxaparin dosing at extremes of weight: literature review and dosing recommendations. Ann Pharmacother. 2018;52:898–909.
92. Sharifi M, Bay C, Skrocki L, Rahimi F, Mehdipour M, et al. Moderate pulmonary embolism treated with thrombolysis (from the "MOPETT" Trial). Am J Cardiol. 2013;111(2):273–7.

93. Shopp JD, Stewart LK, Emmett TW, et al. Findings from 12-lead electrocardiography that predict circulatory shock from pulmonary embolism: systematic review and meta-analysis. Acad Emerg Med. 2015;22:1127–37.
94. Shukla AN, Thakkar B, Jayaram AA, Madan TH, Gandhi GD. Efficacy and safety of tenecteplase in pulmonary embolism. J Thromb Thrombolysis. 2014;38(1):24–9.
95. Sista AK, Horowitz JM, Tapson VF, et al. Indigo aspiration system for treatment of pulmonary embolism: results of the EXTRACT-PE trial. JACC Cardiovasc Interv. 2021;14:319–29.
96. Solanki NN, Tanwar N, Solanki ND. Subacute massive pulmonary embolism treated with streptokinase. Cureus. 2020;12(10):e11157.
97. Stein PD, Matta F. Thrombolytic therapy in unstable patients with acute pulmonary embolism: saves lives but underused. Am J Med. 2012;125(5):465–70.
98. Stein PD, Beemath A, Matta F, et al. Clinical characteristics of patients with acute pulmonary embolism: data from PIOPED II. Am J Med. 2007;120:871–9.
99. Stevens SM, Woller SC, Kreuziger LB, et al. Antithrombotic therapy for VTE disease: second update of the CHEST guideline and expert panel report. Chest. 2021;160:e545–608.
100. Streiff MB, Holmstrom B, Angelini D, et al. NCCN guidelines insights: cancer-associated venous thromboembolic disease, version 2.2018. J Natl Compr Cancer Netw. 2018;16(11):1289–303.
101. Tapson VF. Pulmonary embolism. In: Fuster V, Narula J, Vaishnava P, et al., editors. Fuster and Hurst's the heart. 15th ed. McGraw Hill; 2022. Available at https://accesscardiology. mhmedical.com/content.aspx?bookid=3134§ionid=265683652.
102. Tapson VF, Sterling K, Jones N, et al. A randomized trial of the optimum duration of acoustic pulse thrombolysis procedure in acute intermediate-risk pulmonary embolism: the OPTALYSE PE trial. JACC Cardiovasc Interv. 2018;11(14):1401–10.
103. Tsikouris JP, Jackson KC, Fike DS, et al. Thrombolytic fibrin specificity influences activated partial thromboplastin time prolongation in vitro. Blood Coagul Fibrinolysis. 2002;13(8):725–31.
104. Tu A. FDA information on medication errors involving Activase and TNKase. FDA News for Health Professionals; 2015. Available from: https://fda.report/media/93606/FDA-Information-on-Medication-Errors-Involving-Activase-and-TNKase.pdf.
105. Tu T, Toma C, Tapson VF, et al. A prospective, single-arm, multicenter trial of catheter-directed mechanical thrombectomy for intermediate-risk acute pulmonary embolism: the FLARE study. JACC Cardiovasc Interv. 2019;12(9):859–69.
106. van Belle A, Büller HR, Huisman MV, et al. Effectiveness of managing suspected pulmonary embolism using an algorithm combining clinical probability, D-dimer testing, and computed tomography. JAMA. 2006;295:172–9.
107. van der Hulle T, Cheung WY, Kooij S, et al. Simplified diagnostic management of suspected pulmonary embolism (the YEARS study): a prospective, multicentre, cohort study. Lancet. 2017;390(10091):289–97.
108. van der Pol LM, Tromeur C, Bistervels IM, et al. Pregnancy-adapted YEARS algorithm for diagnosis of suspected pulmonary embolism. N Engl J Med. 2019;380(12):1139–49.
109. van Oosterom N, Winckel K, Barras M. Evaluation of weight based enoxaparin dosing on anti-Xa concentrations in patients with obesity. J Thromb Thrombolysis. 2019;48(3):387–93.
110. Vyas V, Goyal A. Acute pulmonary embolism. [Updated 2022 May 1]. In: StatPearls [Internet]. StatPearls Publishing; 2022. Available at www.ncbi.nlm.nih.gov/books/NBK560551/.
111. Wells PS, Ginsberg JS, Anderson DR, et al. Use of a clinical model for safe management of patients with suspected pulmonary embolism. Ann Intern Med. 1998;129:997–1005.
112. Wells PS, Anderson DR, Rodger M, et al. Excluding pulmonary embolism at the bedside without diagnostic imaging: management of patients with suspected pulmonary embolism presenting to the ED by using a simple clinical model and d-dimer. Ann Intern Med. 2001;135:98–107.

113. Wendelboe AM, Raskob GE. Global burden of thrombosis: epidemiologic aspects. Circ Res. 2016;118:1340–7.
114. Wilson SJ, Wilbur K, Burton E, et al. Effect of patient weight on the anticoagulant response to adjusted therapeutic dosage of low-molecular- weight heparin for the treatment of venous thromboembolism. Haemostasis. 2001;31(1):42–8. https://pubmed.ncbi.nlm.nih.gov/11408748/.
115. Yang J, Madani MM, Mahmud E, Kim NH. Evaluation and Management of Chronic Thromboembolic Pulmonary Hypertension. Chest. 2023;164(2):490–502.
116. Young AM, Marshall A, Thirlwall J, et al. Comparison of an Oral factor Xa inhibitor with low molecular weight heparin in patients with cancer with venous thromboembolism: results of a randomized trial (SELECT-D). J Clin Oncol. 2018;36(20):2017–23.
117. Zagoridis K, Karatisidis L, Mprotsis T, et al. Apixaban reduces the risk of major and clinically relevant non-major bleeding compared to warfarin in patients with end stage renal disease; a systematic review and meta-analysis of ten studies. Thromb Res. 2023;231:17–24.
118. Zghouzi M, Mwansa H, Shore S, et al. Sex, racial, and geographic disparities in pulmonary embolism-related mortality Nationwide. Ann Am Thorac Soc. 2023;20(11):1571–7.

Chapter 9
Extracorporeal Membrane Oxygenation

Stephanie Davis, Alana Ciolek, and Atul Dilawri

9.1 ECMO Overview and History

Extracorporeal membrane oxygenation (ECMO) is a technique that provides temporary pulmonary and/or cardiac support by offering circulation and perfusion outside of the body [88]. Short-term ECMO was first used in the 1950s during the first open-heart procedure; subsequently, it was used throughout the 1960s in pediatric respiratory failure and during the repair of congenital heart conditions [88]. In the 1970s, long-term ECMO was successfully utilized for a patient with severe respiratory distress syndrome (ARDS) [88]. It then gained momentum in subsequent years, particularly with the publication of the CESAR trial, demonstrating positive outcomes 6 months after randomization, and then with its successful use during the H1N1 influenza epidemic [88, 145].

There are two types of ECMO circuits that consist of several components: cannulas, centrifugal blood pump, tubing, oxygenator, and heat exchanger (see Fig. 9.1a, b) [48]. In short, venovenous ECMO (VV-ECMO) supports the pulmonary system, and venoarterial ECMO (VA-ECMO) provides respiratory and cardiac support [88]. In VV-ECMO, the circuit is connected in series to the heart and lungs, and in VA-ECMO, the circuit is connected in parallel [88]. Deoxygenated blood is removed from the venous system through the inflow cannula and then passed

S. Davis (✉)
Cardiovascular Surgical ICU and Clinical Nutrition, The Johns Hopkins Hospital, Baltimore, MD, USA
e-mail: sdavis87@jh.edu

A. Ciolek
New York-Presbyterian Hospital/Weill Cornell Medical Center, New York, NY, USA

A. Dilawri
Cardiothoracic Intensive Care, New York-Presbyterian Hospital, Columbia University Irving Medical Center, New York, NY, USA

219

Y. Alzaidi, M. A. Gebily (eds.), *The Pharmacist's Expanded Role in Critical Care Medicine*, https://doi.org/10.1007/978-3-031-77335-8_9

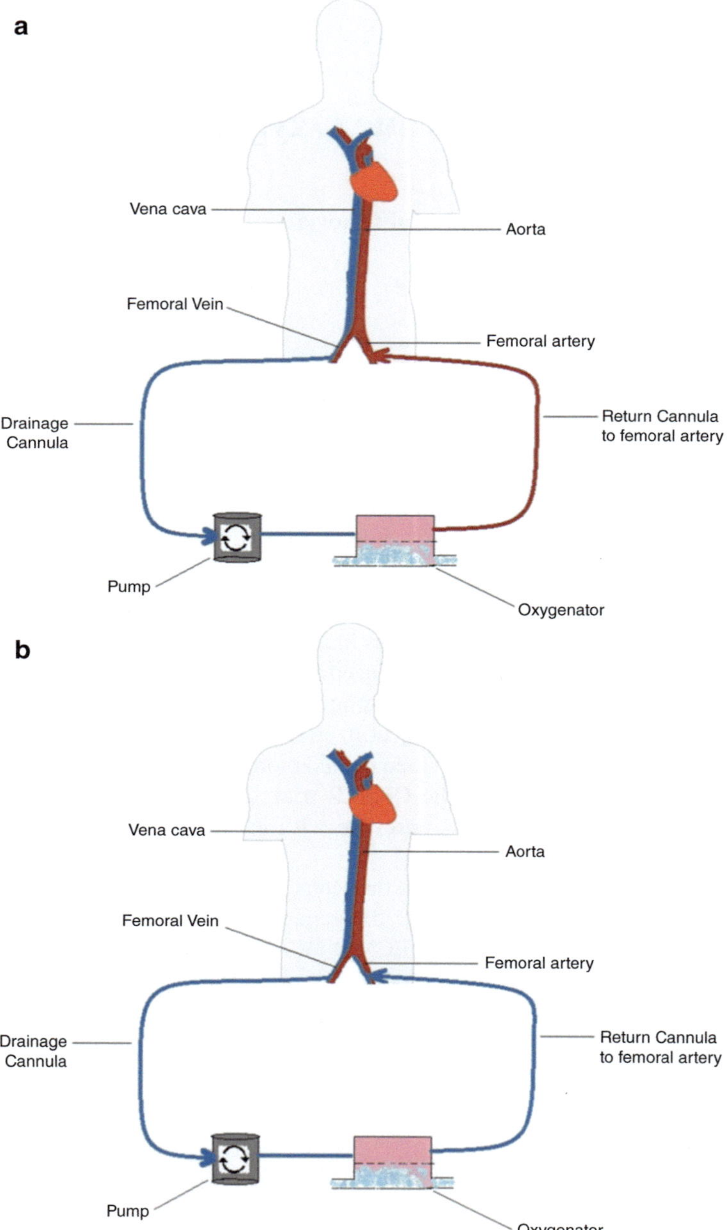

Fig. 9.1 VV- and VA-ECMO configurations. (**a**) Simplified visualization of peripheral VV-ECMO cannulation. The right femoral vein is cannulated to the inflow cannula, which drains to a blood pump and then to an oxygenator (blood becomes oxygenated as depicted by the red color), and then the outflow cannula drains blood back into the left femoral artery via the outflow cannula. (**b**) Simplified visualization of peripheral VA-ECMO cannulation. In this figure, the right femoral vein is cannulated to the inflow cannula, which proceeds to a blood pump and oxygenator. Oxygenated blood is returned to the left femoral artery via the outflow cannula [115]. *VV-ECMO* veno-venous extracorporeal membrane oxygenation, *VA-ECMO*, venoarterial extracorporeal membrane oxygenation

through a blood pump to a membrane oxygenator, where carbon dioxide is removed and hemoglobin is replenished with oxygen [145]. The oxygenators typically have integrated heat exchangers to replace heat loss as blood circulates outside of the body [82, 88]. In VV-ECMO, the newly oxygenated blood is returned back to the patient's venous system via the outflow cannula, where it passes through the lungs (albeit the lungs need to do minimal work because the blood is already oxygenated). Contrary to VV-ECMO, in VA-ECMO, newly oxygenated blood is returned back to the patient's arterial system via the outflow cannula [88]. In both configurations, the ECMO circuit can be peripherally or centrally placed, depending on where the cannulation occurs. Peripheral ECMO cannulation typically involves the internal jugular vein, femoral vein/artery, or axillary artery, and central ECMO cannulation involves the vena cava, right atrium, and ascending aorta.

9.1.1   Indications, Contraindications, and Patient Selection

ECMO is primarily indicated as rescue therapy in the management of critically ill patients with severe cardiac and/or respiratory failure, refractory to optimal conventional therapies. ECMO is neither a definitive treatment nor a destination therapy. Instead, it is commonly employed as a bridge to recovery, transplant, or destination therapy with mechanical circulatory support (MCS). The Extracorporeal Life Support Organization (ELSO) guidelines suggest that ECMO should be considered when the risk of mortality is 50% or greater and is indicated when the risk of mortality is >80% [49]. Given the complexity and multiple facets involved in the care of patients receiving ECMO support, decisions regarding the initiation of ECMO should involve an experienced multidisciplinary team, inclusive of pharmacists [40]. When critically ill adult patients are being assessed for ECMO support, it is important to establish whether the underlying cause of severe cardiac and/or pulmonary dysfunction is potentially reversible, refractory to conventional therapies, and without formal contraindications to ECMO support. Additionally, consideration of the patient's age, comorbidities, severity of circulatory dysfunction, and degree of multiple organ system dysfunction should be incorporated into the risk-benefit assessment. For cases of irreversible cardiopulmonary disease, candidacy for ECMO may be suitable as a bridge to transplant or a durable MCS device.

Although there is an absence of widely accepted standards for indications of ECMO support, consensus statements provide recommendations for the use of ECMO in critically ill adult patients [12, 120]. Indications for ECMO are broadly classified by the ELSO registry into three categories: cardiac failure, respiratory failure, and cardiopulmonary resuscitation. VA-ECMO helps support patients with cardiac failure, characterized as low cardiac output (cardiac index <2 L/min/m^2) and hypotension (systolic blood pressure <90 mmHg) despite adequate fluid resuscitation, inotropic support, and intra-aortic balloon pump support [53]. Common cardiac indications for VA-ECMO support include cardiogenic shock, inability to wean from cardiopulmonary bypass support, primary graft dysfunction after heart transplantation, and periprocedural support for high-risk percutaneous cardiac interventions (Fig. 9.2) [4, 88]. VA-ECMO as a bridge to recovery is initiated for reversible cardiac conditions such as acute myocardial infarction, myocarditis, pulmonary embolism, postcardiotomy shock, and refractory ventricular arrhythmias [40]. VA-ECMO also provides a bridge to, or can be used in addition to, other forms of temporary MCS (e.g., percutaneous left ventricular assist device or intra-aortic balloon pump) for refractory cardiac conditions and a bridge to heart transplantation or long-term ventricular assist device for end-stage heart failure [40]. In the setting of cardiac arrest, extracorporeal cardiopulmonary resuscitation in the form of VA-ECMO support can serve as a salvage treatment option in patients who have failed to achieve a sustained return of spontaneous circulation with conventional cardiopulmonary resuscitation [36].

VV-ECMO is indicated for patients with acute respiratory failure and refractory hypoxemia (PaO2/FiO2 < 80 mmHg) or severe hypercapnic respiratory failure (pH <7.25 with a PaCO2 $\geq$ 60 mm Hg), despite optimal conventional mechanical ventilation and medical management. Common respiratory indications for VV-ECMO support include ARDS, acute lung injury secondary to trauma or toxic inhalation, diffuse alveolar or pulmonary hemorrhage, pulmonary embolism, status asthmaticus, and primary graft dysfunction after lung transplantation (Fig. 9.2) [145]. Echocardiography should be performed prior to cannulation onto VV-ECMO to rule out cardiac etiologies of respiratory failure and severe cardiac dysfunction which otherwise would necessitate the need for VA-ECMO support. Importantly, the incidence of right ventricular dysfunction in patients with isolated respiratory failure is approximately 10% secondary to hypoxemia, hypercarbia, and acidosis with ARDS [106]. Concomitant right ventricular dysfunction in the setting of respiratory failure can oftentimes be managed with diuretics, pulmonary vasodilators, inotropes, and optimization of acid-base status without the need for VA-ECMO. For isolated respiratory failure, ECMO serves as a bridge to recovery for reversible pulmonary conditions and a bridge to transplant for irreversible pulmonary conditions.

There are no universally accepted contraindications to ECMO support. Absolute contraindications are rare and limited to patients with non-recoverable cardiac or respiratory failure who are not candidates for transplantation or permanent MCS [40]. Most contraindications are relative and balance the risk of the procedure versus the potential benefit. At the time of initial presentation, the clinical outlook or prognosis may remain uncertain, and ECMO can be used as a temporary bridge to decision, if it is believed that the patient may be a transplantation or MCS candidate. Relative contraindications are summarized in Fig. 9.2. The ultimate decision to withhold ECMO support should be based on an evaluation of the prognosis and an assessment of whether ECMO will improve or worsen the overall prognosis.

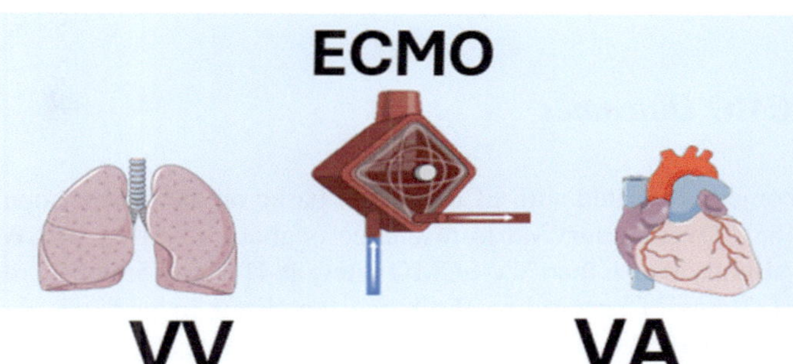

Fig. 9.2 ECMO indications and contraindications. Adapted from Refs. [4, 145]. *CNS* central nervous system, *CPB* cardiopulmonary bypass, *CPR* cardiopulmonary resuscitation, *ECMO* extracorporeal membrane oxygenation, *MCS* mechanical circulatory support, *VA* venoarterial, *VV* veno-venous

9.1.2 ECMO Outcomes

Patient outcomes associated with ECMO differ based on the patient population and indication [88]. Overall, survival to discharge is about 45–50%, with VA-ECMO rates being slightly worse than VV-ECMO rates, at 41% and 55–63%, respectively [48, 71, 88]. Rates of survival to discharge are better in pediatric versus adult patients, at 74% and 57% for neonates and pediatrics, respectively [88]. The landmark CESAR trial randomized adult ARDS patients to receive VV-ECMO compared to conventional ARDS management (positive-pressure ventilation ± high-frequency oscillatory ventilation) [114]. The primary outcome of death or disability at 6 months was significantly decreased in the ECMO group, and ECMO was also associated with a gain of 0.03 quality life-adjusted years. Critiques of this trial include the following: a long recruitment period (5 years) during which conventional therapies for ARDS progressed, 24% of patients randomized to the ECMO group never received ECMO (potentially due to transfer to a center with more resources for conventional therapy), and the study was powered for an expected mortality rate of 70% with an actual mortality rate of 50% [114, 130]. The second landmark VV-ECMO trial was not until 2018 when the EOLIA study randomized ARDS patients on <7 days of mechanical ventilation to VV-ECMO or standard of care (high positive end-expiratory pressure, high recruitment) [32]. There was no significant difference found in the primary outcome of 60-day mortality, though the secondary endpoints of death or crossover to ECMO by day 60, ventilator-free days, renal failure, and cardiac failure all favored the VV-ECMO group. Critiques of the EOLIA trial include the inclusion of non-ECMO centers, early cessation of recruitment when a 20% decrease in mortality was not met, a long recruitment period (10 years), and a 28% crossover rate for patients with refractory hypoxia [32, 42].

Rates of survival in VA-ECMO vary significantly based on the indication. Use of VA-ECMO for primary graft failure after heart transplantation or for acute fulminant myocarditis has the highest rates of survival at 70–80% [48]. Largely, the survival data for VA-ECMO use in various etiologies of cardiogenic shock stems from small, retrospective studies, and the data is often conflicting. Bréchot et al. found that in severe sepsis-induced cardiogenic shock, the use of VA-ECMO significantly improved survival compared to conventional treatment [19]. Another study, however, found no difference in outcomes in patients with severe cardiogenic shock who immediately received VA-ECMO versus those who only received it downstream, if hemodynamics worsened [107].

9.2 ECMO During Cardiopulmonary Resuscitation (eCPR)

The use of VA-ECMO during cardiac arrest (eCPR) has potentially the worst survival outcomes at only 20–30%, and in the subset who experienced out-of-hospital cardiac arrest, survival outcomes are even worse at 15–22% [48, 88]. In the EOLIA trial, six patients required crossover to VA-ECMO for eCPR, and this group had a mortality rate of 57% [32]. Despite the worse outcomes, studies have demonstrated improved survival and neurologic outcomes compared to conventional cardiopulmonary resuscitation (CPR) [27, 129]. The ARREST trial randomized adult patients with out-of-hospital cardiac arrest due to ventricular fibrillation or pulseless ventricular tachycardia to VA-ECMO or standard advanced cardiac life support (ACLS) resuscitation [146]. The trial ended early after 30 patients were enrolled due to the superiority of the VA-ECMO resuscitation strategy.

Given the emergent and high-risk nature, patient selection for eCPR should be well defined as to ensure an acceptable risk-benefit balance. The ELSO Guidelines for Adult eCPR recommend utilizing this strategy in patients under 70 years of age, who have witnessed arrest, and with absence of previously known life-limiting comorbidities, arrest to first CPR of less than 5 minutes, arrest to ECMO cannulation and flow less than 60 minutes, an initial cardiac rhythm that does not include asystole, and no known aortic valve incompetence [119]. Conventional ACLS measures should continue during ECMO cannulation, with interruptions in chest compressions only done when absolutely necessary [119]. Only once the ECMO is cannulated, clamps have been removed, and adequate ECMO blood flow is achieved should chest compressions be discontinued [119]. Of note, vasopressors or inotropes that may have been started during the arrest should be weaned, as full support will be provided by the ECMO circuit [119]. If the patient remains in a refractory, non-perfusing rhythm, all attempts should be made to restore a perfusing rhythm, which may be more successful once acid-base balance and coronary perfusion pressure are improved by ECMO [119]. Targeted temperature management is allowable and possible through the heat exchanger [119]. There is no consensus as to the amount of time a patient should remain on ECMO after cardiac arrest, and it should be assessed based on the underlying etiology of the cardiac arrest and what is deemed acceptable cardiac recovery; an average of 3–4 days of ECMO is reported for eCPR [119].

9.2.1 Extracorporeal Carbon Dioxide Removal

Although beyond the scope of this chapter, for completeness, the use of extracorporeal carbon dioxide removal ($ECCO_2R$) will be briefly discussed here. The major benefit of $ECCO_2R$ is that it is less invasive than standard ECMO [105]. $ECCO_2R$ can be done at much lower blood flow rates because of the CO_2 dissociation curve and its higher threshold for removal; therefore, the cannula sizes can be much smaller, reducing the complexity of care [105]. There are two different ways in which CO_2 can be removed from the blood through this circuit—via arteriovenous or venovenous removal ($AVCO_2R$ and $VVCO_2R$, respectively) [105]. In $AVCO_2R$, the native arteriovenous pressure gradient drives blood flow through the circuit and has no external pump [105]. The circuit is set up by creating an arteriovenous shunt through the cannulation of the femoral artery and vein and placing the oxygenator (which removes the CO_2) in between [105]. In $VVCO_2R$, the setup is similar, except that blood is drawn out and returned via the venous side, and a pump and oxygenator are connected to the circuit (Fig. 9.3) [105]. Of note, $ECCO_2R$ can only be a potential replacement for VV-ECMO, as it does not offer cardiac support.

$ECCO_2R$ was first used in the 1980s primarily for ARDS. In 1994, the first randomized controlled trial on $ECCO_2R$ was published that compared $ECCO_2R$ to conventional therapy (mechanical ventilation) and found no differences in outcomes between both groups [99]. Of note, patients in this trial used practices that involved high airway pressures as lung-protective ventilation was not standardized yet. Since then, other studies in patients with ARDS have explored outcomes associated with $ECCO_2R$ and found overall no difference in mortality with the use of $ECCO_2R$ versus various types of mechanical ventilation strategies; however, there are significant flaws in the study designs [33, 93]. One small study did find that $ECCO_2R$ can be effective in facilitating the use of ultra-protective lung ventilation [34, 35]. Case series in patients with COPD have reported success in the use of $ECCO_2R$ to facilitate weaning from mechanical ventilation as well as significantly decrease the risk of mechanical ventilation in individuals on $ECCO_2R$ plus noninvasive ventilation [2, 136].

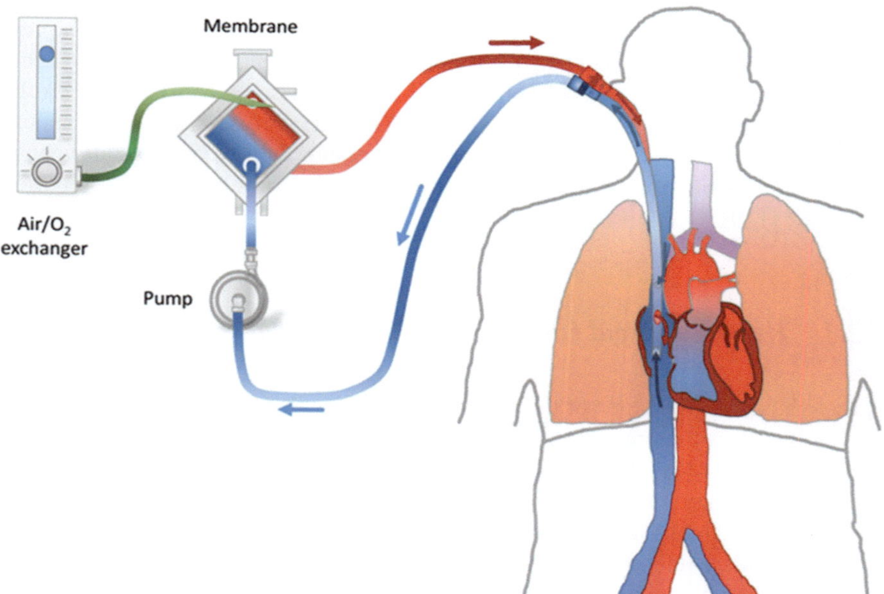

Fig. 9.3 Example of $VVCO_2R$ configuration. In this version of $VVCO_2R$, the dual-lumen single catheter removes deoxygenated blood from the right atrium where it then flows through a pump (necessary as blood flow is very low) and into a membrane that removes CO_2 from the blood, and it is then returned back to the right atrium [57]. *$VVCO_2R$ veno-venous carbon dioxide removal*

9.3 ECMO Management

9.3.1 Circuit Priming

Prior to ECMO initiation, the assembled circuit is primed with an isotonic electrolyte solution resembling normal extracellular fluid [49]. Priming solutions serve several purposes including preventing air from entering the circuit, providing anti-thrombotic properties, and ensuring that the system is properly filled. Depending on institutional protocols, patient clinical factors, and available resources, circuits are primed with crystalloid solutions and/or blood products under sterile conditions. The typical priming volumes vary depending on the oxygenator size, ranging from 80 mL in smaller pediatric-specific oxygenators to 250 mL in larger adult-specific oxygenators [54]. For adults and large children, priming with crystalloid solutions is a common and safe practice [54]. Many institutions add 50 mL of 25% albumin to the crystalloid primed circuit to "coat" the plastic surfaces and to potentially add oncotic properties [54]. As is discussed in more detail in the Anticoagulation section, when blood comes into contact with artificial surfaces within the ECMO circuit, it leads to the formation of a layer of fibrinogen, albumin, and other serum hematologic proteins which coat these artificial surfaces. As a result, this process can trigger platelet activation and inflammation. Incorporating albumin within the priming solution may result in decreased platelet activation by decreasing the early adsorption of fibrinogen [131]. In infants, smaller children (weight less than 10–15 kg), and anemic patients, blood products including packed red blood cells, fresh frozen plasma, and albumin are often required, if time permits, to prime the circuit to avoid excessive hemodilution [54]. For blood-primed solutions, heparin is also added (1 unit/mL of prime) to maintain anticoagulation; calcium is also added to replace citrate-bound calcium in the banked blood [20]. Additional additives may include sodium bicarbonate to overcome acidosis and hyperkalemia. If time permits, it is advisable to check the electrolyte composition of the blood prime before initiating ECMO. For emergency use or eCPR, where the goal is to establish ECMO support as soon as possible, priming with crystalloid solutions is recommended.

After the onset of support, the effects of hemodilution by the priming solution can be treated with diuretics and/or transfusions. Circuits can be primed at the time of cannulation, or several days before. Many institutions keep ECMO circuits preassembled and filled with a crystalloid solution due to the time required for assembly and priming. This approach, which involves assembling and priming the circuit under sterile conditions, is preferable to priming at the bedside in an emergency. By using sterile techniques and no glucose, and no albumin or crystalloid solutions that contain no substrates for bacterial growth (e.g., glucose or albumin), the circuit is unlikely to develop bacterial contamination over time [20]. According to ELSO Infection Control Guidelines, it is considered safe to maintain pre-primed circuits for up to 30 days [49].

9.3.2 Circuit and Patient Maintenance and Monitoring

Once the patient is cannulated, frequent management of the circuit is necessary to prevent complications. Complications can be either medical or mechanical in nature and are associated with significant increases in morbidity and mortality [88, 145]. Medical complications are reported in approximately 40% of patients and can include most commonly bleeding (30%) followed by thrombosis, thrombocytopenia, infection, and neurologic issues [88, 145]. Mechanical complications may entail thrombi within the circuit or oxygenator, or cannula malposition or misplacement [145].

Monitoring of the circuit and the patient involves several factors. The ECMO components themselves are at risk of malfunction or failure. Adequate circulating volume must be maintained to avoid circuit "chatter" at the site of the inflow cannula. In VA-ECMO, blood flows should be provided at the lowest rate possible to maintain organ support and keep the arterial pulse pressure at least 10 mm Hg to ensure adequate ventricular ejection and reduce the risk of ventricular thrombosis [49]. In VV-ECMO, flow rates should be set to maintain an arterial saturation greater than 80% [49].

The flow rate of blood through the ECMO circuit determines the degree of oxygenation. Elimination of carbon dioxide is controlled through the oxygenator device, through what is referred to as sweep gas flow rates [49, 88]. Flow rates should be maintained between 3 and 6 L/min to ensure adequate oxygenation in VV-ECMO; however, the degree of oxygenation is also dependent on the native cardiac output because blood infuses back into the patient from the venous side [88]. This is unlike VA-ECMO, where blood oxygenated by the circuit mixes directly with natively perfused blood to provide adequate oxygenation [88]. In VA-ECMO, the proportion of natively versus artificially perfused blood is controlled by the flow rates. The ECMO system has a control panel, where providers can adjust these flow rates depending on the clinical status of the patient.

Assuming that flow rates are set appropriately for the membrane oxygenator being used, the oxygen saturation at the outlet of the oxygenator should be at least 95% [49]. The venous saturation should be 20–30% less than the arterial saturation to maintain an appropriate proportion of oxygen delivery to oxygen consumption [49]. The sweep gas flow rate to blood flow rate is initially set in a 1:1 ratio and then titrated based on PCO_2 [49]. The oxygenator's transmembrane pressure gradients, commonly referred to as Delta P, should be maintained at <50 mm Hg; if larger, then it may indicate thrombi in the oxygenator [145]. Additionally, the oxygenator should be visually inspected with a flashlight for any sign of thrombi [145]. A patient with refractory hypoxemia on VV-ECMO, despite high pre-oxygenator oxygen saturations, should be evaluated for recirculation; in these instances, the inflow and outflow cannulas should be separated, or the circuit reconfigured to a single dual-lumen catheter [145]. VV-ECMO flows should be maintained at a minimum of 60% of the total native systemic flow to avoid poor systemic oxygenation from occurring [145]. This situation may occur if a patient goes into septic shock, as the patient's native cardiac output could then potentially exceed the ECMO flow rates due to this highly vasodilatory state [145].

In VA-ECMO, a right radial arterial line can be used as a surrogate marker for cerebral perfusion as it is farthest from the site of the outflow cannula; this arterial line should ensure that oxygen saturations are maintained >88% [48]. This is also particularly important to monitor in peripheral VA-ECMO, where a mixture of less oxygenated blood ejected from the patient's left ventricle and oxygenated blood from the circuit (delivered via retrograde flow) creates a "mixing point" that moves depending on the patient's native heart function [145]. This mixing point can lead to Harlequin syndrome, or a differential hypoxemia between the lower and upper body, increasing the risk of hypoxic blood flow to the brain and heart [145]. VA-ECMO may also cause pulmonary edema and/or left ventricular distension, and serial chest X-rays should be obtained and evaluated for the possible need for left ventricular venting strategies [145]. Providers must also serially evaluate adequate perfusion of the arterial cannulated leg if utilizing femoral arterial access and consider the placement of a distal perfusion cannula to prevent limb ischemia or compartment syndrome [145].

Finally, the pressures in the inflow and outflow cannulas must be monitored regularly, as high pressures in either area may be a signal for an underlying complication. For example, high inflow pressures may be caused by cannula kinking, thrombosis, or an undersized cannula, and a high outflow pressure may be secondary to kinks, systemic hypertension, or thrombosis [100].

9.3.3 Fluid Management

During the initial phases of ECMO, patients frequently require large-volume fluid resuscitation to maintain adequate ECMO blood flow and treat the underlying disease process contributing to severe cardiopulmonary failure. Liberal fluid resuscitative efforts are further amplified by the fact that the majority of patients being initiated on ECMO support are already in a state of intravascular hypovolemia, aggravated by systemic capillary leakage. Additionally, the administration of blood products to correct anemia or coagulopathy accompanying ECMO cannulation also plays a role in aggravating fluid overload in ECMO-supported patients. Intravenous fluids used during intravenous drug administration can also contribute greatly to a patient's positive fluid balance over a 24-h period. These challenges in maintaining normal extracellular fluid volumes result in fluid overload, which has implications for clinical outcomes. In critically ill patients with sepsis, positive fluid balance is associated with a higher risk of mortality [96]. Among patients with ARDS, the FACTT and FACTT Lite studies both demonstrated that conservative fluid management, compared to liberal fluid management, improved lung function and shortened ICU length of stay and duration of mechanical ventilation, albeit without a significant impact on mortality [58, 143]. Since ARDS is a common indication for ECMO initiation, the assessment of fluid management strategies in these patients was also evaluated in a retrospective study of 152 patients with severe ARDS requiring ECMO support. The study found that higher cumulative fluid balance (CFB) during the first 3 days of ECMO was independently associated with increased hospital mortality [28]. Similarly, observational studies evaluating CFB and clinical outcomes in patients receiving VA- or VV-ECMO support for cardiopulmonary diseases have also demonstrated poor survival outcomes among patients with higher CFB, particularly notable on day 3 following ECMO initiation [73, 124]. Overall, fluid overload in patients receiving ECMO has been associated with negative impacts on organ function, impaired oxygenation, increased duration of ECMO support, and mortality.

Fluid therapy management in patients receiving ECMO is usually driven by clinical endpoints such as maintaining a mean arterial pressure greater than 60–65 mmHg. Volume resuscitation is also initiated in response to the chattering of the ECMO circuit, decreased urinary output, and hyperlactatemia. Monitoring and maintaining ECMO drainage pressures also serve as a surrogate for fluid status since higher negative pressures predispose patients to a greater degree of hemolysis and should be avoided.

9.4 Anticoagulation Considerations in ECMO

9.4.1 Coagulation Changes

The exposure of large volumes of blood to the polyvinyl chloride tubing and polymethylpentene oxygenator of the ECMO circuit results in inflammation, with subsequent changes and disruption to platelets and the coagulation system [131]. The four main changes that occur include platelet activation and dysfunction, contact activation, pro-inflammatory cytokine response, and decreased levels of natural anticoagulants (Fig. 9.4) [98]. Shortly after blood contacts the artificial surfaces of the ECMO circuit, blood proteins, mainly albumin and fibrinogen, adhere to the tubing. These blood proteins then act as anchors for platelets, resulting in platelet activation, aggregation, and consumption at the site. In addition, von Willebrand factor (vWF) is activated by the high shear stress of the blood flow through the circuit and binds to platelets, causing subsequent platelet activation through the release of platelet granules. This high shear stress may also cause the loss of platelet receptors needed for platelet adhesion, leading in part to platelet dysfunction [131]. The shear stress also causes the loss of high-molecular-weight multimers of vWF, making it more difficult for platelets to bind to the surfaces of these smaller multimers [131].

The contact activation pathway is activated through factor XII's attachment to the foreign surface of the ECMO tubing within 10 minutes of starting ECMO [98]. The contact activation pathway activates the rest of the intrinsic pathway of the coagulation cascade and also plays a significant role in inflammation through its production of bradykinin [98]. There is a strong relationship between the inflammatory and coagulation responses that occur during ECMO. In addition to the contact

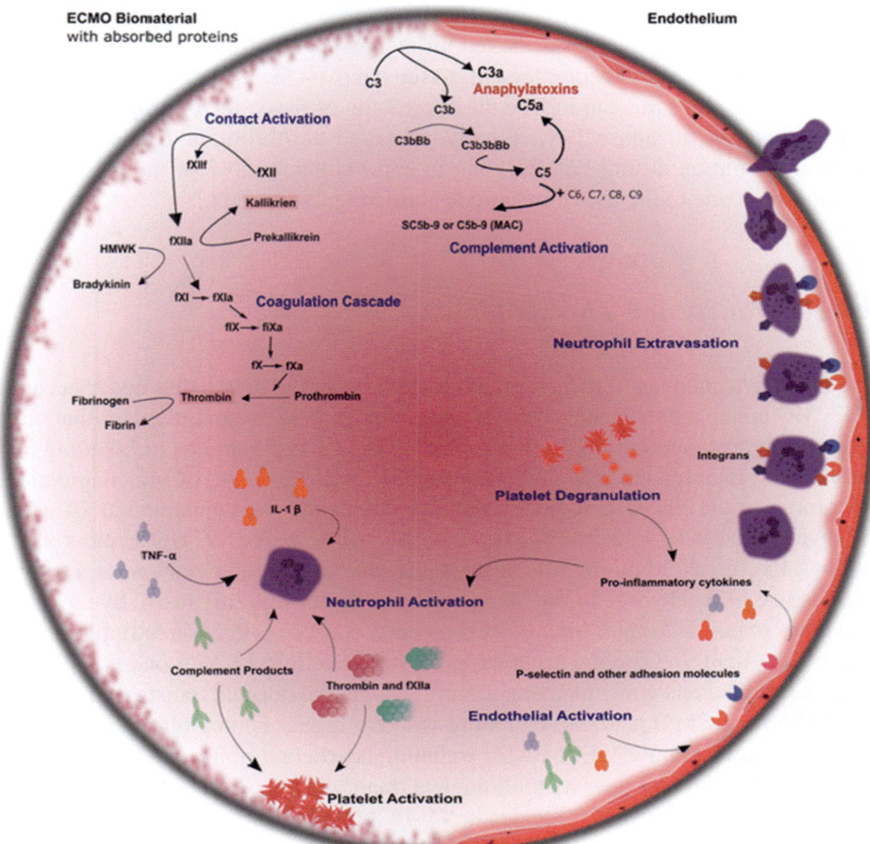

Fig. 9.4 Coagulation and inflammatory responses to ECMO. During ECMO, major coagulation and inflammatory changes occur: (1) Contact activation: FXII attaches to the foreign surface of the ECMO tubing and is subsequently converted to FXIIa, which cleaves PK to kallikrein and HMWK to bradykinin. The contact activation pathway then goes on to activate the intrinsic pathway of the coagulation cascade. The contact activation pathway plays a significant role in inflammation through its production of bradykinin. (2) Pro-inflammatory cytokines: There is a strong relationship between the inflammatory and coagulation responses that occur during ECMO. Complement is activated through the complement activation pathway when blood contacts the ECMO circuit. Products C3a and C5a promote the activation of T cells and other pro-inflammatory cytokines. Activated complement also plays a role in coagulation by inducing the expression of TF on endothelial cells and directly activating platelets [98]. *ECMO* extracorporeal membrane oxygenation, *FXII* factor XII, *FXIIa* activated factor XII, *PK* pre-kallikrein, *HMWK* high-molecular-weight kininogen, *TF* tissue factor

activation pathway's contributions to a pro-inflammatory response, the immune system's complement pathway is activated through exposure to the foreign material of the circuit [98]. Activated complement, tissue necrosis factor-α (TNF-α), and interleukin-6 (IL-6), in turn, can induce the expression of tissue factor, triggering a further coagulation response [98]. Finally, acquired antithrombin III deficiency is relatively common during ECMO, seen in approximately 50% of individuals, and thought to be due to the use of heparin for anticoagulation [116].

9.4.2 Transfusion Thresholds

The extensive changes to the coagulation cascade and platelets that occur because of ECMO create a fine balance between hemorrhagic and thrombotic risks that must be carefully mitigated through monitoring of signs and symptoms of bleeding and thrombosis, maintenance of goal hemoglobin levels, and use of anticoagulation. According to the ELSO guidelines, hemoglobin should be maintained at 14–15 g/dL or hematocrit of >40% [92]. The majority of surveyed ECMO centers use a hemoglobin threshold of 10 g/dL, followed by 8 g/dL for other centers, as a trigger to transfuse [92]. There is limited data on the safety of utilizing restrictive transfusion goals in patients on ECMO; however, expert consensus deems restrictive strategies of less than 7–7.5 g/dL acceptable for non-bleeding ECMO patients [92]. A recent meta-analysis concluded uncertainty in what the optimal transfusion strategy should be for ECMO patients, including whether higher hemoglobin goals should be used in patients on VA-ECMO for ischemic heart conditions, due to a high risk of publication bias and poor methodological quality [1].

The data for transfusion strategies in VV-ECMO patients, however, is beginning to become clearer. Patients on VV-ECMO tend to require less transfusions due to lower-intensity anticoagulation and lack of arterial cannulation. Small, retrospective studies of patients with ARDS on VV-ECMO support transfusion triggers of <7 g/dL [1, 72]. A retrospective study in VV-ECMO for patients with ARDS found no difference in 28-day survival for transfusion thresholds of 8 versus 10 g/dL; however, the more restrictive goal was associated with a lower chance of successful ventilator weaning [68]. Finally, in the recently published multicenter, prospective cohort PROTECMO study, a hemoglobin of less than 7 g/dL was associated with a higher risk of mortality, and subsequently, transfusions for this threshold were associated with improved mortality [91].

9.4.3 Anticoagulation Strategies in ECMO

Anticoagulation is a pivotal part of ECMO management. The ELSO guidelines recommend the routine use of anticoagulation for VA- and VV-ECMO, although the literature is emerging that suggests that low intensity to no anticoagulation may be safe for VV-ECMO [92]. There are no established, standardized dosing and monitoring protocols for anticoagulation for several reasons. First, ECMO technology continues to evolve, with older circuits requiring greater anticoagulation intensity compared to contemporary circuits [47]. Data regarding optimal monitoring using the anti-factor Xa assay (anti-Xa) or activated partial thromboplastin time (aPTT) varies, and therefore, different centers prefer different monitoring and targets (see Sect. 9.4.4). Centers also vary in the level of anticoagulation intensity targeted, which differs based on patient risk factors for bleeding versus thrombosis. The retrospective nature of currently published literature makes it difficult to control for these various risk factors and how they impact optimal management [47].

9.4.3.1 Heparin

Unfractionated heparin (UFH) is the most common anticoagulant utilized and is also recommended as the anticoagulant of choice by the International Society on Thrombosis and Haemostasis, primarily due to its many advantages (Table 9.1) [64]. UFH is a large polysaccharide molecule that binds to antithrombin III (ATIII), increasing its activity 1000-fold [66]. This complex inactivates factors IIa (thrombin), Xa, IXa, XIa, and XIIa, leading to decreased coagulation [66]. It also binds proteins from platelets and endothelial cells and doubles levels of tissue factor pathway inhibitor, specifically in ECMO patients, leading to inter-patient variability in response [64]. Heparin is administered via continuous infusion with or without boluses and, kinetically, has an immediate onset of action and a short half-life of 60–90 minutes [64]. Additionally, it is fully reversible with protamine [64]. It is easy to monitor by using either aPTT, activated clotting time (ACT), or anti-Xa [64] (see Sect. 9.4.4). Finally, heparin requires no dose adjustments for liver or renal dysfunction [101]. Given the kinetic and monitoring benefits of heparin as well as its reversibility and familiarity, heparin is by far the most common anticoagulant used, reported as the anticoagulant of choice at 96% of ECMO centers [101]. Despite its popularity, heparin does have limitations that must be considered. One of the most serious adverse effects of heparin is the risk of heparin-induced thrombocytopenia (HIT), which can be fatal; furthermore, as discussed previously, the ECMO circuit itself can cause platelet consumption and thrombocytopenia as well as thrombotic complications, often making it difficult to diagnose true HIT versus thrombocytopenia from other causes [69]. Additionally, heparin use can deplete intrinsic stores of ATIII, leading to an acquired ATIII deficiency and subsequent heparin resistance [69].

While heparin resistance due to ATIII deficiency can become problematic for achieving therapeutic aPTT or anti-Xa levels, there is limited data to suggest that replacement of ATIII improves outcomes [92]. Additionally, data suggests that heparin resistance is not associated with increased rates of thrombosis, hemorrhage, or survival; however, these studies tend to be small and retrospective in nature [116]. Concerns remain that increasing doses of heparin in the setting of heparin resistance can increase the risk of bleeding, and using ATIII supplementation to better control

Table 9.1 Pros and cons of heparin and direct thrombin inhibitors [24, 64]

Anticoagulant	Pros	Cons
Heparin	Quick onset of action Short half-life Reversible Easily monitored No dose adjustments are required for liver or renal dysfunction Extensive experience, familiarity Inexpensive Easily titratable	Inter-patient variability in response Risk of HIT Heparin resistance possible due to acquired ATIII deficiency
Direct thrombin inhibitors	Anticoagulant effects independent of ATIII No risk of HIT High efficacy Easily monitored Easily titratable	No reversal agent Expensive Risk of clotting in static blood
Bivalirudin	Anticoagulant effects independent of ATIII No risk of HIT High efficacy Easily monitored Easily titratable	Prolonged half-life in renal dysfunction
Argatroban	Anticoagulant effects independent of ATIII No risk of HIT High efficacy Easily monitored Easily titratable	Prolonged half-life in hepatic dysfunction and critical illness

Each anticoagulant has its benefits and drawbacks. Heparin remains the most commonly used anticoagulant in ECMO, primarily due to its familiarity. Limited data exist to guide the choice of anticoagulant, and the choice often is based on provider preference, local ECMO center protocols, and patient factors

ATIII antithrombin III, *HIT* heparin-induced thrombocytopenia

anticoagulation targets can improve outcomes, although emerging data does not support this strategy [110]. The ELSO guidelines note that ATIII can be monitored anywhere from daily to as needed, highlighting that there is currently no standardized approach to how or when ATIII supplementation should be given [92]. Literature has recommended various thresholds for repleting ATIII, including when ATIII is less than 50%, when ATIII is less than 100% and heparin requirements are higher than 45 units/kg/hour, or when aPTT, anti-Xa, and ATIII are subtherapeutic and heparin requirements are higher than 25 units/kg/hour in adults or 35–40 units/kg/hour in pediatric patients [29, 31].

9.4.3.2 Direct Thrombin Inhibitors

In a minority of ECMO centers or in situations where heparin is contraindicated (e.g., HIT), direct thrombin inhibitors (DTIs) are used as either the primary or the secondary choice of anticoagulation, respectively. As the name implies, DTIs bind directly to thrombin, inhibiting the conversion of fibrin to fibrinogen and the activation of factors V, VIII, and XI [24]. The DTIs most used in ECMO are argatroban and bivalirudin, and they have several advantages over heparin, including a predictable anticoagulant effect independent of antithrombin III and no risk for HIT (Table 9.1) [24]. Additionally, bivalirudin and argatroban bind circulating and clot-bound thrombin, suggesting that they may be more effective than heparin, which only binds circulating thrombin [24]. Argatroban and bivalirudin are monitored with aPTT or ACT and can markedly increase the INR disproportionate to their actual anticoagulant effects [24]. Despite these advantages, there are limitations that exist within the class and each specific agent. Unlike heparin, DTIs do not have a reversal agent and have considerations in organ dysfunction [24]. Bivalirudin has a short half-life (25 minutes), but is renally cleared, and requires significant dose reductions in renal dysfunction [24]. Argatroban is hepatically metabolized, and dose reductions are necessary with hepatic dysfunction; argatroban has demonstrated a prolonged half-life in critical illness and should be dose adjusted accordingly [24]. Bivalirudin is unique in that it is locally metabolized by proteases and therefore can disassociate from thrombin in static blood, increasing the risk of clotting, which can be of concern in low-flow ECMO states or in areas of the circuit where blood may pool (e.g., the oxygenator) [24]. Finally, DTIs are significantly more expensive than heparin; for a 70 kg patient receiving starting dose infusions of heparin, argatroban, and bivalirudin at wholesale acquisition pricing, the cost per day would be $12.50, $800, and $2200, respectively [6, 14].

The data for use of bivalirudin or argatroban in ECMO patients is largely limited to retrospective studies, case series, and case reports. Overall, the data for bivalirudin suggests that bivalirudin is comparable to heparin in terms of bleeding or thrombotic complications [24]. Patients in the studies were switched to bivalirudin, due to either HIT, heparin resistance, or intolerance to heparin (e.g., persistent clotting or bleeding). In one retrospective study of eight patients receiving ECMO postcardiotomy, there was significantly less blood loss associated with bivalirudin with no difference in thrombosis compared to heparin [117]. Of note, a more recent study did report thrombosis in the oxygenator and a 28% bleeding incidence as well as wide variation in dosing for patients who received bivalirudin [141]. Nearly all patients in the study received VV-ECMO for ARDS, except for two patients who received VA-ECMO post-cardiac surgery [141]. In one of the largest retrospective studies to date, 52 patients received either VV- or VA-ECMO for various indications, including respiratory failure, cardiogenic shock, or post-heart and/or lung transplant, and were anticoagulated with either heparin or bivalirudin [69]. At 7 days, the composite endpoints of thrombosis, major bleeding, in-hospital mortality, and 30-day mortality were no different between patients who received heparin versus bivalirudin, and the aPTT remained in the therapeutic range significantly longer for patients on bivalirudin versus heparin (85.7% vs. 50%; $p = 0.007$) [69].

Similarly, the data for argatroban overall suggests that its use in VV- and VA-ECMO may be safe and effective. In one large retrospective study of patients on VV-ECMO for ARDS with HIT or heparin resistance, 39 patients received argatroban, and a matched cohort of 39 patients received heparin as a comparator group [95]. The study found no differences in bleeding, thrombosis, rates of transfusion, and device-related complications [95]. Like bivalirudin, the aPTT was less likely to be subtherapeutic for argatroban compared to heparin [95]. In another propensity-matched cohort study of patients, specifically without HIT on VV-ECMO, thrombotic and bleeding events were similar between the argatroban and heparin groups; of note, the cost of using each anticoagulant was also similar, primarily driven by the higher number of blood products used (e.g., platelets) and HIT diagnostic tests sent in the heparin group [51]. When it comes to choosing between bivalirudin and argatroban, there are currently no head-to-head studies comparing the two agents, and the decision is often based on patient-specific factors.

9.4.4 Monitoring Anticoagulation

As mentioned previously, there are no standardized protocols regarding dosing and monitoring of anticoagulation in ECMO. Monitoring of heparin can be done utilizing aPTT, ACT, or anti-Xa, and DTIs can be monitored with aPTT or ACT. The ELSO guidelines make no recommendations as to the preferred laboratory monitoring parameter for heparin or DTIs, and note that each method has its advantages and disadvantages (Table 9.2) [92]. In addition to considering the various pros and cons of each method, patient factors also play a role in deciding the optimal method to choose including the patient's age, comorbidities, and other coagulation deficiencies the patient may have [29]. It is important to note that while these methods as a whole help to guide the clinician in determining the patient's response to anticoagulation, their results do not always correlate to outcomes; bleeding and thrombotic events can happen at subtherapeutic, therapeutic, or supratherapeutic levels [29]. In addition, these methods do not give a full picture of what is going on within the coagulation cascade and platelet activation, as they are only able to measure pieces of this very complex system [29].

The ACT is a whole blood test that is initiated through the stimulation of the contact activation pathway and measures the time to fibrin formation [29]. While ACT is a bedside test with a quick turnaround time and is relatively inexpensive, it has disadvantages. ACT assesses the coagulation response to many factors that impact hemostasis, which can be a benefit; however, this also means that ACT is affected by many different variables including high C-reactive protein levels, consumptive coagulopathies, hypothermia, platelet function, hypofibrinogenemia, and hemodilution [29, 101]. One of the largest concerns with the use of ACT in ECMO is its potential insensitivity to lower heparin ranges [29, 101]. While ACT for

Table 9.2 Advantages and disadvantages of anticoagulation monitoring methods [92]

Monitoring method	Pros	Cons
ACT	Bedside test Easy to use Quick turnaround time Inexpensive Assesses hemostasis response on a bigger picture level	Insensitive to low heparin ranges Affected by many factors (high CRP, consumptive coagulopathies)
aPTT	Widely available Familiar Sensitive to low heparin doses	Not immediately available results Affected by many factors (acute-phase reactants, fibrinogen, FVIII) High inter- and intra-patient variability Therapeutic range dependent upon the reagent used
Anti-Xa	Reliable accuracy Therapeutic range transferrable across institutions Correlates well with heparin concentrations	Affected by high plasma free hemoglobin and hyperbilirubinemia Assesses small part of overall hemostatic picture Not immediately available results Expensive

ACT activated clotting time, *aPTT* activated partial thromboplastin time
Several different monitoring methods may be employed for monitoring anticoagulants, depending on which anticoagulant is used. Choice of method should be based on turnaround time, cost, sensitivity, and specificity. A mixed monitoring method is often utilized

cardiopulmonary bypass targets high ranges of 400–800 seconds, for ECMO, targets are much lower at 180–200 seconds [29]. Studies have shown that there can be discordance between ACT and anti-Xa, particularly in patients with hemorrhagic complications, where ACT was <180 seconds but anti-Xa was >0.7 IU/mL [13, 84]. Other studies have shown poor correlation between the ACT result and the heparin dosing [7].

The aPTT measures time from factor XII activation via the contact activation pathway to fibrin formation specifically through the intrinsic pathway; however, unlike ACT, it uses plasma and not whole blood [29]. There are many different methods for measuring the aPTT, and its therapeutic range is highly dependent on calibration to the reagent used; this dependency makes the range of therapeutic aPTT levels widely variable, and therefore, the therapeutic range used in one ECMO center's protocols cannot necessarily be used at another center [29]. In general, the therapeutic range is 1.5–2.5 times the patient's baseline aPTT prior to starting anticoagulation; however, this range is not validated specifically in patients on ECMO [92]. The aPTT is one of the most commonly used methods for monitoring heparin or DTIs due to its wide availability and familiarity and correlates well with lower concentrations of heparin [92, 101]). The largest disadvantage to using aPTT is that in critically ill patients, the baseline aPTT may not be comparable to the baseline aPTT of a control population, which can impact the interpretation of the aPTT's measure of heparin's effects [92]. Additionally, the aPTT is affected by many variables, including factor VIII, fibrinogen levels, presence of antiphospholipid syndrome, and acute-phase reactants [92]. These variables can also change throughout the course of the patient's illness, leading to a high risk of intrapatient variability in aPTT levels, and they should therefore be interpreted within the clinical context of each patient [92].

The anti-Xa test directly measures the inhibition of factor Xa via heparin's effect on ATIII [29, 92]. While one of the major benefits of the anti-Xa level is that it correlates best with heparin concentrations versus ACT or aPTT, its major critique is that it only assesses a small part of heparin's impact on hemostasis [29]. Anti-Xa gives no insight into the prothrombotic state of a patient, including the amount of fibrin and thrombin being generated or the functionality of platelets [29, 92]. Additionally, anti-Xa can be impacted by high levels of plasma-free hemoglobin or hyperbilirubinemia [29, 92]. Despite these disadvantages, anti-Xa appears to be quite reliable and maintains a therapeutic range of 0.3–0.7 IU/mL universally [29].

As stated previously, there is no recommendation on the optimal lab method to use for monitoring anticoagulants in patients on ECMO; however, more ECMO centers are moving towards utilizing anti-Xa levels as the primary monitoring method due to their accuracy [29]. All methods have advantages and disadvantages, and limited studies are comparing these methods in a head-to-head fashion. In one single-center retrospective study of adult patients on ECMO, ACT, aPTT, anti-Xa, antithrombin level, and heparin dose were collected simultaneously on 37 patients for a total of 129 lab values [102]. Patients were on VV- or VA-ECMO for a median of 7 days for indications including ARDS, myocardial infarction, and acute myocarditis [102]. The study showed that the ACT was falsely elevated in patients with ATIII deficiency [102]. The aPTT and anti-Xa were well correlated (correlation coefficient 0.72) and were better correlated in patients with ATIII deficiency compared to those who did not have deficiency [102]. The study also found that the heparin dose was moderately correlated with anti-Xa and aPTT values but had no correlation with ACT in patients without ATIII deficiency (correlation coefficient 0.57, 0.62, and 0.16, respectively), and in patients with ATIII deficiency, the heparin dose moderately correlated with anti-Xa level only [102].

One large meta-analysis of 26 studies in VA-ECMO was conducted to determine the optimal targets and strategies for anticoagulation management in relation to complications such as bleeding and thrombosis [133]. Overall, the meta-analysis noted that the majority of studies were of low quality [133]. The study found that the prevalence of bleeding events was 50% in patients monitored solely by aPTT and that this prevalence decreased to 24% when patients were monitored by a mixture of methods [133]. Similarly, in patients with thromboembolic complications, the study found the prevalence to be 9–12% with ACT monitoring, 3% with aPTT monitoring, and 6% with a mixture of methods [133]. This suggests that perhaps it is best to not rely on one lab methodology when monitoring anticoagulation in patients on ECMO, as different methods may help to paint a fuller clinical picture when assessed together.

9.5 Pharmacokinetic Alterations in Patients on ECMO

9.5.1 Pharmacokinetic Changes in Critically Ill Patients

During a critical illness, the body undergoes a plethora of changes related to how drugs are absorbed, distributed, metabolized, and excreted (Table 9.3). These changes may require empiric dose alterations or more frequent monitoring for efficacy and safety. In addition to the changes occurring in the body, the use of support therapies, such as renal replacement or ECMO, provides unique challenges to the adequate dosing of medications.

Acute kidney injury (AKI) is a frequent complication of both critical illness and ECMO support (see Acute Kidney Injury and Renal Replacement Therapies section). Continuous renal replacement therapy (CRRT) is the most common renal replacement modality used in critically ill patients and provides another mechanism to alter drug pharmacokinetics. Similar to critically ill patients not on CRRT, patients on CRRT exhibit increased Vd, diminished clearance of renally eliminated medications, alterations in protein binding, and added complexity of drug adsorption to the dialyzer membrane [8].

Table 9.3 Selected pharmacokinetic changes in critical illness

Pharmacokinetic parameter	Physiologic change	Pharmacokinetic changes
Absorption	Increased gastric pH from PPI/H_2RA use	Decreased absorption of basic drugs
	Reduced perfusion to GI tract	Decreased absorption of oral formulations resulting in reduced concentrations
	Reduced perfusion to peripheral tissues	Decreased absorption of transdermal, sublingual, and intramuscular formulations
Distribution	Decreased albumin	Increased free concentration of acidic drugs
	Increased alpha-1-acid glycoprotein	Decreased concentration of basic drugs
	Volume resuscitation and fluid shifts (e.g., third spacing)	Increased volume of distribution
Metabolism	Induction or inhibition of hepatic enzymes	Increased or decreased clearance of low hepatic-cleared drugs
	Reduced hepatic blood flow	Decreased clearance of high hepatic-cleared drugs
Elimination	Acute kidney injury	Reduced drug clearance
	Renal replacement therapy	Variable effect on drug clearance

GI gastrointestinal, *H₂RA* histamine-2 receptor antagonist, *PPI* proton pump inhibitor
Adapted from Ref. [26]

9.5.2   Properties of the ECMO Circuit Affecting Pharmacokinetics

As previously mentioned, the ECMO circuit is composed of cannulas, tubing, oxygenator, heat exchanger, and blood pump. These components have undergone several technologic improvements since their inception to improve efficacy as well as temper potential complications. These changes include heparin-coated polyvinyl chloride tubing and cannulas to reduce drug adsorption and inflammatory response, silicone-based oxygenators replaced with polymethylpentene oxygenators with integrated heat exchangers for increased durability and reduced circuit changes, and conversion from roller to centrifugal pumps to decrease shear stress and hemolysis [26]. Despite these improvements, the ECMO circuit provides physical and chemical changes to drug distribution, which can result in profound therapeutic alterations.

The ECMO circuit and resultant priming add notable volume into the system and result in an increased Vd [59]. This increased Vd primarily affects hydrophilic drugs and results in decreased plasma concentrations and potentially therapeutic failure of the drug [59]. The increased volume from priming may also result in the hemodilution of plasma proteins, which can impact drugs that exhibit high protein binding, particularly to albumin. This can lead to toxicity caused by an increased free fraction of the drug that can exert its pharmacologic effect. Additionally, it is possible that certain blood components may compete with drugs for binding sites within the ECMO circuit. An ex vivo study demonstrated that the sequestration of certain drugs in blood-primed circuits was significantly less than in circuits that have been primed with crystalloid solutions [94].

9.5.3   Properties of the Drug Affecting Pharmacokinetics

In addition to the properties of the circuit materials, properties of the drug itself play a large role in whether the drug is susceptible to sequestration in the circuit. The most important characteristics are the amount of protein binding and lipophilicity of the drug molecule [59].

Drugs exhibit a wide variability of binding to plasma proteins such as albumin. Protein-bound drugs are not available for distribution into tissues or able to exert a pharmaceutical effect; however, the ECMO circuit can sequester both protein-bound and unbound medications, effectively removing them from circulation [128]. Protein binding >70% is considered to be "high," and protein binding <30% is considered to be "low" [113]. Highly protein-bound drugs will be too large to fit through the pores of the oxygenator membrane and will be sequestered out of circulation, while low protein-bound drugs will pass easily through the circuit membrane and remain in the blood. An ex vivo study showed that among medications with similar lipophilicity (discussed below), concentrations of high-protein-bound medications were significantly reduced in the ECMO circuit cohort [128].

Lipophilicity is expressed as the logarithm of the ratio of unionized drug dispersed in octanol (lipid layer) to unionized drug dispersed in water (i.e., the partition coefficient or logP). A positive logP indicates lipophilicity (a drug with a logP of 2 partitions 100 times more into octanol than into water), and a negative logP indicates hydrophilicity (a drug with a logP of −2 partitions 100 times more into water than octanol). Drugs with both high protein binding and high lipophilicity are most likely to be sequestered in the ECMO circuit [59]. In general, a logP >2 is considered to be "high" lipophilicity, and logP <1 is considered to be "low" lipophilicity (Patel et al. 2023). High-lipophilicity drugs will be attracted to and trapped in the membrane oxygenator fibers, while hydrophilic drugs will pass easily through the membrane and be more attracted to the hydrophilic blood plasma.

Upon initiation of ECMO, large amounts of drug adsorb onto the new, "clean" circuit. This results in a low concentration of drugs back to the body. Over time, once the circuit components are fully saturated, the adsorbed drug will be released back into circulation based on concentration gradients in the blood versus on the membrane and will potentially contribute more to the therapeutic effect. This cycle will repeat with each circuit change. In light of these pharmacokinetic changes with the ECMO in addition to the changes seen in critically ill patients and with CRRT, medication dosing in critically ill patients on ECMO (with and without CRRT) can be quite complex. Details and considerations for dosage will be addressed in the individual medication sections that follow.

9.6 Analgesia and Sedation Considerations in ECMO

9.6.1 Assessment of Pain and Sedation

The provision of analgesia and sedation to patients undergoing ECMO support is a standard of practice aimed at achieving various clinical goals. These goals include ensuring adequate pain control, preventing and addressing agitation, enhancing ventilator synchrony, optimizing ECMO flows, maintaining catheter positioning, reducing metabolic demands, enabling effective patient communication, promoting early liberation from ECMO, and ultimately improving long-term functional outcomes. Fundamental principles of managing pain and sedation should align with those applied to other critically ill patients of equal severity of illness, in accordance with international guidelines [43]. There are no specific sedation and analgesia guidelines tailored to patients undergoing ECMO support, and therefore, deviations from existing guidelines are anticipated in this complex patient population. For example, contrary to guideline recommendations advocating for light sedation, the initial 24–48 hours following ECMO cannulation may often necessitate deeper levels of sedation, especially if coupled with neuromuscular blockade, to optimize ECMO support and ventilatory support and prevent potential harm from cannula dislodgement. Deeper levels of sedation beyond the initial cannulation period may still be necessary to maintain appropriate ECMO support. Consequently, there is often a heightened need for more frequent utilization of benzodiazepines and increased doses of other analgesic and sedative medications compared to patients with equal severity of illness not receiving ECMO support. Nonetheless, following guideline-supported practices that advocate for targeting light levels of sedation and avoiding benzodiazepines when clinically suitable plays a vital role in promoting successful endotracheal extubation, preventing physical deconditioning, and enabling regular neurological assessment in ECMO-supported patients [47].

Monitoring of pain and sedation is essential to ensure the effectiveness of treatment and minimize medication overuse. In line with guideline recommendations, it is critical to define, measure, and perform routine daily reassessments of pain and sedation goals in order to adjust doses based on the individual needs of the patient at different stages of critical illness. Clinical monitoring involves subjective bedside assessment and objective evaluations using validated scoring instruments including the Behavioral Pain Scale (BPS), Critical-Care Pain Observation Tool (CPOT), and Richmond Agitation-Sedation Scale (RASS). In an international survey of 221 bedside clinicians caring for adult VV-ECMO patients, pain was primarily assessed using CPOT (42%) and BPS (36%), and level of sedation was assessed using RASS (90%). When clinical monitoring is unreliable in noncommunicative, deeply sedated, and paralyzed patients, the use of electrophysiological techniques in the form of electroencephalography (EEG), electromyography (EMG), and evoked potential signals may be employed [60]. However, the validity and reliability of these methods have not been investigated in ECMO patients [60].

9.6.2 Analgesic and Sedative Agents

9.6.2.1 Opioids

Critical care analgesia and sedation guidelines support an analgesia-first approach (i.e., analgosedation) to minimize the use of sedatives, with opioids remaining as the mainstay for pain management. For most mechanically ventilated ECMO patients, parenteral opioids are the cornerstone for pain management and sedative effects. Opioids are recommended to be used at the lowest effective dose with judicious titration as part of a multimodal analgesia regimen. The decision regarding which opioid to use and frequency of dosing (e.g., intermittent vs. continuous infusion) varies based on clinical goals, anticipated pharmacokinetic alterations during ECMO, and patient-specific factors such as hemodynamics and renal and hepatic function. In two international surveys, fentanyl was the most frequently reported opioid used by clinicians caring for VV-ECMO patients, followed by hydromorphone and morphine [25, 46].

Fentanyl, due to its rapid onset of action and ease of titration, is frequently utilized as the primary analgesic in critically ill patients. However, because fentanyl is both highly lipophilic and extensively protein bound (Table 9.4), its use among patients receiving ECMO support is less desirable due to the high probability of being sequestered within the ECMO circuit. Ex vivo studies have shown that >70% of the fentanyl dose is sequestered in the circuit as compared to ~20% of the hydromorphone dose [63, 126, 127]. To overcome this substantial loss, higher doses of fentanyl may be required to provide adequate pain relief in ECMO patients, or alternatively, other opioids (e.g., hydromorphone) may be considered. A comparison of hydromorphone or fentanyl-based sedation in 148 ECMO patients found a fourfold greater utilization of fentanyl equivalents in the fentanyl-based group as a secondary outcome [79]. The primary outcome of delirium-free, coma-free days, however, was also significantly less in the fentanyl-based group. These results were also demonstrated in a study of 52 ECMO patients receiving either fentanyl or hydromorphone continuous infusions. Opioid requirements, defined as morphine milligram equivalents, were significantly lower in the hydromorphone-based group at 24 and 48 hours with no change in pain or sedation scores or sedative use compared to the fentanyl-based group [90].

Hydromorphone, a hydrophilic and low protein-bound opioid (Table 9.4), may be considered as the preferred agent in patients receiving ECMO or as a second-line agent for patients who have inadequate pain control despite high doses of fentanyl (≥400 mcg/hour) [139]. Contrary to the increased fentanyl requirements seen in the Landoff and Martin studies discussed above, Browder and colleagues found no difference in opioid requirements between fentanyl- and hydromorphone-based regimens in predominately VV-ECMO patients [21]. Limitations of this study included clinician unfamiliarity with hydromorphone doses and titration and inclusion of patients receiving hydromorphone only within 24 hours of cannulation, which limits generalizability to patients who are switched to hydromorphone-based analgosedation after 24 hours of cannulation due to inadequacy of pain control with fentanyl.

Morphine, a hydrophilic and moderately protein-bound opioid (Table 9.4), has a low propensity for sequestration within the ECMO circuit. An ex vivo study evaluating morphine concentrations at 24 hours following administration of a single dose in blood-, crystalloid-, and albumin-primed ECMO circuits demonstrated no significant loss compared to baseline [126, 127]. Although morphine displays favorable physicochemical properties, it has not been as widely studied in adult ECMO

Table 9.4 Physiochemical properties of select opioids and sedatives used in ECMO

Opioids/sedatives	Protein binding	LogP
Dexmedetomidine	94%	2.8
Fentanyl	80–85%	4.05
Hydromorphone	10–20%	1.06
Ketamine	27%	3.12
Midazolam	97%	2.73
Morphine	20–35%	0.87
Lorazepam	85–90%	2.39
Propofol	99%	3.79

LogP log of partition coefficient
Information adapted from Lexicomp and DrugBank Online

patients. Furthermore, the use of morphine in the ICU for analgosedation is limited by risks of adverse effects that outweigh the benefits in critically ill patients. These adverse effects include hypotension associated with histamine release as well as prolonged sedation and risk of neurotoxicity in patients with renal dysfunction.

9.6.2.2 Ketamine

Ketamine, because of its N-methyl-d-aspartate (NMDA) receptor-blocking properties, provides both sedative and analgesic effects and is recommended in guidelines to be used at low doses as an adjunct to opioid therapy to improve wakefulness and reduce hyperalgesia and opioid consumption [43]. Since ketamine is moderately lipophilic but exhibits a low degree of protein binding (Table 9.4), it remains uncertain whether high doses are required to attain adequate sedation and reduce total opioid consumption in patients receiving ECMO. In a retrospective observational study, Tellor and colleagues evaluated opioid and sedative requirements among 26 ECMO patients concomitantly receiving a ketamine infusion at a median starting dose of 50 mg/hour (max 150 mg/hour). Within 2 hours of ketamine initiation, a meaningful reduction (defined as a change of at least dexmedetomidine 0.2 mcg/kg/hour, fentanyl 25 mcg/hour, midazolam 1 mg/hour, or propofol 10 mcg/kg/min) in sedative and opioid infusion doses was observed in more than a third of patients, without a change in the median RASS score at 24 hours [135]. Conversely, in a small randomized trial involving 20 VV-ECMO patients with ARDS, low-dose ketamine infusion did not lead to a reduction but instead increased the need for opioids or sedatives [45]. However, these findings could potentially be attributed to the titration of opioid and sedative dosages based on parameters other than the sedation goal, absence of a standardized sedation protocol, and inadequacy of ketamine dosing. There is limited data supporting changes in ketamine pharmacokinetic parameters during ECMO. In two case reports, ketamine administered at doses of 2 mg/kg/hour compared to 0.625 mg/kg/hour reached sufficient mean steady-state plasma concentrations, similar to critically ill patients not receiving ECMO support [50, 77]. Although the benefits of ketamine among ECMO patients remain to be elucidated, studies have not indicated significant harm associated with its use. Initiating ketamine at low-to-moderate doses as an adjunctive agent may be reasonable in patients on ECMO failing to achieve target pain and sedation goals, despite the use of opioids and other sedative agents.

9.6.2.3 Propofol

Propofol is a highly lipophilic and extensively protein-bound agent that possesses sedative, hypnotic, and anxiolytic properties (Table 9.4). Propofol is a frequently used sedative in the ICU owing to its immediate onset, ease of titration, and short duration of action, much like fentanyl. Among patients receiving ECMO support, concerns have been raised regarding the lipophilic nature of propofol and its potential impact on adsorption and oxygenator failure. Several studies evaluating propofol-based sedation strategies among ECMO patients found no difference in the rate of oxygenator exchange in those receiving propofol versus those who did not [21, 67, 78]. Not surprisingly, higher median daily doses of propofol were required in patients who did not require oxygenator exchanges [67]. Despite evidence indicating that propofol likely does not increase oxygenator exchanges, the loss of propofol in the ECMO circuit can be significant. An ex vivo study reported a 70% decrease in propofol concentrations within only 30 minutes of administration [81]. In regard to dosing of propofol, a retrospective study showed that the use of propofol to achieve light levels of sedation in predominantly VV-ECMO patients with ARDS showed no significant increases in median daily doses throughout the duration of ECMO support [112]. On the contrary, propofol doses increased to peak levels on day 3 of ECMO support in a cohort of VV-ECMO patients with ARDS requiring deep sedation [37]. Most clinicians report using propofol when caring for VV-ECMO patients requiring deep levels of sedation [46]. Since propofol is prone to significant circuit sequestration, higher than recommended doses may be necessary to achieve target sedation, especially deeper levels of sedation. Use of propofol at high doses for a prolonged period of time may be limited by hypotension, propofol-related infusion syndrome, or hypertriglyceridemia [10, 132].

9.6.2.4 Benzodiazepines

While non-benzodiazepine sedatives are the preferred agents to improve short- and long-term outcomes in mechanically ventilated critically ill patients, the use of benzodiazepines as an alternative or concomitant therapy may be necessary in ECMO patients when sedation goals are unmet or deep sedation is desired. When targeting deep sedation for VV-ECMO patients, 24% and 41% of clinicians reported using benzodiazepines as a first- and second-line agent, respectively. Benzodiazepines, such as midazolam and lorazepam, are highly lipophilic and extensively protein-bound sedatives, which render them highly susceptible to sequestration within the ECMO circuit (Table 9.4).

Significant sequestration of midazolam was observed in two ex vivo ECMO circuitry experiments with losses at 24 hours of 87% and 89% [81, 126, 127]. To corroborate these findings of circuitry loss, Shekar and colleagues demonstrated a 10% increase (average 18 mg/day) in the daily dose of midazolam after ECMO cannulation to maintain deep sedation [126, 127]. Several observational studies in patients receiving ECMO support for severe ARDS demonstrated high sedative requirements when a deep level of sedation is targeted. DeBacker and colleagues found a need for high midazolam doses, with a median requirement of 202 mg in the first 48 hours following ECMO cannulation (DeBacker et al. 2018). Similarly, a retrospective study of patients with ARDS managed with and without ECMO support demonstrated a twofold increase in the maximum 6-hour sedative exposure in the ECMO-supported group; however, an adjusted analysis found that the ECMO circuit did not have a significant effect on the cumulative sedative doses administered from the start of ECMO to the point at which the maximum 6-hour sedative exposure was achieved [41]. DeGrado and colleagues [39] reported significantly lower sedative requirements compared to previous trials in a mixed cohort of VV- and VA-ECMO patients. Benzodiazepine continuous infusions were administered on less than half of the ECMO days, with a median daily dose (expressed in midazolam equivalents) of 24 mg. Moreover, there were no increased requirements throughout the duration of ECMO support. These reduced sedative requirements could be attributed to lower sedation goals, use of non-benzodiazepine infusions, and variable ECMO indications.

Lorazepam, being comparatively less lipophilic than midazolam yet extensively protein bound, is an appealing alternative agent that has demonstrated a lower degree of loss within the ECMO circuit at 24 hours compared to midazolam (59% vs. 83%) [62]. However, routine use of lorazepam as a sedative in critically ill patients with and without ECMO support is limited by the risk of propylene glycol toxicity in parenteral and enteral solution forms of lorazepam that can result in metabolic acidosis, seizures, respiratory depression, and renal insufficiency. Only 18% of clinicians reported using lorazepam as the preferred benzodiazepine among adult VV-ECMO patients in an international survey [25]. Although the superiority of a specific benzodiazepine has not been established, midazolam has been subject to more extensive in vivo research and, as a result, may be the preferred choice as a sedative.

9.6.2.5 Dexmedetomidine

Dexmedetomidine, a highly lipophilic and extensively protein-bound sedative, has been associated with significant losses in the ECMO circuit (Table 9.4), as demonstrated in an in vitro study observing 24-hour losses between 67% and 93% and 67% and 88% for new and old circuits, respectively [140]. This study also found no difference in pre- and post-oxygenator concentrations, suggesting that the polyvinyl chloride tubing contributes to dexmedetomidine loss. Dexmedetomidine's mechanism of alpha-2 receptor agonism exerts sedative and anxiolytic effects without inducing respiratory depression. Despite concerns of circuit sequestration, these pharmacologic characteristics make dexmedetomidine an ideal sedative when aiming for lighter levels of sedation or when weaning midazolam or propofol. For patients on VV-ECMO with lighter sedation goals (e.g., RASS 0 to −1), clinicians often reported dexmedetomidine as their preferred choice for both initial and secondary sedation when aiming for a lighter level of sedation [46]. While limited clinical data exists on the use of dexmedetomidine in ECMO patients, a small retrospective study of 26 ECMO patients reported 92% receiving dexmedetomidine at a median dose of 0.7 mcg/kg/hour. The authors observed no significant increases in median daily dose of dexmedetomidine throughout the duration of ECMO support [112].

9.7 Infection Considerations in ECMO

ELSO registry data reports nosocomial infection prevalence of up to 21% in adults and a culture positivity rate of up to 65% with an associated increase in mortality [3, 16]. Bizzarro and colleagues reported that an indication of eCPR and VA cannulation was associated with the highest rates of infection. Coagulase-negative staphylococci were the most common organisms, followed by *Candida, Pseudomonas aeruginosa, Staphylococcus aureus*, and other gram-negative organisms [16]. In a meta-analysis by Li and colleagues, the prevalence of nosocomial infections was 8.8–64% with a relative 32% increased risk of death compared to noninfected ECMO patients [83]. Independent risk factors for infection included duration of ECMO, high severity of illness score (e.g., sequential organ failure assessment), age, time on ventilator prior to ECMO, and use of VV cannulation [83]. The most common causative organisms were gram negative (*Acinetobacter baumannii*, enteric bacilli, and *Klebsiella pneumoniae*); however, gram-positive and fungal organisms were also reported [83]. Early infections in ECMO are usually the result of gram-positive skin flora and gram-negative organisms found in the femoral cannulation site; late ECMO infections may result from these same pathogens or fungal pathogens, particularly yeast [123]. Given the variety of potential organisms associated with nosocomial infections during ECMO, a broad-spectrum antimicrobial strategy is often employed.

9.7.1 Aminoglycosides

As a class, aminoglycosides are minimally protein bound and hydrophilic (Table 9.5). The effect of the ECMO circuit sequestration on this class is expected to be minimal, though increased Vd in critically ill patients, with or without ECMO, may result in the need for higher aminoglycoside doses. An observational, case-control study of 46 ECMO patients showed no significant difference in peak concentrations of amikacin compared to non-ECMO critically ill patients [56]. There was also no difference in the prevalence of subtherapeutic, therapeutic, and supratherapeutic levels between the groups; however, 50% of ECMO patients and 64% of non-ECMO patients had amikacin levels outside of the therapeutic range. A prospective, observational study of 44 ECMO patients found that in eight patients receiving aminoglycosides, gentamicin, and tobramycin, therapeutic peaks were achieved in all patients, but only 37.5% of amikacin peak levels were therapeutic [18]. Therapeutic drug monitoring (TDM) is routinely performed for aminoglycosides, and this data emphasizes the importance of TDM in critically ill patients, especially in those on either ECMO, CRRT, or both.

9.7.2 Beta-Lactams

Beta-lactams with or without beta-lactamase inhibitors generally have low protein binding and low logP across the class, with the exception of ceftriaxone being 85–90% protein bound (Table 9.5). Given these characteristics, these agents do not bind significantly to the ECMO circuit and are cleared with the same frequency as a non-ECMO patient. In a study of 105 ECMO patients (majority VV) receiving either piperacillin, ceftazidime, meropenem, or linezolid, there was no difference in total serum concentrations of ceftazidime and high-dose (6 g/day) meropenem compared to non-ECMO patients [76]. Serum concentrations of piperacillin/tazobactam and standard-dose (3 g/day) meropenem were significantly reduced in patients on ECMO; however, all median values met therapeutic targets. There was also an association between increased ceftazidime and meropenem concentrations with prolonged use of the same ECMO circuit membrane, indicating that once the membrane is saturated, sequestration subsides and serum concentrations increase [76]. Other studies have shown 80–100% of therapeutic level attainment with ceftolozane/tazobactam, cefepime, ceftazidime, meropenem, and piperacillin/tazobactam [5, 18, 61]. Overall, ECMO does not have a significant effect on the pharmacokinetics and pharmacodynamic profiles of beta-lactam antibiotics. Use of continuous-infusion antimicrobials has been shown to improve cure rates and mortality in critically ill patients and should be utilized, along with TDM when possible, to optimize antimicrobial efficacy.

Table 9.5 Physiochemical properties of select antibiotics used in ECMO

Antibiotic	Protein binding	LogP
Amikacin	10%	−3.2
Ceftaroline	20%	−0.79
Ceftolozane/tazobactam	20%/30%	−6.17/−1.8
Ceftriaxone	85–90%	−1.7
Cefepime	20%	−0.37
Daptomycin	84–93%	−0.47
Gentamicin	<30%	−3.1
Imipenem/cilastatin	20%/40%	−0.19/−0.29
Linezolid	31%	0.9
Meropenem	2%	−0.6
Piperacillin/tazobactam	30%/30%	0.3/−1.8
Tobramycin	<30%	−5.8
Vancomycin	55%	−3.1

LogP log of partition coefficient
Information adapted from Lexicomp and DrugBank Online

9.7.3 Glycopeptides, Lipopeptides, and Oxazolidinones

Daptomycin, linezolid, and vancomycin exhibit variable protein binding but relatively low lipophilicity (Table 9.5). Data for daptomycin in ECMO is limited to ex vivo studies, which demonstrate no significant decrease in daptomycin concentrations or sequestration in the circuit [30, 70]. In a case report of three patients on ECMO who received standard-dose linezolid (1200 mg/day), adequate concentrations were achieved if the MIC was ≤1 for methicillin-resistant *Staphylococcus aureus* pneumonia [38]. Ex vivo studies demonstrate minimal sequestration of vancomycin in the ECMO circuit [94, 126, 127]. An observational study of 11 ECMO patients (55% VV) matched with 11 control patients demonstrated similar vancomycin concentrations between ECMO and non-ECMO patients when administered as a loading dose over 4 hours followed by a daily continuous infusion [44]. However, in a study of 20 patients (55% VA), 95% were found to require a dose increase after initial non-steady-state trough levels were obtained on standard dosing (mean 16 mg/kg q12h) [111]. It is important to note that patients in this study did not receive a loading dose of vancomycin, and the low initial trough results are likely due to the increased Vd of vancomycin in critically ill ECMO patients and lack of a loading dose rather than due to ECMO circuit sequestration of vancomycin. A recent study of 116 patients on ECMO (61% VA) treated with vancomycin (25 mg/kg load followed by 15 mg/kg q12h) found that only 18% of patients had >50% of levels in the therapeutic range (Marella et al. 2020). The highest proportion of subtherapeutic levels was noted in patients on ECMO for <6 days, and levels for patients on ECMO for 6–13 days were significantly more likely to be therapeutic. Conversely, patients on CRRT were more likely to have supratherapeutic levels. While physiochemical properties have shown that vancomycin is not prone to circuit sequestration, the conflicting data with in vivo studies underlines the importance of TDM monitoring for vancomycin in critically ill ECMO patients.

9.7.4 Antifungals

Azole derivatives have moderate-to-high protein binding and high lipophilicity, with the exception of fluconazole, and therefore would be more likely to sequester into the ECMO circuit components (Table 9.6). In a study of 85 patients on ECMO, of the 10 who received fluconazole, 9 had adequate serum concentrations [125]. Eighty percent of the fluconazole patients were on concomitant RRT, including the one patient who had concentrations below target. In a retrospective study of 132 patients receiving voriconazole, first trough concentrations were significantly lower in the ECMO group compared to non-ECMO patients. The ECMO patients were significantly younger and had a higher SOFA score at baseline. This study found the use of ECMO to be an independent risk factor of below target voriconazole exposure [147]. Another retrospective study of 69 patients (74% VV-ECMO) did not find

Table 9.6 Physiochemical properties of select antifungals used in ECMO

Antifungal	Protein binding	LogP
Caspofungin	97%	0.17
Fluconazole	12%	0.5
Isavuconazole	>98%	3.46
Micafungin	>99%	−1.5
Posaconazole	>99%	5.5
Voriconazole	58%	1.65

LogP log of partition coefficient
Information adapted from Lexicomp and DrugBank Online

a difference in median trough concentrations on ECMO versus non-ECMO days; however, 48% of all samples were subtherapeutic despite a median trough concentration within the goal range [137, 138].

Contrary to what the physiochemical properties might predict, isavuconazole and posaconazole pharmacokinetics show minimal changes during ECMO. A prospective study of seven ECMO patients (86% VV) receiving isavuconazole for aspergillosis prophylaxis found no difference between serum, pre-oxygenator, or post-oxygenator levels. Target plasma levels were obtained within 24 hours and maintained for the duration of the study utilizing standard doses. No breakthrough fungal infections were observed [74]. In a study of six ECMO patients (100% VV) receiving posaconazole, all trough levels achieved the target range for prophylaxis ($\geq$0.7 mg/L), and 69% achieved the target for treatment ($\geq$1 mg/dL) [137, 138]. Since these studies are small, robust conclusions cannot be made, and further ex vivo studies will elucidate the true effect of the ECMO circuit on isavuconazole and posaconazole. It is hypothesized that since the Vd of the agents in critically ill patients is large at baseline, further increases in Vd from the ECMO circuit may not have a clinically meaningful effect [137, 138]. Based on these results, empiric dose changes may not be warranted with the use of azole antifungals in ECMO patients; however, TDM should be implemented when possible, especially if treating invasive fungal infections.

Echinocandins as a class have a very high degree of protein binding (>90%) and low lipophilicity (Table 9.6). An observational, prospective study in 12 ECMO patients receiving micafungin for prophylaxis found no difference in micafungin concentrations pre- and post-oxygenator membrane. No breakthrough fungal infections were observed [85]. Studies and case reports have also found no effect of ECMO on anidulafungin and caspofungin [87]. No studies have yet evaluated the effect of ECMO on rezafungin. No empiric dose adjustments seem to be necessary with the use of echinocandin agents on ECMO.

9.8 Fluid Management Considerations in ECMO

As mentioned in the prior section on fluid management, maintaining euvolemia with adequate perfusion in the setting of ECMO can be very challenging. Euvolemia can be achieved through the use of loop diuretics with or without additional agents

Table 9.7 Physiochemical properties of select diuretics used in ECMO

Diuretic	Protein binding	LogP
Bumetanide	96%	2.6
Chlorothiazide	40%	−0.24
Furosemide	99%	2.09
Metolazone	95%	2.5
Torsemide	>99%	3.36

LogP log of partition coefficient
Information adapted from Lexicomp and DrugBank Online

(e.g., thiazide diuretics) for fluid removal. A paucity of data exists on appropriate dosing of diuretics in ECMO. The suitable dose required to achieve the desired urine output is often determined through a process of trial and error by clinicians. Limited data in pediatric patients suggest that there may be a need to administer higher initial bolus doses of bumetanide and furosemide [122, 142].

Bumetanide and furosemide have high lipophilicity and are highly protein bound (Table 9.7), which may make them susceptible to circuit sequestration. An in vitro analysis of furosemide disposition within four neonatal ECMO circuits demonstrated 63–87% reduction in serum concentrations over a 4-hour observation period when doses of 5 mg and 10 mg were administered [23]. While intermittent and continuous infusion dosing of loop diuretics is a common practice in many institutions, limited data exists to guide practice in patients on ECMO. Some institutions prefer the use of continuous infusions over intermittent doses to prevent fluctuations in diuretic serum concentrations and to potentially overcome drug sequestration. Nevertheless, there is no available comparative data to endorse one dosing strategy over the other in ECMO patients. Thiazide diuretics display widely variable physiochemical properties, with chlorothiazide being the least protein bound and lipophilic. There are no studies evaluating the effect of ECMO on thiazide diuretics. Standard doses can be initiated and titrated for clinical response. For cases of refractory diuresis or overt renal failure, renal replacement therapy (RRT) can be initiated.

9.8.1 Acute Kidney Injury and Renal Replacement Therapies

Acute kidney injury (AKI) is a frequent complication in patients receiving ECMO treatment, resulting in increased morbidity and mortality [108]. The incidence of AKI in ECMO-supported patients is widely variable and ranges from 26% to 85% due to differences in AKI definition, patient characteristics, ECMO modes, and clinical setting [121]. The combined estimated incidence of severe AKI necessitating RRT is approximately 45%. The prevalence of AKI is greater with VA-ECMO compared to VV-ECMO at 61% and 46%, respectively, and is most often observed on the day of ECMO cannulation [108]. Patient-specific factors prior to ECMO initiation that contribute to AKI include hemodynamic instability, reduced cardiac output, elevated intrathoracic and intra-abdominal pressures, exposure to nephrotoxic agents, sepsis, bleeding, coagulopathy, severe hypoxemia, and hypercapnia.

Following cannulation, ECMO-related factors that contribute to AKI include ischemia–reperfusion injury, continuous flow during VA-ECMO, hemolysis, malposition of cannulas, higher pump speeds, and release of inflammatory cytokines induced by blood exposure to artificial surfaces. Several standardized definitions including the Risk, Injury, Failure, Loss, End-stage (RIFLE) criteria, the Acute Kidney Injury Network (AKIN) criteria, and the Kidney Disease Improving Global Outcomes (KDIGO) guidelines have been validated in non-ECMO-supported patients and allow for the classification of AKI by both serum creatinine and urine output. Fluid overload is another manifestation of kidney dysfunction and, as previously mentioned, is associated with negative clinical outcomes. Since AKI and fluid overload are both linked to higher mortality rates, treatment of these comorbidities is recommended to improve ECMO outcomes.

Fluid overload and AKI are the most common indications for RRT on ECMO. According to an international survey, the primary reasons for initiating RRT during ECMO were the management of fluid overload (43%) and prevention (16%) of fluid overload (16%). This was followed by AKI (35%) and electrolyte disturbances (4%) [52]. Early initiation of continuous renal replacement therapy (CRRT) while on ECMO has demonstrated beneficial outcomes in neonates [108]; however, similar data in adult patients receiving ECMO are lacking, and optimal timing to initiate CRRT is not well defined. Several randomized controlled trials conducted in critically ill adult patients with AKI have failed to demonstrate a survival benefit of the early (<12 hours) strategy for RRT initiation compared to delayed (>48–72 hours) strategy. Instead, earlier initiation increased the risk of dialysis dependence at 90 days and adverse events [9, 11, 55]. A retrospective study using propensity score matching of 94 adult patients on ECMO compared early initiation of CRRT to delayed initiation (median time to CRRT initiation, 1.1 vs. 14.6 days) and found no benefit on hospital length of stay (LOS) or mortality benefit with early initiation [109]. Given that serum creatinine, urine output, and staging of AKI have been proven to be unreliable markers for guiding initiation of RRT, a concept known as "demand-capacity" has been suggested to assist in the decision-making process. This concept proposes that RRT should be considered if the extent of AKI-related metabolic disturbances and fluid overload are going to surpass the kidney's ability to compensate and when conventional pharmacological interventions like diuretics and sodium bicarbonate are going to be ineffective. Therefore, RRT should be initiated in adult ECMO patients in situations where fluid overload is refractory to diuretic therapies and when AKI-related metabolic derangements impede chances of cardiopulmonary failure recovery.

While on ECMO, various modalities of RRT can be administered including intermittent hemodialysis (IHD), sustained low-efficiency dialysis (SLED), peritoneal dialysis, and any CRRT modality such as hemofiltration (CVVH), hemodialysis (CVVHD), and hemodiafiltration (CVVHDF). Each RRT modality has advantages and disadvantages. Three main techniques exist for delivering RRT with ECMO: (1) RRT device connected using independent access from ECMO circuit (parallel system), (2) in-line hemofilter, and (3) RRT device connected within the ECMO circuit (integrated system) (Fig. 9.5). For parallel systems, a separate vascular access point ensures that the RRT machine does not interfere with ECMO flows. While this technique is a simple approach in patients who have vascular access prior to ECMO cannulation, a potential disadvantage is an increased risk of bleeding when introducing a new dialysis catheter since ECMO patients commonly receive anticoagulation to minimize clot formation in the ECMO circuit. With this configuration, CRRT is managed similarly to patients not on ECMO, with the exception that additional anticoagulation for the CRRT circuit may not be necessary. In-line hemofilters are inserted by creating a shunt post-pump and pre-oxygenator within the ECMO circuit. In-line hemofilters are mainly used for ultrafiltration using SCUF mode; however, CVVH or CVVHD can be delivered through standard infusion pumps (Fig. 9.5). In-line hemofilters were the first method to provide CRRT during ECMO, with the advantages of being inexpensive, less resource intensive, and simple to set up. However, multiple disadvantages include inaccurate fluid removal, ECMO recirculation, and absence of a pressure monitor to detect hemolysis, filter rupture, or thrombus formation. Integrating a commercially available CRRT machine in-line with the ECMO circuit provides superior control of fluid balance and clearance of solutes compared to an in-line hemofilter. This technique requires a thorough understanding of circuit pressures since pre-ECMO pump pressures are negative (-20 to -100 mmHg) and post-ECMO pump pressures are positive ($+150$ to $+350$ mmHg), and these pressure differences might interfere with the CRRT circuit [108]. There are many ways to integrate the CRRT device into the ECMO circuit, and the optimal connection depends on multiple factors, including ECMO circuit design, type of ECMO pump, and CRRT device. Risks associated with introducing additional catheters to the ECMO circuit for RRT delivery include hemolysis and thrombosis because of ECMO circuit manipulation. The effectiveness of any specific RRT technique is not well supported by existing evidence, and therefore, clinical practices rely on expert opinion, local expertise, and availability of machines and resources. A 2012 international survey of 65 ECMO centers revealed that most centers (50.8%) use independent CRRT circuits within the ECMO circuit, compared to in-line hemofilters (21.5%) [52]. In general, many centers prefer to perform CRRT through venous access independent of the ECMO circuit.

As with ECMO support, the addition of RRT does not resolve the underlying cause of organ failure, and providing effective pharmacotherapy is imperative to treat these causes. The presence of extracorporeal therapies (e.g., ECMO and RRT), especially when combined, can further exacerbate existing pathophysiological changes from critical illness. Consequently, the interplay between critical illness, ECMO, and RRT significantly alters the pharmacokinetics (i.e., volume of distribution and drug clearance) of important medications such as antibiotics, opioids, and sedatives. Conventional dosing strategies seldom consider the impact of altered pharmacokinetics and thus may lead to variations in drug concentrations resulting in therapeutic failure or drug toxicity in a considerable portion of critically ill patients receiving ECMO and RRT. Literature supporting optimal dosing strategies in patients receiving both ECMO and RRT is lacking, which can be explained by difficulties in estimating pharmacokinetic parameters in the presence of two

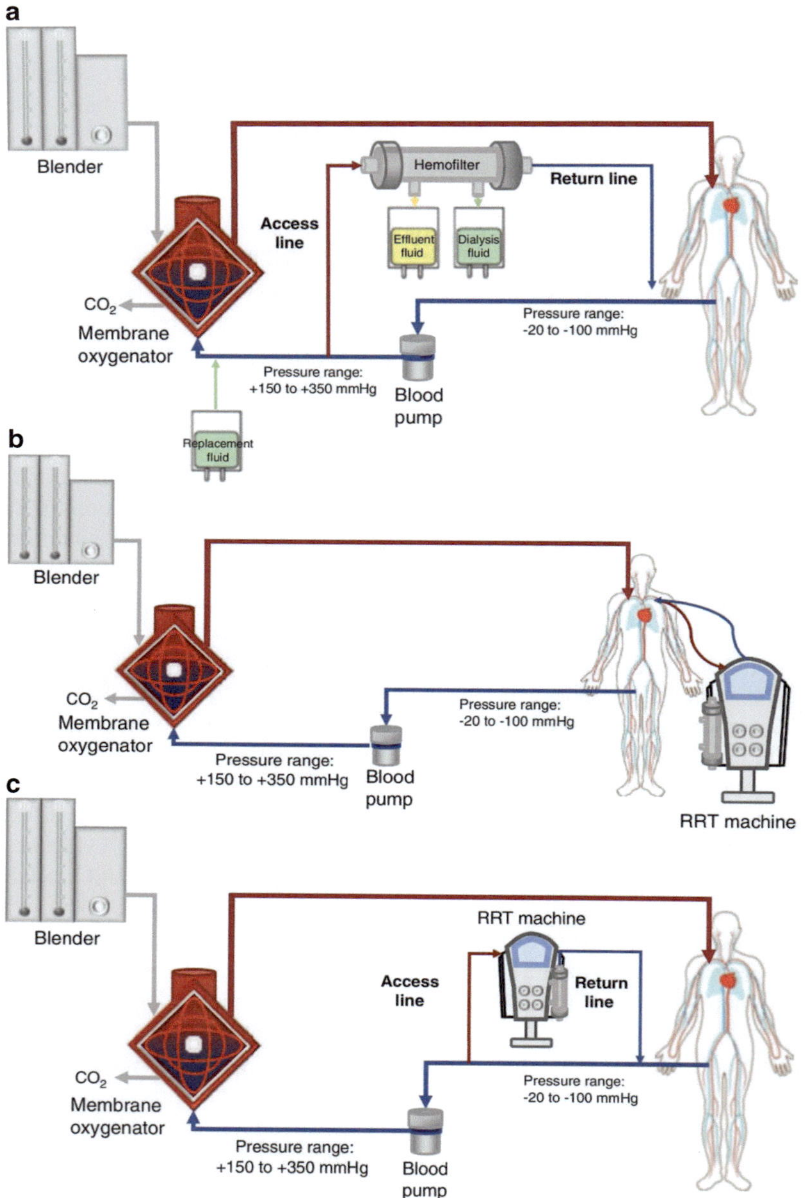

Fig. 9.5 Continuous renal replacement therapy with ECMO. Various options of combining ECMO and CRRT: (1) An in-line hemofilter is integrated into the ECMO circuit. Replacement fluid is directly administered into the ECMO circuit. Alternatively, dialysis fluid can be supplied in a countercurrent position. Replacement/dialysis fluid rates and ultrafiltration rates can be controlled via infusion pumps. (2) The CRRT device is connected to the patient through a separate catheter independent of the ECMO circuit. The access (inlet) and the return (outlet) lines of the CRRT device are connected before the centrifugal blood pump (low-pressure part) of the ECMO circuit [108]. *CRRT*, continuous renal replacement therapy, *ECMO* extracorporeal membrane oxygenation

extracorporeal circuits. To make informed decisions in the absence of robust data, an in-depth understanding of physicochemical properties of medications must be considered when assessing the impact both ECMO and RRT have on pharmacokinetic changes (see "Properties of the Drug Affecting Pharmacokinetics" section). For RRT, serum concentrations and half-life of medications depend on blood/dialysate flow and sieving coefficient of the hemodialyzer. In general, modifying conventional RRT dosing strategies based on pharmacokinetic changes from ECMO and patient-specific factors can be employed until more data becomes available.

9.9 Other Complications

9.9.1 Bleeding

Bleeding is the most common medical complication of ECMO, with an incidence ranging between 30% and 60% [103]. Data shows that the risk of major bleeding is similar between VA- and VV-ECMO and can be contributed to the use of anticoagulation, platelet dysfunction, underlying comorbidities, critical condition of the patient during ECMO, or supratherapeutic aPTT [103]. Bleeding can happen at any site, including surgical, cannulation, intrathoracic, abdominal, intracerebral, retroperitoneal, or pulmonary [88]. Bleeding is associated with worse outcomes; studies have shown that major bleeding on the first day of ECMO is associated with a two- to three-fold increase in the risk of in-hospital or 90-day mortality as well as longer ECMO durations [103].

Management of bleeding may vary slightly depending on the site of the bleeding; however, there is consensus that anticoagulation should be temporarily held until bleeding is controlled [88, 92]. While anticoagulation is held, serial monitoring for circuit thrombosis is essential [92]. If bleeding occurs at the surgical or cannulation site, topical hemostatics may suffice, with consideration for systemic aminocaproic acid or tranexamic acid [92]. Internal bleeding or more severe surgical or cannulation site bleeding may require transfusions; however, studies are lacking in regard to best practices. Table 9.8 outlines recommended goals per the ELSO guidelines.

Reversal agents for severe hemorrhage, such as prothrombin complex concentrates or activated recombinant factor VII (rFVIIa), have limited use and data in the ECMO population. One small case series in pediatric patients on ECMO showed successful hemostasis with no thromboembolic events following the use of rFVIIa; however, a larger case series showed success in bleeding cessation but a major stroke, circuit thrombosis, and a high mortality rate [118, 144]. The use of these agents should only be considered at this time for intractable bleeding where the benefits outweigh the risks.

Steps have been taken to prevent bleeding complications including improvements in surgical techniques and changes in the coatings of ECMO cannulas and tubing [103]. A small, retrospective study showed that the use of prophylactic anticoagulation with subcutaneous enoxaparin 40 mg daily resulted in no fatal or

Table 9.8 Blood product and goals for bleeding and non-bleeding patients [49]

Blood product	Goal
Platelets	>100,000 × 10⁹/L (bleeding) 50,000 – 100,000 × 10⁹/L (non-bleeding)
Fibrinogen	>150 mg/L (bleeding) >100 g/L (non-bleeding)
Hemoglobin	>7–9 g/dL

intracranial hemorrhage, 18% incidence of clinically relevant bleeding, and 6.5% incidence of thrombosis resulting in pump exchange [75]. Other studies demonstrated that the use of no anticoagulation resulted in a similar prevalence of bleeding events as those who were anticoagulated and meeting ACT or aPTT targets, with either a significantly higher or a similar prevalence of thromboembolic events [104, 133].

9.9.2 Thrombosis

Thrombotic complications typically occur within the circuit and are less likely to occur compared to bleeding complications, with an incidence of 10–20% [88, 104]. The pathogenesis of thrombotic complications stems paradoxically from many of the same factors that cause bleeding, including critical illness, underlying comorbidities, and aspects of the ECMO circuit itself such as its nonpulsatile blood flow and exposure of blood to the circuit tubing [104]. Thrombosis is more likely to occur in VV- versus VA-ECMO at 22.1% and 15.6%, respectively, potentially due to lower flow states with VV-ECMO [104].

Thrombosis most commonly occurs within the circuit itself, and particularly within the oxygenator of the circuit [88, 104]. Circuit thrombosis only becomes clinically relevant when it requires circuit/oxygenator exchange, or when high levels of hemolysis are present, as measured by plasma free hemoglobin [92]. Hemolysis leading to high plasma free hemoglobin levels can cause hemoglobinuria nephropathy, endothelial dysfunction, and vasoconstriction and increases the risk of death [92]. Circuit thrombosis can cause malfunction or reduced efficiency of the device [104]. Thrombosis is prevented and treated with the use of anticoagulation and serial visual inspections of the circuit and oxygenator [88]. One small case report shows success with the use of low-dose tissue plasminogen activator (5–20 mg) to treat life-threatening oxygenator thrombosis [134]. Of note, HIT is a possible underlying cause of thrombosis in the ECMO population treated with heparin and should be considered as part of the thrombotic workup [88].

Outside of circuit thrombosis, leg ischemia is also a possible thrombotic complication with an incidence of 10% and has primarily been reported in VA-ECMO due to cannulation of the femoral artery, although it is still possible in VV-ECMO [104]. The use of distal perfusion catheters helps to ensure perfusion and potentially prevent limb ischemia [17, 104]. Conservative strategies, including removal and repositioning of the cannula, maintaining anticoagulation on the high end of the therapeutic range, optimizing peripheral temperature, and limiting the use of vasoconstrictors, are often enough to reverse limb ischemia; however, fasciotomy or amputation may be necessary in severe or irreversible cases [17].

9.9.3 Neurologic

The indications and cannulation techniques of ECMO are commonly associated with alterations in perfusion, which can frequently result in neurologic injury. Neurologic injury increases mortality in hospitalized patients, and this trend continues in ECMO patients with neurologic complications [148]. Neurologic injury has been reported more frequently in patients on VA-ECMO compared to VV-ECMO; however, when excluding eCPR, the incidence is similar between VA- and VV-ECMO [97, 148].

Patients undergoing VA-ECMO may experience reduced blood flow to the left heart and thrombosis in the circuit or cannula, resulting in a neurologic event, most typically acute ischemic stroke (AIS). A meta-analysis of 878 VA-ECMO patients found a 7.4% overall rate of brain injury with 5.3% acute ischemic stroke and 2.8% intracranial bleeding [80]. Risk factors for AIS identified in this study were central cannulation and platelets >350 K/cu mm at the time of cannulation. AIS was not associated with anticoagulant use, fibrinogen level, or platelet counts during ECMO. Risk factors for intracranial bleeding were female sex, central cannulation, and platelets <100 K/cu mm at the time of cannulation. Platelet count <100 K/cu mm at the time of cannulation was also associated with mortality in this study [80]. North VV-ECMO is most often associated with intracranial hemorrhage, including subarachnoid and petechial intraparenchymal hemorrhage [148]. A retrospective analysis of the ELSO database found that 7.1% of VV-ECMO patients experienced a neurologic injury, most often intracranial hemorrhage (42.5%). Neurologic injury was associated with a 75.8% in-hospital mortality compared to 37.8% in VV-ECMO patients without neurologic injury [86]. Despite advances in ECMO and medical therapy over the study time period (1992–2015), the prevalence of neurologic injury did not change. Risk factors associated with neurologic injury included pre-ECMO cardiac arrest, hyperbilirubinemia during ECMO, and use of CVVH [86].

Routine neurologic exams should be performed on all patients receiving ECMO therapy. Exams should include at minimum Glasgow coma scale assessment, pupil examinations, and brainstem, tendon, and pathologic reflex testing [148]. Other high-sensitivity methods, such as neurological pupil index, near-infrared spectroscopy (NIRS), transcranial Doppler (TCD), and EEG, may be considered; however, data is conflicting on their routine use in ECMO patients [148]. The ELSO guidelines recommend holding sedation and analgesia daily to assess neurological status and note that eCPR is associated with the highest rate of neurologic injury, but do not make a recommendation on any specific neuroprognostication tools [119].

9.10 Conclusion

VV- and VA-ECMO are important strategies in the management of ARDS, cardiogenic shock, and post-cardiac arrest. Use of these strategies improves mortality outcomes compared to conventional management, but overall mortality is high for these patient populations. The use of this potentially lifesaving intervention requires constant monitoring, as both VV- and VA-ECMO remain associated with many complications, including, but not limited to, coagulopathy (bleeding and thrombosis), hypervolemia, infection, limb ischemia, renal failure, intracerebral hemorrhage, and stroke. Medication dosing in ECMO is complicated by the increased volume of distribution, renal failure, and potential sequestration of drug in the circuit. Clinicians should carefully consider the effects that ECMO may have on various medications to guide optimal choice and dosing. Use of therapeutic drug monitoring should be used when possible to ensure that appropriate drug concentrations are achieved. Despite the significant advances made in the use of ECMO, there are still many areas of uncertainty and limited data that require further research to ensure continued improved outcomes with its use.

References

1. Abbasciano RG, Yusuff H, Vlaar APJ, et. al. Blood Transfusion Threshold in Patients Receiving Extracorporeal Membrane Oxygenation Support for Cardiac and Respiratory Failure-A Systematic Review and Meta-Analysis. J Cardiothorac Vasc Anesth. 2021;35:1192–202.
2. Abrams DC, Brenner K, Burkart KM, et al. Pilot study of extracorporeal carbon dioxide removal to facilitate extubation and ambulation in exacerbations of chronic obstructive pulmonary disease. Ann Am Thorac Soc. 2013;10(4):307–14. https://doi.org/10.1513/AnnalsATS.201301-021OC.
3. Abrams D, Grasselli G, Schmidt M, et al. ECLS-associated infections in adults: what we know and what we don't yet know. Intensive Care Med. 2020;46:182–91.
4. Ali J, Vuylsteke A. Extracorporeal membrane oxygenation: indications, technique and contemporary outcomes. Heart. 2019;105:1437–43.
5. Arena F, Marchetti L, Henrici de Angelis L, et al. Ceftolozane-tazobactam pharmacokinetics during extracorporeal membrane oxygenation in a lung transplant recipient. Antimicrob Agents Chemother. 2019;63:1–3.
6. Argatroban. Lexi-Drugs. Hudson, OH: Lexicomp; 2023. Updated July 11, 2023. Accessed October 16, 2023.
7. Atallah S, Liebl M, Fitousis K, Bostan F, Masud F. Evaluation of the activated clotting time and activated partial thromboplastin time for the monitoring of heparin in adult extracorporeal membrane oxygenation patients. Perfusion. 2014;29(5):456–61. https://doi.org/10.1177/0267659114524264.
8. Atkinson AJ. Atkinson's principles of clinical pharmacology. 4th ed. Academic Press; 2022. p. 73–90. https://doi.org/10.1016/B978-0-12-819869-8.00018-5.
9. Bagshaw SM, Wald R, Adhikari NKJ, et al. Timing of initiation of renal-replacement therapy in acute kidney injury. N Engl J Med. 2020;383:240–51.
10. Bakdach D, Akkari A, Gazwi K, et al. Propofol safety in anticoagulated and nonanticoagulated patients during extracorporeal membrane oxygenation. ASAIO J. 2021;67:201–7.

11. Barbar SD, Clere-Jehl R, Bourredjem A, Hernu R, Montini F, Bruyere R, et al. Timing of renal-replacement therapy in patients with acute kidney injury and sepsis. N Engl J Med. 2018;379:1431–42.
12. Beckmann A, Benk C, Beyersdorf F, et al. Position article for the use of extracorporeal life support in adult patients. Eur J Cardiothorac Surg. 2011;40:676–80.
13. Bembea MM, Schwartz JM, Shah N, et al. Anticoagulation monitoring during pediatric extracorporeal membrane oxygenation. ASAIO J. 2013;59(1):63–8. https://doi.org/10.1097/MAT.0b013e318279854a.
14. Bertini P, Guarracino F, Flacone M, et al. ECMO in COVID-19 patients: a systematic review and meta-analysis. J Cardiothorac Vasc Anesth. 2022;36:2700–6.
15. Bivalirudin. Lexi-Drugs. Hudson, OH: Lexicomp; 2023. Updated September 30, 2023. Accessed October 16, 2023.
16. Bizzarro MJ, Conrad SA, Kaufman DA, et al. Infections acquired during extracorporeal membrane oxygenation in neonates, children, and adults. Pediatr Crit Care Med. 2011;12:277–81.
17. Bonicolini E, Martucci G, Simons J, et al. Limb ischemia in peripheral veno-arterial extracorporeal membrane oxygenation: a narrative review of incidence, prevention, monitoring, and treatment. Crit Care. 2019;23(1):266. https://doi.org/10.1186/s13054-019-2541-3.
18. Bouglé A, Dujardin O, Lepère V, et al. PHARMECMO: therapeutic drug monitoring and adequacy of current dosing regimens of antibiotics in patients on extracorporeal life support. Anaesth Crit Care Pain Med. 2019;38:493–7.
19. Bréchot N, Hajage D, Kimmoun A, et al. Venoarterial extracorporeal membrane oxygenation to rescue sepsis-induced cardiogenic shock: a retrospective, multicentre, international cohort study. Lancet. 2020;396(10250):545–52. https://doi.org/10.1016/S0140-6736(20)30733-9.
20. Brogan TV, Lequier L, Lorusso R, MacLaren G, Peek GJ. Extracorporeal life support: the ELSO red book. 5th ed. Ann Arbor, MI: Extracorporeal Life Support Organization; 2017.
21. Browder KL, Ather A, Pandya KA. The effects of propofol on extracorporeal membrane oxygenation oxygenator exchange. Int J Artif Organs. 2021;44:938–43.
22. Browder K, Wanek M, Wang L, et al. Opioid and sedative requirements in extracorporeal membrane oxygenation patients on hydromorphone versus fentanyl. Artif Organs. 2022;46:378–86.
23. Buck ML. Pharmacokinetic changes during extracorporeal membrane oxygenation: implications for drug therapy of neonates. Clin Pharmacokinet. 2003;42:403–17.
24. Burstein B, Wieruszewski PM, Zhao YJ, Smischney N. Anticoagulation with direct thrombin inhibitors during extracorporeal membrane oxygenation. World J Crit Care Med. 2019;8(6):87–98. https://doi.org/10.5492/wjccm.v8.i6.87.
25. Buscher H, Vaidiyanathan S, Al-Soufi A, et al. Sedation practices in veno-venous extracorporeal membrane oxygenation: an international survey. ASAIO J. 2013;59:636–41.
26. Castro DM, Dresser L, Granton J, et al. Pharmacokinetic alterations associated with critical illness. Clin Pharmacokinet. 2023;62:209–20.
27. Chen YS, Lin JW, Yu HY, et al. Cardiopulmonary resuscitation with assisted extracorporeal life-support versus conventional cardiopulmonary resuscitation in adults with in-hospital cardiac arrest: an observational study and propensity analysis. Lancet. 2008;372:554–61.
28. Chiu LC, Chuang LP, Lin SW, et al. Cumulative fluid balance during extracorporeal membrane oxygenation and mortality in patients with acute respiratory distress syndrome. Membranes. 2021;28(11):567.
29. Chlebowski MM, Baltagi S, Carlson M, Levy JH, Spinella PC. Clinical controversies in anticoagulation monitoring and antithrombin supplementation for ECMO. Crit Care. 2020;24(1):19. https://doi.org/10.1186/s13054-020-2726-9.
30. Cies JJ, Moore WS II, Giliam N, et al. Impact of ex-vivo extracorporeal membrane oxygenation circuitry on daptomycin. Perfusion. 2018;33:624–9.
31. Ciolek A, Lindsley J, Crow J, Nelson-McMillan K, Procaccini D. Identification of cost-saving opportunities for the use of antithrombin III in adult and pediatric patients. Clin Appl Thromb Hemost. 2018;24(1):186–91. https://doi.org/10.1177/1076029617693941.

32. Combes A, Hajage D, Capellier G, et al. Extracorporeal membrane oxygenation for severe acute respiratory distress syndrome. N Engl J Med. 2018;378:1965–75.
33. Combes A, Fanelli V, Pham T, Ranieri VM. European Society of Intensive Care Medicine Trials Group and the "strategy of ultra-protective lung ventilation with extracorporeal CO_2 removal for new-onset moderate to severe ARDS" (SUPERNOVA) investigators. Feasibility and safety of extracorporeal CO_2 removal to enhance protective ventilation in acute respiratory distress syndrome: the SUPERNOVA study. Intensive Care Med. 2019;45(5):592–600. https://doi.org/10.1007/s00134-019-05567-4.
34. Combes A, Peek GL, Hajage D, et al. ECMO for severe ARDS: systematic review and individual patient data meta-analysis. Intensive Care Med. 2020a;46:2048–57.
35. Combes A, Auzinger G, Capellier G, et al. $ECCO_2R$ therapy in the ICU: consensus of a European round table meeting. Crit Care. 2020b;24(1):490. https://doi.org/10.1186/s13054-020-03210-z.
36. Conrad SA, Broman LM, Taccone FS, et al. The extracorporeal life support organization Maastricht treaty for nomenclature in extracorporeal life support. A position paper of the extracorporeal life support organization. Am J Respir Crit Care Med. 2018;198:447–51.
37. deBacker J, Tamberg E, Munshi L, et. al. Sedation Practice in Extracorporeal Membrane Oxygenation-Treated Patients with Acute Respiratory Distress Syndrome: A Retrospective Study. ASAIO J. 2018;64:544–51.
38. De Rosa F, Corcione S, Baietto L, et al. Pharmacokinetics of linezolid during extracorporeal membrane oxygenation. Int J Antimicrob Agents. 2013;41:590–7.
39. DeGrado JR, Hohlfelder B, Ritchie BM, Anger KE, Reardon DP, Weinhouse GL. Evaluation of sedatives, analgesics, and neuromuscular blocking agents in adults receiving extracorporeal membrane oxygenation. J Crit Care. 2017;37:1–6.
40. DellaVolpe J, Barbaro RP, Cannon JW, et al. Joint society of critical care medicine-extracorporeal life support organization task force position paper on the role of the intensivist in the initiation and management of extracorporeal membrane oxygenation. Crit Care Med. 2020;48:838–46.
41. Der-Nigoghossian C, Dzierba AL, Etheridge J, et al. Effect of extracorporeal membrane oxygenation use on sedative requirements in patients with severe acute respiratory distress syndrome. Pharmacotherapy. 2016;36:607–16.
42. Desai M, Dalton HJ. Half-empty or half-full?-interpretation of the EOLIA trial and thoughts for the future. J Thorac Dis. 2018;10:s3248–51.
43. Devlin JW, Skrobik Y, Gélinas C, et al. Clinical practice guidelines for the prevention and management of pain, agitation/sedation, delirium, immobility, and sleep disruption in adult patients in the ICU. Crit Care Med. 2018;46:e825–73.
44. Donadello K, Roberts JA, Cristallini S, et al. Vancomycin population pharmacokinetics during extracorporeal membrane oxygenation therapy: a matched cohort study. Crit Care. 2014;18:632–41.
45. Dzierba AL, Brodie D, Bacchetta M, et al. Ketamine use in sedation management in patients receiving extracorporeal membrane oxygenation. Intensive Care Med. 2016;42:1822–3.
46. Dzierba AL, Abrams D, Madahar P, Muir J, Agerstrand C, Brodie D. Current practice and perceptions regarding pain, agitation and delirium management in patients receiving venovenous extracorporeal membrane oxygenation. J Crit Care. 2019;53:98–106.
47. Dzierba A, Muir J, Dilawri A, et al. Optimizing pharmacotherapy regimens in adult patients receiving extracorporeal membrane oxygenation: a narrative review for clinical pharmacists. J Am Coll Clin Pharm. 2023;6:621–31.
48. Eckman PM, Katz JN, El Banayosy A, Bohula EA, Sun B, van Diepen S. Veno-arterial extracorporeal membrane oxygenation for cardiogenic shock: an introduction for the busy clinician. Circulation. 2019;140(24):2019–37. https://doi.org/10.1161/CIRCULATIONAHA.119.034512.
49. ELSO Guidelines for Cardiopulmonary Extracorporeal Life Support Extracorporeal Life Support Organization, Version 1.4. August 2017. Ann Arbor, MI. www.elso.org.

50. Farrokh S, Kim BS, Cho SM. Ketamine infusion for sedation in a patient on extracorporeal membrane oxygenation (ECMO). Perfusion. 2024;39(1):223–6. https://doi.org/10.1177/02676591221134941.
51. Fisser C, Winkler M, Malfertheiner MV, et al. Argatroban versus heparin in patients without heparin-induced thrombocytopenia during venovenous extracorporeal membrane oxygenation: a propensity-score matched study. Crit Care. 2021;25(1):160. https://doi.org/10.1186/s13054-021-03581-x.
52. Fleming GM, Askenazi DJ, Bridges BC, et al. A multicenter international survey of renal supportive therapy during ECMO: the kidney intervention during extracorporeal membrane oxygenation (KIDMO) group. ASAIO J. 2012;58:407–14.
53. Fraser JF, Shekar K, Diab S, et al. ECMO—the clinician's view. ISBT Sci Ser. 2012;7:82–8.
54. Gajkowski EF, Herrera G, Hatton L, et al. ELSO guidelines for adult and pediatric extracorporeal membrane oxygenation circuits. ASAIO J. 2022;68:133–52.
55. Gaudry S, Hajage D, Schortgen F, Martin-Lefevre L, Pons B, Boulet E, et al. Initiation strategies for renal-replacement therapy in the intensive care unit. N Engl J Med. 2016;375:122–33.
56. Gélisse E, Neuville M, de Montmollin E, et al. Extracorporeal membrane oxygenation (ECMO) does not impact on amikacin pharmacokinetics: a case-control study. Intensive Care Med. 2016;42:946–8.
57. Giraud R, Banfi C, Assouline B, De Charrière A, Cecconi M, Bendjelid K. The use of extracorporeal CO_2 removal in acute respiratory failure. Ann Intensive Care. 2021;11(1):43. https://doi.org/10.1186/s13613-021-00824-6.
58. Grissom CK, Hirshberg EL, Dickerson JB, et al. Fluid management with a simplified conservative protocol for the acute respiratory distress syndrome. Crit Care Med. 2015;43:288–95.
59. Ha MA, Sieg AC. Evaluation of altered drug pharmacokinetics in critically ill adults receiving extracorporeal membrane oxygenation. Pharmacotherapy. 2017;37(2):221–35.
60. Hajat Z, Ahmad N, Andrzejowski J. The role and limitations of EEG-based depth of anaesthesia monitoring in theatres and intensive care. Anaesthesia. 2017;72(Suppl 1):38–47.
61. Hanberg P, Obrink-Hansen K, Thorsted A, et al. Population pharmacokinetics of meropenem in plasma and subcutis from patients on extracorporeal membrane oxygenation treatment. Antimicrob Agents Chemother. 2018;62:1–13.
62. Harthan AA, Buckley KW, Heger ML, et al. Medication adsorption into contemporary extracorporeal membrane oxygenator circuits. J Pediatr Pharmacol Ther. 2014;19:288–95.
63. Heith CS, Hansen LA, Bakken RM, et al. Effects of an *ex vivo* pediatric extracorporeal membrane oxygenation circuit on the sequestration of mycophenolate mofetil, tacrolimus, hydromorphone, and fentanyl. J Pediatr Pharmacol Ther. 2019;24:290–5.
64. Helms J, Frere C, Thiele T, et al. Anticoagulation in adult patients supported with extracorporeal membrane oxygenation: guidance from the scientific and standardization committees on perioperative and critical care haemostasis and thrombosis of the international society on thrombosis and haemostasis. J Thromb Haemost. 2023;21(2):373–96. https://doi.org/10.1016/j.jtha.2022.11.014.
65. Heparin. Lexi-Drugs. Hudson, OH: Lexicomp; 2023. Updated October 7, 2023. Accessed October 16, 2023.
66. Hirsh J, Anand SS, Halperin JL, Fuster V, American Heart Association. Guide to anticoagulant therapy: Heparin : a statement for healthcare professionals from the American Heart Association. Circulation. 2001;103(24):2994–3018. https://doi.org/10.1161/01.cir.103.24.2994.
67. Hohlfelder B, Szumita PM, Lagambina S, et al. Safety of propofol for oxygenator exchange in extracorporeal membrane oxygenation. ASAIO J. 2017;63:179–84.
68. Hunsicker O, Materne L, Bünger V, et al. Lower versus higher hemoglobin threshold for transfusion in ARDS patients with and without ECMO. Crit Care. 2020;24(1):697. https://doi.org/10.1186/s13054-020-03405-4.
69. Kaseer H, Soto-Arenall M, Sanghavi D, et al. Heparin vs bivalirudin anticoagulation for extracorporeal membrane oxygenation. J Card Surg. 2020;35(4):779–86. https://doi.org/10.1111/jocs.14458.

70. Kato T, Enokiya T, Morikawa Y, et al. Sequestration of antimicrobial agents in Xcoating and heparin-coated extracorporeal membrane oxygenation circuits: an in vitro study. ASAIO J. 2023;69:23–7.

71. Kaushal M, Schwartz J, Gupta N, et al. Patient demographics and extracorporeal membranous oxygenation (ECMO)-related cations associated with survival to discharge or 30-day survival in adult patients receiving Venoarterial (VA) and Venovenous (VV) ECMO in a Quaternary Care Urban Center. J Cardiothorac Vasc Anesth. 2019;33(4):910–7. https://doi.org/10.1053/j.jvca.2018.08.193.

72. Kim HS, Park S. Blood transfusion strategies in patients undergoing extracorporeal membrane oxygenation. Korean J Crit Care Med. 2017;32(1):22–8. https://doi.org/10.4266/kjccm.2016.00983.

73. Kim H, Paek JH, Song JH, et al. Permissive fluid volume in adult patients undergoing extracorporeal membrane oxygenation treatment. Crit Care. 2018;22:270.

74. Kriegl L, Hatzl S, Zurl C, et al. Isavuconazole plasma concentrations in critically ill patients during extracorporeal membrane oxygenation. J Antimicrob Chemother. 2022;77:2500–5.

75. Krueger K, Schmutz A, Zieger B, Kalbhenn J. Venovenous extracorporeal membrane oxygenation with prophylactic subcutaneous anticoagulation only: an observational study in more than 60 patients. Artif Organs. 2017;41(2):186–92. https://doi.org/10.1111/aor.12737.

76. Kühn D, Metz C, Seiler F, et al. Antibiotic therapeutic drug monitoring in intensive care patients treated with different modalities of extracorporeal membrane oxygenation (ECMO) and renal replacement therapy: a prospective, observational single-center study. Crit Care. 2020;24:664–74.

77. Lam E, Rochani A, Kaushal G, et al. Pharmacokinetics of ketamine at dissociative doses in an adult patient with refractory status asthmaticus receiving extracorporeal membrane oxygenation therapy. Clin Ther. 2019;41:994–9.

78. Lamm W, Nagler B, Hermann A, et al. Propofol-based sedation does not negatively influence oxygenator running time compared to midazolam in patients with extracorporeal membrane oxygenation. Int J Artif Organs. 2019;42:233–40.

79. Landoff KM, Rivosecchi RM, Gómez H, et al. Comparison of hydromorphone versus fentanyl-based sedation in extracorporeal membrane oxygenation: a propensity-matched analysis. Pharmacotherapy. 2020;40:389–97.

80. Le Guennec L, Cholet C, Huange F, et al. Ischemic and hemorrhagic brain injury during venoarterial-extracorporeal membrane oxygenation. Ann Intensive Care. 2018;8:129–38.

81. Lemaitre F, Hasni N, Leprince P, et al. Propofol, midazolam, vancomycin and cyclosporine therapeutic drug monitoring in extracorporeal membrane oxygenation circuits primed with whole human blood. Crit Care. 2015;19(1):40.

82. Lequier L, Horton SB, McMullan DM, Bartlett RH. Extracorporeal membrane oxygenation circuitry. Pediatr Crit Care Med. 2013;14(5 Suppl 1):S7–S12. https://doi.org/10.1097/PCC.0b013e318292dd10.

83. Li X, Wang L, Wang H, et al. Outcome and clinical characteristics of nosocomial infection in adult patients undergoing extracorporeal membrane oxygenation: a systematic review and meta-analysis. Front Public Health. 2022;10:1–11.

84. Liveris A, Bello RA, Friedmann P, et al. Anti-factor Xa assay is a superior correlate of heparin dose than activated partial thromboplastin time or activated clotting time in pediatric extracorporeal membrane oxygenation*. Pediatr Crit Care Med. 2014;15(2):e72–9. https://doi.org/10.1097/PCC.0000000000000028.

85. López-Sánchez M, Moreno-Puigdollers I, Rubio- López MI, et al. Pharmacokinetics of micafungin in patients treated with extracorporeal membrane oxygenation: an observational prospective study. Rev Bras Ter Intensiva. 2020;32:277–83.

86. Lorusso R, Gelsomino S, Parise O, et al. Neurologic injury in adults supported with venovenous extracorporeal membrane oxygenation for respiratory failure: findings from the extracorporeal life support organization database. Crit Care Med. 2017;45:1389–97.

87. Lyster H, Shekar K, Watt K, et al. Antifungal dosing in critically ill patients on extracorporeal membrane oxygenation. Clin Pharmacokinet. 2023;62:931–42.
88. Makdisi G, Wang IW. Extra corporeal membrane oxygenation (ECMO) review of a lifesaving technology. J Thorac Dis. 2015;7:E166–76.
89. Marella P, Roberts J, Hay K, et. al. Effectiveness of vancomycin dosing guided by therapeutic drug monitoring in adult patients receiving extracorporeal membrane oxygenation. Antimicrob Agents Chemother. 2020;64:1–7.
90. Martin NJ, Peitz GJ, Olsen KM, et al. Hydromorphone compared to fentanyl in patients receiving extracorporeal membrane oxygenation. ASAIO J. 2021;67:443–8.
91. Martucci G, Schmidt M, Agerstrand C, et al. Transfusion practice in patients receiving VV ECMO (PROTECMO): a prospective, multicentre, observational study. Lancet Respir Med. 2023;11(3):245–55. https://doi.org/10.1016/S2213-2600(22)00353-8.
92. McMichael ABV, Ryerson LM, Ratano D, Fan E, Faraoni D, Annich GM. 2021 ELSO adult and pediatric anticoagulation guidelines. ASAIO J. 2022;68(3):303–10. https://doi.org/10.1097/MAT.0000000000001652.
93. McNamee JJ, Gillies MA, Barrett NA, et al. Effect of lower tidal volume ventilation facilitated by extracorporeal carbon dioxide removal vs standard care ventilation on 90-day mortality in patients with acute hypoxemic respiratory failure: the REST randomized clinical trial. JAMA. 2021;326(11):1013–23. https://doi.org/10.1001/jama.2021.13374.
94. Mehta NM, Halwick DR, Dodson BL, et al. Potential drug sequestration during extracorporeal membrane oxygenation: results from an ex vivo experiment. Intensive Care Med. 2007;33:1018–24.
95. Menk M, Briem P, Weiss B, et al. Efficacy and safety of argatroban in patients with acute respiratory distress syndrome and extracorporeal lung support. Ann Intensive Care. 2017;7(1):82. https://doi.org/10.1186/s13613-017-0302-5.
96. Messmer AS, Zingg C, Müller M, et al. Fluid overload and mortality in adult critical care patients-a systematic review and meta-analysis of observational studies. Crit Care Med. 2020;48:1862–70.
97. Migdady I, Rice C, Deshpande A, et al. Brain injury and neurologic outcome in patients undergoing extracorporeal cardiopulmonary resuscitation: a systematic review and meta-analysis. Crit Care Med. 2020;48:e611–9.
98. Millar JE, Fanning JP, McDonald CI, McAuley DF, Fraser JF. The inflammatory response to extracorporeal membrane oxygenation (ECMO): a review of the pathophysiology. Crit Care. 2016;20(1):387. https://doi.org/10.1186/s13054-016-1570-4.
99. Morris AH, Wallace CJ, Menlove RL, et al. Randomized clinical trial of pressure-controlled inverse ratio ventilation and extracorporeal CO_2 removal for adult respiratory distress syndrome. Am J Respir Crit Care Med. 1994;149(2 Pt 1):295–305. https://doi.org/10.1164/ajrccm.149.2.8306022.
100. Mossadegh C. Monitoring the ECMO. In: Mossadegh C, Combes A, editors. Nursing care and ECMO. Cham: Springer; 2016. p. 45–70. https://doi.org/10.1007/978-3-319-20101-6_5.
101. Mulder MMG, Fawzy I, Lancé MD. ECMO and anticoagulation: a comprehensive review. Neth J Crit Care. 2018;26(1):6–13.
102. Nguyen TP, Phan XT, Huynh DQ, et al. Monitoring unfractionated heparin in adult patients undergoing Extracorporeal Membrane Oxygenation (ECMO): ACT, APTT, or ANTI-XA? Crit Care Res Pract. 2021;2021:5579936. https://doi.org/10.1155/2021/5579936.
103. Nguyen TP, Phan XT, Nguyen TH, et al. Major bleeding in adults undergoing peripheral Extracorporeal Membrane Oxygenation (ECMO): prognosis and predictors. Crit Care Res Pract. 2022;2022:5348835. https://doi.org/10.1155/2022/5348835.
104. Olson SR, Murphree CR, Zonies D, et al. Thrombosis and bleeding in extracorporeal membrane oxygenation (ECMO) without anticoagulation: a systematic review. ASAIO J. 2021;67(3):290–6. https://doi.org/10.1097/MAT.0000000000001230.

105. Omecinski K, Cove M, Duggal A, Federspiel W. Extracorporeal carbon dioxide removal (ECCO$_2$R): a contemporary review. Appl Eng Sci. 2022;10:1–7. https://doi.org/10.1016/j.apples.2022.100095.
106. Osman D, Monnet X, Castelain V, et al. Incidence and prognostic value of right ventricular failure in acute respiratory distress syndrome. Intensive Care Med. 2009;35:69–76.
107. Ostadal P, Rokyta R, Karasek J, et al. Extracorporeal membrane oxygenation in the therapy of cardiogenic shock: results of the ECMO-CS randomized clinical trial. Circulation. 2023;147:454–64.
108. Ostermann M, Connor M Jr, Kashani K. Continuous renal replacement therapy during extracorporeal membrane oxygenation: why, when and how? Curr Opin Crit Care. 2018;24:493–503.
109. Paek JH, Park S, Lee A, et al. Timing for initiation of sequential continuous renal replacement therapy in patients on extracorporeal membrane oxygenation. Kidney Res Clin Pract. 2018;37:239–47.
110. Panigada M, Cucino A, Spinelli E, et al. A randomized controlled trial of antithrombin supplementation during extracorporeal membrane oxygenation. Crit Care Med. 2020;48(11):1636–44. https://doi.org/10.1097/CCM.0000000000004590.
111. Park SJ, Yang JH, Park HJ, et al. Trough concentrations of vancomycin in patients undergoing extracorporeal membrane oxygenation. PLoS One. 2015;10:1–10.
112. Patel M, Altshuler D, Lewis TC, et al. Sedation requirements in patients on venovenous or venoarterial extracorporeal membrane oxygenation. Ann Pharmacother. 2020;54:122–30.
113. Patel JS, Kooda K, Igneri LA. A Narrative Review of the Impact of Extracorporeal Membrane Oxygenation on the Pharmacokinetics and Pharmacodynamics of Critical Care Therapies. Ann Pharmacother. 2023;57:706–26.
114. Peek GJ, Mugford M, Tiruvoipati R, et al. Efficacy and economic assessment of conventional ventilatory support versus extracorporeal membrane oxygenation for severe adult respiratory failure (CESAR): a multicentre randomized controlled trial. Lancet. 2009;374(9698):1351–63.
115. Rabah H, Rabah A. Extracorporeal Membrane Oxygenation (ECMO): what we need to know. Cureus. 2022;14(7):e26735. https://doi.org/10.7759/cureus.26735.
116. Raghunathan V, Liu P, Kohs TCL, et al. Heparin resistance is common in patients undergoing extracorporeal membrane oxygenation but is not associated with worse clinical outcomes. ASAIO J. 2021;67(8):899–906. https://doi.org/10.1097/MAT.0000000000001334.
117. Ranucci M, Ballotta A, Kandil H, et al. Bivalirudin-based versus conventional heparin anticoagulation for postcardiotomy extracorporeal membrane oxygenation. Crit Care. 2011;15(6):R275. https://doi.org/10.1186/cc10556.
118. Repessé X, Au SM, Bréchot N, et al. Recombinant factor VIIa for uncontrollable bleeding in patients with extracorporeal membrane oxygenation: report on 15 cases and literature review. Crit Care. 2013;17(2):R55. https://doi.org/10.1186/cc12581.
119. Richardson ASC, Tonna JE, Nanjayya V, et al. Extracorporeal cardiopulmonary resuscitation in adults. Interim guideline consensus statement from the extracorporeal life support organization. ASAIO J. 2021;67(3):221–8. https://doi.org/10.1097/MAT.0000000000001344.
120. Rihal CS, Naidu SS, Givertz MM, et al. 2015 SCAI/ACC/HFSA/STS clinical expert consensus statement on the use of percutaneous mechanical circulatory support devices in cardiovascular care: endorsed by the American Heart Assocation, the Cardiological Society of India, and Sociedad Latino Americana de Cardiologia Intervencion; Affirmation of Value by the Canadian Association of Interventional Cardiology-Association Canadienne de Cardiologie d'intervention. J Am Coll Cardiol. 2015;65:e7–e26.
121. Roberts JA, Bellomo R, Cotta MO, et al. Machines that help machines to help patients: optimising antimicrobial dosing in patients receiving extracorporeal membrane oxygenation and renal replacement therapy using dosing software. Intensive Care Med. 2022;48:1338–51.
122. Robinson B, Eshaghpour E, Ewing S, et al. Hypertrophic obstructive cardiomyopathy in an infant of a diabetic mother: support by extracorporeal membrane oxygenation and treat-

ment with beta-adrenergic blockade and increased intravenous fluid administration. ASAIO J. 1998;44:845–7.

123. Rosas MM, Sobieszczyk MJ, Warren W, et al. Outcomes of fungemia in patients receiving extracorporeal membrane oxygenation. Open Forum Infect Dis. 2022;9:1–4.

124. Schmidt M, Bailey M, Kelly J, et al. Impact of fluid balance on outcome of adult patients treated with extracorporeal membrane oxygenation. Intensive Care Med. 2014;40:1256–66.

125. Shekar K, Abdul-Aziz MH, Cheng V, et. al. Antimicrobial Exposures in Critically Ill Patients Receiving Extracorporeal Membrane Oxygenation. Am J Respir Crit Care Med. 2023;207:704–20.

126. Shekar K, Roberts JA, Mcdonald CI, et al. Sequestration of drugs in the circuit may lead to therapeutic failure during extracorporeal membrane oxygenation. Crit Care. 2012a;16:194–200.

127. Shekar K, Roberts JA, Mullany DV, et al. Increased sedation requirements in patients receiving extracorporeal membrane oxygenation for respiratory and cardiorespiratory failure. Anaesth Intensive Care. 2012b;40:648–55.

128. Shekar K, Roberts JA, Mcdonald CI, et al. Protein-bound drugs are prone to sequestration in the extracorporeal membrane oxygenation circuit: results from an *ex vivo* study. Crit Care. 2015;19:164–70.

129. Shin TG, Choi JH, Jo IJ, et al. Extracorporeal cardiopulmonary resuscitation in patients with in-hospital cardiac arrest: a comparison with conventional cardiopulmonary resuscitation. Crit Care Med. 2011;39:1–7.

130. Sidebotham D. Extracorporeal membrane oxygenation - understanding the evidence: CESAR and beyond. J Extra Corpor Technol. 2011;43:23–6.

131. Sniderman J, Monagle P, Annich GM, et al. Hematologic concerns in extracorporeal membrane oxygenation. Res Pract Thromb Haemost. 2020;4:455–68.

132. Stallworth S, Ohman K, Schultheis J, et al. Propofol-associated hypertriglyceridemia in adults with acute respiratory distress syndrome on extracorporeal membrane oxygenation. ASAIO J. 2023;69:856–62.

133. Sy E, Sklar MC, Lequier L, Fan E, Kanji HD. Anticoagulation practices and the prevalence of major bleeding, thromboembolic events, and mortality in venoarterial extracorporeal membrane oxygenation: a systematic review and meta-analysis. J Crit Care. 2017;39:87–96. https://doi.org/10.1016/j.jcrc.2017.02.014.

134. Taccone FS, Nobile L, Annoni F. Thrombolysis for ECMO oxygenator thrombosis. Crit Care. 2023;27(1):142. https://doi.org/10.1186/s13054-023-04433-6.

135. Tellor B, Avidan M. Ketamine infusion for patients receiving extracorporeal membrane oxygenation support. JHLT. 2015;34:S144.

136. Tiruvoipati R, Buscher H, Winearls J, et al. Early experience of a new extracorporeal carbon dioxide removal device for acute hypercapnic respiratory failure. Crit Care Resusc. 2016;18(4):261–9.

137. Van Daele R, Bekkers B, Lindsfors M, et al. A large retrospective assessment of voriconazole exposure in patients treated with extracorporeal membrane oxygenation. Microorganisms. 2021a;9:1543–56.

138. Van Daele R, Bruggemann RJ, Dreesen E, et al. Pharmacokinetics and target attainment of intravenous posaconazole in critically ill patients during extracorporeal membrane oxygenation. J Antimicrob Chemother. 2021b;76:1234–41.

139. Verkerk BS, Dzierba AL, Muir J, et al. Opioid and benzodiazepine requirements in obese adult patients receiving extracorporeal membrane oxygenation. Ann Pharmacother. 2020;54:144–50.

140. Wagner D, Pasko D, Phillips K, et al. In vitro clearance of dexmedetomidine in extracorporeal membrane oxygenation. Perfusion. 2013;28:40–6.

141. Walker EA, Roberts AJ, Louie EL, Dager WE. Bivalirudin dosing requirements in adult patients on extracorporeal life support with or without continuous renal replacement therapy. ASAIO J. 2019;65(2):134–8. https://doi.org/10.1097/MAT.0000000000000780.

142. Watt K, Li JS, Benjamin DK Jr, et al. Pediatric cardiovascular drug dosing in critically ill children and extracorporeal membrane oxygenation. J Cardiovasc Pharmacol. 2011;58:126–32.
143. Wiedemann HP, Wheeler AP, Bernard GR, et al. Comparison of two fluid-management strategies in acute lung injury. N Engl J Med. 2006;354:2564–75.
144. Wittenstein B, Ng C, Ravn H, Goldman A. Recombinant factor VII for severe bleeding during extracorporeal membrane oxygenation following open heart surgery. Pediatr Crit Care Med. 2005;6(4):473–6. https://doi.org/10.1097/01.PCC.0000162449.55887.B9.
145. Wrisinger WC, Thompson SL. Basics of extracorporeal membrane oxygenation. Surg Clin North Am. 2022;102:23–35.
146. Yannopoulous D, Bartos J, Raveendran G, et al. Advanced reperfusion strategies for patients with out of hospital cardiac arrest and refractory ventricular fibrillation (ARREST): a phase 2, single centre, open-label, randomised controlled trial. Lancet. 2020;396:1087–16.
147. Ye Q, Yu X, Chen W, et al. Impact of extracorporeal membrane oxygenation on voriconazole plasma concentrations: a retrospective study. Front Pharmacol. 2022;13:1–12.
148. Zhang H, Xu J, Yang X, et al. Narrative review of neurologic complications in adults on ECMO: prevalence, risks, outcomes, and prevention strategies. Front Med. 2021;8:713333. https://doi.org/10.3389/fmed.2021.713333.

Part III
Cardiovascular Critical Care

Chapter 10
Acute Coronary Syndrome (ACS)

Nicholas Barker, Dusty Lisi, and Adele Robbins

Cardiovascular disease (CVD) is the leading cause of death globally, representing 32% of all deaths [1]. Eighty percent of all CVD deaths globally are related to myocardial infarction (MI) and stroke [1]. In the United States, over 40% of CVD deaths are attributed to myocardial infarction [2]. Acute coronary syndrome (ACS) encompasses a number of conditions associated with acute myocardial ischemia caused by an acute reduction in coronary blood flow and is one of the most common.

It is important to note that myocardial infarction can occur from a number of different causes. The type of myocardial infarction is classified based on a number of characteristics, such as pathophysiology, clinical presentation, and electrocardiographic (ECG) changes.

10.1 Type 1–5 Myocardial Infarctions

Myocardial infarctions (MIs) are categorized into five distinct types based on the underlying etiology [3]. This has helped triage patients who have significant elevations in cardiac troponin, a sensitive and specific biomarker for cardiac damage. Type 1 and 2 MIs account for the majority of MI cases.

N. Barker (✉)
Cardiovascular Intensive Care Unit, Emory Saint Joseph's Hospital, Atlanta, GA, USA
e-mail: nicholas.barker@emoryhealthcare.org

D. Lisi
Heart Failure, Emory Saint Joseph's Hospital, Atlanta, GA, USA

A. Robbins
Advanced Heart Failure and Transplant, Piedmont Hospital, Atlanta, GA, USA

Y. Alzaidi, M. A. Gebily (eds.), *The Pharmacist's Expanded Role in Critical Care Medicine*, https://doi.org/10.1007/978-3-031-77335-8_10

Type 1 MI occurs when atherosclerotic plaque is dislocated, typically rupture or erosion, resulting in thrombus formation in one or more coronary arteries. Plaque rupture is a result of plaque integrity disruption allowing more contact with the platelet-rich interior of the plaque. In response, multiple pro-thrombotic substances are released and promote platelet activation/aggregation and thrombus formation, leading to coronary artery occlusion (partial or complete). Type 1 MI is further classified based on 12-lead ECG interpretation into ST-segment elevation myocardial infarction (STEMI) and NSTE-ACS. NSTE-ACS is classified as either non-ST-segment elevation myocardial infarction (NSTEMI) or unstable angina (UA) [4, 5]. Type 1 MI will be the primary focus of this chapter. Duration of ischemia and damaged tissue location correlate with the degree of damage and potential complications, which will be discussed later in this chapter.

Type 2 MI occurs when there is an oxygen supply/demand mismatch instead of coronary artery occlusion. A number of conditions such as hypertension, hypoxia, anemia, and tachyarrhythmias may precipitate type 2 MI. Atrial fibrillation (AF) is the most common cause of type 2 MI, and tachyarrhythmias are responsible for as much as 47% of occurrences [6].

Type 3 MI references sudden cardiac death with a high suspicion for myocardial ischemia believed to be a result of new thrombus. Death occurs prior to appropriate testing that includes defining diagnoses such as cardiac biomarkers.

Type 4 MI is associated with percutaneous coronary intervention (PCI). This is further divided into two subcategories. Type 4a is diagnosed based on the elevation of cardiac biomarkers following PCI. Type 4b signifies stent thrombosis, a potential risk after stent placement.

Type 5 MI occurs when there is an elevation of cardiac biomarkers following coronary bypass grafting (CABG). This may be related to graft thrombosis.

10.2   Acute Coronary Syndrome (Type 1 MI)

Type 1 MI is classified as either STEMI or NSTE-ACS (NSTEMI or UA). This is determined by the presence of elevated troponin and evidence on a 12-lead ECG. Understanding the various types of MI is important for appropriate diagnosis, treatment, and future management.

STEMI accounts for up to 40% of all myocardial infarctions [7]. STEMI occurs when resulting thrombus from plaque rupture completely blocks one or more coronary arteries, resulting in ischemia and significant damage to cardiac tissue. This is evidenced by ST-segment elevation on a 12-lead ECG and elevated troponin. Due to the severity of complication and high risk for mortality, it is considered a medical emergency. NSTE-ACS is another frequent type 1 MI. This is a result of partial blockage of a coronary artery, which is evident by the lack of ST-segment elevation on a 12-lead ECG.

10.3 Clinical Presentation/Evaluation

Patients may present in a varying degree of symptoms. While the most common symptom is chest discomfort, up to 60% of all MIs are asymptomatic or unrecognized. Approximately one-third of patients will present with symptoms other than chest pain/discomfort [8]. This is more common in women, elderly adults, and patients with diabetes. Chest pain can be persistent or increasing and radiate to other locations such as the jaw, neck, and arms. The less common/more atypical symptoms include diaphoresis, syncope, unexplained fatigue, indigestion, and nausea/vomiting. More extreme symptoms include acute decompensated heart failure, cardiogenic shock, and cardiac arrest.

Most evaluation and treatment strategies use first medical contact (FMC) as the guiding point in time. This is the time at which trained medical personnel who can interpret an ECG assess a patient. FMC should include an initial evaluation of vital signs, personal history, physical examination, troponin level collection, and ECG. 12-Lead ECG recording and interpretation should be completed as soon as possible, with a target of less than 10 min from FMC [4].

STEMI is diagnosed based on 12-lead ECG findings. STEMI is diagnosed when two contagious leads have ST elevation of $\geq$2.5 mm in men <40 years, $\geq$2 mm in men $\geq$40 years, or $\geq$1.5 mm in women regardless of age in leads V2–V3 and/or $\geq$1 mm in the other leads (in the absence of left ventricular hypertrophy or left bundle branch block) [4]. In patients who present with a left bundle branch block or a ventricular paced rhythm, Sgarbossa Criteria may be used to assist in diagnosis, which has a high specificity but low sensitivity [10]. Location of ST elevation on ECG has a high predictive value for the location of coronary artery occlusion and guides reperfusion strategies. Objective findings of NSTEMI/UA may include ST depression, T-wave inversion, or no ECG changes [4].

Figure 10.1 illustrates ST elevation in the anterior and lateral leads. Lateral leads consist of I, aVL, V5, and V6 [9]. These typically correlate with blockage of the circumflex artery. The anterior leads consist of V3 and V4, which correlate with the left anterior descending (LAD) artery. Figure 10.2 provides an example of an inferior STEMI. Inferior leads consist of II, III, and aVF and are characteristic of right coronary artery occlusion. ST elevation found in septal leads (V1, V2) also correlates with LAD occlusion. Figure 10.3 is an example of a recent or evolving STEMI. This is evident by the negative deflection of the Q wave.

Serial troponin levels should be collected at FMC and at 3–6 h as the initial troponin may not be positive [4]. Cardiac troponins are detectable within 6 h of insult and may remain elevated for approximately 10 days [11].

Early therapies can be initiated to manage ischemia and treat pain. The common acronym associated with these therapies is "MONA." Morphine (M) is the most common analgesic utilized in the management of chest pain, in part due to potential vasodilatory effects. Morphine has a IIb recommendation by ACC/AHA guidelines due to at least one trial finding an association between morphine administration and

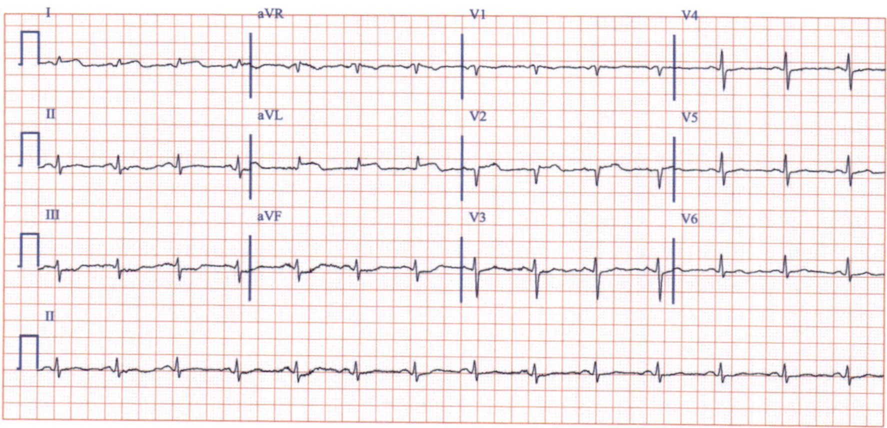

Fig. 10.1 ECG of acute/evolving ST-elevation anterolateral MI (STEMI) [9]

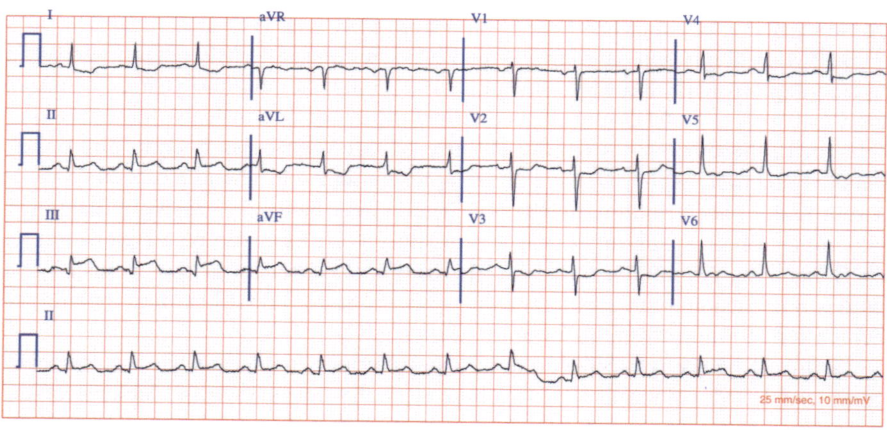

Fig. 10.2 ECG of acute inferior STEMI [9]

increased mortality [12–15]. The European Society of Cardiology (ESC) guidelines do not specifically comment on this but do state a concern for decrease in antiplatelet absorption and no evidence of increased risk of adverse effects with concomitant use of morphine and antiplatelet agents [4]. This association with supplemental oxygen (O) has been shown to be beneficial in patients with arterial oxygen saturation less than 90% or signs/symptoms of significant hypoxia. Nitroglycerin (N) is converted into nitric oxide, which activates guanylate cyclase increasing cyclic guanosine monophosphate (c-GMP). This leads to dilation of coronary arteries, improving collateral flow to ischemic regions, and may decrease cardiac demand via a decrease in preload. Nitroglycerin is contraindicated in patients who received oral phosphodiesterase inhibitors within the past 24-48 h depending on agent. In

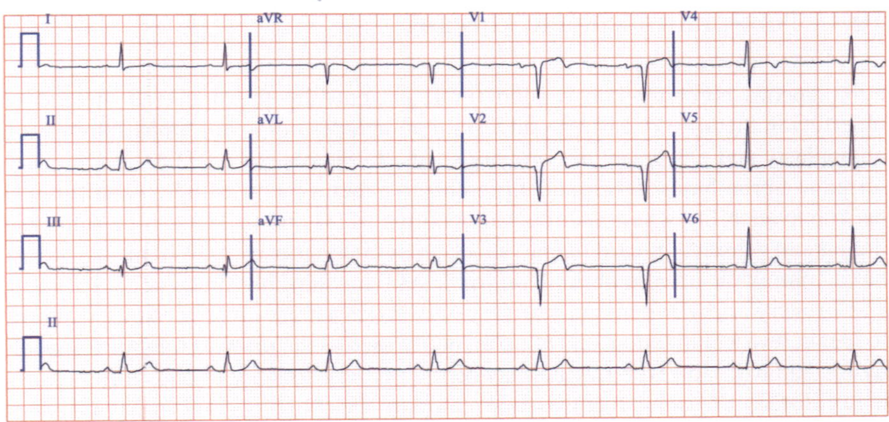

Fig. 10.3 ECG of anterior ST-elevation/Q-wave myocardial infarction, possibly recent or evolving [9]

addition, ACC/AHA guidelines provide contraindication criteria for hypotension (SBP <90 mmHg or ≤30 mm Hg from baseline), marked bradycardia/tachycardia, and right ventricular infarction [12]. Sublingual nitroglycerin may be used for up to three doses. After three doses, an intravenous infusion is recommended and titrated to chest pain. Prolonged nitroglycerin administration may result in decreasing effects due to tachyphylaxis, which can occur within 24 h of use. Aspirin (A), discussed later in this chapter with other antiplatelet agents, should be chewed at a dose of 324 mg (chewable) or 325 mg (non-enteric coated). The use of beta-blockers should be initiated within the first 24 h unless there is evidence of acute decompensated heart failure, heart block, or risk/evidence of shock.

Short-term goals of treatment in ACS consist of reperfusion to the narrowed or blocked artery and minimization of infarct size. Other treatment goals include prevention of death and other complications, relief of ischemic symptoms, and prevention of current ischemia. The AHA/ACC recommend that patients be quickly elevated and strategized based on their risks [12]. Current risk calculators for NSTE-ACS include the TIMI risk score and the GRACE risk model [4]. Both are used to evaluate the risk of recurrent MI and mortality. During evaluation, factors such as time from onset of symptoms, risk of bleeding, and availability of interventional cardiology facilities should also be considered when determining reperfusion therapy. Early invasive strategies are indicated in case of recurrent angina/ischemia at rest with low-level activities despite intensive medical therapy, new ST-segment depression, presence of cardiac troponin, signs/symptoms of heart failure (including reduced left ventricular function), new/worsening mitral regurgitation, high-risk findings from noninvasive testing, sustained ventricular tachycardia, signs of hemodynamic instability, PCI within 6 months or prior to CABG, and high-risk stratification scoring (4+ TIMI, >140 GRACE) [4, 16].

10.4 Non-pharmacologic Therapy

Percutaneous coronary intervention (PCI) is generally the preferred method of reperfusion therapy. PCI is a broad term that includes but is not limited to balloon angioplasty and placement of coronary stents. In the case of a STEMI, PCI is preferred to fibrinolytics if the patient presents to a facility with 24-h PCI and surgical backup availability where door-to-balloon time of 90 min or less can be achieved, the patient presents in cardiogenic shock, if symptom onset is >3 h, or the patient has a contraindication to fibrinolytics or is at high risk of bleeding [12].

Coronary artery bypass graft surgery (CABG) is a more invasive strategy, slower to regain revascularization, and not commonly used as the primary treatment modality for STEMI. However, CABG may be the primary strategy of choice for a number of different reasons. It consists of removing a viable blood vessel from another part of the body and connecting it to bypass the artery blockage. Urgent CABG may be indicated if unsuccessful PCI/fibrinolysis, recurrent/persistent ischemia, mechanical complications of MI, life-threatening ventricular arrhythmias, multivessel disease as an alternative to other delayed strategies, or coronary anatomy more suitable for CABG [4, 17].

10.5 Pharmacologic Therapy

10.5.1 Fibrinolytics

Fibrinolytic therapy is indicated for reperfusion therapy if patient with a STEMI cannot receive a PCI within 120 min of first medical contact [12]. While fibrinolytics have the best efficacy if received within the first 4 h of the onset of symptoms, it should ideally be given within 12 h of the onset of symptoms [18]. Fibrinolytics break down clots by binding to fibrin within the clot and by activating plasminogen into plasmin. Use of fibrinolytics comes with an increased risk of bleeding, and therefore, each patient who may be a candidate for fibrinolytic therapy must be reviewed for the risks and benefits of its use. Some contraindications to fibrinolytics are active bleeding; history of intracranial hemorrhage; recent history of major bleeding, trauma, or surgery; severe uncontrolled hypertension; known intracranial aneurysm; and pregnancy. With any of the fibrinolytic therapy used for STEMI, adjunctive therapy with an anticoagulant and antiplatelets should also be given. A pharmacologic comparison of fibrinolytics available in the United States can be seen in Table 10.1 [19–21].

Table 10.1 Fibrinolytics used in MI [19–21]

	Alteplase	Tenecteplase	Reteplase
STEMI dose	≥67 kg: 15 mg bolus, 50 mg over 30 min, 35 mg over 60 min <67 kg: 15 mg bolus, 0.75 mg/kg over 30 min, 0.5 mg/kg over 60 min (max dose 100 mg)	~0.5 mg/kg IV once rounded to nearest 5 mg • <60 kg: 30 mg • 60–69 kg: 35 mg • 70–79 kg: 40 mg • 80–89 kg: 45 mg • ≥90 kg: 50 mg	10 units IV push every 30 min ×2 doses
Onset	30–60 min	60 min	30–90 min
Duration	Up to 6 h	Up to 6 h	Up to 6 h
Half life	26–46 min	20–24 min	13–16 min
Excretion	Hepatic	Hepatic	Renal

10.5.2 Anticoagulants

Regardless of the reperfusion method, adjunctive therapy with an anticoagulant should be used in all patients who present with acute coronary syndrome (ACS) unless a contraindication exists. Options for parenteral anticoagulation to inhibit propagation of the clotting cascade include unfractionated heparin (UFH), low-molecular-weight heparins (LMWHs), and direct thrombin inhibitors (DTIs). While fondaparinux can be used in ACS, it is not recommended as the sole anticoagulant for primary PCI in STEMI and, therefore, not commonly used [4, 12]. Heparin products use antithrombin as a cofactor to bind factor Xa and thrombin (factor IIa). LMWHs have a greater binding affinity to factor Xa than IIa. Direct thrombin inhibitors bind directly and irreversibly to both circulating and clot-bound thrombin (factor IIa).

10.5.2.1 Heparins

While heparin products remain the most commonly used anticoagulant for ACS, they differ greatly in their pharmacokinetic profiles. Unfractionated heparin (UFH) has less predictable and highly variable pharmacokinetics but is still widely used due to familiarity of dosing and monitoring, as well as a known antidote, protamine, if a bleeding event were to occur. UFH is given as a bolus of 60 units/kg (maximum dose of 4000 units) followed by a continuous infusion titrated to a goal PTT or anti-Xa level. More recently, the ESC guidelines recommend an initial bolus dose of 70–100 units/kg. UFH is typically continued until the time of PCI or up to 48 h for medical management [4, 12].

On the other hand, LMWHs, such as enoxaparin, have a slightly better safety and efficacy profile when compared directly to UFH. This is thought to be due to its highly predictable pharmacokinetics. While it is given subcutaneously, with the exception of an IV bolus for STEMI patients or if the additional dose is needed during a PCI, it does not require routine monitoring or IV access, but it does require dose adjustments for renal function and for those greater than or equal to 75 years of age experiencing ACS [4].

10.5.2.2 Direct Thrombin Inhibitors

The use of direct thrombin inhibitors is frequently reserved for patients with active or a history of heparin-induced thrombocytopenia. Cost may also prohibit their use in clinical practice. The half-lives of both bivalirudin and argatroban are shorter than heparins, therefore requiring more frequent monitoring. There is also no specific reversal agent for DTIs. Table 10.2 shows dosing strategies and pharmacokinetic considerations [22, 23].

10.5.3 Antiplatelets

All patients diagnosed with ACS should be treated with two antiplatelet agents, commonly referred to as dual-antiplatelet therapy or DAPT, which includes aspirin (ASA) in combination with a P2Y12 inhibitor. The duration of DAPT is dependent on various factors such as the type of stent placed, bleeding risk, concomitant oral anticoagulation therapy, and recurrent ischemic events.

10.5.3.1 Aspirin

Aspirin is an irreversible cyclooxygenase (COX)-1 inhibitor that blocks the formation of thromboxane A2, which is one pathway responsible for platelet aggregation. All patients should receive a loading dose of 162–325 mg as early as possible once ACS is suspected. After an initial loading dose, subsequent dose of 81 mg daily is appropriate.

Table 10.2 Direct thrombin inhibitors used in MI [22, 23]

	Bivalirudin	Argatroban
Dosing	ACS: 0.1 mg/kg IV bolus followed by 0.25 mg/kg/h, titrated to PTT goal PCI: 0.75 mg/kg bolus prior to PCI followed by 1.75 mg/kg/h during the procedure and may be continued for up to 4 h after PCI • Requires renal dose adjustment	ACS: 0.5–2 mcg/kg/min titrated to PTT goal PCI: 350 mcg/kg bolus followed by 25 mcg/kg/min infusion, titrated to ACT • Requires hepatic dose adjustment
Metabolism	Renal	Hepatic
Half-life	25–34 min, longer in renal impairment	39–50 min, longer in hepatic impairment

10.5.3.2 P2Y12 Inhibitors

In addition to aspirin, patients should also receive a second oral antiplatelet. The combination of aspirin and a P2Y12 inhibitor is what makes up the mainstay of ACS therapy. P2Y12 inhibitors affect the adenosine diphosphate receptors on platelets, decreasing the amplification of platelet activation. The choice of P2Y12 inhibitors depends mainly on pharmacokinetic differences, patient characteristics, if PCI is performed, and provider preference. However, the ESC guidelines recommend the use of ticagrelor or prasugrel over clopidogrel. Considerations related to long-term therapy will be discussed later in this chapter. Table 10.3 includes dosing information and important considerations related to oral P2Y12 inhibitors.

Table 10.3 Oral P2Y12 inhibitors [24–26]

	Clopidogrel	Prasugrel	Ticagrelor
Mechanism of action	Prodrug *Irreversibly* binds to the P2Y12 component of ADP receptors on the platelet	Prodrug *Irreversibly* binds to the P2Y12 component of ADP receptors on the platelet	Active parent compound and metabolites *Reversibly and noncompetitively* binds to the P2Y12 component of ADP receptors on the platelet
Dosing	*Medical management:* 1. LD 300 mg; 75 mg daily *PCI:* 4. LD 600 mg (unless fibrinolytic past 24 h = 300 mg); 75 mg daily	*PCI:* 60 mg LD; 10 mg daily	*PCI/medical management:* 180 mg LD followed by 90 mg BID • **Must be used with ASA ≤ 101 mg**
Contraindications	Active bleeding	Active bleeding, **history of TIA or stroke**	Active bleeding, **h/o intracranial hemorrhage; hepatic impairment**
Precautions	Poor clopidogrel metabolizer due to CYP2C19 genetic variation	**Caution in patients who weigh <60 kg** (could use 5 mg daily) **Not recommended in patients >75 years old**	Hyperuricemia; dyspnea; bradycardia; creatinine levels may rise during therapy; 3A4 inducers/ inhibitors
Adverse events	Bruising; bleeding	Hypertension; headache; hyperlipidemia; nausea; back pain; epistaxis; dyspnea	**Dyspnea**; ventricular pauses; HA; dizziness; creatinine increase; bleeding; epistaxis
Onset after loading dose	2–4 h	<30 min	<30 min
CABG	Stop 5 days prior	Stop 7 days prior	Stop 5 days prior

Clopidogrel

Clopidogrel is an inactive thienopyridine that requires oxidation with CYP2C19 by a two-step process to generate an active metabolite, which irreversibly binds to the P2Y12 receptor on platelets blocking aggregation. A loading dose of 300 mg should be given with concomitant fibrinolytic therapy or 600 mg for PCI. There are genetic polymorphisms of the PGY2C19 that can be tested for if there is concern that patients are poor metabolizers.

Prasugrel

Prasugrel is also an inactive thienopyridine prodrug that also requires hepatic activation, although with a faster onset of action than clopidogrel. It irreversibly binds to P2Y12 receptors with a higher binding affinity compared to clopidogrel. Due to these pharmacokinetic aspects, there is a higher bleeding risk with prasugrel. Use of prasugrel is only indicated with coronary stents and not for medication management of ACS [4, 12]. Its use is contraindicated in patients with a history of transient ischemic attack (TIA) or stroke (both hemorrhagic and ischemic) [24]. Use is also generally not recommended in patients who are 75 years old or greater or those who weigh under 60 kilograms. If used, a dose reduction may be appropriate.

Ticagrelor

Ticagrelor is a cyclopentyl-triazolo-pyrimidine that reversibly binds to the P2Y12 receptor with more rapid onset and offset than clopidogrel. It can be used both for medical management of ACS and with PCI. Its use is contraindicated in patients with a history of intracranial hemorrhage or severe hepatic impairment. There is also a Black Box Warning by the US Food and Drug Administration to use only with maintenance doses of aspirin ≤ 100 mg daily. Side effects include dyspnea and ventricular pauses, both of which may be related to the ticagrelor's inhibition of adenosine reuptake.

Intravenous Antiplatelets

Intravenous antiplatelet agents are primarily used in patients who cannot take oral medications (i.e., altered mental status, severe nausea/vomiting), when there is a significant delay in oral therapy, or in specific high-risk scenarios, including high clot burden seen at the time of PCI.

10.5.3.3   Glycoprotein IIb/IIIa Receptor Inhibitors

There are three glycoprotein (GP) IIb/IIIa inhibitors available in the United States. Most of the clinical trials using these agents in ACS for invasive strategies were in combination with UFH and prior to the routine use of oral P2Y12 inhibitors. All have a fast onset of action but differ in the half-lives and reversibility, which makes tirofiban and eptifibatide preferred options if a GP IIb/IIIa receptor inhibiter is needed. Both tirofiban and eptifibatide have shorter half-lives, which will allow platelet aggregation to return to normal a few hours after the medication is discontinued. However, abciximab's antiplatelet effect may last days after discontinuation, although this effect may be reversed with platelet transfusions, which is not the case for tirofiban and eptifibatide. A bolus-only option during PCI has been adopted in clinic practice, but not in practice guidelines. Besides bleeding, GP IIb/IIIa receptor inhibitors may also cause thrombocytopenia. Table 10.4 provides dosing and pharmacokinetics considerations for intravenous GP IIb/IIIa inhibitors.

10.5.3.4   Cangrelor

Cangrelor is an intravenous P2Y12 inhibitor with an almost immediate on/off effect. It is primarily used during PCI or when oral P2Y12 therapy is delayed or has to be withheld for various reasons. Dosing consists of a 30 mcg/kg bolus followed by a 4 mcg/kg/min infusion for a minimum of 2 h or the duration of procedure (whichever is longer). When transitioning to an oral P2Y12 inhibitor, important notice should be taken as to when to initiate [4, 27].

Table 10.4 Intravenous GP IIb/IIIa inhibitors [23]

	Abciximab (ReoPro)	Eptifibatide (Integrilin)	Tirofiban (Aggrastat)
PCI dosing	0.25 mg/kg bolus, 0.125 mg/kg/min	180 mcg/kg bolus, 2 mcg/kg/min	0.4 mcg/kg/min for 30 min, then 0.1 mcg/kg/min
Chemical structure	Monoclonal antibody	Peptide	Nonpeptide
Inhibition	Steric hindrance	Competitive binding	Competitive binding
Onset	~30 min	Within 1 h	~30 min
Renal elimination	No	Yes, dose reduced if CrCl <50 mL/min	Yes, dose reduced if CrCl <30 mL/min
Return of platelet function	~48–72 h (up to 7 days)	~2–4 h	~2–4 h
Side effect	Thrombocytopenia		

10.5.3.5   Management of Antithrombotics Prior to CABG

Patients admitted for ACS may and often do receive some form of an oral P2Y12 inhibitor loading dose either at the time of hospitalization prior to or following left heart catheterization. As previously discussed, the platelet inhibitory effects of these medications can range from 5 to 7 days depending on the agent used [24–26]. Due to the high risk of bleeding associated with CABG, P2Y12 inhibitors are not recommended within 5 days in most cases. In patients who did not receive any form of a stent, it is prudent to withhold the P2Y12 inhibitor and consider continuing an anticoagulant infusion. The P2Y12 inhibitor effect may be evaluated using platelet reactivity testing to demonstrate appropriate medication clearance/platelet activity. Many of these patients may have a new cardiac stent placed during PCI that is high risk for thrombosis requiring some form of antiplatelet agent in conjunction with aspirin. Holding aspirin has been observed to increase the risk for major adverse ischemic events by threefold [4, 27]. If the ASA is held due to surgeon preference, then ASA should be stopped 7 days or less prior to the surgery date. In this scenario, IV antiplatelet agents are the drugs of choice. Initiation of IV antiplatelet agents is dependent on the choice of P2Y12 inhibitor but typically should be initiated at approximately 48 h from the last dose [28]. IV antiplatelet agents can then be discontinued within 2–6 h prior to surgery depending on the agent's pharmacokinetic and patient-specific factors. Cangrelor has a shorter half-life than the GP IIb/IIIa inhibitors, and platelet reactivity testing can be used to demonstrate appropriate clearance. However, cangrelor lacks the potency of an antiplatelet effect that may be warranted in high-risk patients.

Following surgery, P2Y12 inhibitor therapy can be restarted within 24 h. In patients who are undergoing minor surgery including dermatologic or dental procedures, antiplatelet therapy with a single agent can be continued, and patients receiving DAPT should hold the P2Y12 inhibitor (5 days for clopidogrel/ticagrelor and 7 days for prasugrel).

10.6   Complications of ACS

Complications occurring after a patient experiences acute coronary syndrome with STEMI, NSTEMI, or UA can include pericarditis, arrhythmias, mechanical complications, or heart failure (HF) with or without cardiogenic shock.

Pericarditis is generally defined as inflammation of the pericardium. After myocardial infarction, pericarditis can develop early (within 4 days), related to the infarct, or late (1–2 weeks after infarction), which is known as Dressler syndrome [4]. The risk for early post-MI pericarditis is due to delayed/incomplete reperfusion or large infarct size. Early pericarditis is due to necrosis of the cardiac muscle damaged by the MI and inflammation of the surrounding pericardium. The criteria used for diagnosis of early or late pericarditis are the same and include at least two of the following: cardiac rub, chest pain that is pleuritic in nature, pericardial effusion that is new or worsening, and characteristic ECG changes (e.g., diffuse ST-segment elevations with associated PR interval depressions). There may also be detectable increased levels of troponin and other inflammatory markers [29–31]. Treatment of early post-infarct pericarditis is aspirin 500 mg every 8–12 h for up to 7 days. Aspirin is also used for late post-infarct pericarditis at 500–1000 mg every 6–8 h until patients start to have resolution of symptoms; then decrease dose every 2 weeks by 250 mg–500 mg. Colchicine can also be used as an adjunct anti-inflammatory agent for 3 months with 0.5 mg every 12 h [4, 29]. Patients with post-infarct pericarditis have also demonstrated that antiplatelet and anticoagulant therapy can safely be continued [4, 29–31].

Arrhythmias are common after acute myocardial infarction. They are more common in patients who have delayed or incomplete reperfusion, especially if the left ventricular ejection fraction (LVEF) is ≤40% [4, 29]. The most common type of supraventricular arrhythmia is AF. Patients can have a history of AF or experience new onset during the management of ACS [32, 33]. For patients with new-onset AF with early detection affecting hemodynamic stability of the patient, electrical cardioversion is the preferred method for re-establishing normal sinus rhythm. For patients who remain otherwise hemodynamically stable, controlling the heart rate is preferred with the use of beta-blockers. For patients who have HF and LVEF ≤40%, the beta-blockers that are preferred include metoprolol succinate, carvedilol, or bisoprolol. In patients who are unable to receive beta-blockers due to hypotension, amiodarone, digoxin, or both in combination can be used. Chronic oral anticoagulation with warfarin or direct oral anticoagulants should be added for patients with AF and underlying risk factors, including history of thromboembolism, hypertension, diabetes, heart failure, or age 65 years or greater [4, 29, 32, 33].

Ventricular arrhythmias can also occur in about 6–8% of patients following acute coronary syndrome. The occurrence has significantly declined in the setting of early revascularization. Early after the occurrence of ACS, patients most frequently experience non-sustained monomorphic ventricular tachycardia (NSVT). Treatment is typically not required for the management of NSVT. Arrhythmias may also present initially as ventricular tachycardia that is unstable and polymorphic and has a high risk for progressing into ventricular fibrillation. Beta-blocker initiation provides an early reduction of the risk for ventricular arrhythmias. In the setting of polymorphic ventricular arrhythmias, amiodarone should be initiated, followed by lidocaine and lastly procainamide. Long-term pharmacotherapy for prevention of ventricular arrhythmias can include amiodarone with or without mexiletine. Class IC antiarrhythmics such as flecainide and propafenone are contraindicated in patients with structural heart disease based on findings from the CAST trial [34] and should not be used. Long-term management of post-MI ventricular arrhythmia with an implantable cardioverter defibrillator (ICD) has demonstrated improved outcomes and survival benefit over pharmacotherapy [4, 29, 32].

Mechanical complications can include ventricular septal rupture, papillary muscle rupture, and free wall rupture. Mechanical complications have a high rate of mortality, 10–40% specifically in elderly patients, but the incidence remains low [35, 36]. Mechanical complications can occur within 3–7 days of experiencing

ACS. Symptoms can include cardiogenic shock, chest pain, and pulmonary edema. For free wall rupture, patients may also have cardiac arrest and develop cardiac tamponade [4, 29]. Free wall rupture is managed through urgent surgical repair. Pre- and perioperative mechanical circulatory support may be needed to reduce left ventricular end diastolic pressure. Management of ventricular septal or papillary muscle rupture involved a combination of pharmacotherapy to maintain blood pressure and cardiac output (e.g., vasopressors and inotropes) as well as surgical repair, ideally 7 days or more from the event [29, 35, 36]. Mechanical circulatory support may be required for both complications. It is also recommended to incorporate palliative care due to the nature and severity of the complications [29, 35].

Heart failure can also develop as a complication of acute coronary syndrome. HF can be preexisting and can develop at the time of MI, during hospitalization, or following discharge. The risk factors for development of HF include female gender, hypertension, diabetes, chronic kidney disease, atrial fibrillation, history of previous MI, and age greater than 75 years. Symptoms of excess fluid and resting shortness of breath are usually present in patients who present with MI and acute onset of HF. Urgent concomitant management of both ACS and HF is essential to improve patient outcomes. Intravenous diuretics (furosemide or bumetanide) are utilized for fluid management. Decreased cardiac output and symptoms of cardiogenic shock are managed with the addition of inotropes (dobutamine and/or milrinone) and vasopressors (norepinephrine or epinephrine). In some patients, temporary mechanical circulatory support (MCS) with or without respiratory and/or renal replacement may be required. MCS can include intra-aortic balloon pump (IABP), heart pump, or extracorporeal membrane oxygenation (ECMO). MCS has not consistently demonstrated consistent reduction in morbidity and mortality and, therefore, should be evaluated on a case-by-case basis. Patients who have cardiogenic shock in the setting of MI should be managed at a PCI-capable hospital. Once patients who have ACS and HF are stabilized, pharmacotherapy demonstrating the benefit for patients with HF should be initiated [4, 29, 37].

10.7 Long-Term Management

Long-term pharmacotherapy for stabilization of cardiac disease and prevention of ACS recurrence and further morbidity and mortality includes DAPT, statins, beta-blockers, angiotensin-converting enzyme (ACE) inhibitors or angiotensin receptor blockers (ARBs), and mineralocorticoid receptor antagonists.

DAPT with aspirin and P2Y12 inhibitor post-acute coronary syndrome has demonstrated reduced rates of stent restenosis, myocardial infarction, death from cardiovascular causes, or stroke. DAPT-initiated post-acute coronary syndrome should continue in ideal circumstances for 12 months. Premature discontinuation or interruption of DAPT can increase the risk for stent thrombosis and mortality. Stent thrombosis can result in mortality rates up to 45% [4, 29, 38, 39]. Aspirin should be continued lifelong in all patients unless otherwise contraindicated.

Ticagrelor and prasugrel are recommended over clopidogrel as the P2Y12 of choice in DAPT. In the results of the PLATO trial, patients receiving ticagrelor had a significant reduction in the combined primary efficacy end point evaluating the occurrence of myocardial infarction, death from cardiovascular causes, or stroke without experiencing increased fatal or TIMI major bleeding [40]. In the results of the TRITON TIMI 38 study, patients undergoing PCI who received prasugrel in comparison to clopidogrel demonstrated a significant reduction in the rates of the primary combined efficacy end point of myocardial infarction, death from cardiovascular causes, or stroke. However, patients receiving prasugrel also experienced increased rates of fatal and nonfatal TIMI major hemorrhage. Patients demonstrating the greatest benefit from prasugrel include patients with diabetes or who had in-stent thrombosis. Subgroup analysis of TRITON TIMI 38 also defined three patient groups that would not benefit from prasugrel [41]. There is a risk for net harm when prasugrel is used in patients with a history of stroke (ischemic or hemorrhagic). There is no net benefit observed in patients who are 75 years of age or greater or who weigh less than 60 kg [42]. Overall, in these three patient groups, there is an increased risk of bleeding with prasugrel. The updated ESC guidelines for ACS provide a class I recommendation for ticagrelor or prasugrel (when available and tolerated) over clopidogrel in patients undergoing PCI [4, 29, 38, 39].

For patients who underwent ischemia-guided therapy without intervention, the aspirin can be combined with either clopidogrel or ticagrelor. TRITON-TIMI did not include patients who received medical management for acute coronary syndrome [39]. TRIOLOGY ACS evaluated patients receiving medical management with prasugrel in comparison to clopidogrel in patients with unstable angina or NSTEMI. There was not a statistically significant difference in the occurrence of the primary end point of myocardial infarction, death from cardiovascular causes, or nonfatal stroke or the safety end point of major bleeding events in patients receiving prasugrel. Therefore, prasugrel is not recommended as part of DAPT in patients with acute coronary syndrome receiving medical/ischemia-guided management [4, 29, 38, 39].

DAPT may be stopped at 6 months in patients who have stable ischemic heart disease and elective PCI with stent placement. (Class I ACS) Shorter duration of DAPT may also be considered in patients who have a lower ischemic risk, and the risk of morbidity and bleeding with continuation exceeds the benefits of therapy. In patients who have an increased risk for bleeding, proton pump inhibitors can be considered to reduce risk. While esomeprazole and omeprazole may decrease response to clopidogrel, there is not enough evident to demonstrate increased risk of ischemic events [4, 29, 38, 39]. Table 10.5 provides details regarding DAPT de-escalation following a minimum of 1 month of DAPT therapy.

Table 10.5 DAPT de-escalation [4]. Adapted from ESC ACS guidelines 2023

Time (months)	Abbreviated DAPT options			DAPT de-escalation
0	HBR	HBR and non-HBR patients		Potent P2Y12 DAPT ASA + ticagrelor or prasugrel
1	1 month	3 months	6 months	P2Y12 inhibitor de-escalation Change to ASA + clopidogrel
3				
6				
9	P2Y12 or ASA monotherapy			
12				

10.7.1 High Bleed Risk (HBR)

Pharmacists should counsel patients about the role and benefit of taking DAPT and the potential increased risk for stent thrombosis and mortality with noncompliance or premature discontinuation.

10.7.2 Statins

Atherosclerotic coronary vascular disease is known to be related to circulating levels of cholesterol; in particular, the most atherogenic form is known to be low-density lipoprotein (LDL). High-density lipoprotein (HDL) cholesterol is not atherogenic and may confer protective benefits, and very-low-density lipoprotein (VLDL) cholesterol is known to be both atherogenic and the primary transporter for triglycerides. Apolipoprotein B, or apoB, is the main atherogenic component of both LDL-C and VLDL-C and therefore may be a better measure of atherogenic risk than cholesterol levels alone. High-intensity or maximally tolerated statin therapy is recommended for secondary prevention in all patients who have ASCVD. Statins inhibit 3-hydroxy-3-methylglutaryl coenzyme A (HMG-CoA) reductase, which is the rate-limiting enzyme in cholesterol synthesis. This results in increased expression of LDL receptors on hepatic tissue and breakdown of LDL. Statin therapy is usually well tolerated but does have a 5–20% occurrence of subjective statin-associated muscle symptoms (SAMSs), which can lead to noncompliance or avoidance of statin therapy. The guidelines recommend considering SAMS as a side effect rather than an intolerance because patients will oftentimes be able to tolerate therapy with an alternative statin or dose [4, 43–45].

High-intensity statin therapy includes atorvastatin 40 or 80 mg daily or rosuvastatin 20 or 40 mg daily. The definition of ASCVD includes patients who have experienced acute coronary syndrome, e.g., STEMI, NSTEMI, unstable or stable angina, and coronary revascularization, as well as symptomatic peripheral arterial disease or previous revascularization or amputation, stroke, and transient attack. Low-density lipoprotein (LDL) cholesterol is reduced 50% by high-intensity statin therapy. LDL and non-high-density lipoprotein (non-HDL) cholesterol treatment targets

Table 10.6 Statin dosing and intensity. Adapted from 2018 Cholesterol Guidelines [43]

Intensity	LDL reduction (%)	Statins	Doses validated in RCT
High	≥50	Atorvastatin	40 or 80 mg daily
		Rosuvastatin	20 or 40 mg daily
Moderate	30–49	Atorvastatin	10 mg daily
		Fluvastatin	40 mg twice daily
		Lovastatin	40 mg daily
		Pravastatin	40 mg daily
		Simvastatin	20 or 40 mg daily
		Rosuvastatin	10 mg daily
Low	<30	Lovastatin	20 mg daily
		Pravastatin	10 or 20 mg daily

were removed in the 2013 ACC/AHA cholesterol guideline, as many patients with ASCVD may still benefit from reduction of LDL cholesterol levels by 50% or greater than baseline levels even when already at prior target levels before therapy [4, 43–45]. Table 10.6 illustrates comparative statin potency and LDL reduction.

In the 2018 ACC/AHA multidisciplinary guideline for management of cholesterol, the addition of non-statin therapy with ezetimibe for LDL cholesterol reduction can be considered for patients who are considered to have a very-high-risk ASCVD [43]. Very-high-risk ASCVD includes patients with multiple major ASCVD events or ASCVD in combination with multiple high-risk conditions (e.g., diabetes, hypertension, current smoking, persistent LDL elevation of 70 mg/dL or greater despite high-intensity statin therapy) [43, 45]. Ezetimibe inhibits the absorption of cholesterol at the brush border of the small intestine [43–45]. Addition of ezetimibe to statin therapy further improves cardiovascular outcomes and reduces LDL cholesterol. Ezetimibe has a low risk for side effects and can lower LDL-C by 15–30% [4, 43–46]. Furthermore, proprotein convertase subtilisin/kexin type 9 (PCSK9) inhibitor therapy could be considered for very-high-risk ASCVD patients who are already receiving statin therapy at the maximum tolerated dose in combination with ezetimibe and when LDL remains 70 mg/dL or greater [4, 43–45]. PCSK9 binds to LDL receptors and promotes degradation within the liver. Circulating LDL is primarily cleared when bound to the LDLR; therefore, lower levels of LDLR result in increased levels of LDL-C. There are three agents available in the United States that reduce PCSK9 activity, which include alirocumab, evolocumab, and inclisiran. These agents have been observed to reduce LDL-C by 45–70%. Adverse effects observed are typically mild and include injection-site reactions and nasopharyngitis. These are not usually therapies that are initiated during hospitalization due to cost and require insurance review and approval to confirm that patients will be able to obtain and afford them [4, 47].

Statin doses provided in the table were validated in the RCT and 2010 meta-analysis, which demonstrated reduced risk for major cardiovascular events. Although higher doses of simvastatin (80 mg) were previously studied and demonstrated benefit, due to the increased risk for myopathy and rhabdomyolysis, the FDA does not recommend initiation or titration of simvastatin to 80 mg dosing.

10.7.3 Beta-Blockers

Long-term pharmacotherapy for acute coronary syndrome aims to decrease the risk for stent thrombosis, mortality, chest pain, and recurrence of cardiac events. Data supports the use of beta-blockers in patients who have chronic heart failure with reduced ejection fraction (HFrEF, LVEF $\leq$40%); it reduces mortality as well as cardiovascular events. The beneficial effects of beta-blockers do not appear to be dose dependent in this population. There is less data and experience regarding the effects of beta-blockers in patients without previous heart failure or acute coronary syndrome [4, 29, 48, 49]. Side effects associated with beta-blocker therapy are dose related and include fatigue, bradycardia, and postural hypotension [4, 29, 48].

Cardiovascular death or complications at 30 days and 3-year follow-up were not reduced in retrospective evaluation of 755,215 national registry patients 65 years of age or older with coronary artery disease undergoing elective PCI without a previous history of heart failure or acute coronary syndrome [49]. Reduction in mortality and cardiovascular events was observed in patients undergoing CABG either with or without a history of acute coronary syndrome [4, 29, 48–50]. The recommended duration of beta-blocker therapy is still unclear [4, 50, 51]. There is questionable benefit for the use of beta-blocker therapy for greater than 1 year in patients experiencing STEMI or NSTEMI [4, 52–54]. For patients who have left ventricular ejection fraction $\leq$40%, specific beta-blockers are recommended based upon data demonstrating reduced mortality and improved cardiac function.

10.7.4 Angiotensin-Converting Enzyme Inhibitors/Angiotensin Receptor Blockers

Outcomes in post-MI patients who have hypertension, LVEF $\leq$40%, chronic kidney disease, or diabetes have also been improved by ACE inhibitors. In particular, initiation of ACE inhibitors post-MI has demonstrated a significant reduction in mortality at 30 days and ventricular remodeling [4, 12]. Valsartan, losartan, and candesartan are the ARBs determined to have benefit in patients with HF or LVEF $\leq$40%, whereas all ACE inhibitors provide similar benefit. Although ACE inhibitor or ARB transition to angiotensin receptor neprilysin inhibitor (ARNI, valsartan/sacubitril) is recommended through guideline-directed medication therapy for heart failure patients with LVEF $\leq$40%, trial data has not supported greater benefit in post-MI patients. A recent trial failed to demonstrate that valsartan/sacubitril reduced the risk of death from cardiovascular causes or hospitalization due to symptomatic HF compared to ACE inhibitors. No difference was observed in the ARNI vs. ACE inhibitor group [55]. As a result, the guidelines recommend ACE inhibitor initiation in patients post-MI who have LVAD $\leq$40% over ARNI [4, 29].

10.7.5   *Mineralocorticoid Receptor Antagonists*

Mineralocorticoid receptor antagonists (MRAs) block aldosterone binding to receptors in the distal renal tubules. As a result, sodium and water excretion is increased without loss of potassium and hydrogen ions. In addition, effects on arterial smooth muscle may also be blocked. Spironolactone administration in combination with ACE inhibitor early post-myocardial infarction was found to reduce left ventricular remodeling post-myocardial infarction [4, 12, 56]. There are two MRAs available, spironolactone and eplerenone. Side effects associated with MRAs include hyperkalemia and impotence. Spironolactone is associated with a 10% risk of gynecomastia, whereas eplerenone is not. For patients who have experienced acute coronary syndrome and LVEF $\leq$40%, MRAs reduce collagen formation and remodeling of the ventricles of the heart [4, 12, 56, 57]. In patients who had experienced recent ACS and had LVEF $\leq$40% with heart failure symptoms, eplerenone has demonstrated reduced all-cause and cardiovascular mortality or cardiovascular-related hospitalizations [57]. Spironolactone or eplerenone is started at 25 mg daily and titrated up to 50 mg daily, if tolerated. Eplerenone was further studied evaluating the safety and efficacy of early treatment in patients with acute MI without previous heart failure or reduced LVEF. The results demonstrated a reduction in the composite end point for rehospitalization, sustained ventricular arrhythmia, elevated natriuretic peptides, cardiovascular mortality, LVEF $\leq$40%, or extended hospitalization due to heart failure diagnosis [58].

The prevalence and consequences of ACS constitute the consideration of a medical emergency. Immediate medical attention is vital to survival and improved outcomes in many cases. While non-pharmacological therapies are the primary form of management, concomitant pharmacological treatment is vital to preventing disease progression and improving outcomes. A variety of complications can occur or be exacerbated in relation to ACS. Management of these complications is often dynamic depending on the severity of ischemia experienced and preexisting medical conditions. Long-term medication management with goal-directed therapy improves survival and cardiac outcomes. These therapies are often started in the intensive care unit and should be considered early in management as tolerated by the patient. Timely recognition, treatment, and secondary prevention are fundamental to patient outcomes.

References

1. Cardiovascular Diseases Fact Sheet. World Health Organization (WHO). June 2021. https://www.who.int/news-room/fact-sheets/detail/cardiovascular-diseases-(cvds).
2. Heart Disease and Stroke Statistics 2023 Update. American Heart Association (AHA). January 2023. https://professional.heart.org/en/science-news/heart-disease-and-stroke-statistics-2023-update.
3. Thygesen K, et al. Fourth universal definition of myocardial infarction. Circulation. 2018;38(20):e618–51.

4. Byrne RA, et al. ESC guidelines for the management of acute coronary syndromes. Eur Heart J. 2023;2023(44):3720–826.

5. Gulati M, et al. 2021 AHA/ACC/ASE/CHEST/SAEM/SCCT/SCMR guideline for the evaluation and diagnosis of chest pain: a report of the American College of Cardiology/American Heart Association Joint Committee on Clinical Practice Guidelines. Circulation. 2021;144(22):e368–454.

6. Sandoval Y, et al. Type 1 and 2 myocardial infarction and myocardial injury: clinical transition to high-sensitivity cardiac troponin I. Am J Med. 2017;130:1431–9.

7. Mozaffarian D, et al. Heart disease and stroke statistics-2016 update: a report from the American Heart Association. Circulation. 2016;133(4):e38–360.

8. Kolesova MV, Minor S. Silent myocardial infarction: a case report. Cureus. 2023;15(8):e43906.

9. Nathanson L A, McClennen S, Safran C, Goldberger AL. ECG wave-maven: self-assessment program for students and clinicians. http://ecg.bidmc.harvard.edu

10. Cai Q, et al. The left bundle-branch block puzzle in the 2013 ST-elevation myocardial infarction guideline: from falsely declaring emergency to denying reperfusion in a high-risk population. Are the Sgarbossa criteria ready for prime time? Am Heart J. 2013;166(3):409–13.

11. Kontos MC, Turlington JS. High-sensitivity troponins in cardiovascular disease. Curr Cardiol Rep. 2020;22(5):30.

12. Levine G, et al. 2015 ACC/AHA/SCAI focused update on primary percutaneous coronary intervention for patients with ST-elevation myocardial infarction: an update of the 2011 ACCF/AHA/SCAI guideline for percutaneous coronary intervention and the 2013 ACCF/AHA guideline for the management of ST-elevation myocardial infarction. JACC. 2016;67(10):1235–50.

13. Montalescot G, et al. Prehospital ticagrelor in ST-segment elevation myocardial infarction. N Engl J Med. 2014;371:1016–27.

14. Meine TJ, et al. Association of intravenous morphine use and outcomes in acute coronary syndromes: results from the CRUSADE quality improvement initiative. Am Heart J. 2005;149(6):1043–9.

15. Bonin M, et al. Effect and safety of morphine use in acute anterior ST-segment elevation myocardial infarction. J Am Heart Assoc. 2018;7(4):e006833.

16. Jobs A, et al. Optimal timing of an invasive strategy in patients with non-ST-elevation acute coronary syndrome: a meta-analysis of randomised trials. Lancet. 2017;390:737–46.

17. Lawton JS, et al. 2021 ACC/AHA/SCAI guideline for coronary artery revascularization: executive summary: a report of the American College of Cardiology/American Heart Association Joint Committee on Clinical Practice Guidelines. Circulation. 2022;145(3):e4–e17.

18. Indications for fibrinolytic therapy in suspected acute myocardial infarction: collaborative overview of early mortality and major morbidity results from all randomised trials of more than 1000 patients. Fibrinolytic Therapy Trialists' (FTT) Collaborative Group. Lancet. 1994;343(8893):311–22.

19. Activase [prescribing information]. South San Francisco, CA: Genentech, Inc.

20. TNKase [prescribing information]. South San Francisco, CA: Genentech, Inc.

21. Retavase [prescribing information]. Cary, NC: Chiesi, Inc.

22. Bivalirudin [prescribing information]. Princeton, NJ: Sandoz, Inc.

23. Argatroban [prescribing information]. Princeton, NJ: Sandoz, Inc.

24. Effient [prescribing information]. Indianapolis, IN: Eli Lilly & Company.

25. Plavix [prescribing information]. Bridgewater, NJ: Bristol-Meyers Squibb/Sanofi, Inc. Partnership.

26. Brilinta [prescribing information]. Wilmington, DE: AstraZeneca Pharmaceuticals LP.

27. Kangreal [prescribing information]. Cary, NC: Chiesi, Inc.

28. Sullivan AE, et al. Bridging antiplatelet therapy after percutaneous coronary intervention: JACC review topic of the week. JACC. 2021;78(15):1550–63.

29. Byrne RA, et al. ESC guidelines for the management of acute coronary syndromes supplementary data. Eur Heart J. 2023;2023(00):1–52.

30. Rodevic G, et al. Acute pericarditis after percutaneous coronary intervention: a case report. Medicina. 2021;57:490.
31. Imazio M, et al. Incidence and prognostic significance of new onset atrial fibrillation/flutter in acute pericarditis. Heart. 2015;101:1463–7.
32. Frampton J, et al. Arrhythmias after acute myocardial infarction. Yale J Biol Med. 2023;96:83–94.
33. Thomsen AF, et al. Risk of arrhythmias after myocardial infarction in patients with left ventricular systolic dysfunction according to mode of revascularization: a cardiac arrhythmias and risk stratification after myocardial infarction (CARSIMA) study. Europace. 2021;23:616–23.
34. Echt DS, et al. Mortality and morbidity in patients receiving encainide, flecainide, or placebo. The Cardiac Arrhythmia Suppression Trial. NEJM. 1991;324(12):781-8.
35. Damluji AA, et al. Mechanical complications of acute myocardial infarction. Circulation. 2021;144:e16–35.
36. Mahtta D, Ibrahim M, Elgendy IY. Overview of prevalence, trends, and outcomes of post myocardial infarction mechanical complications. Ann Cardiothorac Surg. 2022;11(3):322–4.
37. Jenca D, et al. Heart failure after myocardial infarction: incidence and predictors. ESC Heart Fail. 2021;8:222–37.
38. Smith SC, et al. AHA/ACCF secondary prevention and risk reduction therapy for patients with coronary and other atherosclerotic vascular disease: 2011 update. JACC. 2011;58(23):2432–46.
39. Virani SS, et al. 2023 AHA/ACC/ACCP/ASPC/NLA/PCNA guideline for the management of patients with chronic coronary disease: a report of the American Heart Association/American College of Cardiology Joint Committee on Clinical Practice Guidelines. Circulation. 2023;148:e9–e119.
40. Wallentin L, et al. Ticagrelor versus clopidogrel in patients with acute coronary syndromes. N Engl J Med. 2009;361(11):1045–57.
41. Wiviott SD, et al. Prasugrel versus clopidogrel in patients with acute coronary syndromes. N Engl J Med. 2007;357(20):2001–15.
42. Roe MT, et al. Prasugrel versus clopidogrel for acute coronary syndromes without revascularization. N Engl J Med. 2012;367:1297–309.
43. Grundy SM, et al. AHA/ACC/AACVPR/AAPA/ABC/ACPM/ADA/AGS/APhA/ASPC/NLA/PCNA guideline on the management of blood cholesterol. Circulation. 2019;139:e1082–143.
44. Stone NJ. Statins in secondary prevention, intensity matters. J Am Coll Cardiol. 2017;69(22):2707–9.
45. Smith SC Jr, et al. AHA/ACCF secondary prevention: 2011 update. JACC. 2011;23:2432–46.
46. Pokhrel B, Yuet WC, Levine SN. PCSK9 inhibitors. [Updated 2022 May 13]. In: StatPearls [Internet]. Treasure Island, FL: StatPearls Publishing; 2024. https://www.ncbi.nlm.nih.gov/books/NBK448100/.
47. Cannon CP, et al. Ezetimibe added to statin therapy after acute coronary syndromes. N Engl J Med. 2015;372(25):2387–97.
48. Collete JP, et al. 2020 ESC guidelines for the management of acute coronary syndromes in patients presenting without persistent ST-segment elevation: supplementary data. Eur Heart J. 2020;00:1–35.
49. Li C, et al. Relationship between b-blocker therapy at discharge and clinical outcomes in patients with acute coronary syndrome undergoing percutaneous coronary intervention. J Am Heart Assoc. 2016;5:E004190.
50. Gibson CM, et al. Prevention of bleeding in patients with atrial fibrillation undergoing PCI. N Engl J Med. 2016;375:2423–34.
51. Windecker S, et al. Antithrombotic therapy in patients with atrial fibrillation and acute coronary syndrome treated medically or with percutaneous coronary intervention or undergoing elective percutaneous coronary intervention: insights from the AUGUSTUS trial. Circulation. 2019;140:1921–32.

52. Steg PG, et al. Low-dose vs standard-dose unfractionated heparin for percutaneous coronary intervention in acute coronary syndromes treated with fondaparinux: the FUTURA/OASIS-8 randomized trial. JAMA. 2010;304:1339–49.
53. Lopes RD, et al. Antithrombotic therapy after acute coronary syndrome or PCI in atrial fibrillation. N Engl J Med. 2019;380:1509–24.
54. Dewilde WJ, et al. Uninterrupted oral anticoagulation versus bridging in patients with long-term oral anticoagulation during percutaneous coronary intervention: subgroup analysis from the WOEST trial. EuroIntervention. 2015;11:381–90.
55. Pfeffer MA, et al. Angiotensin receptor-neprilysin inhibition in acute myocardial infarction. N Engl J Med. 2007;357(20):1845–55.
56. Hayashi M, et al. Immediate administration of mineralocorticoid receptor antagonist spironolactone prevents post-infarct left ventricular remodeling associated with suppression of a marker of myocardial collagen synthesis in patients with first anterior acute myocardial infarction. Circulation. 2003;107:2559–65.
57. Pitt B, et al. Eplerenone, a selective aldosterone blocker, in patients with left ventricular dysfunction after myocardial infarction. N Eng J Med. 2003;348(14):1309–21. EPHESUS.
58. Montalescot G, et al. Early eplerenone treatment in patients with acute ST-elevation myocardial infarction without heart failure: the randomized double-blind reminder study. Eur Heart J. 2014;35:2295–302. REMINDER.

Chapter 11
Acute Decompensated Heart Failure

Caitlin E. Kulig

11.1 Introduction

Heart failure (HF) is an extremely common disease state with an overall poor prognosis, despite advancements in guideline-directed medical therapy (GDMT). With an aging population, the incidence of heart failure continues to grow in the United States and worldwide. An estimated 6.5 million Americans over the age of 20 have heart failure, with an estimated 960,000 new heart failure cases per year. Heart failure is a progressive disease and, by some estimates, contributes to roughly 36% of all cardiovascular deaths, with some studies citing that heart failure is mentioned in one in every eight death certificates [1]. Heart failure hospitalization, due to acute decompensated heart failure (ADHF), is a sentinel event associated with a worse prognosis and a negative disease trajectory and remains a huge burden on both patients and the healthcare system [2]. Heart failure hospitalizations remain the number one cause of hospitalizations in Medicare patients and the most common cause of hospitalization in the United States for patients greater than 65 years of age [3]. Heart failure hospitalization has the highest 30-day rehospitalization rate among all medical and surgical conditions, accounting for up to 26.9% of total readmission rates. HF costs the US healthcare system nearly 31 billion dollars per year, and the costs are projected to increase by 50 billion by 2030 [4].

The landscape of heart failure therapy has changed drastically in the past 30 years, with a number of medication classes now found to decrease the incidence of mortality and morbidity in these patients. However, heart failure hospitalizations are still extremely common, and the practitioner must be prepared and familiar with the nuances of management of this specialized patient.

C. E. Kulig (✉)
Ernest Mario School of Pharmacy, Rutgers the State University of New Jersey, Piscataway New Jersey and St. Joseph's University Medical Center, Paterson, NJ, USA
e-mail: Caitlin.kulig@pharmacy.rutgers.edu

Y. Alzaidi, M. A. Gebily (eds.), *The Pharmacist's Expanded Role in Critical Care Medicine*, https://doi.org/10.1007/978-3-031-77335-8_11

11.2 Definitions

11.2.1 Heart Failure

Heart failure can present in many different ways and is an umbrella term. Two patients may both have the diagnosis of "heart failure" but have vastly different cardiac structural changes and require different treatments.

In order to really understand heart failure, it is best to first strip this term down to a bare-bones definition.

Heart failure is a condition where, for a variety of reasons that may differ from patient to patient, **the heart is unable to pump enough blood out to meet the demands of the body.**

The two historic definitions of heart failure are systolic heart failure, also known as heart failure with *reduced* ejection fraction (HFrEF), and diastolic heart failure, also known as heart failure with *preserved* ejection fraction (HFpEF). However, more recently, new categories of heart failure have emerged, leaving us with some new acronyms in our bowl of alphabet soup: heart failure with *improved* ejection fraction (HFimpEF) and heart failure with *mildly reduced* ejection fraction (HFmrEF) [2].

To better understand this terminology, it is important to first have a clear grasp of the term **ejection fraction** (EF). Take a moment and ask yourself:

11.2.2 What is Ejection Fraction?

As the name suggests, ejection fraction is a fraction, one number over another, and is defined as stroke volume divided by the ventricular end-diastolic volume (VEDV).

$$\text{Ejection fraction} = \frac{\overbrace{\left(\begin{array}{l}\text{The amount of blood pumped out of the}\\ \text{ventricle in 1 contraction}\end{array}\right)}^{\text{Stroke volume}}}{\underbrace{\text{Ventricular end diastolic volume}}_{\left(\text{The vloume of blood in the ventricle at its fullest}\right)}}$$

Stroke volume (SV) is the amount of blood that the ventricle pumps out per each beat (aka in 1 contraction).

Ventricular end-diastolic volume (VEDV) is the total amount of blood in the ventricle at the end of diastole (relaxation)—when the ventricle is at its fullest point immediately prior to contraction.

Test Your Knowledge
At the end of diastole (relaxation), a patient's left ventricle holds 100 mL. During systole (contraction), the left ventricle pumps 50 mL of blood out to the aorta.

What is the patient's:

A. Stroke volume
B. LVEDV
C. EF

The patient's stroke volume is 50 mL. The LVEDV is 100 mL. Therefore the EF is 50/100 = 0.5 = 50%.

There are two phases of the cardiac cycle: systole (squeeze) and diastole (relaxation). Systole is the part of the cardiac cycle when both ventricles contract (and the atria relax), and diastole is when both ventricles undergo relaxation (and the atria contract).

Systolic heart failure, also known as **HFrEF**, occurs when there is an issue with the force of *contraction* of the ventricle. As the name suggests, there is an issue with the *systole*, or the squeeze, of the ventricle. The ventricular muscle is weakened and can no longer squeeze as hard as it used to, to push that blood out of the ventricle. Systolic heart failure is defined by an EF of <40% [2].

Diastolic heart failure, also known as **HFpEF**, occurs when there is an issue with the relaxation of the ventricles. As the name suggests, there is an issue with *diastole* or the relaxation of the ventricle. The ventricular wall can become stiff and rigid, and no longer be elastic enough to relax and accommodate a normal blood volume; in other patients, the left ventricular wall can hypertrophy and grow thicker and thicker, decreasing the amount of space available to hold blood within the ventricle. In this way, diastolic heart failure is really an issue with the amount of blood volume the ventricle can hold.

But what differentiates a healthy person from a patient with HFpEF? After all, both ejection fractions are considered "normal" in both patients.

This can be best illustrated in an example.

Test Your Knowledge (*note: the volumes used in these examples are for illustrative purposes only)
Patient A: Patient A's left ventricle is able to hold 80 mL at the end of diastole. During systole, the LV pumps 40 mL of blood out to the aorta.

Patient B: Patient B's left ventricle is able to hold 30 mL at the end of diastole. During systole, the LV pumps 15 mL of blood out to the aorta.

What is each patient's:

A. LVEDV
B. SV
C. EF

*Patient A's LVEDV is 80 mL. Patient B's LVEDV is 30 mL. Patient A's SV is 40 mL, and Patient B's SV is 80 mL. **However, both patients have an EF of 50%.***

As illustrated in the case above, although both these patients have an EF of 50%, there is a big difference between the amount of blood that the body is receiving.

Patient B illustrates a case of a patient with heart failure with a "normal" EF. Keep in mind that ejection fraction is a *relative* term (because it is a fraction!), which is why a patient with a healthy heart can have the same EF as a person with HFpEF.

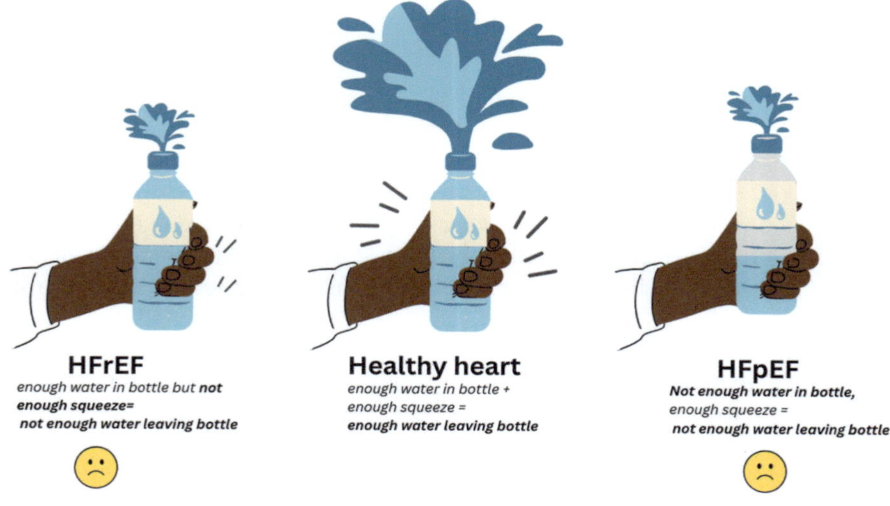

Fig. 11.1 Analogy: the difference between HFrEF and HFpEF

For the visual learners, another way to visualize systolic vs. diastolic heart failure is by the visual analogy of a hand squeezing a water bottle filled with water, where the water bottle represents the ventricle, the hand squeeze represents the force of contraction, and the water leaving the bottle represents stroke volume (Fig. 11.1).

In a healthy heart, there is a good amount of water in that bottle—and there is also a good squeeze. The end result is a lot of water exiting and spewing out of that water bottle.

In a heart with reduced ejection fraction (aka HFrEF, aka systolic heart failure), there is a good amount of water in that bottle—but the hand squeezing it is very weak, unable to generate a good contracting force. The end result is less water leaving out that bottle.

In a heart with preserved ejection fraction (aka HFpEF, aka diastolic heart failure), there is not enough water in that bottle. You have a great squeeze, but because there is not enough volume to begin with, and you end up with the same result as you do in the HFrEF example, with less water leaving that bottle.

Let us delve into the different definitions of heart failure that were released with the new 2022 American guidelines [2]. As stated earlier, HFrEF is defined as an EF of <40%. Heart failure with *mildly* reduced ejection fraction (HFmrEF) is defined by an EF of 40–49%; HFpEF is defined as an EF of ≥50%; and heart failure with *improved* ejection fraction (HFimpEF), is defined as a patient with an previous EF of <40%, but has since recovered.

11.3 Common Causes of HFrEF vs. HFpEF

HFrEF is often caused by ischemia [2]. In other words, it is heart failure caused by a lack of blood flow to the myocytes within the heart. If there is not enough blood flow to the myocytes, the myocytes will start dying. The more muscle cells that die, the larger the extent of the damage, and the less squeeze that ventricle is capable of. A common cause of HFrEF is a patient with a myocardial infarction. Other causes of nonischemic HFrEF include autoimmune conditions, chemotherapy, cardiotoxic medications, myocarditis, and substance abuse [2].

HFpEF can be caused by heart rhythm abnormalities, chronic hypertension, severe aortic stenosis, and anemia, among others [2]. Keep in mind that your heart is a muscle, just like other muscles within your body. If you went to the gym every day and started lifting heavy weights, what would happen to your biceps? They would grow. Your heart is no different. If your heart has to deal with a high chronic afterload (aka the amount of pressure your left ventricle has to fight against to ensure forward flow), your heart will also start to grow and hypertrophy. The greater the amount of hypertrophy, the thicker the ventricle wall, and the smaller the area in the ventricle that can fill with blood.

11.4 Understanding Blood Pressure

To understand acute decompensated heart failure (ADHF), a general overview of the determinants of blood pressure would also be helpful. The easiest way to break this idea down is by thinking of the garden hose sitting in your backyard. The higher the pressure of the water leaving that hose, the further it will shoot out, right?

But how to make the water shoot further? Let us say the spout is completely off, and you tweak the spout *just a tad* to let some water start going into that hose. At the end of your hose, that water is barely going to go anywhere. It is just going to start trickling out, and basically fall right onto the ground right next to the end of that hose.

But if we go back to that spout, and crank it all the way up to the max, that water at the end of the hose will start picking up pace and shoot out in an arc and go much farther.

In other words, the more the water - the more volume-, the higher the water pressure.

Now, let us say the spout is already maxed out—you have a nice arc of water flowing from the end of the hose, but let us say you want to spray your unsuspecting sibling who is across the yard. The hose is extended fully, so you cannot drag it out anymore, and the water spout is already maxed out. What can you do to increase that water pressure and get that water to shoot out farther?

For all those with siblings, you might know that putting your thumb to cover the end of that open hose and blocking a lot of the water flow will allow the water exiting that hose to *shoot* out much farther in a smaller stream, now able to be flung across the yard and soak the unsuspecting victim.

In other words, the smaller the space we allow water to go through, the higher the pressure of the water leaving it.

Believe it or not, your body is not that different. In this analogy, the water represents your blood and the hose represents the vessels of your body.

The more **blood volume**, the higher the blood pressure. By giving patients fluids, we can help increase their pressure. Luckily for us, our body has built-in systems to help increase blood volume if patients have low blood pressure (I am looking at you, aldosterone).

Fig. 11.2 Blood pressure equation

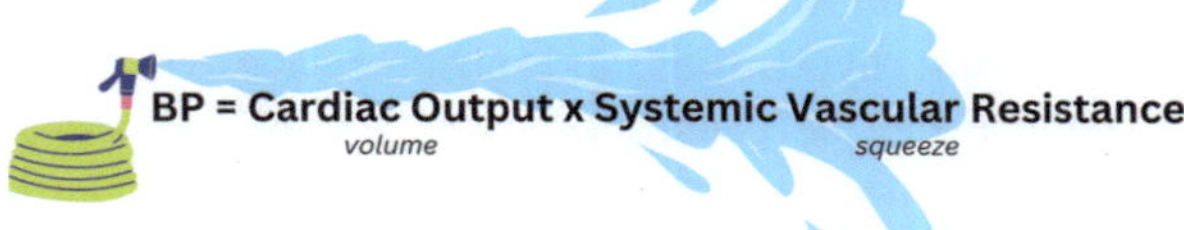

The **smaller** the vessels, the higher the blood pressure. Luckily for us, our body is able to self-regulate by vasoconstricting or vasodilating our vessels. We can also use medications to help us achieve these goals.

The variable we use to represent volume is **cardiac output**—or the amount of blood volume that the body receives from our heart per unit of time. We use the term **systemic vascular resistance** to represent the amount of squeeze (or size of) our vessels are exerting (Fig. 11.2).

11.5   Preload vs. Afterload

An integral part of understanding heart failure and the treatment of acute decompensated heart failure is having a clear idea of what the terms "**preload**" and "**afterload**" mean.

Let us start with afterload, which I think can be a little easier to visualize. Afterload is defined as the amount of pressure the heart has to exert in order to eject blood out during ventricular contraction. For those who are visual, I would like you to picture yourself inside of a patient's left ventricle (LV). To orient you, on one side, you have the **mitral valve**, where blood enters the LV from the left atrium (LA). And looking ahead of you, you can see the **aortic valve**, which is where blood must pass through in order to get out of the ventricle and into the **aorta** and systemic circulation.

Now keep in mind that your aorta and arteries carry their own baseline pressure even when the heart is relaxing (this is what we call your diastolic pressure). The *higher* that pressure, the *harder* your heart will have to *squeeze* and *contract* in order to ensure forward flow of blood. In other words, in order to get forward flow, your heart—specifically your left ventricle—must exert a pressure that is *higher* than the pressure in your arteries/aorta.

In patients who are hypertensive with high systemic vascular resistance (SVR) or have stenosis of their aortic valve, afterload will be higher, and your heart will have to squeeze extra hard to get forward flow of blood.

In the context of left-sided heart failure, factors such as arterial vascular resistance (the size of your arteries) will determine that left ventricle's afterload. Patients with high arterial SVR will make forward flow harder for that left ventricle, while patients with lower SVR with arterial dilation will make forward flow easier on that left ventricle.

The second term to understand is **preload**. The technical definition of preload is **ventricular end-diastolic pressure (VEDP)** or the amount of stretch the ventricle experiences at the end of diastole, prior to contraction. Two main factors can determine preload. The first is volume. The more volume your patient has, the higher the amount of pressure and stretch your ventricle will experience. Giving patients fluids will increase preload; diuresing patients will decrease preload. Besides volume (since after all, most of the time patients remain with a fairly fixed volume unless we are actively giving them fluids or if they are being diuresed or have blood loss), the other thing that can influence preload is the amount of pressure the blood enters the heart with. This is influenced by **venous** vascular resistance. For example, if we **vasodilate** the veins, the pressure entering the heart will be **decreased**. A lot of times, this may be confusing, but keep in mind that in a patient with *constant* volume, dilation will cause decrease in pressure (think back to your hose analogy). If we **constrict** the veins, the pressure of the blood entering your heart will **increase** and preload will be increased.

11.6 Acute Decompensated Heart Failure

11.6.1 Definition

In chronic heart failure, the heart has issues keeping up with the demands of the body; however, with the use of medications, it is still able to meet the demands of the body. However, in acute decompensated heart failure, the heart can no longer meet those demands, and hospitalization may be needed to get that patient back to their "baseline."

11.6.2 Etiology

It is important when your patient comes in with a new decompensated heart failure event that you assess for any precipitating causes and interview your patient. Some of the common causes of acute decompensated heart failure (ADHF) include ischemia, infection, atrial fibrillation or other arrhythmias, pulmonary embolism, renal failure, anemia, valvular issues, and aortic dissection, among others. Medications can also precipitate ADHF. In HFrEF, any medication that has negative inotropic effects (aka decreases the force of contraction of the heart) can induce an ADHF event. A common example is the initiation of non-DHP calcium channel blockers, such as verapamil or diltiazem [2]. Additionally, the use of high-dose NSAIDs can also induce ADHF. In patients who come in with ADHF, these medications should be discontinued and avoided [2].

11.6.3 Presentation and Classification

Forrester's classification is often used to classify the main ways a patient with ADHF can present (Fig. 11.3). The classification system is broken up into two main concepts: What is my patient's **volume** status? What is their **perfusion** status?

Let us start with the assessment of volume status. The "gold standard" of volume assessment in terms of Forrester's classification is known as **pulmonary capillary wedge pressure** or PCWP [2].

Pulmonary capillary wedge pressure is a measurement taken by using an invasive catheter. The physician will make an incision at a major vein (usually the internal jugular vein, though there are other access options) and insert a long, thin, and flexible tube known as a catheter into the vein. They will then guide the tube up through the vena cava, into the right side of the heart, through the right atria, through the right ventricle, and out through the pulmonary artery. Once in the pulmonary artery, the physician will place the tip of that catheter into a small pulmonary arterial branch. The tip of that catheter has an inflatable balloon on it; once in position, the team will inflate that balloon for a few seconds and "wedge" that branch closed while reading the pressure at that moment in time. That pressure—the **pulmonary capillary wedge pressure**—is a marker of volume status and left atrial pressure.

A typical PCWP in a "dry" or euvolemic ADHF patient is <18 mmHg. Any measurement greater than 18 mmHg is one marker that your patient may be presenting with volume overload [2].

The other parameter of Forrester's classification focuses on perfusion. The "gold standard" marker of perfusion in terms of Forrester's is **cardiac index** [2].

Cardiac index is a method of standardizing **cardiac output**, which, as we said above, is the amount of blood that leaves the heart per unit of time. In other words, it tells you how much blood your body is getting from the heart over a period of time.

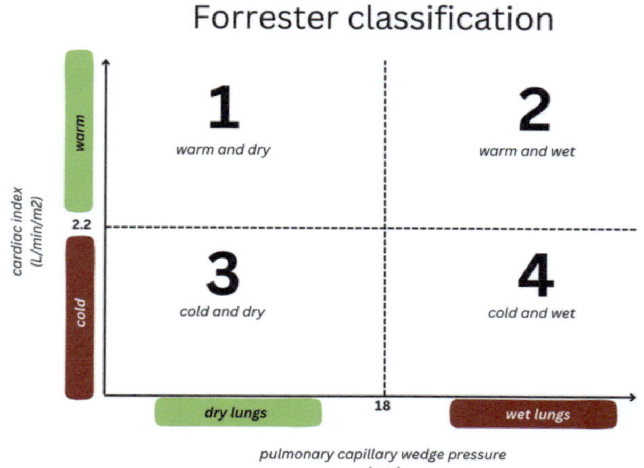

Fig. 11.3 Forrester's classification system

However, if we only looked at cardiac output, it would be very tricky to quickly discern what a patient's normal cardiac output should be for them. After all, a super-muscular 6′4″ male would likely require more blood per unit of time than let us say a frail, small grandmother.

In order to "standardize" this term for any given patient, cardiac output is divided by a patient's body surface area. This means that a cardiac index (CI) of 2.0 L/min/m^2 means approximately the same thing whether you are talking about a body-builder or someone's Nana.

The "gold standard" for a patient that is adequately perfusing is a CI >2.2 L/min/m^2. Anything below indicates that the patient may not be getting adequate perfusion to their body [2].

11.6.4   Pulmonary Artery Catheters (PACs) for All?

Now, not every patient is going to have invasive monitoring. In fact, most patients *do not* require invasive monitoring. Surprisingly, despite the fact that we as clinicians love our data and values, there is not a lot of data supporting better outcomes with the use of PACs in ADHF.

The 2022 AHA/ACC/HFSA Heart Failure Guidelines only recommend right heart catheterization in the setting of persistent congestion despite treatment due to the lack of compelling data [2].

If we do not have a PAC available, what are some other markers of either volume overload or low perfusion?

Markers of volume overload to look out for include shortness of breath, rales, pulmonary edema, pitting edema, and elevated BNP, among others. Ultrasound can even be used to visualize the vena cava and assess if it is plump (volume up) or collapsible (volume down).

When we are thinking about perfusion, keep in mind what the whole point of your heart is—to supply blood to the vital organs. Let us start with the brain—if the brain is not getting enough blood supply, patients may present with confusion and altered mental status. If the kidneys (which tend to be very sensitive to changes in perfusion) are not getting enough blood flow, we can see increased serum creatinine and decreased urine output in our patients. For the liver, we can see elevated liver function tests. Lastly, if our extremities are not perfusing, we can see cold extremities to the touch, increased capillary filling time, and even ischemic digits.

11.7   Goals of ADHF Hospitalization

The first thing to keep in mind with heart failure hospitalizations is that hospitalization is really a sentinel event in these patients, and we want to avoid hospitalizations at all costs in these patients.

Heart failure is very similar to chronic obstructive pulmonary disease (COPD) in that once a patient has an exacerbation, they often never return to their true baseline prior to hospitalization [2]. Besides triggering negative overall outcomes for our patients, ADHF hospitalizations are also a huge burden on both a patient's quality of life and the healthcare system. Rehospitalizations within 90 days of discharge are unfortunately very common, and the frequency of hospitalizations increases as the patient's heart function deteriorates [2].

A big goal of ADHF hospitalizations, besides stabilizing the patient, is to get "guideline-directed medical therapy," also known as GDMT, onboard for these patients [2]. These agents are extremely effective at preventing death and hospitalizations in these patients. We will be focusing on GDMT at the end of this chapter.

Lastly, another goal of hospitalization is to try to determine the patient's euvolemic weight, relieve their decongestion, and treat their symptoms.

11.7.1 Treatment of ADHF

When thinking about treating acute decompensated heart failure, it is important to gauge which of Forrester's classification your patient falls into and assess wet vs. dry and warm vs. cold. This classification will help guide treatment.

11.8 Treating Volume Overload

If your patient is volume overloaded—they come in with rales, shortness of breath, pitting edema, pleural edema on chest X-ray, elevated CVPs, pro-BNP, and PCWPs—it is important to help patients take this excessive volume off the heart and also to reduce symptoms such as dyspnea.

11.8.1 Loop Diuretics

The long-time mainstay decongestion in these patients, which is echoed in the 2022 AHA/ACC/HFSA Heart Failure Guidelines, continues to be intravenous **loop diuretics** [2]. IV loop diuretics provided the most rapid and effective method of decongestion in these patients, and although they are not associated with clinical outcomes such as mortality, they are extremely effective at improving symptoms of volume overload in these patients [2]. Every patient coming in for a heart failure hospitalization should have a discharge plan that includes the adjustment of their diuretics [2].

Because of the phenomenon of "diuretic resistance" that involves nephron remodeling causing resistance with a need to continue escalating doses to reach the "diuretic threshold," loop diuretic dosing is not a "one-size-fits-all" approach [2].

The 2011 DOSE trial investigated the question of optimal dosing in these patients as well as examined whether or not it is more effective to administer these doses as IV boluses or continuous infusions at a low dose [5]. The trial showed that "high"-dose diuretics (defined as 2.5× the home dose administered as IV) was more effective than "low-dose" diuretics and found no difference between the routes of administration (e.g., bolus dosing was no different than the continuous infusion dosing) [5].

A few things are important to note about this trial:

1. The trial did not account for the bioavailability of PO:IV furosemide (which is 2:1). For example, if a patient was on 40 mg PO QD at home, they would receive 100 mg IV furosemide. This really does support the claim that we should be aggressive and use "high-dose" diuretics.
2. The trial did not give an initial bolus prior to starting continuous infusion diuretics. Keep in mind that in order to see diuresis in these patients, the concentration of the diuretic must be above that patient's own "diuretic threshold." Because continuous infusion diuretics are given at such a low dose per time, it would take a long time to reach that threshold without the help of an initial bolus. **If considering starting a continuous infusion, always keep in mind to give an initial bolus up front to prevent this delay in effect.** Additionally, **continuous infusion may be beneficial in patients sensitive to quick fluid shifts, as it causes slow but prolonged diuresis and prevents things like hypotension.**

We have three loop diuretic agents: furosemide, torsemide, and bumetanide. These agents all differ in potency so need to be converted if interchanging between drugs. Tables 11.1 and 11.2 illustrate both oral and intravenous diuretic options; Table 11.3 illustrates equivalent diuretic doses.

Table 11.1 Commonly used oral diuretics [2]

Drug	Starting dose	Max daily dose	Duration of action
Loop diuretics			
Bumetanide	0.5–1.0 mg QD or BID	10 mg	4–6 h
Furosemide	20–40 mg QD or BID	600 mg	6–8 h
Torsemide	10–20 mg QD	200 mg	12–16 h
Thiazide diuretics			
Chlorothiazide	250–500 mg QD or BID	1000 mg	6–12 h
Chlorthalidone	12.5–25 mg QD	100 mg	24–72 h
Hydrochlorothiazide	25 mg QD or BID	200 mg	6–12 h
Indapamide	2.5 mg QD	5 mg	36 h
Metolazone	2.5 mg QD	20 mg	12–24 h

Table 11.2 Intravenous diuretics

Drug	Dose	Onset of action
Loop diuretics		
Bumetanide	1 mg IV load, then 0.5–2 mg/h infusion	5 min
Furosemide	40 mg IV load, then 10–40 mg/h infusion	5 min
Torsemide	20 mg IV load, then 5–20 mg/h infusion	10 min
Thiazide diuretics		
Chlorothiazide	500 mg—1000 mg IV	15 min

Table 11.3 Equivalent doses of diuretics

Equivalent doses
Furosemide 40 mg PO
Furosemide 20 mg IV
Torsemide 20 mg PO/IV
Bumetanide 1 mg PO/IV

11.8.2 Reassessing Diuresis and Adding Thiazides

If there is no response or the response is suboptimal, it is recommended to double the dose of loop diuretic at 2-h intervals as needed until the maximum recommended dose is reached [2]. For context, a furosemide bolus of up to 160–200 mg may be given. Higher doses of loop diuretics should be avoided due to the very real risk of ototoxicity [2].

It is important to note that in patients with renal insufficiency, higher doses of loop diuretics may be required as less of the medication gets to the site of action in the loop of Henle [2].

If diuretic resistance remains an issue despite escalating doses, *thiazide* diuretics may be added on in combination to the existing loop diuretics [2]. These diuretics work *distal* to the loop of Henle where additional sodium and water reabsorption can take place, so by inhibiting this later step, the body does not have that opportunity and more water is excreted. This recommendation is supported by the 2022 AHA/ACC/HFSA guidelines as well [2]. Recently, data looking at the effect of oral vs. IV adjuncts to loop diuretics in those with ADHF found no difference in weight loss between oral metolazone and IV chlorothiazide [6].

11.8.3 Side Effects of Loop Diuretics

Whenever a patient is undergoing diuresis, it is imperative that laboratory evaluation is conducted routinely, with particular attention to electrolytes and renal function. The most commonly seen electrolyte abnormalities with aggressive diuresis are hypokalemia and hyponatremia. Diuretics can also cause acute kidney injury, and so blood urea nitrogen (BUN), serum creatinine (SCr), and overall urine output should be assessed daily.

11.8.4 Adjuncts to Loop Diuretics

Though loop diuretics are the mainstay of diuresis, diuretic resistance can often be an issue, and adjunct agents can be considered. As mentioned previously, the addition of thiazide diuretics in addition to loop diuretics is commonly used, and guideline endorsed [2].

If cardiac output and perfusion are an issue, diuresis may be augmented by the use of inotropes [2]. Inotropes increase the force of contraction of the cardiac muscle and can increase perfusion, thus getting more blood to the kidneys and aiding in diuresis. Other considerations may include plasma ultrafiltration, aquapheresis, or renal dose dopamine [2]. Since the publication of the guidelines, new studies have also been published investigating the role of SGLT2-is or acetazolamide in these patients [7, 8].

11.8.5 Clinical Pearls Associated with Diuresis

11.8.5.1 Clinical Pearl #1: Always Look at the Whole I/Os Picture

It is a common scenario—you might be on rounds, and you find out that your patient has had "poor" diuresis overnight and is only net negative 250 mL.

Before you go increasing their diuretic regimen, it is important to get the whole picture, instead of being reactive to a suboptimal net negative number.

Ask Yourself the Following Questions
We know that the patient was only net negative 250 mL. But what were the ins and what were the outs?

For example, it is very possible that the patient had great diuresis, with an impressive urine output, but is getting a lot of fluids in. Is the patient volume restricted? How much fluid are they getting through their medications? Is it possible to concentrate any of the medications or switch from IV to oral? *Is this truly a diuresis issue or is it an intake issue?*

Let Us Solidify with a Case
Patient A is net positive 103 mL (not including insensible losses) in the past 24 h. The team would like to increase their diuretic regimen, but you first look at their I/Os. Table 11.4 shows their I/Os in the past 24 h. For reference, Patient A weighs 92 kg.

The first thing to assess is urine output for your given patient. A good rule of thumb is to look at 24-h output and translate it in terms of mL/kg/h.

Table 11.4 I/Os

Outs	Total:	2050 mL
	Urine output (24 h)	2050 mL
Ins		
	Oral intake (24 h)	946 mL
	Medication A (24 h)	432 mL
	Medication B (24 h)	150 mL
	Medication C (24 h)	250 mL
	Medication D (24 h)	250 mL
	Medication E (24 h)	125 mL
Net (24 h)		+103 mL

In this patient—>2050 mL total/92 kg/24 h = 0.93 mL/kg/h.

A urine output of >0.5/mL/kg/h is generally considered "good," with values closer to 1 or above being excellent. In this case, the patient appears to be having adequate diuresis on their current regimen.

But why is the patient still net positive? The answer lies in the amount of volume the patient is getting through medications and oral intake. Ensure that the patient is on a volume-restricted diet. Next, assess the indications and concentrations of all medications the patient is getting.

Do they truly need every IV medication? Is there an appropriate indication? Or can we discontinue any IV medications in the interim?

Are you able to concentrate any of the current medications? Check with your hospital IV room. Keep in mind that if concentrating any IV medications, make sure that they are still compatible to run in the type of line that the patient has (e.g., if currently running through a peripheral line, is a higher concentration still compatible with a peripheral line? Or would a central line be required?). These are all considerations to make.

11.8.5.2 Clinical Pearl #2: Keep in Mind That It Is Possible to Be Volume Overloaded as a Whole, But Still Be Intravascularly Dry

Another common scenario in these patients: they have a day or two of fantastic diuresis, and then all of a sudden, urine output drops and serum creatinine and BUN rise. What is going on here? Should we increase the diuretic regimen?

It is important to understand and be aware of the concept that even though a patient still has volume overload—they still have pitting edema, are above their euvolemic weight, etc.,—they can still be *intravascularly* dry.

This can happen if we are diuresing too aggressively, too quickly. When patients diurese their excess volume, volume from the "third space" such as the tissues slowly gets pulled back into the vasculature and into blood volume where it can be diuresed out. However, if we are too aggressive with our diuretic regimen, what can happen is that we diurese these patients too quickly and do not allow enough time for volume in the third space to reenter the vasculature. This can lead to decreased blood volume, hypotension, and acute kidney injury.

In this case, you may see soft blood pressures, an increase in SCr and BUN (with a BUN:SCr ratio > 20), and, in the days/hours preceding, a very high urine output (in this case, too high!).

The last thing we would want to do in this scenario is escalate the diuretics. Instead, in this case, you would want to slow down the diuresing process, allowing time for that volume to reenter the vasculature. The solution here would be to increase the frequency and possibly decrease the dose of diuretics.

Remember that each patient has their own unique diuretic threshold at which lower doses will not produce adequate diuresis. In these patients who are already on their personal lowest dose, increasing the frequency would be effective at slowing net diuresis.

11.9 Intravenous Vasodilators

Depending on a patient's hemodynamics, intravenous vasodilators can be considered; however, the role for directed vasodilators in ADHF is still unclear and does not affect outcomes in ADHF [2]. Vasodilators that cause venodilation and decrease preload may target pulmonary congestion and help more acutely with symptoms such as dyspnea while waiting for significant diuresis [2].

Intravenous nitroglycerin and nitroprusside are commonly utilized in ADHF (Table 11.5).

Nitroglycerin can be considered in those with hypertension, significant mitral regurgitation, or coronary ischemia.

Nitroprusside has the ability to cause potent blood pressure reduction, and so invasive hemodynamic monitoring (such as with an arterial line) is often required and used in an intensive care setting only. It can be considered in those with hypertension or severe mitral valve regurgitation complicating left ventricle dysfunction.

An issue with both nitroglycerin and nitroprusside is that tachyphylaxis can occur within a period of 24 h, and 1 in 5 patients may be resistant even at high doses.

Nitroprusside has an additional concern of thiocyanate and cyanide toxicity, especially in those with renal or hepatic disease and so caution should be taken in these patients.

Importantly, there is no data suggesting that IV vasodilators improve outcomes in these patients; therefore, their use is limited to relieving dyspnea in those with intact or high blood pressure [2].

Table 11.5 IV vasodilator comparison in ADHF

	IV nitroglycerin	IV sodium nitroprusside
Clinical effect	Venous dilation >> arterial dilation; arterial dilation can be seen at high doses Has more preload reduction than afterload reduction	Potent venous *and* arterial dilator = potent preload and afterload reduction
Dosing	Initial: 5–10 mcg/min; titrate as needed based on response and tolerability in increments of 5–10 mcg/min every 3–5 min up to 200 mcg/min	Initial: 0.1–0.3 mcg/kg/min; titrate as needed every 5–15 min to achieve desired hemodynamic effect; usual dosage range: 1–3 mcg/kg/min; maximum dose: 5 mcg/kg/min for an 80 kg patient
Adverse effects	Hypotension, tachyphylaxis (within 24–48 h of continuous infusion), headache, reflex tachycardia	Hypotension (more potent than seen with nitroglycerin), tachyphylaxis, reflex tachycardia, cyanide toxicity
Clinical pearls	Duration of therapy is usually short term due to tachyphylaxis	Caution in renal dysfunction—Can accumulate. Patients with renal impairment are at higher risk of cyanide toxicity Invasive monitoring generally required due to risk of hypotension (potent afterload reducer) May be particularly useful in an ADHF patient with HFrEF and dyspnea who is hemodynamically stable due to afterload reduction Duration of therapy is usually short term due to tachyphylaxis and the risk of cyanide toxicity

11.10 Cardiogenic Shock

Cardiogenic shock has a high mortality rate and is characterized by low cardiac output and hypotension.

In those who have progressed from ADHF to cardiogenic shock, intravenous inotropic support should be utilized to preserve end-organ function and maintain perfusion [2].

Despite their common use, there are few prospective trials or randomized controlled evidence to guide their use. Additionally, there is also a lack of robust data to guide the choice of one agent over another; factors such as blood pressure and presence of concomitant arrhythmia tend to guide agent selection [2].

Although all agents that have beta-1 agonism can be considered inotropes, in the context of heart failure, generally the "true" inotrope agents include milrinone and dobutamine (Table 11.6).

Key factors to consider between the agents are their effects on blood pressure and their route of elimination. Milrinone is renally excreted and can accumulate in those with renal failure. Table 11.6 reviews key differences between these agents.

Table 11.6 Inotrope comparison in ADHF

	IV dobutamine	IV milrinone
Mechanism of action	Beta-1 agonist	PDE-3 inhibitor
Renally cleared/ renal dose adjustment	No	Yes
Side effects	Tachyarrhythmias	Tachyarrhythmias and hypotension
Effect on cardiac output	Increase	Increase
Effect on SVR	Minimal	Decrease
Clinical pearls	Do not co-administer with beta-blockers as mechanisms of action cancel each other out	Caution in renal dysfunction as accumulation and prolonged hypotension can occur

11.10.1 Inotrope Clinical Pearl

Oftentimes, patients in ADHF may require vasopressors in addition to inotropes due to hypotension. A commonly seen scenario is a patient with ADHF in acute kidney injury on milrinone who has become hypotensive and was started on a vasopressor such as norepinephrine to keep mean arterial pressures (MAP) up. Because milrinone can cause hypotension and is renally eliminated, it can accumulate in those with renal dysfunction. Oftentimes, this accumulation can be part of the reason why hypotension occurs. Instead of relying on the addition of vasopressors which can increase afterload making it harder for a struggling HFrEF heart to push blood out, switching from milrinone to dobutamine may eliminate the need for pressors.

11.11 Management of Patients with ADHF and Atrial Fibrillation (AF)

As heart failure progresses and the heart continues to remodel, arrhythmias can become increasingly prominent. Chronic atrial fibrillation can become increasingly common in these patients as these structural changes occur. However, even in those without chronic AF and mild structural changes, ADHF may precipitate acute episodes of AF due to volume overload. As a patient becomes volume overloaded, the volume of blood that the left atrium needs to handle increases, and may cause stretching of the atrial wall, thus precipitating acute atrial fibrillation. In this patient, the need for diuresis is the underlying treatment of the acute atrial fibrillation episode.

In general, cardioversion should be considered in those with *new-onset* atrial fibrillation and in those with hemodynamic instability.

However, in patients with long-standing heart failure and chronic atrial fibrillation, cardiac structural changes are advanced and the chance of meaningful and successful rhythm control is oftentimes low; oftentimes, these patients are best managed with rate control strategies such as beta-blockers and/or digoxin. Keep in mind that any medications such as non-DHP calcium channel blockers should be avoided in those with systolic heart failure due to their negative inotropic properties [2].

Other precipitating causes for atrial fibrillation should also be investigated such as hormonal (e.g., hyperthyroidism), toxicologic, acute infection, or other medications (e.g., inotropes) [2].

11.12 Digoxin

11.12.1 The Role of Digoxin

The role of digoxin in heart failure is somewhat controversial, as there is conflicting data on whether or not it benefits patients with heart failure, and it is not included in the "pillars" of guideline-directed medical therapy (GDMT) management for these patients [2]. However, digoxin is often considered as a rate control agent, especially in those in the intensive care setting who cannot tolerate the potential blood pressure-lowering effects of other rate control agents, such as beta-blockers, and who are not candidates for non-dihydropyridine calcium channel blockers (e.g., those with HFrEF).

Digoxin can be theoretically beneficial to patients with heart failure given its positive inotropic properties and has two main mechanisms of action. For rate control, digoxin has an indirect effect on both the sinoatrial and atrioventricular nodes by stimulating the vagus nerve and vagal tone, thus decreasing the heart rate.

11.12.2 Mechanism of Action

Digoxin exerts its positive inotropic activity indirectly by inhibiting the Na+/K+ ATPase pump on the surface of the myocytes. To truly understand its action, you must first understand the function of two key pumps on the surface of the myocytes.

The Na+/K+ ATPase is present on the surface of myocytes (Fig. 11.4). As the name "ATPase" suggests, this pump requires energy (in the form of ATP) to actively pump ions across its channel. In other words, this pump must move ions *against* a concentration gradient.

At baseline, there is a high level of sodium *extra*cellularly (aka outside the cells) and a high level of potassium *intra*cellularly (within the cells) (this is why if blood samples are shaken or mishandled and the red blood cells lyse, you can end up with false hyperkalemia).

The Na+/K+ ATPase pumps 3Na+ out of the cell for every 2 K+ it pumps into the cell, thus leaving the cellular membrane with a net negative charge.

Mechanism of Action of Digoxin

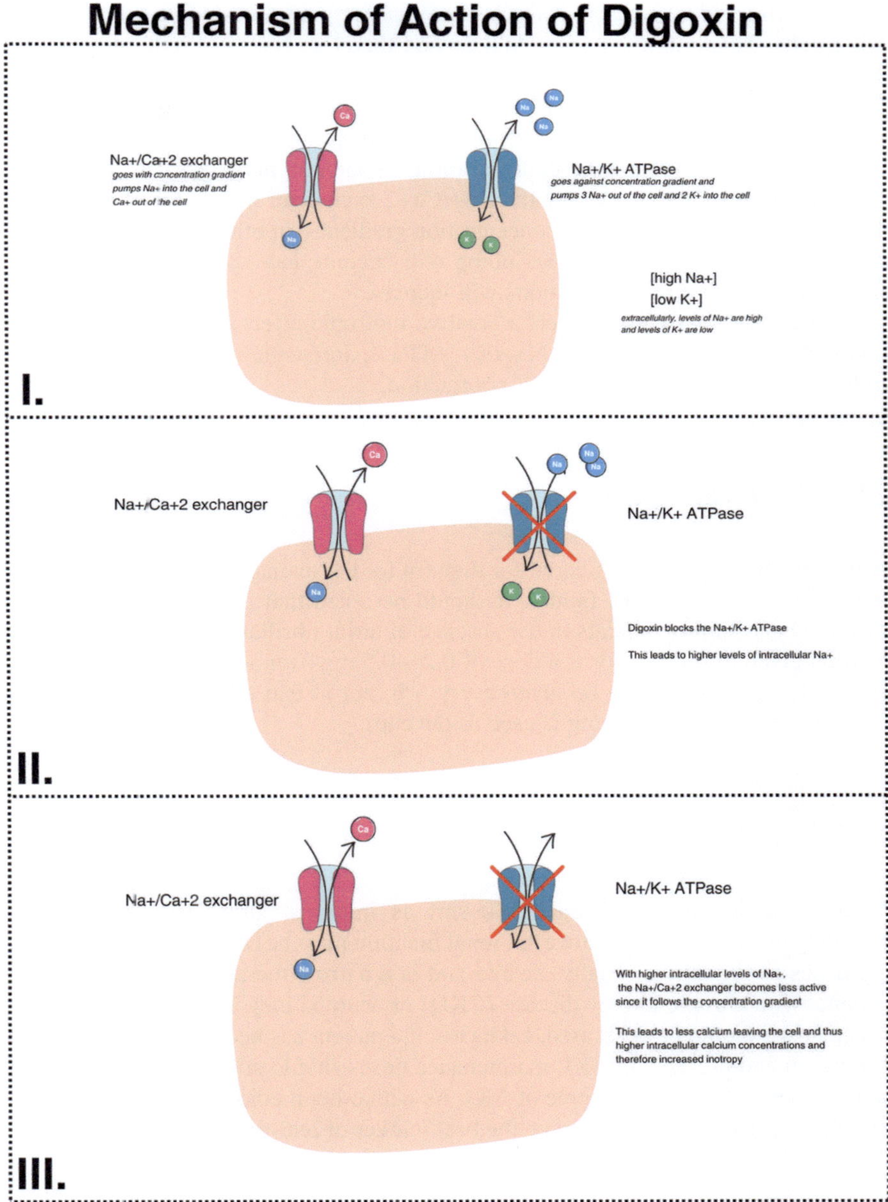

Fig. 11.4 Digoxin's mechanism of action

Meanwhile, there is also a Na+/Ca+2 exchanger pump located on the surface of these cells. This pump is *not* an ATPase and therefore does not require energy to work. In other words, this pump works *with* the concentration gradient and pumps Ca+2 *out* of the cell in exchange for Na+ based on the concentration gradient.

When digoxin inhibits the Na+/K+ ATPase, the pump no longer pumps Na+ out of the cell—thus, intracellular concentrations of sodium increase.

As mentioned above, usually the Na+/Ca+2 exchanger pumps Ca+2 **out** of cell and Na+ in to the cell *with* the concentration gradient—in other words, when intracellular Na+ levels are *high*, this pump will become less active, and as a result, intracellular calcium concentrations will increase.

This is how digoxin can exert a positive inotropic effect and increase force of contraction. By inhibiting the Na+/K+ ATPase, intracellular calcium levels rise indirectly causing a higher force of contraction.

11.12.3   Loading Dose

A loading dose can be considered for digoxin for the management of atrial fibrillation in patients with heart failure. It should be noted that loads are generally not given in heart failure patients in the absence of atrial fibrillation. Dosing varies but is often given intravenously at a dose of 0.25–0.5 mg over several minutes. Repeat doses of 0.25 mg IV may be given every 6 h, not to exceed 1.5 mg within 24 h (though often in practice 1 mg is used as the cap).

11.12.4   Maintenance Dosing

After initial loading, maintenance dosing is initiated. Oral doses range from 62.5 mcg to 250 mcg daily; however, renal function must be considered when selecting doses as digoxin is renally cleared and is a narrow therapeutic index drug. In patients with chronic kidney disease (CKD) or acute kidney injury (AKI), maintenance doses should be decreased. Likewise, if a patient has been on digoxin prior to admission and presents in AKI, maintenance doses should still be adjusted or even stopped depending on the degree of AKI. As with other medications in the critically ill, oftentimes urine output may be the best marker of real-time kidney function.

11.12.5   Monitoring

As mentioned above, digoxin is a narrow therapeutic index drug—this means that small differences in dose or blood concentrations may lead to either drug failures (subtherapeutic) or toxicities (supratherapeutic).

Digoxin levels should be taken as **troughs**, ideally immediately prior to the next dose; however, levels at least 6 h after an oral dose can be considered acceptable. Prior to 6 h after dosing, digoxin is still undergoing redistribution into target tissues (e.g., it will likely be falsely high). It is important to note that in patients with heart failure as a comorbidity, goal digoxin levels are 0.5–0.9 ng/mL, which are significantly lower than goal ranges for patients without heart failure (e.g., 0.8–2.0 ng/mL) [2].

11.12.6 When to Get a Level?

The half-life of digoxin is fairly long, 36–48 h in adults with healthy renal function, and can be as high as 3.5–5 days in those with renal impairment. Because it takes four to five half-lives for a drug to reach steady state, this means that digoxin levels will not represent steady-state levels for a minimum of 6 days. Early levels can be considered if toxicity is expected but, in general, will be falsely low if taken prior unless loading doses have been given recently.

11.12.7 Distribution

Digoxin primarily distributes into the heart, liver, kidneys, and skeletal muscle. Therefore, caution should be taken in giving high doses to obese patients, and digoxin does not distribute extensively into fat. Patients with extremes of skeletal muscle (e.g., elderly malnourished patients vs. bodybuilders) may require different doses.

11.12.8 Drug-Drug Interactions

Digoxin has multiple drug-drug interactions and is a substrate of p-glycoprotein. Always assess a patient's profile for drug-drug interactions when starting digoxin or when starting new medications.

11.12.9 Digoxin Toxicity

Aside from renal function, potassium levels are important to monitor during digoxin therapy. Hypokalemia may predispose a patient to digoxin toxicity; once digoxin toxicity occurs, hyperkalemia may occur. Other signs and symptoms of digoxin toxicity include bradycardia, GI upset and diarrhea (these are the most common symptoms), visual disturbances (yellow-green disturbances), and syncope.

11.13   ADHF Clinical Pearls

11.13.1   Liver Metabolism

Due to liver congestion, there may be altered liver metabolism when a patient is in ADHF, which may affect drug dosing. A common co-administered medication is warfarin. Patients in ADHF may present with supratherapeutic INRs, which may not be a true indicator of their warfarin dosing. For example, a patient on warfarin in ADHF that presents with a supratherapeutic INR may not necessarily require a warfarin dose adjustment on discharge as their liver congestion decreases and blood flow returns to normal.

11.13.2   Volume of Distribution

Also keep in mind that as peripheral edema and water retention increase, so does the volume of distribution in patients. This may affect drug dosing and considerations.

11.13.3   Avoid Phenylephrine

In the circumstance that vasopressors are needed, a general rule of thumb is that phenylephrine should be avoided. Phenylephrine is a pure alpha-1 agonist and increases vasoconstriction in the peripheries and therefore increases afterload, without any increase in heart contraction (inotropy). This may exacerbate an ADHF episode as the heart needs to compensate as it fights against the increased afterload. Phenylephrine can also increase pulmonary pressures making it more difficult for the heart to pump blood effectively.

11.13.4   Use Mean Arterial Pressure (MAP)

As we do in most of our critically ill patients, consider using MAP in evaluating these patients, as systolic/diastolic pressures may be misleading. Patients with severe HFrEF often are unable to generate high systolic pressures due to weakened ventricular squeeze. Because of this, they may at first glance incorrectly appear to be hypotensive if MAP is not utilized.

11.14 Guideline-Directed Medical Therapy

Guideline-directed medical therapy is extremely important in chronic heart failure and should be continued during ADHF whenever possible, with a class 1 recommendation in those with HFrEF to continue and **optimize** all preexisting GDMT unless contraindicated [2]. True contraindications are fairly rare, but include advanced-degree heart block without pacemaker for beta-blockers, angioedema for ACE-I or ARNI, and cardiogenic shock [2].

Acute kidney injury and hypotension can be common during ADHF, and in those who have a mild decrease in renal function or asymptomatic hypotension, GDMT should be continued [2].

If GDMT is discontinued or decreased, it should be restarted or optimized, respectively, as soon as possible once stable [2].

Why is there such an emphasis on GDMT in these patients? Apart from GDMT being extremely important in reducing mortality and morbidity in chronic heart failure, data supports that continuation of oral GDMT during hospitalization lowers postdischarge death and readmission vs. patients in which GDMT was discontinued [2]. Despite the importance of GDMT, the rate of GDMT prescribing after hospitalization is staggeringly low, with 42% of patients not on any GDMT or GDMT monotherapy within 1 year post-hospitalization [2]. As the 2022 AHA/ACC/HFSA guidelines put perfectly: "it cannot be assumed that oral GDMT will be initiated or optimized after hospitalization with HFrEF" [2].

Keep in mind that all GDMT in heart failure should be increased until target dose is reached or at the highest tolerated dose. Importantly, asymptomatic hypotension is not an indication to stop uptitrating these medications. See Table 11.7 for target doses.

Implementing and optimizing GDMT are one of the most important goals of ADHF hospitalization and one that should not be overlooked.

11.15 Venous Thromboembolism (VTE) Prophylaxis

In patients hospitalized with heart failure, VTE prophylaxis is recommended and is guideline supported with a class 1 recommendation.

11.16 Conclusion

ADHF is a complex but interesting disease state that every critical care practitioner will likely encounter at one time or another. Treatment of these patients is extremely nuanced, and an understanding of the underlying cardiac issues of each patient is of utmost importance.

Table 11.7 Commonly used medications in heart failure

Drug	Initial daily dose(s)	Target dose(s)
Angiotensin-converting enzyme inhibitors (ACEis)[a]		
Captopril	6.25 mg TID	50 mg TID
Enalapril	2.5 mg BID	10–20 mg BID
Fosinopril	5–10 mg QD	40 mg QD
Lisinopril	2.5–5 mg QD	20–40 mg QD
Perindopril	2 mg QD	8–16 mg QD
Quinapril	5 mg BID	20 mg BID
Ramipril	1.25–2.5 mg QD	10 mg QD
Trandolapril	1 mg QD	4 mg QD
ARB[a]		
Candesartan	4–8 mg QD	32 mg QD
Losartan	25–50 mg QD	50–150 mg QD
Valsartan	20–40 mg QD	160 mg BID
ARNi[a]		
Sacubitril/valsartan	24/26 mg BID	97/103 mg BID
Beta-blockers[a]		
Bisoprolol	1.25 mg QD	10 mg QD
Carvedilol	3.125 mg BID	25–50 mg BID
Carvedilol CR	10 mg QD	80 mg QD
Metoprolol succinate	12.5–25 mg QD	200 mg QD
Mineralocorticoid receptor antagonists[a]		
Spironolactone	12.5–25 mg QD	25–50 mg QD
Eplerenone	25 mg QD	50 mg QD
SGLT2i[a]		
Dapagliflozin	10 mg QD	10 mg QD
Empagliflozin	10 mg QD	10 mg QD
Sotagliflozin	200 mg QD	200 mg QD
Isosorbide dinitrate and hydralazine		
Fixed dose combination	20 mg and 37.5 mg TID	40 mg and 75 mg TID
Isosorbide dinitrate and hydralazine	20–30 mg and 25–50 mg TID-QID	120 mg and 300 mg in divided doses
Other		
Ivabradine	5 mg BID	7.5 mg BID
Vericiguat	2.5 mg QD	10 mg QD

[a] Indicates GDMT

References

1. Heart Failure Society of America. HFSA. 2024. https://hfsa.org/patient-hub/heart-failure-facts-information. Accessed 20 Dec 2023.
2. Heidenreich PA, Bozkurt B, Aguilar D, et al. 2022 AHA/ACC/HFSA guideline for the management of heart failure: a report of the American College of Cardiology/American Heart Association Joint Committee on Clinical Practice Guidelines. J Am Coll Cardiol. 2022;79(17):e263–421.

3. Nair R, Lak H, Hasan S, Gunasekaran D, Babar A, Gopalakrishna KV. Reducing all-cause 30-day hospital readmissions for patients presenting with acute heart failure exacerbations: a quality improvement initiative. Cureus. 2020;12(3):e7420. Published 2020 Mar 25. https://doi.org/10.7759/cureus.7420.

4. Wang SY, Valero-Elizondo J, Ali HJ, et al. Out-of-pocket annual health expenditures and financial toxicity from healthcare costs in patients with heart failure in the United States. J Am Heart Assoc. 2021;10(14):e022164. https://doi.org/10.1161/JAHA.121.022164.

5. Felker GM, Lee KL, Bull DA, et al. Diuretic strategies in patients with acute decompensated heart failure. N Engl J Med. 2011;364(9):797–805. https://doi.org/10.1056/NEJMoa1005419.

6. Cox ZL, Hung R, Lenihan DJ, Testani JM. Diuretic strategies for loop diuretic resistance in acute heart failure: the 3T trial. JACC Heart Fail. 2020;8(3):157–68. https://doi.org/10.1016/j.jchf.2019.09.012.

7. Schulze PC, Bogoviku J, Westphal J, et al. Effects of early empagliflozin initiation on diuresis and kidney function in patients with acute decompensated heart failure (EMPAG-HF). Circulation. 2022;146(4):289–98. https://doi.org/10.1161/CIRCULATIONAHA.122.059038.

8. Meekers E, Dauw J, Martens P, et al. Renal function and decongestion with acetazolamide in acute decompensated heart failure: the ADVOR trial. Eur Heart J. 2023;44(37):3672–82. https://doi.org/10.1093/eurheartj/ehad557.

Chapter 12
Right Ventricular Failure and Pulmonary Hypertension in the ICU

Ada Selina Jutba

12.1 Introduction

Right ventricular (RV) failure is a heterogeneous syndrome with various etiologies. The syndrome involves dysfunction of the heart, lungs, or a combination of both. While the left ventricle is often the center of attention with respect to cardiac function and systemic circulation, the RV is also essential for maintaining hemodynamics. RV failure was noted to be the primary cause of hospitalizations for 2.2% of heart failure admissions within the CHARITEM registry by Mockel and colleagues, so it is relatively uncommon compared to LV failure. However, RV failure was present secondary to acute LV failure in over 20% of the cases highlighting the interdependence of the ventricles [1].

Many situations in the critical care setting, whether it is the underlying disease state or through an iatrogenic cause, may progress to RV failure. Unlike other shock states that generally have a protocolized approach to treatment, understanding the etiology is imperative to guide management of critically ill patients with RV failure. Treatment involves a nuanced balance between preload optimization, afterload reduction, and contractility augmentation. Pharmacists play a vital role in ensuring safe and appropriate use of high-risk and specialty medications used in RV failure and pulmonary hypertension specifically; therefore, it is essential for them to be knowledgeable on the complexities of this disease state.

A. S. Jutba (✉)
Department of Pharmacy, Memorial Hermann Memorial City Medical Center, Houston, TX, USA
e-mail: AdaSelina.Jutba@memorialhermann.org

Y. Alzaidi, M. A. Gebily (eds.), *The Pharmacist's Expanded Role in Critical Care Medicine*, https://doi.org/10.1007/978-3-031-77335-8_12

317

12.2 Pathophysiology of Right Ventricular Failure

The right ventricle of the heart is connected to systemic venous return and pulmonary circulation. Compared to the left ventricle, the right ventricle is thinner and has less muscle fibers because the pressure in pulmonary circulation is significantly lower than the pressure in systemic circulation. Furthermore, the right ventricle is slightly larger and more compliant. This makes the right ventricle very sensitive to changes in afterload, and it will hypertrophy and dilate to preserve stroke volume. While an increase in afterload in the left ventricle will undoubtedly decrease stroke volume, the same increase will reduce the stroke volume in the right ventricle even further [2]. Sagawa and colleagues defined RV failure as a state in which the RV is unable to meet the demands for blood flow without excessive use of the Frank-Starling mechanism [3]. The underlying mechanisms of right ventricular failure can be described as altered preload, increased RV afterload, decreased RV contractility, altered ventricular interdependence, and arrhythmias. None of the aforementioned mechanisms are mutually exclusive but rather concomitant.

Group 2 PH (discussed below) is caused by left ventricular dysfunction, valvular insufficiency, and congenital abnormalities. Collectively, their hemodynamics are represented by elevated mean pulmonary artery pressure (mPAP) and elevated pulmonary capillary wedge pressure (PCWP), or RV preload. This can lead to chronic excessive RV preload. The passive backward flow of filling pressures, either through loss of atrial compliance, diastolic dysfunction, or regurgitation, results in excessive RV preload. The worsening of pulmonary vascular remodeling over time precipitates RV failure.

Pulmonary diseases play a role in the development of RV failure due to the outflow of the RV to the lungs via the pulmonary artery. A high-risk pulmonary embolism (PE) occurs when over 50% of the pulmonary vasculature is occluded by thrombosis [4]. The degree of occlusion, coupled with hemodynamic instability, increases RV afterload. Chronic respiratory disorders can also cause acute RV failure. In chronic thromboembolic pulmonary hypertension (CTEPH), secondary remodeling of the arterioles and myocardium over time causes a gradual increase in RV afterload [5]. In chronic obstructive pulmonary disease (COPD), pulmonary hyperinflation, airway resistance, chronic CO_2 retention, hypoxia, endothelial dysfunction, and rarefaction of the vascular bed are all mechanisms that increase RV afterload [2].

Cardiac diseases involving the right side of the heart, such as RV ischemia or infarction, lead to decreased perfusion in the right side of the heart, which decreases RV contractility and progresses to RV failure. Cardiomyopathies can alter the structure of the RV. Dilated cardiomyopathy involves the enlargement of the left ventricle. Hypertrophic obstructive cardiomyopathy is the muscle thickening of the interventricular septum. Both structural abnormalities affect the RV's contractility and may lead to RV failure. Pericardial diseases (e.g., tamponade) may alter ventricular interdependence. Tachyarrhythmias can also precipitate RV failure. For instance, atrial fibrillation increases LV filling pressures, subsequently causing PH and eventually RV failure [2, 6].

An iatrogenic cause of right ventricular failure common in critically ill patients is the use of mechanical ventilation. Humans normally breathe through negative-pressure respiration. During inhalation, the chest cavity and rib cage expand while the diaphragm contracts causing a decrease in intrathoracic pressure. Air enters the lungs through negative pressure. During exhalation, the diaphragm relaxes and creates positive pressure to flow air out of the lungs. Conversely, mechanical ventilation administers positive pressure to the upper airways, thereby increasing intrathoracic pressure. Increased intrathoracic pressure can subsequently increase right atrial pressure and consequently decrease venous return (i.e., right ventricular preload) and cardiac output. Furthermore, prolonged mechanical ventilation may lead to atelectatic and overdistended alveoli, both of which compress alveolar vessels and increase RV afterload [2, 7–9].

12.3 Diagnostic Findings

Signs of RV failure are the downstream effects of systemic congestion and hypoperfusion. Systemic congestion can present as jugular venous distension and peripheral edema. Hypoperfusion can lead to organ dysfunction like acute kidney injury, hepatic congestion, and impairment of the intestinal barrier in the gastrointestinal tract. If collected, elevated brain natriuretic peptides may be sensitive but not specific for diagnosing right ventricular failure. Patients may endorse symptoms of dyspnea, fatigue, lower extremity edema, exercise intolerance, and right upper quadrant tenderness [7–10].

Echocardiography can provide comprehensive information regarding the right heart's morphology, right ventricular function, valvular abnormalities, and estimated hemodynamics. The American Society of Echocardiography and the European Association of Cardiovascular Imaging recommend quantitative assessment of RV function using at least one of the following parameters: fractional area change, tricuspid annular plane systolic excursion, systolic S′ velocity of the tricuspid annulus by Doppler tissue imaging (DTI), and right ventricular index of myocardial performance (Table 12.1) [10–12]. A more invasive diagnostic tool is a pulmonary artery (PA) catheter, or Swan-Ganz catheter. The PA catheter measures continuous hemodynamic parameters about right and left atrial pressures,

Table 12.1 Echocardiographic findings in RV failure

Parameter	Abnormality threshold
Fractional area change	<35%
Tricuspid annular plane systolic excursion	<17 mm
DTI-derived systolic S′ velocity of the tricuspid annulus	<9.5 cm/s
RV index of myocardial performance	>0.54

Table 12.2 Pulmonary artery catheter measurements

Parameter	Normal values
Right atrial pressure (RAP)	2–6 mmHg
Right ventricular systolic pressure (RVSP)	15–25 mmHg
Right ventricular diastolic pressure (RVDP)	0–8 mmHg
Mean pulmonary artery pressure (mPAP)	8–20 mmHg
Pulmonary capillary wedge pressure (PCWP)	$\leq$15 mmHg
Cardiac output (CO)	4–8 L/min
Cardiac index (CI)	2.5–4.0 L/min.m^2

pulmonary vascular resistance, and cardiac output (Table 12.2). The pressures on the right side of the heart, the mPAP, or the PCWP can be elevated in RV failure depending on the etiology. The cardiac output and index will likely be reduced in decompensated RV failure.

12.4 Management of Acute Decompensated Right Ventricular Failure

12.4.1 Oxygen Therapy

Oxygen therapy should be used to maintain arterial oxygen saturation greater than 90%. Hypoxia, hypercapnia, and acidosis promote vasoconstriction in the pulmonary vasculature, which further increases RV afterload. Patients with respiratory failure and hypercapnia may benefit from noninvasive ventilation. Positive-pressure ventilation with intubation should be avoided if possible because it can also increase RV afterload. Furthermore, intravenous sedation that may be required during mechanical ventilation may lead to systemic hypotension, thereby decreasing LV preload [10].

12.4.2 Pharmacological Management

Treatment of acute right ventricular failure is determined by the underlying insult and can be either optimizing preload, reducing afterload, or increasing right ventricular contractility [2, 8, 12]. Patients with RV failure may be preload dependent, but volume loading should be done cautiously and only in the setting of low arterial pressure without elevated filling pressures. Volume loading can potentially overdistend the right ventricle, decrease contractility, and ultimately reduce systemic cardiac output. Rather, patients may benefit from volume removal to normalize preload to decrease stress on the right ventricle [2, 9, 10]. Volume reduction can be done through the use of loop diuretics. Loop diuretics inhibit the sodium-potassium-chloride cotransporter in the thick ascending loop of Henle. The net result is a reduction in the reabsorption of the ions and consequently water through osmosis. Examples of loop diuretics are furosemide, bumetanide, torsemide, and ethacrynic acid. Diuresis can be augmented with concomitant use of thiazide diuretics through sequential nephron blockade as they work more distally in the nephron at the distal convoluted tubule. Thiazide diuretics inhibit the sodium-chloride cotransporter to also decrease sodium reabsorption but to a lesser degree than loop diuretics. Examples include metolazone, hydrochlorothiazide, and chlorothiazide. In some instances, ultrafiltration or renal replacement therapy may be necessary to reduce preload.

Afterload reduction is beneficial in scenarios with elevated right ventricular afterload or elevated pulmonary vascular resistance (PVR). In the setting of an intermediate-high or high-risk PE, thrombolytics with alteplase or tenecteplase may be indicated to decrease RV afterload [5]. Group 1 PH, or pulmonary arterial hypertension (PAH), has the most well-established therapies to reduce afterload. The three main pathways in pharmacologic management of PAH are endothelin, nitric oxide, and prostacyclin [13–15]. Endothelin-1 normally acts on endothelin receptor A to cause vasoconstriction and cell proliferation and on endothelin receptor B to cause vasodilation and antiproliferation. Endothelin receptor antagonists such as bosentan, ambrisentan, and macitentan competitively inhibit endothelin-1. Phosphodiesterase type 5 inhibitors include sildenafil and tadalafil. They prevent the breakdown of cyclic guanosine monophosphate (cGMP) in pulmonary vascular smooth muscle, thereby potentiating pulmonary vascular smooth muscle relaxation and pulmonary vascular bed vasodilation. Riociguat is a soluble guanylate cyclase stimulator and sensitizes endogenous soluble guanylate cyclase by stabilizing nitric oxide-soluble guanylate cyclase binding. The resultant effect increases cyclic guanosine monophosphate, which influences vascular tone, proliferation, fibrosis, and inflammation. Riociguat is also approved for the treatment of group 4 PH patients who have residual CTEPH after surgical treatment or are deemed inoperable [16]. Prostacyclins mimic endogenous prostacyclin (PGI$_2$) and cause direct vasodilation of pulmonary and systemic arterial vascular beds, inhibition of platelet aggregation, and antiproliferative effects. Prostacyclins are available in different dosage formulations and can be administered intravenously [epoprostenol (Flolan®, Veletri®), treprostinil (Remodulin®)], subcutaneously [treprostinil (Remodulin®), orally [epoprostenol (Iloprost®), treprostinil (Orenitram®)], or inhaled [treprostinil (Tyvaso®)]. Initial combination therapy is now the standard of care for PAH to ideally target the different pathways [17, 18].

Lastly, augmentation of right ventricular contractility can also be utilized. Addressing the underlying insult of right ventricular failure is important; however, inotropic support may be utilized in the interim. Inotropes will increase forward flow in situations of inadequate cardiac output [2, 9, 10]. Milrinone is a phosphodiesterase III (PDE III) inhibitor. Inhibition of PDE III prevents the breakdown of cyclic adenosine monophosphate (cAMP) and guanosine monophosphate (cGMP). cAMP leads to phosphorylation of calcium ion channels in the sarcoplasmic reticulum and increasing calcium availability in the myocytes. This manifests as increased cardiac contractility. Subsequently, PDE III inhibition increases calcium reuptake into the sarcoplasmic reticulum and improves myocardial relaxation. Additionally, PDE III inhibition prevents cGMP metabolism in the vascular smooth muscle, resulting in dilation of the arteries and veins. Dobutamine stimulates beta-1 adrenergic receptors in the myocardium to increase contractility and heart rate. It also stimulates beta-2 receptors in the peripheral vasculature, causing vasodilation. Milrinone has more potent pulmonary and systemic vasodilatory effects compared to dobutamine, leading to more profound reductions in right ventricle end-diastolic pressures. Consequently, due to milrinone's potent vasodilatory effects and longer half-life, it is more likely to incite hypotension.

12.4.3 Mechanical Circulatory Support (MCS)

If all pharmacological options have been optimized and exhausted, MCS can be considered. Patient criteria for eligibility vary by institution. Timing of cannulation or implantation and device selection are crucial to minimize end-organ damage and maximize the chances of recovery. Device selection also depends on the anticipated duration of support. Extracorporeal membrane oxygenation (ECMO) is a form of life support where deoxygenated blood from the vasculature is circulated outside of the body by a mechanical pump, gets saturated with oxygen through an oxygenator, and then gets recirculated back into the body. Venoarterial (VA) ECMO bypasses the heart and lungs and provides respiratory and hemodynamic support. The typical recommended duration of ECMO is 5–10 days due to its associated complications such as infection, thrombus formation, and limb hypoperfusion [10, 13]. A right ventricular assist device (RVAD) is a device surgically or percutaneously implanted to assist with right ventricular contractility to the pulmonary artery. RVADs have more data for prolonged use up to months, though they are only approved for up to 4 weeks [19]. Due to the temporary nature of MCS, these devices only serve as a bridge therapy to either recovery or cardiac transplantation.

12.5 Pulmonary Hypertension

Pulmonary hypertension, among many other diseases, can progress to right ventricular (RV) failure. Pulmonary hypertension (PH) is a complex disease state that has a direct impact on the RV. The gold standard for diagnosing PH is a right heart catheterization. The 2022 European Society of Cardiology and European Respiratory Society Guidelines for the Diagnosis and Treatment of Pulmonary Hypertension define PH as a mPAP 20 mmHg at rest. Other pertinent hemodynamic measurements include PVR and PCWP, both of which are utilized to differentiate between precapillary PH and isolated postcapillary PH [13–15].

12.5.1   Classification of Pulmonary Hypertension

The World Health Organization (WHO) classifies pulmonary hypertension under five different clinical subgroups (Table 12.3) based on the underlying pathophysiology, clinical presentation, and hemodynamics. Understanding the different classifications of PH is imperative as it will guide the course of treatment. Group 1 PH is known as pulmonary arterial hypertension (PAH). PAH is the most aggressive form of PH with the most targeted pharmacologic therapies to slow its progression. The World Symposium on Pulmonary Hypertension proposed that the following medications and toxins have definitive association with PAH: anorexigens (e.g., aminorex, dexfenfluramine, fenfluramine), benfluorex, dasatinib, methamphetamines,

Table 12.3 Clinical classification of pulmonary hypertension

Group		Subclassifications
1	Pulmonary arterial hypertension (PAH)	• Idiopathic • Heritable • Associated with drugs and toxins • Associated with connective tissue disease, HIV infection, portal hypertension, congenital heart disease, schistosomiasis • PAH with features of venous/capillary (PVOD/PCH) involvement • Persistent PH of the newborn
2	PH associated with left heart disease	• Heart failure with preserved ejection fraction • Heart failure with reduced or mildly reduced ejection fraction • Valvular heart disease • Congenital/acquired cardiovascular conditions leading to postcapillary PH
3	PH associated with lung diseases and/or hypoxia	• Obstructive lung disease or emphysema • Restrictive lung disease • Lung disease with mixed restrictive/obstructive pattern • Hypoventilation syndromes • Hypoxia without lung disease (e.g., high altitude) • Developmental lung disorders
4	PH associated with pulmonary artery obstructions	• Chronic thromboembolic PH • Other pulmonary artery obstructions (sarcomas, malignant and nonmalignant tumors, arteritis without connective tissue disease, congenital pulmonary arterial stenosis, hydatidosis)
5	PH with unclear and/ or multifactorial mechanisms	• Hematological disorders (inherited and acquired chronic hemolytic anemia, chronic myeloproliferative disorders) • Systemic disorders (sarcoidosis, pulmonary Langerhans cell histiocytosis, neurofibromatosis) • Metabolic disorders (glycogen storage disease, Gaucher disease) • Chronic renal failure with or without hemodialysis • Pulmonary tumor thrombotic microangiopathy • Fibrosing mediastinitis

and toxic rapeseed oil. Certain genetic mutations may also predispose a patient to develop PAH. Bone morphogenetic protein receptor 2 (BMPR2) mutations have been identified in approximately 75% of patients with familial PAH. Other rare mutations include activin-like receptor kinase 1 (ALK-1), endoglin (ENG), and mothers against decapentaplegic homolog 9 (SMAD9). The pathophysiology of PAH involves narrowing of the pulmonary arteries caused by an imbalance of prostacyclin, nitric oxide (NO), and endothelin 1 (ET1).

Group 2 PH is associated with left heart disease. Patients in this group typically have concomitant heart failure with preserved or reduced ejection fraction. Abnormalities on the left side of the heart increase PCWP to >15 mmHg and cause passive backflow of filling pressures on the right side, thereby increasing mPAP. Group 3 PH is associated with lung diseases and/or hypoxia. Lung diseases associated with this group include COPD, interstitial lung diseases, and developmental lung diseases. Hypoxia releases molecules such as endothelin that lead to smooth muscle cell vasospasm, proliferation, and vasoconstriction. Other pathophysiologic changes are arteriolar neo-muscularization, intimal thickening, and adventitial collagen deposition. These changes will eventually obliterate the pulmonary vasculature.

Group 4 PH is associated with pulmonary artery obstructions. Pulmonary emboli and prolonged obstruction of the pulmonary arteries will increase mPAP over time. These patients may have underlying hematological disorders contributing to their hypercoagulable state. Lastly, group 5 captures PH secondary to unclear causes or multifactorial mechanisms. Sickle cell disease (SCD) in particular is a hallmark disorder associated with group 5 PH. SCD patients have a component of group 2 PH with left ventricular dysfunction but also characteristics of group 4 due to vasculopathy from intravascular hemolysis.

The severity of disease and its impact on a patient's daily activities are classified based on the WHO functional status, which was modeled after the New York Heart Association functional class (Table 12.4). WHO functional class is one of the strongest predictors of survival. A patient's worsening functional status is an indicator of disease progression [15].

12.6   The Pharmacist's Role

Pharmacists are key healthcare team members in the ICU with pulmonary hypertension management. Pulmonary hypertension medications are highly specialized. The pharmacist must be well versed in knowing which medications are indicated for a specific WHO group and which have been studied as combination therapies. Responsibilities of the pharmacist include regulatory compliance, medication safety, medication reconciliation, transitions of care, and side effect management [20].

Endothelin receptor antagonists and soluble guanylate cyclase stimulators are highly teratogenic. All prescribers and patients must be enrolled in a Risk Evaluation and Mitigation Strategy (REMS) program to prescribe and receive the medication,

Table 12.4 WHO functional status classification

Class	Description
I	Patients with PH but without resulting limitation of physical activity. Ordinary physical activity does not cause undue dyspnea or fatigue, chest pain, or near syncope
II	Patients with PH resulting in slight limitation of physical activity. They are comfortable at rest. Ordinary physical activity causes undue dyspnea or fatigue, chest pain, or near syncope
III	Patients with PH resulting in marked limitation of physical activity. They are comfortable at rest. Less than ordinary activity causes undue dyspnea or fatigue, chest pain, or near syncope
IV	Patients with PH with an inability to carry out any physical activity without symptoms. These patients manifest signs of right heart failure. Dyspnea and/or fatigue may even be present at rest. Discomfort is increased by any physical activity

respectively. Female patients of childbearing potential are required to be on contraception and take monthly pregnancy tests. Bosentan carries a risk of hepatic impairment; therefore, liver function tests are required at baseline and monthly while a patient is on therapy. Pharmacists are instrumental in ensuring safety and regulatory compliance with the REMS programs when dispensing these medications. Furthermore, these medications are only available through certain outpatient specialty pharmacies to also maintain a limited dispensing process. In the inpatient setting, it is crucial that the pharmacy department has outlined protocols for initiation and continuation of these therapies.

Parenteral prostacyclin analogs are recognized by the Institute for Safe Medication Practices as a high-alert medication. There have been multiple documented medication errors surrounding these therapies. Examples of errors included unintentional bolus administration from flushing the line, incorrect dose calculations, and pump-related errors. Pharmacists can be instrumental in ensuring safe administration of the prostacyclin analogs. First, pharmacists can contact the patient's specialty pharmacy to confirm the patient's dosing weight and dose. Next, pharmacists can double-check the calculations of IV bags and confirm the correct concentration. Pharmacists can collaborate with the physician on dose titrations, which are dependent on the patient's tolerability, and minimize adverse effects. The vasodilatory effects of prostacyclin analogs may lead to flushing, headaches, nasal congestion, nausea, and diarrhea [21]. Lastly, pharmacists can implement policies outlining the entire medication distribution process within the hospital. They can create standardized order sets to prevent medication errors, restrict inpatient administration to units with trained staff, and develop protocols for line exchanges and blood culture draws.

12.7   Conclusion

Acute RV failure is a multifaceted disease state that requires an in-depth understanding of the underlying pathophysiology and disease state for appropriate management. RV failure is commonly encountered in the critically ill population and is associated with poor prognosis if left untreated. Pulmonary hypertension is one of many disease states that can progress to RV failure. Treatment of RV failure involves preload optimization, afterload reduction, and cardiac contractility augmentation.

References

1. Mockel M, Searle J, Muller R, Slagman A, Storchmann H, Oestereich P, Wyrwich W, Ale-Abaei A, Vollert JO, Koch M, Somasundaram R. Chief complaints in medical emergencies: do they relate to underlying disease and outcome? The Charité emergency medicine study (CHARITEM). Eur J Emerg Med. 2013;20(2):103–8.
2. Arrigo M, Huber LC, Winnik S, Mikulicic F, Guidetti F, Frank M, Flammer AJ, Ruschitzka F. Right ventricular failure: pathophysiology, diagnosis and treatment. Card Fail Rev. 2019;5(3):140.
3. Sagawa K, Maughan L, Suga H, Sunagawa K. Cardiac contraction and the pressure-volume relationships. New York, NY: Oxford University Press; 1988.
4. Liu J, Yang P, Tian H, Zhen K, McCabe C, Zhao L, Zhai Z. Right ventricle remodeling in chronic thromboembolic pulmonary hypertension. J Transl Int Med. 2022;10(2):125–33.
5. Konstantinides SV, Meyer G, Becattini C, Bueno H, Geersing GJ, Harjola VP, Huisman MV, Humbert M, Jennings CS, Jiménez D, Kucher N. 2019 ESC guidelines for the diagnosis and management of acute pulmonary embolism developed in collaboration with the European Respiratory Society (ERS) the task force for the diagnosis and management of acute pulmonary embolism of the European Society of Cardiology (ESC). Eur Heart J. 2020;41(4):543–603.
6. Gorter TM, van Melle JP, Rienstra M, Borlaug BA, Hummel YM, Van Gelder IC, Hoendermis ES, Voors AA, Van Veldhuisen DJ, Lam CS. Right heart dysfunction in heart failure with preserved ejection fraction: the impact of atrial fibrillation. J Card Fail. 2018;24(3):177–85.
7. Vieillard-Baron A, Naeije R, Haddad F, Bogaard HJ, Bull TM, Fletcher N, Lahm T, Magder S, Orde S, Schmidt G, Pinsky MR. Diagnostic workup, etiologies and management of acute right ventricle failure: a state-of-the-art paper. Intensive Care Med. 2018;44:774–90.
8. Sanz J, Sánchez-Quintana D, Bossone E, Bogaard HJ, Naeije R. Anatomy, function, and dysfunction of the right ventricle: JACC state-of-the-art review. J Am Coll Cardiol. 2019;73(12):1463–82.
9. Houston BA, Brittain EL, Tedford RJ. Right Ventricular Failure. N Engl J Med. 2023;388(12):1111–25.
10. Harjola VP, Mebazaa A, Čelutkienė J, Bettex D, Bueno H, Chioncel O, Crespo-Leiro MG, Falk V, Filippatos G, Gibbs S, Leite-Moreira A. Contemporary management of acute right ventricular failure: a statement from the heart failure association and the working group on pulmonary circulation and right ventricular function of the European Society of Cardiology. Eur J Heart Fail. 2016;18(3):226–41.
11. Lang RM, Badano LP, Mor-Avi V, Afilalo J, Armstrong A, Ernande L, Flachskampf FA, Foster E, Goldstein SA, Kuznetsova T, Lancellotti P. Recommendations for cardiac chamber quantification by echocardiography in adults: an update from the American Society of Echocardiography and the European Association of Cardiovascular Imaging. Eur Heart J Cardiovasc Imaging. 2015;16(3):233–71.
12. Cherpanath TG, Lagrand WK, Schultz MJ, Groeneveld AB. Cardiopulmonary interactions during mechanical ventilation in critically ill patients. Neth Hear J. 2013;21:166–72.
13. Humbert M, Kovacs G, Hoeper MM, Badagliacca R, Berger RM, Brida M, Carlsen J, Coats AJ, Escribano-Subias P, Ferrari P, Ferreira DS. 2022 ESC/ERS Guidelines for the diagnosis and treatment of pulmonary hypertension: Developed by the task force for the diagnosis and treatment of pulmonary hypertension of the European Society of Cardiology (ESC) and the European Respiratory Society (ERS). Endorsed by the International Society for Heart and

Lung Transplantation (ISHLT) and the European Reference Network on rare respiratory diseases (ERN-LUNG). Eur Heart J. 2022;43(38):3618–731.

14. Bousseau S, Fais RS, Gu S, Frump A, Lahm T. Pathophysiology and new advances in pulmonary hypertension. BMJ Med. 2023;2(1):e000137.

15. Sysol JR, Machado RF. Classification and pathophysiology of pulmonary hypertension. Contin Cardiol Educ. 2018;4(1):2–12.

16. Ghofrani HA, D'Armini AM, Grimminger F, Hoeper MM, Jansa P, Kim NH, Mayer E, Simonneau G, Wilkins MR, Fritsch A, Neuser D. Riociguat for the treatment of chronic thromboembolic pulmonary hypertension. N Engl J Med. 2013;369(4):319–29.

17. Kirtania L, Maiti R, Srinivasan A, Mishra A. Effect of combination therapy of endothelin receptor antagonist and phosphodiesterase-5 inhibitor on clinical outcome and pulmonary haemodynamics in patients with pulmonary arterial hypertension: a meta-analysis. Clin Drug Investig. 2019;39:1031–44.

18. Sitbon O, Jaïs X, Savale L, Cottin V, Bergot E, Macari EA, Bouvaist H, Dauphin C, Picard F, Bulifon S, Montani D. Upfront triple combination therapy in pulmonary arterial hypertension: a pilot study. Eur Respir J. 2014;43(6):1691–7.

19. Makdisi G, Wang IW. Extra corporeal membrane oxygenation (ECMO) review of a lifesaving technology. J Thorac Dis. 2015;7(7):E166.

20. Macaulay TE, Covell MB, Pogue KT. An update on the management of pulmonary arterial hypertension and the pharmacist's role. J Pharm Pract. 2016;29(1):67–76.

21. Torbic H. Management of pulmonary arterial hypertension in the ICU. J Pharm Pract. 2019;32(3):303–13.

Chapter 13
Cardiac Arrhythmias

GwangYee J. Hu and Cavan O'Kane

13.1 Introduction

Cardiac arrhythmias are defined as abnormal rhythms of the heart. The overall estimated prevalence is between 1.5% and 5% of the general population and is associated with significant morbidity and mortality [1]. There are a wide range of classifications and presentations, but these arrhythmias are generally categorized based on their origin (atrial vs. ventricular), conduction rate (tachycardia vs. bradycardia), and/or QRS complex width (narrow vs. wide). Diagnosis is determined and confirmed by the readings on an electrocardiogram (ECG). In a normal conduction pathway, an electrical impulse is first triggered by the sinoatrial (SA) node and travels to the atrioventricular (AV) node, where it then passes through the bundle of His, the left and right bundle branches of the heart, and finally the Purkinje fibers. A departure at any point of this electrical pathway is considered an arrhythmia and may require medical or surgical treatment. This chapter is broken down into the various atrial and ventricular arrhythmias and their respective management.

G. J. Hu (✉)
Ernest Mario School of Pharmacy, Rutgers, the State University of New Jersey, Piscataway, NJ, USA

Robert Wood Johnson University Somerset, Somerville, NJ, USA
e-mail: jessica.hu@pharmacy.rutgers.edu

C. O'Kane
Ernest Mario School of Pharmacy, Rutgers, the State University of New Jersey, Piscataway, NJ, USA

Penn Medicine Princeton Medical Center, Plainsboro Township, NJ, USA

13.2 Atrial Arrhythmias

13.2.1 Sinus Bradycardia

Sinus bradycardia is defined as sinus rhythm with a heart rate ≤50–60 beats per minute (bpm) [2]. Sinus bradycardia may be a result of sinus node dysfunction (SND), historically referred to as sick sinus syndrome. SND carries a prevalence of 403–666 per million individuals with an incidence of 63 per million per year requiring a permanent pacemaker [3]. One of the major causes of SND is idiopathic degeneration associated with aging. In older adult patients ≥65 years of age, SND is present in 1 of every 600 individuals [4]. Other intrinsic and extrinsic risk factors and etiologies for SND are listed in Table 13.1 [2].

Signs and symptoms of sinus bradycardia vary from asymptomatic to symptomatic. Symptomatic presentations often include hypotension, fatigue, weakness, dizziness, lightheadedness, syncope, and exercise intolerance [2]. ECG findings usually consist of a regular rhythm, rate ≤50 bpm, normal QRS duration, and PR interval, and P-wave is usually visible before each QRS complex (Fig. 13.1).

Treatment is only necessary if the patient is symptomatic, as many patients have a heart rate of less than 60 bpm under normal physiological conditions. The patient should be assessed for any reversible causes of sinus bradycardia, such as drugs. For patients who recently had a myocardial infarction (MI) or heart failure with reduced ejection fraction (HFrEF), β-blockers may need to be continued despite sinus bradycardia for their mortality-lowering effects. For most patients, you can monitor and observe the patient without intervention. However, if the patient is

Table 13.1 Select intrinsic and extrinsic causes of SND

Intrinsic causes
Idiopathic degenerative disease associated with aging (most common cause)
Myocardial ischemia
Infiltrative diseases (e.g., sarcoidosis, amyloidosis)
Collagen vascular diseases (e.g., systemic lupus erythematosus, rheumatoid arthritis, scleroderma)
Infection (e.g., infective endocarditis, Lyme disease, Chagas disease, toxoplasmosis)
Surgical trauma (e.g., valve replacement, heart transplantation)

Extrinsic causes
Drug induced
Examples: β-blocker, non-dihydropyridine calcium channel blockers, amiodarone, dronedarone, propafenone, flecainide, ivabradine, clonidine, dexmedetomidine, propofol, cisplatin, fluorouracil, paclitaxel, donepezil, citalopram
Neurologic disorders
Autonomic syndromes
Hypothyroidism
Electrolyte abnormalities (e.g., hyper/hypokalemia, hypomagnesemia)
Hypothermia
Hypoxia
Metabolic acidosis

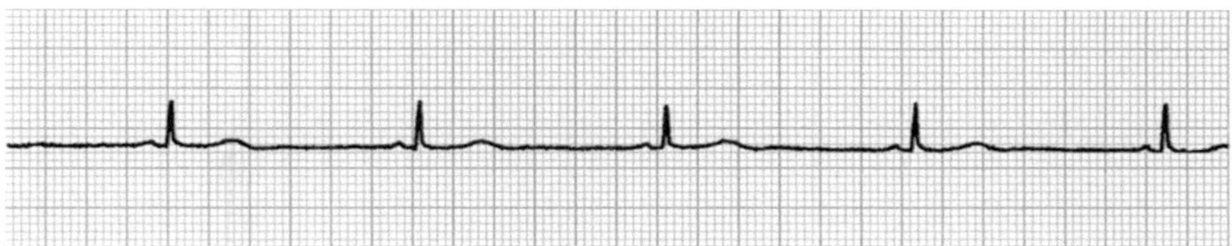

Fig. 13.1 Sinus bradycardia

persistently bradycardic with hypotension, altered mentation, evidence of shock, ischemic chest discomfort, and/or acute heart failure, atropine 1 mg intravenously may be considered [2]. Repeat dosing every 3–5 min may be performed up to a maximum dose of 3 mg. Atropine is a parasympatholytic drug that enhances AV nodal conduction and automaticity [5]. The efficacy of atropine for sinus bradycardia is supported by small nonrandomized studies with small populations [5–7]. Atropine was shown to increase heart rate above 60 bpm for most individuals included in these studies. One study reported that approximately 47% of patients had a complete or partial response to atropine treatment to achieve a heart rate ≥60 bpm and systolic blood pressure ≥90 mmHg [5]. Of note, atropine will not improve AV block at the bundle of His, and some reports suggest worsened AV conduction and hemodynamic compromise [2]. Adverse effects of atropine include dry mouth, blurred vision, urinary retention, and altered mentation. If bradycardia is unresponsive to atropine, then transcutaneous pacing may be initiated and/or dopamine 2–10 mcg/kg/min or epinephrine 2–10 mcg/min continuous infusions titrated to response [2]. In refractory cases, transvenous pacing may be considered. Goals of therapy include correcting heart rate and preventing further hemodynamic instability. Monitor heart rate, blood pressure, electrocardiogram, symptoms, and adverse effects of interventional medications.

13.2.2 Atrioventricular Blocks

The prevalence of atrioventricular blocks is not well characterized. First-degree AV blocks appear to be more common than second-degree or third-degree AV blocks [2]. For first-degree AV block, prevalence has been reported in African American patients compared with Caucasian patients in most age groups [8]. The etiologies of AV block are similar to those described for SND (see Table 13.1). AV block may be classified by the degree of blockage (i.e., first-degree, second-degree, and third-degree) or anatomically by the site of block (i.e., AV node, within the bundle of His, or below the bundle of His) [2]. Anatomic determination of block is usually determined by invasive electrophysiology studies but may be clinically important to guide interventions. For example, AV nodal blocks are typically more responsive to autonomic manipulation, and blocks occurring within or below the bundle of His are less likely to respond to atropine therapy [2]. Conduction delays in the AV node

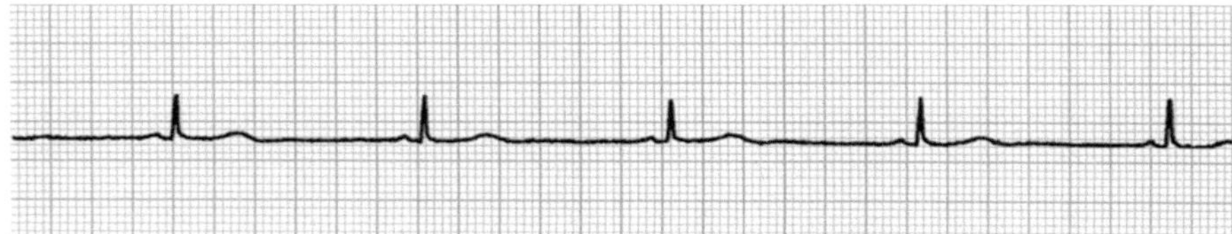

Fig. 13.2 First-degree AV block

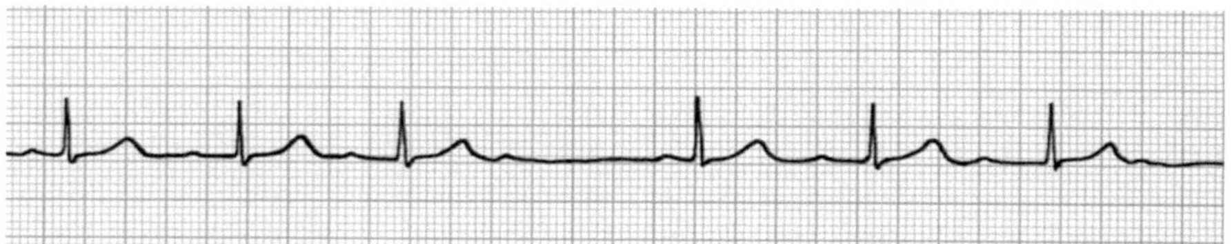

Fig. 13.3 Second-degree AV block, Mobitz I

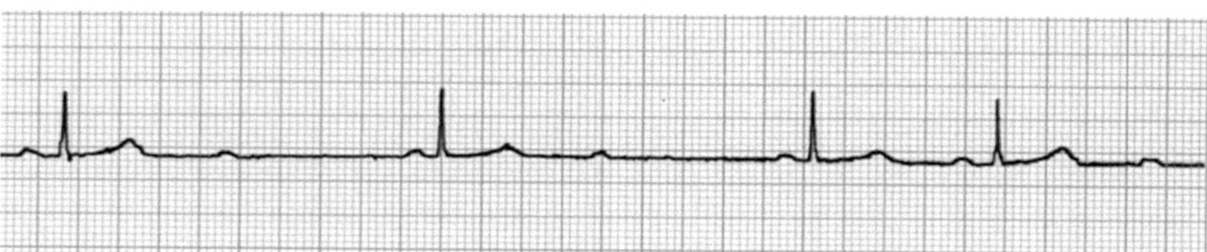

Fig. 13.4 Second-degree AV block, Mobitz II

may be present in all degrees of blocks, while conduction delays within or below the bundle of His may occur in second-degree and third-degree blocks.

First-degree AV block is defined as sinus rhythm with a PR interval >200 milliseconds (ms) (Fig. 13.2). First-degree AV block is not a true block but rather delayed electrical conduction through the AV node [1]. Second-degree AV block is further classified into Mobitz I (Wenckebach conduction) and Mobitz II [9]. In both classifications, the ECG will show group beating as a result of dropped QRS complexes. Mobitz I block occurs after gradual PR prolongation and Mobitz II does not. The PR interval lengthens between successive beats due to increasing delayed conduction through the AV junction until a beat is dropped. At that point, the cycle starts again. The QRS duration is usually narrow unless there is a preexisting bundle branch disease (Fig. 13.3). In Mobitz II, the impulse either passes through the AV junction normally or is blocked completely. Beats are intermittently not conducted and QRS complexes dropped, usually in a repeating cycle of every third (3:1 block) or fourth (4:1 block) P wave [1]. Additionally, Mobitz II AV blocks are commonly located in the bundle of His, which results in widening QRS intervals (Fig. 13.4).

There are some exceptions when a second-degree AV block cannot be classified as Mobitz I or Mobitz II. In the event that the ECG demonstrated second-degree AV block with 2:1 conduction (i.e., two P waves for every QRS complex), then you may

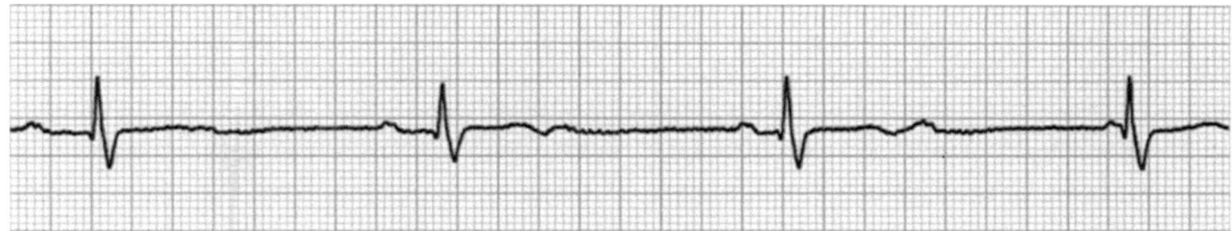

Fig. 13.5 Third AV block

have to concede that further categorization is indeterminate since it is impossible to differentiate between the two classifications based on the P:QRS ratio or the lengthening PR intervals. Additionally, in second-degree high-grade AV blocks, ≥2 consecutive P waves at a normal rate are not conducted without complete loss of AV conduction. High-grade AV block is generally considered to be a block at the level of the bundle of His and typically treated with pacing. It may be difficult to distinguish between high-grade second-degree AV blocks and third-degree AV blocks.

Third-degree AV block (commonly referred to as "complete heart block") is complete AV dissociation (Fig. 13.5). Third-degree AV block implies no conduction at all from atria to ventricles, may be paroxysmal or persistent, and is usually associated with either a junctional or a ventricular escape mechanism. A narrow QRS rhythm suggests a junctional escape focus usually in the AV node. A wide QRS rhythm suggests a ventricular escape focus. The location of the block may be in the AV junction or bilaterally in the bundle of His.

Signs and symptoms of AV blocks vary and depend on the degree of AV block, the ventricular rate, and the frequency of its occurrence. Symptoms may include hypotension, fatigue, weakness, dizziness, lightheadedness, syncope, heart failure-associated symptoms, and exercise intolerances [2]. Patients with first-degree and second-degree AV blocks may be asymptomatic or symptomatic. Patients with third-degree AV blocks are almost always symptomatic.

Treatment of AV blocks is similar to sinus bradycardia described previously. In patients persistently bradycardic with hypotension, altered mentation, evidence of shock, ischemic chest discomfort, and/or acute heart failure, atropine 1 mg intravenously may be considered [2]. Repeat dosing every 3–5 min may be performed up to a maximum dose of 3 mg. For patients with second-degree and third-degree AV blocks with widening QRS intervals, atropine may be avoided as the block is likely below the level of the AV node, which may hinder the efficacy or increase the risk for adverse outcomes as described above. β-Agonists such as isoproterenol, dopamine, dobutamine, and epinephrine may be considered in select patients with second-degree and third-degree AV blocks who carry a low risk for coronary ischemia [2]. β-Agonists exert direct effects to enhance AV node conduction and His-Purkinje conduction. These drugs may also enhance automaticity of secondary junctional and ventricular pacemakers in third-degree AV block. Adverse effects of β-agonist therapy include increased risk for ventricular arrhythmias and induction of coronary ischemia. Isoproterenol may exacerbate hypotension due to its vasodilatory effects [10]. Lastly, aminophylline may be considered for select patients with second-degree and third-degree AV blocks in the setting of acute inferior myocardial infarctions [2]. Aminophylline is a nonselective adenosine receptor antagonist and phosphodiesterase inhibitor. Increased adenosine production may be implicated in the pathophysiology of AV blocks in acute inferior myocardial infarctions [2]. Aminophylline may combat this proposed mechanism to improve AV conduction, increase ventricular rate, and improve symptoms. In refractory cases, transvenous pacing may be considered. Goals of therapy include correcting heart rate and preventing further hemodynamic instability. Monitor heart rate, blood pressure, electrocardiogram, symptoms, and adverse effects of interventional medications.

13.2.3 Atrial Fibrillation

Atrial fibrillation (AF) remains the most common cardiac arrhythmia. The estimated US prevalence of AF was 5.6 million people in 2015 with 11% of these cases being undiagnosed AF [11]. As the incidence of AF increases with advancing age, the estimated prevalence of AF is expected to rise to 12.1 million in 2030 [12]. The overall lifetime risk of AF is 26% for men and 23% for women [13]. There are several comorbidities and risk factors that increase an individual's risk for AF, including smoking, alcohol use, obesity, hypertension, diabetes, heart failure, coronary artery disease, valvular heart disease, obstructive sleep apnea, and hyperthyroidism [14]. The pathophysiology of AF is a multifactorial process that is a result of atrial metabolic, electrical, and structural remodeling. This remodeling is a result of neurohormonal dysfunction, metabolic dysfunction, inflammation, and ischemia, which disrupts synchronized electrical signaling leading to arrhythmogenesis [14]. AF is associated with many adverse outcomes, such as stroke, cognitive impairment, dementia, myocardial infarction, cardiac death, heart failure, chronic kidney disease, and peripheral artery disease. For these reasons, AF is associated with higher healthcare utilization and costs. Investigators examining health insurer data estimated that AF accounted for $28.4 billion (95% CI, $24.6–$33.8 billion) in healthcare spending [15]. The socioeconomic impact of AF in conjunction with chronic cardiovascular disease cannot be understated, as hospitalization rates for AF and AF-associated complications continue to increase.

The diagnosis of AF is suggested by irregularly irregular R-R intervals in the absence of P waves on a 12-lead ECG (Fig. 13.6) [16]. In patients with newly

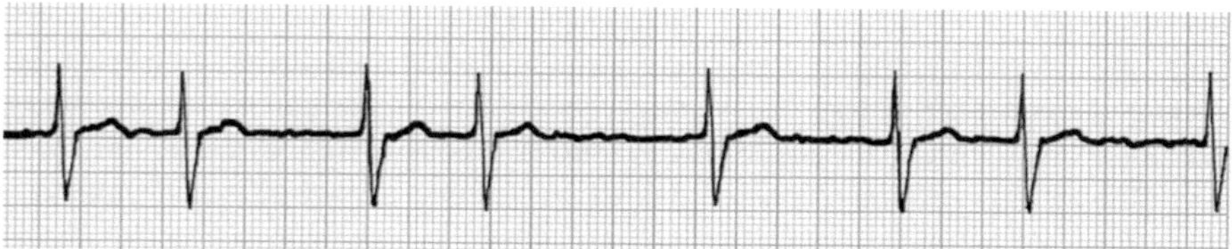

Fig. 13.6 Atrial fibrillation

Table 13.2 Stages of AF

Stage	Category	Description
1	At risk for AF	Presence of modifiable and nonmodifiable risk factors associated with AF
2	Pre-AF	Evidence of structural or electrical findings further predisposing a patient to AF
3A	Paroxysmal AF	AF that is intermittent and terminates ≤7 days of onset
3B	Persistent AF	AF that is continuous and sustains for >7 days and requires intervention
3C	Long-standing persistent AF	AF that is continuous for >12 months in duration
3D	Successful AF ablation	Freedom from AF after percutaneous or surgical intervention to eliminate AF
4	Permanent AF	Shared decision made between patient and clinician to cease attempts to restore normal sinus rhythm (NSR)

diagnosed AF, a transthoracic echocardiogram (TTE) to assess cardiac structure and pertinent laboratory testing, including metabolic panel, complete blood count, and thyroid function, should be performed to determine stroke and bleeding risk and identify underlying conditions that may guide further management [14]. AF is a progressive disease that requires different strategies at different stages. A summary of stages is included in Table 13.2. The foundation of optimal AF management is to treat risk factors and enact behavioral changes. Once AF develops, there are three important pillars that must be addressed with all patients—stroke risk assessment and treatment, optimize all modifiable risk factors, and manage symptoms using rate- and rhythm-controlling strategies. The symptoms of atrial fibrillation include palpitations, shortness of breath, lightheadedness, syncope, angina, heart failure symptoms, fatigue, and hypotension. Many patients may be asymptomatic [15].

13.2.3.1 Stroke Risk Assessment and Bleeding Risk Assessment

AF increases the risk of ischemic stroke and systemic embolism. The risk of stroke can be assessed by calculating the CHA_2DS_2-VASc score or other validated clinical risk scores such as Anticoagulation and Risk Factors in Atrial Fibrillation (ATRIA) and Global Anticoagulant Registry in the Field-Atrial Fibrillation (GARFIELD-AF) [14]. The CHA_2DS_2-VASc is most commonly used in clinical practice and recommended for use with the most updated guidelines. The CHA_2DS_2-VASc score assigns one point each to congestive heart failure, hypertension, diabetes mellitus, history of vascular disease, age ≥65 years, and female sex and two points each to age ≥75 years and history of stroke or transient ischemic attack (TIA). For patients with AF and an estimated annual thromboembolic risk of ≥2% per year (CHA_2DS_2-VASc score ≥2 in men and ≥3 in women), anticoagulation is recommended to prevent stroke and systemic thromboembolism [14]. Risk scores are equally beneficial in quantifying bleeding risk in AF. The HAS-BLED score assigns one point each to hypertension, abnormal liver function or renal function, history of stroke, history of bleeding, labile international normalized ration (INR), age >65 years, concomitant antiplatelet or nonsteroidal anti-inflammatory drugs (NSAIDs), and alcohol use [14]. A score ≥ 3 indicates a high bleeding risk. Other validated bleeding risk scores that are recommended by guidelines include $HEMORR_2HAGES$ and ATRIA. Bleeding risk scores should not be used in isolation to determine the eligibility for anticoagulation but identify and modify bleeding risk factors.

13.2.3.2 Anticoagulation

For patients with AF and an estimated annual thromboembolic risk of $\geq 2\%$ per year (CHA_2DS_2-VASc score ≥ 2 in men and ≥ 3 in women), anticoagulation is recommended to prevent stroke and systemic thromboembolism [14]. For patients with AF and an estimated annual thromboembolic risk of $\geq 1\%$ but $<2\%$ per year (equivalent to a CHA_2DS_2-VASc score of 1 in men and 2 in women), anticoagulation is reasonable to prevent stroke and systemic thromboembolism. Direct oral anticoagulants (DOACs) are preferred over warfarin for stroke prevention in the setting of AF due to convenience of fixed doses, minimal monitoring parameters, and superior safety profiles [17]. Warfarin (target INR 2–3) remains an option for select patients with AF such as those with moderate to severe mitral stenosis, rheumatic mitral stenosis, or mechanical heart valves [14]. A detailed comparison between warfarin and DOAC can be found in Table 13.3. Additionally, oral anticoagulation recommendations and preferences for select patient populations can be found in Table 13.4 [14].

For hemodynamically stable patients undergoing cardioversion, therapeutic anticoagulation should be established before cardioversion and continued for at least 4 weeks afterwards without interruption to prevent thromboembolism [14]. For patients that have been on uninterrupted therapeutic anticoagulation for at least 3 weeks, then they may proceed with cardioversion without imagining for intracardiac thrombus. For patients who were not receiving uninterrupted therapeutic anticoagulation, then it is recommended to undergo imaging to assess the patient for intracardiac thrombi including device-related thrombi prior to cardioversion. This remains a reasonable approach even for patients with left atrial appendage occlusion (LAAO) who are no longer actively on anticoagulation. If intracardiac thrombus is identified on imaging, then treatment with therapeutic anticoagulation for at least 3–6 weeks is recommended before cardioversion. It is also recommended to repeat imaging before cardioversion.

13.2.3.3 Rate vs. Rhythm Control

The primary goal of treatment of AF is to reduce symptoms, such as palpitations and shortness of breath, with rate- or rhythm-controlling strategies. The optimal strategy remains debated, and neither strategy confers definitive mortality benefit

Table 13.3 Comparison of oral anticoagulation for AF [18–22]

Drug	Warfarin	Dabigatran	Apixaban	Edoxaban	Rivaroxaban
Class	Vitamin K antagonist	Direct thrombin inhibitor	Factor Xa inhibitor		
Metabolism	S-isomer: CYP2C9 R-isomer: CYP1A2, CYP2C19, CYP3A4	Minimal P-glycoprotein (P-gp) substrate	CYP3A4 P-gp substrate		CYP3A4/5 P-gp substrate
Excretion	92% renal (only metabolites)	80% renal	27% renal 73% biliary and intestinal	50% renal 50% liver, biliary, and intestinal	66% renal 28% feces
Half-life (h)	20–60	12–17	12	10–14	5–9
Renal dose adjustments	None	CrCl 15–30 mL/min: 75 mg twice daily	If any 2 of the following—Age ≥80 years, body weight ≤60 kg, SCr ≥1.5 mg/day: 2.5 mg twice daily	CrCl 15–50 mL/min: 30 mg daily	CrCl 15–50 mL/min: 15 mg daily
Hepatic dose adjustments	Adjust dose based on INR trends	Child-Pugh B (moderate): Use with caution Child-Pugh C (severe): Avoid use	Child-Pugh B (moderate): Use with caution Child-Pugh C (severe): Avoid use	Child-Pugh B (moderate): Use with caution Child-Pugh C (severe): Avoid use	Child-Pugh B (moderate) and child-Pugh C (severe): Avoid use
CYP3A4 inhibitors/ P-gp **inhibitors** Dose adjustments	Adjust dose based on INR trends	Yes	Yes	No	Yes
CYP3A4 inhibitors/ P-gp **inducers** Dose adjustments	Adjust dose based on INR trends	Avoid use	Avoid use	Avoid use	Avoid use

Table 13.4 Anticoagulation recommendations in select populations [14]

Specific population	Recommendations
AF complication acute coronary syndrome or percutaneous coronary intervention (PCI)	DOACs are preferred over warfarin for most patients with AF who undergo PCI Early discontinuation of aspirin (within 1–4 weeks) and continuation of dual-antithrombotic therapy with oral anticoagulant and P2Y12 inhibitor are preferred over triple therapy (aspirin, oral anticoagulant, and P2Y12 inhibitor)
Chronic coronary disease	Oral anticoagulation monotherapy is recommended over combination therapy (oral anticoagulant and antiplatelet) for patients with AF and chronic coronary disease beyond 12 months after last revascularization
Peripheral artery disease	Oral anticoagulation monotherapy is recommended over combination therapy (oral anticoagulant and antiplatelet) for patients with AF and stable peripheral artery disease
Chronic kidney disease (CKD) including end-stage renal disease (ESRD)	CKD stage 3: Dose-adjusted DOAC[a] or warfarin CKD stage 4: Dose-adjusted DOAC[a] or warfarin ESRD with or without dialysis: Dose-adjusted apixaban[b] or warfarin
Valvular heart disease	Rheumatic mitral stenosis: Warfarin Moderate-to-severe mitral stenosis: Warfarin Mechanical heart valve: Warfarin All other valvular heart disease: DOAC preferred over warfarin
Obesity	Obesity (body mass index ≥ 40 kg/m^2): Rivaroxaban and apixaban are reasonable to select over warfarin Obesity following bariatric surgery: Warfarin may be reasonable to choose over DOAC due to concerns for drug absorption

[a] Dose-adjusted DOAC = labeled dose adjustments (see Table 13.3)
[b] Dose-adjusted apixaban = evidence-based dosing included 2.5 mg or 5 mg twice daily (stroke and bleeding risk assessment should be performed to guide dosing)

compared to the other. Earlier studies comparing the two approaches did not show differences in efficacy endpoints when evaluating cardiovascular death or incidence of adverse cardiovascular outcomes, such as the development of heart failure, or adverse cerebrovascular outcomes, such as incidence of stroke or transient ischemic attack (TIA) [23–25]. Additionally, some of these studies demonstrated that there may be a higher risk for hospitalizations related to AF or incidence of adverse outcomes to treatment with a rhythm-based treatment. However, recent literature suggests that a rhythm-controlling strategy with antiarrhythmic medications, catheter ablation, or cardioversion may confer a reduction in cardiovascular death, stroke, and hospitalizations related to AF [26]. This may be due to advances in rhythm-controlling strategies, increased use of catheter ablation, and availability of newer antiarrhythmic medications with closer monitoring.

For the reasons mentioned above, rate control and rhythm control are both reasonable approaches for managing patients with AF. However, rate control is often the initial strategy for patients with AF due to familiarity and safety of the drugs. Antiarrhythmic medications should be considered if patients remain symptomatic. An up-front rhythm-controlling strategy may be attempted to restore and maintain

NSR in patients with a recent diagnosis of AF to prevent atrial remodeling. Patient factors and preferences should be considered before electing to pursue one strategy over the other. Rate-controlling strategies may be preferred in older patients with longer histories of AF, those with less symptom burden, those with easily controlled heart rates, and those with less left ventricular (LV) or valvular dysfunction [14]. A rhythm-controlling strategy may be preferred in younger patients with newer histories of AF, those with many symptoms of AF, those for whom it is difficult to control heart rate, and those with LV dysfunction or valvular dysfunction [14].

Treatment with Rate Control

Previous recommendations for rate control suggested a heart rate (HR) goal <80 beats/min at rest in symptomatic patients and <110 beats/min at rest in asymptomatic patients [27]. However, more recent literature suggests that lenient HR goals are comparable to strict HR goals [28]. The updated recommendation is that rate control should be guided by underlying patient symptoms, in general aiming for a resting HR <100–110 beats/min [14]. The initial rate control strategy involves a gradual titration of β-blockers or non-dihydropyridine calcium channel blockers (non-DHP CCB) until the HR is adequately controlled and symptoms are manageable. Both classes of medications are equally efficacious at acutely controlling HR [29]. β-Blockers are preferred in patients with a history of HFrEF. Non-DHP CCBs are avoided in this population due to their negative inotropic effects. In patients with heart failure with preserved ejection fraction (HFpEF), a strategy of either diltiazem or β-blockers is acceptable. These agents are initiated during the episode of AF in a hospital or ambulatory care setting. Hemodynamically unstable patients with AF and rapid ventricular rate response (AF with RVR) should undergo emergent cardioversion to restore NSR. Rate control in a hospital setting can be complicated by hypotension or heart failure, precluding the use of a high dose of β-blockers or non-DHP CCB. In these situations, intravenous amiodarone or digoxin may be a reasonable approach. A combination of the agents can be used to achieve adequate rate control. Medications used for rate control are described in Table 13.7.

AV nodal ablation followed by permanent pacemaker placement may be considered in select patients with refractory AF with rapid ventricular rate in whom rate- and rhythm-controlling strategies are not ideal or have been unsuccessful [14]. Considerations to consequences of lifelong pacemaker implantation with respect to age and comorbidities are imperative before electing this type of strategy for rate control.

Treatment with Rhythm Control

After the decision to pursue rhythm control is established, patients must first be converted to NSR with electrical or pharmacological cardioversion. Pharmacological cardioversion is a reasonable alternative to electrical cardioversion for those individuals who are hemodynamically stable or in situations where electrical cardioversion cannot be performed [14]. As previously discussed, appropriate anticoagulation should be established before cardioversion and continued after to reduce the incidence of stroke and systemic embolism. For patients undergoing electrical cardioversion, an initial electrical shock of at least 200 joules (J) should be delivered synchronized to the QRS interval to reduce the risk of inducing ventricular fibrillation [14]. In patients with longer duration AF or unsuccessful initial shock, using higher energy and pretreatment with antiarrhythmic medications can facilitate the success of electrical cardioversion. Patients should be adequately sedated prior to electrical cardioversion. For acute pharmacological cardioversion, ibutilide and intravenous amiodarone are usual options [14]. Ibutilide works rapidly but is associated with severe adverse effects such as QT interval prolongation and torsades de pointes, particularly in patients with HFrEF. For this reason, it should be avoided in patients with known HFrEF and those with long QT syndromes. Intravenous amiodarone requires a longer time for AF cardioversion (8–12 h) compared to ibutilide. Procainamide may also be considered for pharmacological cardioversion of AF but was considered less effective than ibutilide [30, 31]. Outside of the hospital, flecainide and propafenone demonstrated efficacy to support their use in pharmacological cardioversion using the pill-in-the-pocket approach [32]. Dofetilide, oral amiodarone, and oral sotalol can be used for pharmacological cardioversion of AF but require several days and are not practical for acute conversion of AF to NSR [14]. Intravenous sotalol is not supported for pharmacological cardioversion of AF.

The choice of antiarrhythmic drugs to maintain NSR is based upon the patient's underlying comorbidities. Comorbidities of importance include coronary artery disease (CAD), HFrEF, chronic obstructive pulmonary disorders (COPDs), renal dysfunction, and long QT syndromes. In patients with CAD, sodium channel blockers (Vaughan-Williams class I antiarrhythmics) are contraindicated due to increased mortality [33]. Alternative therapies include sotalol, dofetilide, amiodarone, and dronedarone. In patients with HFrEF, sodium channel blockers (Vaughan-Williams class I antiarrhythmics) are also contraindicated due to increased mortality, negative inotropic effects, and increased risk for ventricular arrhythmias [16]. Dronedarone use has been associated with increased mortality in this population, especially with decompensated heart failure, thus leaving dofetilide, sotalol, and amiodarone as options for the maintenance of NSR [34]. Sotalol also possesses β-blocking properties and is often avoided in HFrEF to maintain higher doses of β-blockers as part of guideline-directed medical therapy. Therefore, dofetilide and amiodarone remain preferred options in patients with HFrEF. The choice between dofetilide and amiodarone is based on age, renal function, baseline-corrected QT (QTc) interval, and presence of pulmonary disease [16]. For patients without underlying cardiac comorbidities, sodium channel blockers, particularly the class Ic medications flecainide and propafenone, are commonly used. Once the antiarrhythmic drug is chosen, the patient should be monitored for recurrence of AF and adverse effects. A review of rhythm-controlling medications may be found in Table 13.7. If a patient experiences an adverse event, especially proarrhythmias, the offending agent should be withdrawn. Consideration of an antiarrhythmic drug from a different class may be considered if contraindications are not present, as can catheter-based or surgical ablation.

AF is a disease continuum that requires a variety of strategies at different stages targeting lifestyle and risk factor modification, increased screening, and initiating therapy when necessary. The three important pillars for atrial fibrillation management include thromboembolism assessment and treatment, optimizing modifiable risk factors, and managing symptoms of AF using rate- and/or rhythm-controlling strategies.

13.2.4 Atrial Flutter

Atrial flutter (AFL) is an easily treatable atrial tachycardia related to atrial fibrillation. In fact, the updated guidelines for the management of atrial fibrillation classify atrial flutter under stage 2 pre-AF [14]. ECG findings are consistent with a narrow QRS complex tachycardia with an irregular "sawtooth" pattern (Fig. 13.7). Atrial flutter is an electrical abnormality usually as a result of structural changes in the heart. Atrial flutter typically originates from the right atrium. It typically involves a large circuit around the area of the tricuspid valve, which gives it the name "typical AFL" [35]. Other circuits that form in the right atrium or left atrium resulting in AFL are less common and termed "atypical AFL." Symptoms are similar to those seen in atrial fibrillation. For that reason, treatment modalities are similar to management principles described in atrial fibrillation with regard to rate/rhythm control and anticoagulation. However, many patients are treatable with catheter ablation, specifically cavotricuspid isthmus (CTI) ablation [36]. This is a routine and straightforward procedure used to treat typical AFL.

13.2.5 Supraventricular Tachycardia (SVT)

Supraventricular tachycardia (SVT) is a broad term used to describe tachyarrhythmias originating above the ventricles of the heart. The estimated incidence of SVT is 35 per 100,000 person-years [37]. Examples of these tachyarrhythmias include AV nodal reentrant tachycardia (AVNRT), AV reentrant tachycardia (AVRT,

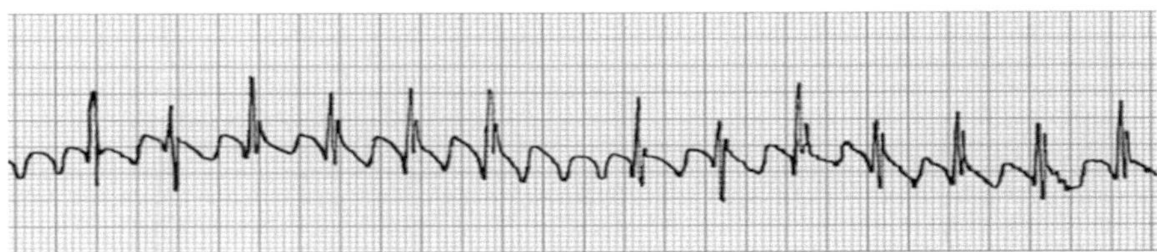

Fig. 13.7 Atrial flutter

including Wolff-Parkinson-White [WPW]), atrial tachycardia, inappropriate sinus tachycardia, and junctional tachycardia. The most common forms of SVT include AVNRT (60% of cases) and AVRT (30% of cases). ECG findings typically show a regular rhythm (may be irregular in some cases), rate between 120 and 220 beats/ min, narrow QRS complex, and absent P waves (Fig. 13.8). Some forms of SVT present with wide QRS complex like WPW syndrome. Signs and symptoms of SVT include a pounding sensation in the neck, palpitations, dizziness, lightheadedness, weakness, syncope, and polyuria due to the release of atrial natriuretic factor which increases diuresis [38].

Reentry refers to an action potential that propagates in a closed-loop-like manner. Reentry may occur within the AV node itself or through an accessory pathway. AVNRT refers to a reentry pathway that occurs in the AV node, while AVRT is usually a result of an accessory pathway. For AVNRT, there will be one impulse that divides into two pathways within the AV node—the fast pathway and the slow pathway [39, 40]. During sinus rhythm, electrical impulses travel down both pathways simultaneously. With discordance of these impulses and refractory periods, impulses can continually cycle around the two pathways activating the bundle of His from above and the atria from below within the AV node. For AVRT, there will be one impulse generated from the sinoatrial node that travels through two pathways—the AV nodal pathway and an accessory pathway [39, 40]. A premature atrial impulse will occur and reach the accessory pathway while it is still refractory. The impulse will also travel through the AV nodal pathway but will take longer, so it will reach the ventricle in an excitable state and conduct the impulse back to the atrium, thus creating a reentry circuit.

Patients who present with SVT will be assessed for hemodynamic stability and underlying cardiac-related causes of arrhythmia. If patients have regular rhythms and are hemodynamically stable, then AV nodal stimulation should be considered using vagal maneuvers such as having the patient cough, gag, instruct them to bear down using the Valsalva maneuver, carotid massage, and using cold stimulation [38]. Increased vagal stimulation causes bradycardia at the level of the AV node. It prolongs the refractoriness of the nodal tissue and disrupts the reentry circuit. If patients do not convert to NSR, then adenosine should be considered. Adenosine is a miscellaneous antiarrhythmic that exerts its activity on purinergic adenosine receptors located in the AV node. Usual dosing of adenosine 6 mg intravenous bolus should be performed, followed by up to two 12 mg intravenous bolus if unresponsive. Initial lower doses of adenosine 3 mg intravenous bolus may be considered when administering via a central venous catheter rather than peripheral venous

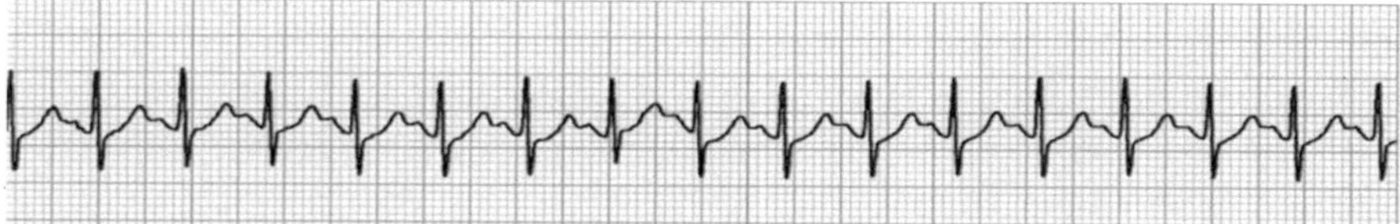

Fig. 13.8 Supraventricular tachycardia

catheters [41, 42]. Adenosine administration is usually recommended to be given through a two-syringe system or stopcock system to administer a 0.9% sodium chloride flush solution following adenosine. However, some observational data suggests that adenosine 6 mg may be diluted in 18 milliliters (mL) of 0.9% sodium chloride solution (20 mL total) and pushed via intravenous bolus using a single-syringe administration method [43]. For narrow QRS complex tachycardia, β-blockers or non-DH CCB may be considered. However, for wide QRS complex tachycardia, procainamide, amiodarone, or sotalol should be considered [38]. You may still use adenosine in wide QRS complex tachycardia as long as the rhythm is regular and monomorphic. For WPW syndrome, preferred agents are ibutilide or procainamide. Adenosine, β-blockers, non-DHP CCB, digoxin, and amiodarone should be avoided as they may accelerate antegrade conduction down the accessory pathway and increase ventricular rate in patients leading to serious ventricular arrhythmias. Prevention of SVT recurrence may include performing catheter ablation if the patient is considered a good candidate or using rate/rhythm-controlling strategies similar to those seen in the management of atrial fibrillation. Goals of therapy include terminating SVT and restoring NSR, preventing the recurrence of SVT, and avoiding adverse effects from medication therapies.

13.3 Ventricular Arrhythmias

Ventricular arrhythmias (VAs) are defined as any abnormal rhythm originating from below the AV node. All ventricular arrhythmias are characterized by a wide QRS complex, greater than or equal to 120 ms in duration, and often require immediate intervention. It is one of the leading causes of sudden cardiac death (SCD) and is estimated to account for 30–75% of all out-of-hospital cardiac arrests [44]. In the United States, around 300,000 deaths annually from SCD are caused by VA [45]. The prognosis is poor as significant anoxic brain injury is often seen in patients with prolonged downtime resulting in lack of oxygenation and perfusion to the brain. In the setting of hemodynamic instability and cardiac arrest, the American Heart Association Advanced Cardiac Life Support (ACLS) algorithm for pulseless ventricular tachycardia and ventricular fibrillation should be initiated and followed. Treatments for non-pulseless ventricular tachycardia and ventricular fibrillation will be discussed later in this section.

Electrical reentry is the most common mechanism for VA in patients with structural heart disease due to the cardiac remodeling that results from myocardial scar tissue. Other mechanisms include enhanced automaticity between the Purkinje fibers and myocytes in the ventricles that occurs often around the area of ischemic damage as well as triggered activity from delayed afterdepolarizations of the action potential [44]. Conversely, early afterdepolarization (EAD) is the most common mechanism for torsades de pointes [46]. Some VAs, such as premature ventricular complexes and non-sustained ventricular tachycardias, can be asymptomatic and self-limiting. But if symptoms are present, they can range widely in severity, from palpitations, shortness of breath, and/or syncope, all the way to the extremes of cardiac arrest and/or death. Physical and emotional stress can also precipitate VA which will often resolve once the underlying cause is addressed and rectified. The most common etiology of VA is ischemic heart disease, specifically myocardial infarction [45]. Patients with acute coronary syndromes are at risk of developing VA within the first 48 h of their infarct and are known to have poorer outcomes than those without coronary artery disease [44]. Other etiologies for ventricular arrhythmias include congenital heart disease, cardiomyopathy, electrolyte disturbances, medications that prolong the QT interval, illicit drug use, and sepsis. Idiopathic presentations of VA are generally seen in patients with no structural heart disease.

13.3.1 Premature Ventricular Complexes

Premature ventricular complexes (PVCs) present as premature heartbeats followed by a full compensatory pause on an ECG (Fig. 13.9). PVCs can be seen in isolation or repetitions; depending on the pattern, they can further be characterized based on the presentation (bigeminy for every other beat, trigeminy for every third beat, etc.). PVCs that present consecutively three or more times in a series are then referred to as ventricular tachycardia.

Some risk factors for PVC include male sex, older age, hypertension, African American race, and ischemic heart disease [47]. PVCs are generally self-resolving and asymptomatic, requiring no pharmacologic treatment, especially in patients with no presence of structural heart damage or ischemia and low PVC burden. However, patients may still experience symptoms like palpitations or dyspnea, and therefore common etiologies such as stimulant ingestion or electrolyte abnormalities should be investigated. If structural damage is present and/or PVC burden is high, β-blockers are considered first-line treatment. Non-dihydropyridines are considered in symptomatic patients with no structural heart disease and high PVC burden as well. But if symptoms persist despite initiating medical therapy, catheter ablation can be pursued. Success rates for PVC resolution with catheter ablations are relatively high, particularly for unifocal or monomorphic targets. For those who may not be good candidates for ablation or experience multifocal PVCs, antiarrhythmic medications such as flecainide, propafenone, or amiodarone can be trialed but are considered off-label uses [47, 48].

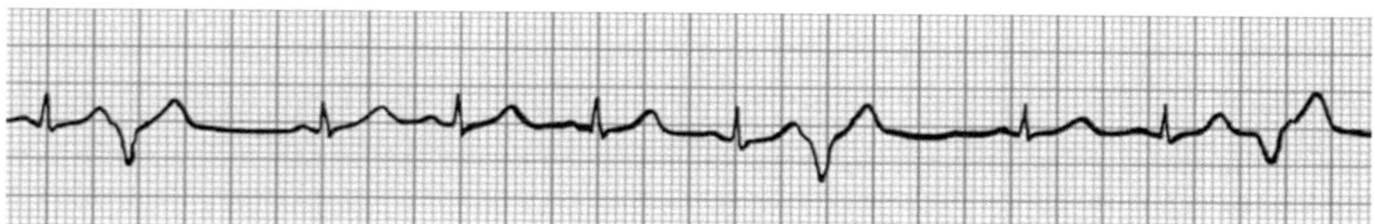

Fig. 13.9 Premature ventricular complexes

13.3.2 Ventricular Tachycardia

Ventricular tachycardia (VT) is defined as three or more consecutive beats at a rate greater than 100 beats per minute and a cycle length <600 ms. VT can be further classified based on duration and QRS morphology and is highlighted in Table 13.5 [44, 49–51]. Electrical storm is defined as having three or more sustained episodes of a ventricular arrhythmia or appropriate shocks from an implantable cardioverter-defibrillator (ICD) within 24 h. In the absence of an ICD, a VT storm can be characterized as subsequent VT recurring within 5 min of the cessation of the initial episode as well as sustained and non-sustained VT resulting in more ventricular ectopic beats than sinus beats over a 24-h period [52]. Electrical storm due to ventricular fibrillation can occur, however, less frequently than VT. Assessment of any reversible causes, such as sepsis and/or electrolyte abnormalities, should be performed as well as interrogation of patients' ICD, if applicable. Treatment in the setting of sustained and pulseless VT with hemodynamic compromise will require initiation of ACLS. Subsequent management or VT that is not pulseless will be addressed in the Treatment Strategies section.

Table 13.5 Ventricular tachycardia definitions

Term	Definition
Sustained	VT lasting ≥30 s or requiring interventions within 30 s of hemodynamic instability
Non-sustained (NSVT)	VT lasting <30 s and terminates spontaneously; not associated with hemodynamic instability
Incessant	Multiple, refractory VT episodes within a 24-h period despite treatment in hemodynamically stable patients
Bidirectional	VT with beat-to-beat alternation in the QRS frontal plan axis; most associated with digoxin toxicity and catecholaminergic polymorphic ventricular tachycardia (CPVT)
Monomorphic	Uniform and stable QRS morphology (Fig. 13.9)
Polymorphic	Multiform and variable QRS morphology (Fig. 13.10)

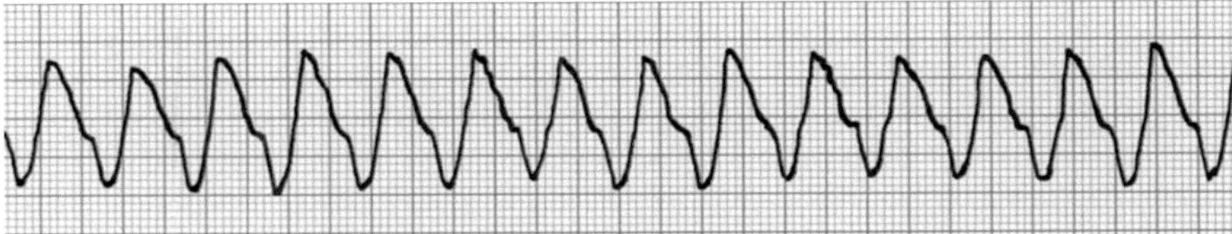

Fig. 13.10 Ventricular tachycardia, monomorphic

13.3.2.1 Torsades de Pointes

Torsades de pointes (TdP) is a form of polymorphic VT that occurs in the setting of QT prolongation. On an ECG, it presents as a gradual change in amplitude and twisting of the QRS complexes or "twisting of the points" around the isoelectric line (Fig. 13.11) [44, 46, 49]. Clinical symptoms are similar to those with VT but often lead to cardiac arrest. This long QT syndrome can be congenital or acquired, with acquired QT prolongation most often being drug induced. A list of various risk factors is given in Table 13.6 [46, 53]. The risk of TdP increases significantly when multiple QT-prolonging agents are used concurrently, and therefore, prompt discontinuation of the offending agents should be performed in addition to a hemodynamic assessment to guide subsequent management.

Regarding treatment strategies, hemodynamically unstable patients will need immediate defibrillation [44]. Adjunctively, intravenous magnesium sulfate 1–2 g can be given as a bolus (over 1–2 min) followed by a continuous infusion to prevent recurrence; however, no benefit has been shown in relation to return of spontaneous circulation (ROSC) or survival to hospital discharge [54]. In hemodynamically stable patients, magnesium can be given over 15 min. It is theorized that magnesium inhibits EAD associated with TdP without shortening the QT interval; however, the exact mechanism remains unknown. Magnesium levels can be monitored with target levels ideally above >2 mmol/L, but administration should occur regardless of the patient's initial serum level. Severe magnesium toxicity can manifest as confusion, coma-like states, and even cardiac arrest; however, these are very rare presentations as magnesium has a relatively wide therapeutic threshold. A continuous infusion of isoproterenol 2–10 mcg/min may also be utilized for bradycardia-associated and acquired TdP as it increases the heart rate while shortening the QT interval [55]. Its use is contraindicated in congenital TdP specifically, as it may actually increase EAD, resulting in a further prolonged QT interval [56]. Rapid pacing through a temporary pacemaker may also be done in patients with bradycardic-associated TdP. Lastly, alkalinization with sodium bicarbonate may also be trialed, especially if patients present with TdP due to quinidine use [57]. Persistent TdP, if inadequately treated, can then quickly progress into ventricular fibrillation.

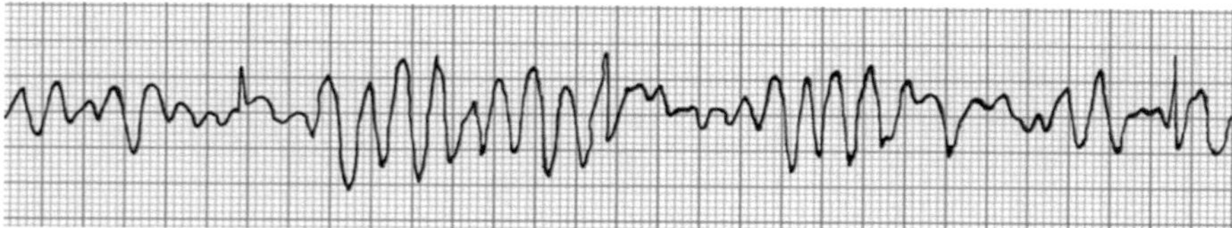

Fig. 13.11 Torsades de pointes, polymorphic VT with prolonged QT interval

Table 13.6 Risk factors for QT prolongation and TdP

Drug induced
Antiarrhythmics
Examples: Amiodarone, disopyramide, dofetilide, dronedarone, ibutilide, procainamide, quinidine, sotalol
Antibiotics/antifungals
Examples: Azithromycin, clarithromycin, erythromycin, fluconazole, levofloxacin, voriconazole
Antidepressants
Examples: Amitriptyline, citalopram, escitalopram, sertraline, venlafaxine
Antiemetics
Examples: Droperidol, metoclopramide, promethazine, ondansetron
Antipsychotics
Examples: Chlorpromazine, haloperidol, olanzapine, quetiapine, risperidone, ziprasidone
Miscellaneous
Examples: Arsenic, methadone, sumatriptan, cocaine
Electrolyte derangements
Examples: Hypocalcemia, hypokalemia, hypomagnesemia
Bradyarrhythmia
Examples: Sinus bradycardia, second- or third-degree AV block
Congenital disease
Examples: Romano-Ward syndrome, Jervell and Lange-Nielsen syndrome
Coronary heart disease
Examples: Myocardial infarction, congestive heart failure
Female sex
Older age

13.3.3 Ventricular Fibrillation

Ventricular fibrillation (VF) is an extremely disorganized VT with varying QRS lengths, morphology, and amplitudes and presents with a ventricular rate of more than 300 beats per minute (Fig. 13.12) [44, 49]. It is one of the shockable rhythms in the ACLS algorithm and is associated with high mortality. Post-myocardial infarction, mortality was found to be significantly higher in patients who developed early-onset VF (less than 24 h) compared to those with late-onset VF [58]. VF is always sustained and life-threatening, which requires immediate defibrillation and compliance with the ACLS algorithm.

13.3.4 Ventricular Arrhythmia Treatment Strategies

Acute management strategies for VA in the setting of cardiac arrest are discussed in a separate chapter. In general, proper adherence to guideline-directed ACLS therapies such as cardiopulmonary resuscitation (CPR), defibrillation, and medications is crucial, with subsequent surgical interventions or revascularization procedures dependent on the underlying cause and/or presence of ischemia postarrest. The

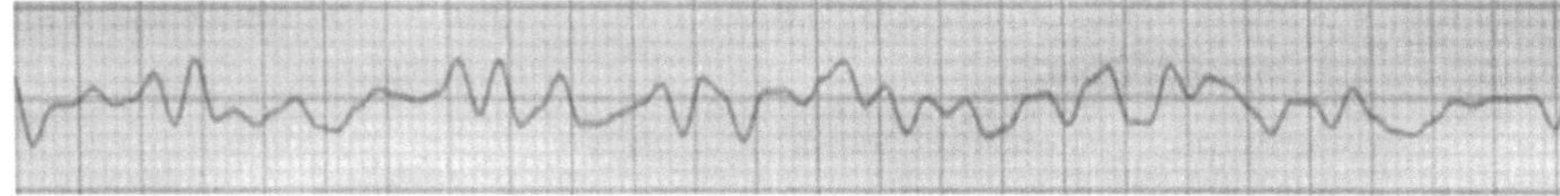

Fig. 13.12 Ventricular fibrillation

interventions listed in this section are for patients with non-pulseless VT/VF or for secondary prevention postarrest.

13.3.4.1 ICD Implantation

For primary prevention of SCD due to life-threatening VT/VF, numerous studies have shown that ICD insertion compared to conventional medication therapies alone improved survival in patients with significant coronary artery disease and ischemic cardiomyopathy, especially those with severe left ventricle systolic dysfunction [59–61]. Secondary prevention with ICD therapy has also shown similar mortality benefits [62–64]. Therefore, the 2017 AHA/ACC/HRS Guidelines recommend ICD therapy for these select patients [44]:

1. Primary prevention in patients with ischemic heart disease:

    (a) Left ventricular ejection fraction (LVEF) ≤40%, receiving guideline-directed medical therapies, and at least 40 days post-myocardial infarct and 90 days post-revascularization with meaningful survival
    (b) LVEF ≤30–35% with New York Heart Association (NYHA) classes I–III heart failure
    (c) LVEF ≤40% with NYHA class IV heart failure who are candidates for advanced cardiac therapies

2. Secondary prevention

    (a) Patients with ischemic heart disease:

        (i) Cardiac syncope and LVEF ≤35%
        (ii) Cardiac syncope with inducible ventricular arrhythmia during electrophysiological studies
        (iii) Resuscitated patients post-cardiac arrest or sustained spontaneous monomorphic VT who do not need revascularization of their ischemia but are good candidates for ICD placement

    (b) Patients with nonischemic cardiomyopathy:

        (i) Resuscitated patients post-cardiac arrest or sustained spontaneous monomorphic VT who are appropriate ICD candidates
        (ii) LVEF ≤35% and NYHA classes II–III heart failure

Other high-risk conditions such as hypertrophic cardiomyopathy, cardiac sarcoidosis, Brugada syndrome, and long QT syndrome may also warrant ICD therapy. It is always important to evaluate for any reversible causes for VT/VF, as these would preclude patients from ICD placement. Other contraindications to therapy include meaningful survival time of less than a year and patients with NYHA class IV heart failure who are not candidates for advanced therapies such as transplantation or mechanical circulatory devices.

13.3.4.2 Pharmacologic Treatments

There are numerous antiarrhythmic agents that can be used to control ventricular arrhythmias, which are listed in Table 13.7. β-Blockers are considered first-line agents in VA and provide mortality benefit in structural heart disease states such as myocardial infarction and systolic heart failure. β-Blockers such as nadolol and propranolol can also be initiated in patients with long QT syndrome. Sodium channel blockers are not typically utilized in VT since specific agents such as propafenone and flecainide have shown increased mortality risk in patients with structural heart disease. However, patients with structural heart disease who present with monomorphic VT and are hemodynamically stable may sometimes receive procainamide as superior outcomes were shown with its use over amiodarone and lidocaine [65, 66]. In the setting of cardiac arrest, both amiodarone and lidocaine can be utilized in pulseless VT/VF. Other specific arrhythmias such as congenital long QT syndrome and Brugada syndrome may also utilize agents with sodium channel blockade like mexiletine and quinidine, respectively [44]. Amiodarone and sotalol may also be trialed in patients with ischemic heart disease presenting with refractory VA due to increased success rates of VT termination, but patient-specific factors, such as having a severely reduced EF (<20%) and/or prolonged QTc interval, may preclude its use. Lastly, non-dihydropyridine calcium channel blockers are only initiated for the treatment of idiopathic interfascicular reentrant left VT. Otherwise, this antiarrhythmic class should not be given for VT management, especially in the setting of systolic heart failure.

13.3.4.3 Catheter Ablation

Catheter ablations can be done for both atrial arrhythmias and ventricular arrhythmias, especially for patients with symptomatic, idiopathic VT. Once cardiac mapping is performed to determine areas of highest arrhythmogenic foci, various energy sources like direct current, radiofrequency, or cryothermal can then be delivered to cardiac tissue to terminate the arrhythmia. Guidelines recommend catheter ablations as adjunctive treatments in patients with structural heart disease who have VT/VF storm despite ICD placement and antiarrhythmic therapy because of the various positive outcomes associated such as lower rates of composite death, VT storm, and ICD shock [44, 67]. Patients with nonischemic cardiomyopathy may also receive a

Table 13.7 Select antiarrhythmic drugs [69–84]

Drug	Vaughan-Williams classification	Indications and dosing	Adverse effects	Additional comments
Procainamide	Ia Sodium channel blockers	Indications: AF, AVRT (including WPW), VT Loading dose (IV) 10–17 mg/kg (IBW) 1000 mg ONCE Maintenance dose (IV) 1–4 mg/min	Infusion-related hypotension Lupus-like reactions VT TdP GI distress	Drug of choice for AF with RVR and WPW Active metabolite NAPA (metabolite) causes QTc prolongation Accumulates in heart failure, renal dysfunction, and hepatic dysfunction
Lidocaine	Ib Sodium channel lockers	Indications: VF, VT Loading dose (IV), ACLS (IV/IO) 1–1.5 mg/kg (IBW), 0.5–0.75 mg/kg as second dose; max 3 mg/kg Maintenance dose (IV): 1–4 mg/min	Bradycardia Hypotension AV block Tremors Delirium Psychosis Seizure GI distress Tinnitus Dyspnea/bronchospasm	Early signs of lidocaine toxicity are tremor or sedation Accumulates in heart failure, renal dysfunction, and hepatic dysfunction Therapeutic monitoring may be performed in patients who are on therapy for >24 h (typically for analgesia indication): 1.5–5.0 mcg/mL (therapeutic) Check levels 8–10 h after the start of infusion, each dose titration, or if toxicity concern is present
Mexiletine		Indications: Ventricular arrhythmias, PVC Maintenance dose (oral) 150–200 mg every 8–12 h, increase by increments of 50–100 mg every 2–3 days; max 1.2 g/day	See above (lidocaine)	Accumulates in heart failure, renal dysfunction, and hepatic dysfunction

Drug	Class	Indications/Dosing	Adverse effects	Notes
Flecainide	Ic Sodium channel blockers	Indications: AF, SVT, PVC, ventricular arrhythmias (with no structural heart disease) Acute cardioversion (oral) 300 mg ONCE (weight ≥ 70 kg) 200 mg ONCE (weight < 70 kg) Maintenance dose (oral) 50 mg every 12 h, max 400 mg/day	Dizziness Visual disturbances Tremor Dyspnea HF exacerbations AV block Atrial flutter VT	Do not use in patients with structural heart disease, prolonged QRS, or bundle branch blocks Should be used in combination with β-blocker or non-DH CCB to reduce the risk for atrial flutter
Propafenone		Indications: AF, SVT, PVC, ventricular arrhythmias (with no structural heart disease) Acute cardioversion (oral IR) 600 mg once (weight ≥ 70 kg) 450 mg once (weight < 70 kg) Maintenance dose (oral) IR: 150 mg every 8 h, max 900 mg/day ER: 225 mg every 12 h, max 900 mg/day	Taste disturbances Dizziness GI distress Angina HF exacerbations AV block Atrial flutter VT	See above (flecainide)
Esmolol	II β-blockers	Indications: AF with RVR, SVT, VT Loading dose (IV) 500 mcg/kg bolus Maintenance dose (IV) 50 mcg/kg/min continuous infusion, max 300 mcg/kg/min	Hypotension Bradycardia Hyperkalemia Extravasation Fluid overload	Titrate rate no faster than every 4 min Due to fluid volume, may consider alternative therapy in HF
Metoprolol		Indications: AF, SVT, NSVT Acute rate control (IV) IR: 2.5–5 mg every 5 min; max 15 mg Maintenance dose (oral) IR: 12.5–50 mg every 6–12 h; max 400 mg/day ER: 50–200 mg every 12–24 h; max 400 mg/day	Hypotension Bradycardia Masking hypoglycemia	IV to PO conversion: 1:2.5 mg
Carvedilol		Indications: AF, SVT, NSVT Maintenance dose (oral) 3.125–25 mg oral twice daily	Hypotension Bradycardia	None

Table 13.7 (continued)

Drug	Vaughan-Williams classification	Indications and dosing	Adverse effects	Additional comments
Amiodarone	III Potassium channel blockers	Indications: AF, SVT, PVC, VT, VF ACLS (IV, IO) 300 mg bolus, followed by 150 mg for second dose, if needed Loading dose (IV, oral) IV: 150 mg bolus, then 1 mg/min for 6 h, then 0.5 mg/min Oral: 400 mg every 8–12 h (target loading dose—6–10 g) Maintenance dose (oral) 200–400 mg daily	Pulmonary fibrosis Hepatotoxicity Photosensitivity Thyroid dysfunction Corneal deposition AV block	Should reserve use for patients who cannot take alternative antiarrhythmic therapies due to toxicities associated with long-term use Many drug-drug interactions due to inhibition of CYP3A4, CYP2D6, and CYP2C9
Dofetilide		Indications: AF, SVT Maintenance dose (oral) 500 mg every 12 h *Dose adjust based on renal function	Headache Dizziness Insomnia Angina TdP	Hospital initiation required Many drug-drug interactions via CYP3A4 and renal tubular secretions (e.g., hydrochlorothiazide) Avoid use in patients with prolonged QTc and discontinue therapy if QTc >500 ms
Ibutilide		Indications: AF Loading dose (IV) 0.01 mg/kg (weight < 60 kg) 1 mg (weight ≥ 60 kg)	Headache GI distress Lupus-like reactions Bradycardia VT TdP AV block	Avoid use in patients with prolonged QT intervals, HFrEF, and those with hypokalemia and hypomagnesemia Avoid in patients with permanent AF as many patients will revert back to AF after pharmacological cardioversion
Dronedarone		Indications: AF Maintenance dose (oral) 400 mg every 12 h	Pulmonary fibrosis Hepatotoxicity AV block Bradycardia	Avoid use in patients with prolonged QT intervals, HFrEF, and patients with permanent AF Discontinue therapy if QTc >500 ms
Sotalol		Indications: AF, SVT, VT Maintenance dose (oral) 80 mg twice daily; max 320 mg/day*	Bradycardia Fatigue Dizziness Dyspnea AV block HF exacerbations Pulmonary edema TdP	Hospital initiation required Avoid use in patients with prolonged QTc and discontinue therapy if QTc >500 ms

Diltiazem	IV Calcium channel blockers	Indications: AF, SVT, NSVT Loading dose (IV) 0.25 mg/kg bolus (may repeat 0.35 mg/kg bolus after 15 min) Maintenance dose (IV, oral) IV: 5–15 mg/h continuous infusion Oral (IR): 30–60 mg every 6 h Oral (ER): 120–480 mg every 12–24 h	Hypotension Bradycardia Peripheral edema Acute decompensated HF	Conversion IV to PO: 5 mg/h = 180 mg/day 10 mg/h = 200–260 mg/day 15 mg/h = 480 mg/day
Verapamil		Indications: AF, SVT, NSVT Loading dose (IV) 0.075–0.15 mg/kg IV bolus over 2 min, may give an additional 10 mg after 30 min if no response Maintenance dose (IV, oral) IV: 0.005 mg/kg/min continuous infusion Oral (ER): 180–480 mg daily	Hypotension Bradycardia Peripheral edema Acute decompensated HF	None
Digoxin	Miscellaneous	Indications: AF, SVT Loading dose (IV, oral) 8–12 mcg/kg (IBW) given as 50% total dose followed by 25% total dose every 6 h for 2 doses Maintenance dose (oral) Oral: 62.5–250 mcg daily	GI distress VT Anorexia Altered mentation AV block Yellow-colored vision	Useful in patients with hypotension since it is hemodynamically neutral Less effective in patients with sepsis or increased sympathetic tone Therapeutic drug monitoring—Digoxin concentrations 0.5–1.2 ng/mL considered therapeutic for AF

AF atrial fibrillation, *AVRT* atrioventricular reentry tachycardia, *AV* atrioventricular, *GI* gastrointestinal, *HF* heart failure, *HFrEF* heart failure with reduced ejection fraction, *IBW* ideal body weight, *IO* intraosseous, *NAPA* N-acetylprocainamide, *Non-DHP CCB* non-dihydropyridine calcium channel blocker, *PVC* premature ventricular contractions, *RVR* rapid ventricular response, *TdP* torsade de pointes, *VF* ventricular fibrillation, *VT* ventricular tachycardia, *WPW* Wolff-Parkinson-White *Dose adjust based on renal function cardiac ablation if they continue to have recurrent sustained monomorphic VT that is refractory to antiarrhythmic therapy, as epicardial ablations were found to be independent predictors for complete short-term success [44, 68]. However, long-term outcomes such as VT-free survival and recurrence were not as prevalent as compared to patients with ischemic cardiomyopathy. Although rare, complications associated with catheter ablation procedures include heart block, thrombosis, new-onset arrhythmias, and even death.

13.4   Conclusion

Early and/or urgent recognition and diagnosis of cardiac arrhythmias are crucial as these may have serious and fatal implications if not treated promptly. Depending on the type of arrhythmia that patients present with, treatments provided will vary. However, the overarching goal remains the same: correct the abnormal rhythm and address any reversible causes. Medication selection is often based on patient-specific factors and may sometimes require hospital admission for therapy initiation. A thorough evaluation of patients' previous interventions can guide appropriate initiation of therapies if they present with persistent or refractory arrhythmias. There is an opportunity for pharmacists to have a significant impact on arrhythmia management for patients. Pharmacists can aid in obtaining prior medication histories, appropriately recommending and dosing medications, and assessing for drug interactions with other concurrent medication use. Especially in emergent situations, pharmacists can advocate for appropriate dosing and timing of medications as well as correct preparations of the medication product. These actions are of tremendous benefit to the medical team and ultimately promote patient safety and efficacy.

References

1. Lakshminarayan K, Anderson DC, Herzog CA, Qureshi AI. Clinical epidemiology of atrial fibrillation and related cerebrovascular events in the United States. Neurologist. 2008;14(3):143–50.
2. Kusumoto FM, Schoenfeld MH, Barrett C, et al. 2018 ACC/AHA/HRS guideline on the evaluation and management of patients with bradycardia and cardiac conduction delay: a report of the American College of Cardiology/American Heart Association Task Force on Clinical Practice Guidelines and the Heart Rhythm Society [published correction appears in Circulation. 2019;140(8):e506-e508]. Circulation. 2019;140(8):e382–482.
3. Brignole M, Menozzi C, Lolli G, Oddone D, Gianfranchi L, Bertulla A. Pacing for carotid sinus syndrome and sick sinus syndrome. Pacing Clin Electrophysiol. 1990;13(12 Pt 2):2071–5.
4. Rodriguez RD, Schocken DD. Update on sick sinus syndrome, a cardiac disorder of aging. Geriatrics. 1990;45(1):26–36.
5. Brady WJ, Swart G, DeBehnke DJ, Ma OJ, Aufderheide TP. The efficacy of atropine in the treatment of hemodynamically unstable bradycardia and atrioventricular block: prehospital and emergency department considerations. Resuscitation. 1999;41(1):47–55.

6. Chadda KD, Lichstein E, Gupta PK, Choy R. Bradycardia-hypotension syndrome in acute myocardial infarction. Reappraisal of the overdrive effects of atropine. Am J Med. 1975;59(2):158–64.

7. Smith I, Monk TG, White PF. Comparison of transesophageal atrial pacing with anticholinergic drugs for the treatment of intraoperative bradycardia. Anesth Analg. 1994;78(2):245–52.

8. Upshaw CB Jr. Comparison of the prevalence of first-degree atrioventricular block in African-American and in Caucasian patients: an electrocardiographic study III. J Natl Med Assoc. 2004;96(6):756–60.

9. Barold SS. Definitions and pitfalls in the diagnosis of atrioventricular block. Heart Lung Circ. 2023;32(12):1413–6.

10. Cossú SF, Rothman SA, Chmielewski IL, et al. The effects of isoproterenol on the cardiac conduction system: site-specific dose dependence. J Cardiovasc Electrophysiol. 1997;8(8):847–53.

11. Turakhia MP, Guo JD, Keshishian A, et al. Contemporary prevalence estimates of undiagnosed and diagnosed atrial fibrillation in the United States. Clin Cardiol. 2023;46(5):484–93. https://doi.org/10.1002/clc.23983.

12. Colilla S, Crow A, Petkun W, Singer DE, Simon T, Liu X. Estimates of current and future incidence and prevalence of atrial fibrillation in the U.S. adult population. Am J Cardiol. 2013;112(8):1142–7.

13. Lloyd-Jones DM, Wang TJ, Leip EP, et al. Lifetime risk for development of atrial fibrillation: the Framingham Heart Study. Circulation. 2004;110(9):1042–6.

14. Joglar JA, Chung MK, Armbruster AL, et al. 2023 ACC/AHA/ACCP/HRS guideline for the diagnosis and management of atrial fibrillation: a report of the American College of Cardiology/American Heart Association Joint Committee on Clinical Practice Guidelines [published correction appears in Circulation. 2024;149(1):e167] [published correction appears in Circulation. 2024 Feb 27;149(9):e936]. Circulation. 2024;149(1):e1–e156.

15. Dieleman JL, Cao J, Chapin A, et al. US health care spending by payer and health condition, 1996–2016. JAMA. 2020;323(9):863–84.

16. Lacoste JL, Szymanski TW, Avalon JC, et al. Atrial fibrillation management: a comprehensive review with a focus on pharmacotherapy, rate, and rhythm control strategies. Am J Cardiovasc Drugs. 2022;22(5):475–96.

17. Kido K, Lee JC, Hellwig T, Gulseth MP. Use of direct oral anticoagulants in morbidly obese patients. Pharmacotherapy. 2020;40(1):72–83.

18. Warfarin. Lexi-drugs. Hudson, OH: Lexicomp; 2024. http://online.lexi.com/. Updated February 24, 2024. Accessed 3 March 2024.

19. Dabigatran. Lexi-drugs. Hudson, OH: Lexicomp; 2024. http://online.lexi.com/. Updated February 29, 2024. Accessed 3 March 2024.

20. Apixaban. Lexi-drugs. Hudson, OH: Lexicomp; 2024. http://online.lexi.com/. Updated February 29, 2024. Accessed 3 March 2024.

21. Rivaroxaban. Lexi-drugs. Hudson, OH: Lexicomp; 2024. http://online.lexi.com/. Updated February 29, 2024. Accessed 3 March 2024.

22. Edoxaban. Lexi-drugs. Hudson, OH: Lexicomp; 2024. http://online.lexi.com/. Updated February 24, 2024. Accessed 3 March 2024.

23. Carlsson J, Miketic S, Windeler J, et al. Randomized trial of rate-control versus rhythm-control in persistent atrial fibrillation: the Strategies of Treatment of Atrial Fibrillation (STAF) study. J Am Coll Cardiol. 2003;41(10):1690–6.

24. Wyse DG, Waldo AL, DiMarco JP, et al. A comparison of rate control and rhythm control in patients with atrial fibrillation. N Engl J Med. 2002;347(23):1825–33.

25. Van Gelder IC, Hagens VE, Bosker HA, et al. A comparison of rate control and rhythm control in patients with recurrent persistent atrial fibrillation. N Engl J Med. 2002;347(23):1834–40.

26. Kirchhof P, Camm AJ, Goette A, et al. Early rhythm-control therapy in patients with atrial fibrillation. N Engl J Med. 2020;383(14):1305–16.

27. January CT, Wann LS, Alpert JS, et al. 2014 AHA/ACC/HRS guideline for the management of patients with atrial fibrillation: a report of the American College of Cardiology/American

Heart Association Task Force on Practice Guidelines and the Heart Rhythm Society [published correction appears in J Am Coll Cardiol. 2014;64(21):2305–7]. J Am Coll Cardiol. 2014;64(21):e1–e76.

28. Van Gelder IC, Groenveld HF, Crijns HJ, et al. Lenient versus strict rate control in patients with atrial fibrillation. N Engl J Med. 2010;362(15):1363–73.

29. Hargrove KL, Robinson EE, Lusk KA, Hughes DW, Neff LA, Fowler AL. Comparison of sustained rate control in atrial fibrillation with rapid ventricular rate: metoprolol vs. diltiazem. Am J Emerg Med. 2021;40:15–9.

30. Volgman AS, Carberry PA, Stambler B, et al. Conversion efficacy and safety of intravenous ibutilide compared with intravenous procainamide in patients with atrial flutter or fibrillation. J Am Coll Cardiol. 1998;31(6):1414–9.

31. Stambler BS, Wood MA, Ellenbogen KA. Antiarrhythmic actions of intravenous ibutilide compared with procainamide during human atrial flutter and fibrillation: electrophysiological determinants of enhanced conversion efficacy. Circulation. 1997;96(12):4298–306.

32. Ibrahim OA, Belley-Côté EP, Um KJ, et al. Single-dose oral anti-arrhythmic drugs for cardioversion of recent-onset atrial fibrillation: a systematic review and network meta-analysis of randomized controlled trials. Europace. 2021;23(8):1200–10.

33. Echt DS, Liebson PR, Mitchell LB, et al. Mortality and morbidity in patients receiving encainide, flecainide, or placebo. The cardiac arrhythmia suppression trial. N Engl J Med. 1991;324(12):781–8.

34. Køber L, Torp-Pedersen C, McMurray JJ, et al. Increased mortality after dronedarone therapy for severe heart failure [published correction appears in N Engl J Med. 2010;363(14):1384]. N Engl J Med. 2008;358(25):2678–87.

35. Boyer M, Koplan BA. Cardiology patient page. Atrial flutter. Circulation. 2005;112(22):e334–6.

36. Christopoulos G, Siontis KC, Kucuk U, Asirvatham SJ. Cavotricuspid isthmus ablation for atrial flutter: Anatomic challenges and troubleshooting. HeartRhythm Case Rep. 2020;6(3):115–20. Published 2020 Mar 16

37. Orejarena LA, Vidaillet H Jr, DeStefano F, et al. Paroxysmal supraventricular tachycardia in the general population. J Am Coll Cardiol. 1998;31(1):150–7.

38. Page RL, Joglar JA, Caldwell MA, et al. 2015 ACC/AHA/HRS guideline for the management of adult patients with supraventricular tachycardia: a report of the American College of Cardiology/American Heart Association Task Force on Clinical Practice Guidelines and the Heart Rhythm Society [published correction appears in Circulation. 2016;134(11):e234–5]. Circulation. 2016;133(14):e506–74.

39. Helton MR. Diagnosis and management of common types of supraventricular tachycardia. Am Fam Physician. 2015;92(9):793–800.

40. Delacrétaz E. Clinical practice. Supraventricular tachycardia. N Engl J Med. 2006;354(10):1039–51.

41. McIntosh-Yellin NL, Drew BJ, Scheinman MM. Safety and efficacy of central intravenous bolus administration of adenosine for termination of supraventricular tachycardia. J Am Coll Cardiol. 1993;22(3):741–5.

42. Chang M, Wrenn K. Adenosine dose should be less when administered through a central line. J Emerg Med. 2002;22(2):195–8.

43. McDowell M, Mokszycki R, Greenberg A, Hormese M, Lomotan N, Lyons N. Single-syringe administration of diluted adenosine. Acad Emerg Med. 2020;27(1):61–3.

44. Al-Khatib SM, Stevenson WG, Ackerman MJ, et al. 2017 AHA/ACC/HRS guideline for management of patients with ventricular arrhythmias and the prevention of sudden cardiac death: a report of the American College of Cardiology/American Heart Association Task Force on Clinical Practice Guidelines and the Heart Rhythm Society [published correction appears in J Am Coll Cardiol. 2018;72(14):1760]. J Am Coll Cardiol. 2018;72(14):e91–e220.

45. Tang PT, Shenasa M, Boyle NG. Ventricular arrhythmias and sudden cardiac death. Card Electrophysiol Clin. 2017;9(4):693–708.

46. Tisdale JE. Drug-induced QT interval prolongation and torsades de pointes: Role of the pharmacist in risk assessment, prevention and management. Can Pharm J (Ott). 2016;149(3):139–52.

47. Simpson RJ Jr, Cascio WE, Schreiner PJ, et al. Prevalence of premature ventricular contractions in a population of African American and white men and women: the Atherosclerosis Risk in Communities (ARIC) study. Am Heart J. 2002;143(3):535–40.

48. Marcus GM. Evaluation and management of premature ventricular complexes. Circulation. 2020;141(17):1404–18.

49. Buxton AE, Calkins H, Callans DJ, et al. ACC/AHA/HRS 2006 key data elements and definitions for electrophysiological studies and procedures: a report of the American College of Cardiology/American Heart Association Task Force on Clinical Data Standards (ACC/AHA/HRS Writing Committee to Develop Data Standards on Electrophysiology). J Am Coll Cardiol. 2006;48(11):2360–96.

50. Srinivasan NT, Schilling RJ. Sudden cardiac death and arrhythmias. Arrhythm. Electrophysiol Rev. 2018;7(2):111–7.

51. Zeppenfeld K, Tfelt-Hansen J, de Riva M, et al. 2022 ESC Guidelines for the management of patients with ventricular arrhythmias and the prevention of sudden cardiac death. Eur Heart J. 2022;43(40):3997–4126.

52. Zaman J, Agarwal S. Management of ventricular tachycardia storm. Heart. 2021;107(20):1671–7.

53. Li M, Ramos LG. Drug-induced QT prolongation and Torsades de Pointes. P T. 2017;42(7):473–7.

54. Tzivoni D, Banai S, Schuger C, et al. Treatment of torsade de pointes with magnesium sulfate. Circulation. 1988;77(2):392–7.

55. Drew BJ, Ackerman MJ, Funk M, et al. Prevention of torsade de pointes in hospital settings: a scientific statement from the American Heart Association and the American College of Cardiology Foundation [published correction appears in Circulation. 2010 Aug 24;122(8):e440]. Circulation. 2010;121(8):1047–60.

56. Shimizu W, Ohe T, Kurita T, et al. Early afterdepolarizations induced by isoproterenol in patients with congenital long QT syndrome. Circulation. 1991;84(5):1915–23.

57. Bruccoleri RE, Burns MM. A literature review of the use of sodium bicarbonate for the treatment of QRS widening. J Med Toxicol. 2016;12(1):121–9.

58. Demidova MM, Smith JG, Höijer CJ, Holmqvist F, Erlinge D, Platonov PG. Prognostic impact of early ventricular fibrillation in patients with ST-elevation myocardial infarction treated with primary PCI. Eur Heart J Acute Cardiovasc Care. 2012;1(4):302–11.

59. Moss AJ, Hall WJ, Cannom DS, et al. Improved survival with an implanted defibrillator in patients with coronary disease at high risk for ventricular arrhythmia. Multicenter Automatic Defibrillator Implantation Trial Investigators. N Engl J Med. 1996;335(26):1933–40.

60. Moss AJ, Zareba W, Hall WJ, et al. Prophylactic implantation of a defibrillator in patients with myocardial infarction and reduced ejection fraction. N Engl J Med. 2002;346(12):877–83.

61. Bardy GH, Lee KL, Mark DB, et al. Amiodarone or an implantable cardioverter-defibrillator for congestive heart failure [published correction appears in N Engl J Med. 2005;352(20):2146]. N Engl J Med. 2005;352(3):225–37.

62. Antiarrhythmics versus Implantable Defibrillators (AVID) Investigators. A comparison of antiarrhythmic-drug therapy with implantable defibrillators in patients resuscitated from near-fatal ventricular arrhythmias. N Engl J Med. 1997;337(22):1576–83.

63. Connolly SJ, Gent M, Roberts RS, et al. Canadian implantable defibrillator study (CIDS): a randomized trial of the implantable cardioverter defibrillator against amiodarone. Circulation. 2000;101(11):1297–302.

64. Kuck KH, Cappato R, Siebels J, et al. Randomized comparison of antiarrhythmic drug therapy with implantable defibrillators in patients resuscitated from cardiac arrest: the Cardiac Arrest Study Hamburg (CASH). Circulation. 2000;102(7):748–54.

65. Gorgels AP, van den Dool A, Hofs A, et al. Comparison of procainamide and lidocaine in terminating sustained monomorphic ventricular tachycardia. Am J Cardiol. 1996;78(1):43–6.

66. Ortiz M, Martín A, Arribas F, et al. Randomized comparison of intravenous procainamide vs. intravenous amiodarone for the acute treatment of tolerated wide QRS tachycardia: the PROCAMIO study. Eur Heart J. 2017;38(17):1329–35.

67. Sapp JL, Wells GA, Parkash R, et al. Ventricular tachycardia ablation versus escalation of antiarrhythmic drugs. N Engl J Med. 2016;375(2):111–21.

68. Dinov B, Fiedler L, Schönbauer R, et al. Outcomes in catheter ablation of ventricular tachycardia in dilated nonischemic cardiomyopathy compared with ischemic cardiomyopathy: results from the Prospective Heart Centre of Leipzig VT (HELP-VT) Study. Circulation. 2014;129(7):728–36.

69. Procainamide. Lexi-drugs. Hudson, OH: Lexicomp; 2024. http://online.lexi.com/. Updated February 24, 2024. Accessed 3 March 2024.

70. Lidocaine. Lexi-drugs. Hudson, OH: Lexicomp; 2024. http://online.lexi.com/. Updated March 1, 2024. Accessed 3 March 2024.

71. Mexiletine. Lexi-drugs. Hudson, OH: Lexicomp; 2024. http://online.lexi.com/. Updated February 28, 2024. Accessed 3 March 2024.

72. Flecainide. Lexi-drugs. Hudson, OH: Lexicomp; 2024. http://online.lexi.com/. Updated February 21, 2024. Accessed 3 March 2024.

73. Propafenone. Lexi-drugs. Hudson, OH: Lexicomp; 2024. http://online.lexi.com/. Updated February 24, 2024. Accessed 3 March 2024.

74. Esmolol. Lexi-drugs. Hudson, OH: Lexicomp; 2024. http://online.lexi.com/. Updated February 29, 2024. Accessed 3 March 2024.

75. Metoprolol. Lexi-drugs. Hudson, OH: Lexicomp; 2024. http://online.lexi.com/. Updated March 2, 2024. Accessed 3 March 2024.

76. Carvedilol. Lexi-drugs. Hudson, OH: Lexicomp; 2024. http://online.lexi.com/. Updated February 29, 2024. Accessed 3 March 2024.

77. Amiodarone. Lexi-drugs. Hudson, OH: Lexicomp; 2024. http://online.lexi.com/. Updated February 28, 2024. Accessed 3 March 2024.

78. Dofetilide. Lexi-drugs. Hudson, OH: Lexicomp; 2024. http://online.lexi.com/. Updated February 23, 2024. Accessed 3 March 2024.

79. Ibutilide. Lexi-drugs. Hudson, OH: Lexicomp; 2024. http://online.lexi.com/. Updated February 23, 2024. Accessed 3 March 2024.

80. Dronedarone. Lexi-drugs. Hudson, OH: Lexicomp; 2024. http://online.lexi.com/. Updated February 29, 2024. Accessed 3 March 2024.

81. Sotalol. Lexi-drugs. Hudson, OH: Lexicomp; 2024. http://online.lexi.com/. Updated February 24, 2024. Accessed 3 March 2024.

82. Diltiazem. Lexi-drugs. Hudson, OH: Lexicomp; 2024. http://online.lexi.com/. Updated February 29, 2024. Accessed 3 March 2024.

83. Verapamil. Lexi-drugs. Hudson, OH: Lexicomp; 2024. http://online.lexi.com/. Updated February 29, 2024. Accessed 3 March 2024.

84. Digoxin. Lexi-drugs. Hudson, OH: Lexicomp; 2024. http://online.lexi.com/. Updated February 29, 2024. Accessed 3 March 2024.

Chapter 14
Shock

Lucas R. Goss, Annette Esper, and Seema S. Tekwani

14.1 Introduction

Shock is a life-threatening condition that requires prompt recognition and treatment, as it is often the final common pathway for which illnesses lead to death. Shock is a state in which the supply of oxygen is inadequate to meet the demand for oxygen by the body's tissues. This results in cellular hypoxia, which subsequently results in cell membrane dysfunction, intracellular edema, leakage of intracellular contents into the extracellular space, and inadequate regulation of intracellular pH. If left untreated, this will result in cell death, organ dysfunction, lactic acidosis, inflammatory cascades, and potentially death. Although shock may be reversible, the longer the shock is present, the more the tissue hypoxia and organ dysfunction occur. This may potentially result in irreversible organ dysfunction and ultimately death [1–4]. This is why identification of shock as well as diagnosing and treating the underlying cause is crucial.

14.2 Pathophysiology of Shock

Shock is a state of global tissue hypoperfusion, leading to an imbalance between oxygen supply to the tissue and its demand. Oxygen delivery depends on the arterial oxygen content of the blood and the cardiac output (Table 14.1). The arterial oxygen content is the sum of the oxygen bound to hemoglobin (product of hemoglobin concentration (Hb) and the percentage of hemoglobin saturated with oxygen (sO_2)

L. R. Goss · A. Esper · S. S. Tekwani (✉)
Division of Pulmonary, Allergy, Critical Care, and Sleep Medicine, Emory University School of Medicine, Atlanta, GA, USA
e-mail: seema.tekwani@emory.edu

Y. Alzaidi, M. A. Gebily (eds.), *The Pharmacist's Expanded Role in Critical Care Medicine*, https://doi.org/10.1007/978-3-031-77335-8_14

359

Table 14.1 Relevant equations in shock physiology

Delivery of oxygen	$DO_2 = CO \times \{(1.39 \times Hb \times sO_2) + (PaO_2 \times 0.003)\}$
Fick	$CO = VO_2/1.34(Hb)\ (10)\ (CA\ O_2\% - CV\ O_2\%)$
Cardiac output	$CO = HR \times SV$
MAP	$CO \times SVR$

DO₂ delivery of oxygen, *CO* cardiac output , *Hb* hemoglobin, *sO₂* arterial oxygen saturation, *PaO₂* arterial partial pressure of oxygen; *VO₂* oxygen consumption, *CAO₂* central arterial oxygen saturation, *CVO₂* central venous oxygen saturation; *HR* heart rate, *SV* stroke volume, *SVR* systemic vascular resistance, *MAP* mean arterial pressure

and the amount of dissolved oxygen in the blood (PaO_2). Cardiac output is determined by the product of stroke volume (SV) and heart rate (HR). Stroke volume is the amount pumped by the heart with each contraction, which further depends on preload/end-diastolic volume, contractility of the heart, and afterload.

The abnormalities in each of these determinants of oxygen delivery can lead to several types of shock (Flowchart 14.1).

Irrespective of the etiology of shock, when the delivery of oxygen (DO_2) decreases, more oxygen is extracted from the hemoglobin to a point of critical DO_2, beyond which the tissue starts producing energy by anaerobic metabolism. In sepsis, the cells may be unable to utilize oxygen despite normal to supranormal oxygen delivery, thus leading to dysoxia and an anaerobic pathway for adenosine triphosphate (ATP) production.

When oxygen extraction is increased, this is seen as a drop in the oxygen saturation of the venous blood. This is often measured in the blood collected from the superior vena cava via a central venous line and reported as central venous oxygen saturation ($ScVO_2$). Normal $ScVO_2$ is 70–75%, and values <70% are indicative of impaired oxygen delivery and increased extraction. In cases of dysoxia with impaired tissue oxygen utilization, $ScVO_2$ may be >80% and may indicate cell death [5].

When anaerobic metabolism ensues, lactate is produced, leading to lactic acidosis. However, high lactate is nonspecific, and high lactate may also be seen in cases of ischemia due to vascular causes like gut ischemia and gangrenous limb and in cases of liver and kidney failure and many other causes like seizures, drug overdose, cyanide poisoning, and thiamine deficiency [6].

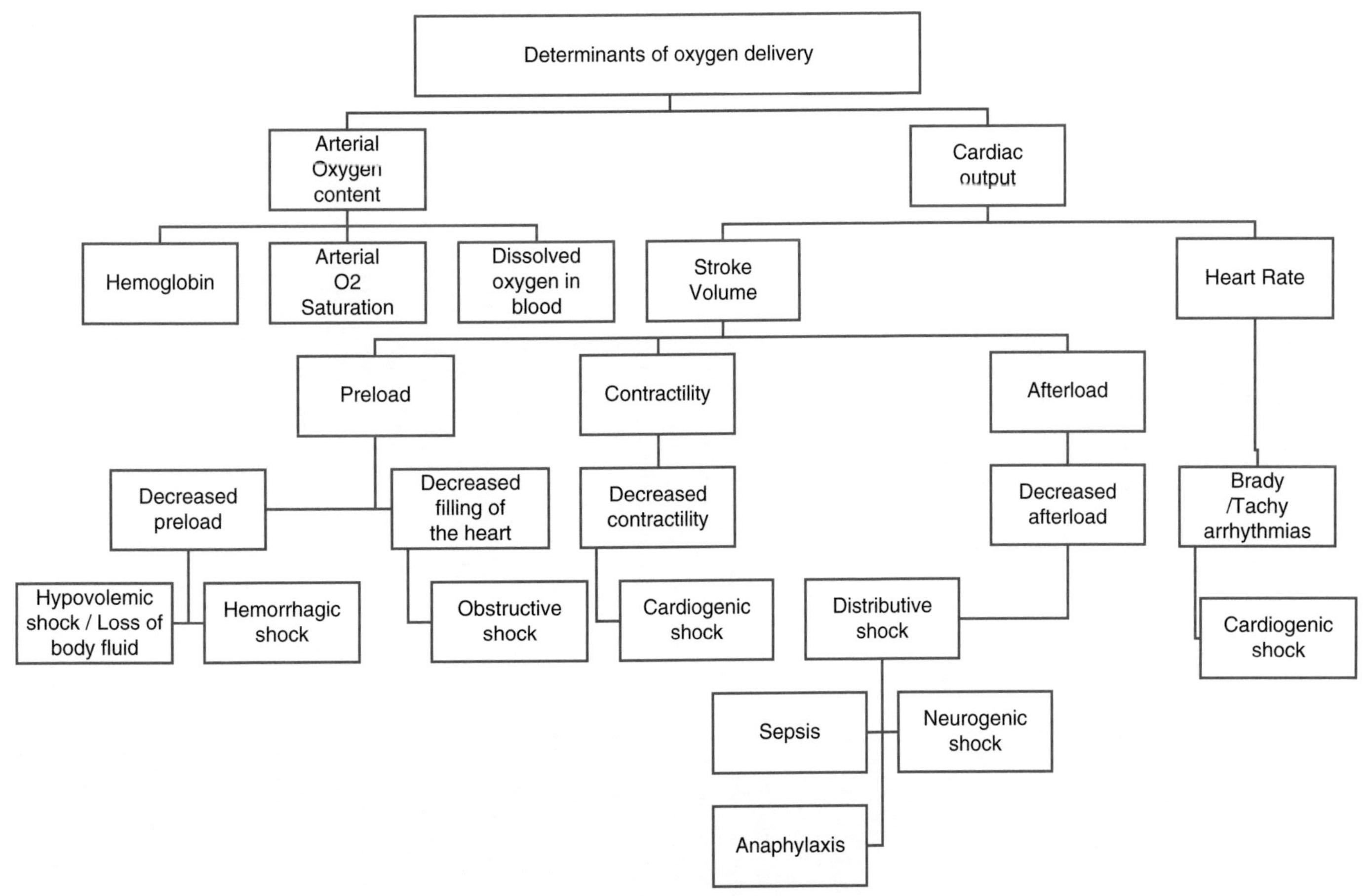

Flowchart 14.1 Determinants of oxygen delivery and its abnormalities leading to several types of shock

14.3 Diagnosis and Evaluation

Shock is a clinical diagnosis, made by incorporating history, physical examination, and laboratory findings. It is important to note that although these tools are used to diagnose shock, shock is not defined by any single vital sign, physical examination finding, or laboratory value. This understanding is crucial, as if misunderstood, it may result in either more or less aggressive treatment than necessary. As an example, consider a patient who presents with symptoms of acute decompensated heart failure, blood pressure of 90/70, heart rate of 112, elevated lactic acid, and cool extremities. Although the mean arterial pressure (MAP) is above 65, it would be a mistake to not diagnose this patient with cardiogenic shock, as it may result in delayed, less aggressive, or inappropriate care. So, although shock is not defined by any single vital sign, physical examination finding, or laboratory value, there are common findings seen in patients with shock.

14.3.1 Vital Signs and Physical Exam

Vital sign abnormalities are common in patients with shock. Most patients have hypotension, tachycardia, and tachypnea. Blood pressure, however, may be normal or rarely elevated, due to sympathetic stimulation. Normotension in a patient that typically has hypertension may be another clinical indication or shock. Tachycardia is commonly present; however, patients on AV nodal blocking medications may not develop tachycardia. The metabolic derangements associated with shock as well as bradyarrhythmias that are the primary source of shock may cause bradycardia. Patients may have tachypnea related to poor diaphragmatic perfusion, acidosis, pulmonary edema, pneumonia, or ARDS. As shock progresses and diaphragmatic weakness worsens, patients may have a normal respiratory rate, bradypnea, or frank respiratory failure [7, 8].

Abnormal physical exam findings in patients with shock are related to inadequate organ perfusion, cause of shock, and sympathetic stimulation. The occurrence of these findings is variable, and not all patients may have them. Table 14.2 summarizes potential physical exam findings one may see in patients with shock. These findings may support the diagnosis of shock and help to determine the shock's cause, but the lack of certain findings does not rule out shock. It is worth noting that decreased urine output is one of the first signs of impaired organ perfusion in shock.

Urine output and capillary refill time are used at the bedside as surrogates for organ perfusion. Decreased urine output reflects renal hypoperfusion and is used as a nonspecific marker of shock and is used to guide fluid resuscitation in the absence of advanced hemodynamic monitoring.

Capillary refill time (CRT) has been used as a sensitive marker of hypovolemia in children and has been recently shown to be useful in adult shock as a prognostic marker and as a guide to resuscitation [9]. Normal CRT is less than 3 s, and more than 5 s is suggestive of impaired perfusion.

Table 14.2 Common physical exam findings in patients with shock

General	Ill appearing Pale Weak Restlessness
Neuro	Altered mental status Agitation Somnolence
Cardiovascular	Tachycardia Bradycardia Arrhythmias Weak pulse Jugular venous distension
Respiratory	Tachypnea Hypoxemia Poor O_2 saturation waveform Bradypnea
Renal	Oliguria or low urine output Anuria or no urine output Dark urine
Skin	Cool skin and extremities Warm skin and extremities Diaphoresis Delayed capillary refill

14.3.2 Laboratory Assessment

Lactic acid is commonly used to evaluate patients for shock and trend for therapy response. The pathophysiology of lactic acidosis in shock is complex and occurs through multiple mechanisms as described above. This includes a shift towards anaerobic metabolism due to ischemia, catecholamine production, and decreased clearance [10]. Unlike in other causes of shock, lactic acidosis in sepsis is mostly due to catecholamine response, impaired cellular metabolism, and microcirculatory dysfunction as opposed to tissue hypoxia [11, 12]. It is also important to note that organ dysfunction in shock is related to elevated lactate due to impaired clearance. This is because lactate clearance is primarily performed by the liver and kidney, which are commonly affected in shock. Lactic acid may be used to aid in diagnosing shock and evaluating response to treatment, particularly in cardiogenic and hemorrhagic shock [13, 14]. Elevated lactic acid has also been associated with increased mortality in many causes of shock [15–17].

Central venous oxygen saturation ($ScVO_2$) is another test used to aid in determining the cause of shock and monitoring response to therapy. Its pathophysiology is described above and is based on the principles of delivery of oxygen (DO_2) equation and Fick equation. By measuring a central venous oxygen saturation, one can calculate the cardiac output; however, one may also presume that cardiac output is low if the central venous oxygen saturation is low (<65%). Typically, a low $ScVO_2$

is associated with cardiogenic or hemorrhagic shock, and a high $ScVO_2$ is associated with septic shock. One can see how this makes sense in both hemorrhagic and cardiogenic shock by analyzing the equations in Fig. 14.1. Conceptually, in cardiogenic shock, tissues have excess time to extract oxygen as flow is sluggish. In hemorrhagic shock, the amount of oxygen delivered is low due to loss of hemoglobin and blood volume. Sepsis instead typically presents with vasodilatory shock, minimizing the ability of tissues to extract oxygen, which results in normal to high $ScVO_2$. However, there are many variables in this equation that limit its accuracy and can make the interpretation of a single $ScVO_2$ value prone to error. For instance, in a patient who is mechanically ventilated and has an elevated partial pressure of oxygen in arterial blood (PaO_2), this would result in a higher $ScVO_2$. In this scenario, ruling out cardiogenic shock by that value alone may be a mistake. $ScVO_2$ may provide value when trending, particularly in cardiogenic shock and evaluating response to therapies. In sepsis, there have been multiple trials that have demonstrated limited utility in determining outcomes and response to therapy as opposed to utilizing lactic acid and clinical assessment [18–22].

Hematologic derangements are also common in shock. Leukocytosis is commonly seen in both sepsis and other causes of shock [23]. Decreased hemoglobin and platelets may be seen due to hemorrhagic shock. Increased blood urea nitrogen (BUN) and creatinine are commonly seen due to impaired renal perfusion. In severe shock, significant elevation of AST and ALT may occur. If severe enough, patients may develop acute liver failure. Elevated troponin is common, especially when utilizing high-sensitivity troponin assays. This occurs even in the absence of acute coronary occlusion [24]. Metabolic acidosis, most commonly due to lactic acid and/or renal failure, may be present.

14.3.3 Imaging

Imaging is an essential aspect in diagnosing the cause of shock. Bedside ultrasound assessing for cardiac function, signs of tamponade, pneumothorax, free intraperitoneal fluid, and aortic abnormalities may immediately help clinicians narrow down the primary etiology of shock [25–28]. A chest X-ray may help identify pneumonia, aortic abnormalities, cardiomegaly, pneumothorax, or other findings to help determine a cause as well. CT imaging can be highly sensitive for foci of infection, pulmonary embolism, aortic pathology, and more.

14.3.4 Invasive Hemodynamic Monitoring

Although no invasive hemodynamic monitoring device has demonstrated sufficient evidence that their use improves mortality in shock in randomized controlled trials, they are commonly used [29, 30]. Arterial lines are helpful to obtain accurate and timely blood pressure measurements, as noninvasive blood pressure cuffs may provide inaccurate measurements in patients with vasoconstriction. Central venous pressure (CVP) monitoring may be helpful in identifying right heart dysfunction and signs of venous congestion. Pulmonary arterial catheters (PACs) are used to determine cardiac output and other hemodynamic variables, which may aid in determining the hemodynamic profile of a patient's shock state. PACs are now less commonly used, as multiple studies have failed to demonstrate mortality benefit for most cases of shock [31–42]. Point-of-care cardiac ultrasound (POCUS) has now been used in place of PACs in many cases; however, they remain useful, especially in cases where echocardiography is limited or in patients with cardiogenic shock.

14.4 Classification

Although there are distinct classifications and phenotypes of shock, it is clinically important to recognize that shock is frequently multifactorial, and certain causes of shock often have phenotypic components of more than one type of shock. Going forward, we will categorize and describe the phenotypes of the several types of shock as detailed in Table 14.3. In the clinical scenarios, however, at the bedside, it can be difficult to determine the exact cause or type of shock. By understanding this, we can improve our ability to diagnose certain types of shock, as well as avoid the pitfall of not considering more than one etiology of shock.

14.4.1 Distributive

Distributive shock is caused by pathologic peripheral vasodilation. Loss of systemic vascular resistance (SVR) without adequate fluid resuscitation causes a decrease in left ventricular (LV) filling pressures and cardiac index due to decreased venous blood volume. However, after fluid resuscitation, these parameters may normalize, and patients commonly have high cardiac output due to decreased systemic vascular resistance. Despite cardiac output being high, there is ineffective tissue perfusion due to excessive vasodilation and microcirculatory dysfunction. Clinically, these patients often have warm, well-perfused extremities, decreased diastolic blood pressure, and increased pulse pressure. Other signs of shock commonly exist, including tachycardia, tachypnea, and oliguria.

Sepsis is the most common cause of distributive shock and is one of the most common causes of mortality in the intensive care unit [43]. Sepsis is caused by a dysregulated host immune response to infection [44]. It is important to point out that sepsis is not only caused by bacteria, as other forms of infection such as viruses and fungi can also result in sepsis. This results in inflammatory mediators including cytokines, kinins, complement, coagulation factors, and eicosanoids that cause vasodilation and multisystem organ dysfunction [45–51]. Sepsis may commonly present with signs and symptoms of other forms of shock as well. Cardiogenic shock

Table 14.3 Classification of the several types of shock and their common causes

Distributive	• Sepsis • SIRS • Neurogenic • Anaphylactic • Drug or toxin induced • Adrenal crisis • Myxedema coma or decompensated hypothyroidism • Thyroid storm • Liver failure

Cardiogenic	• Myopathic
	  – Myocardial infarction
	  – Myocarditis
	  – Nonischemic cardiomyopathy
	  – Sepsis-induced cardiomyopathy
	  – Drug toxicity
	  – Myocardial contusion
	  – Hypertrophic obstructive cardiomyopathy
	• Arrhythmic
	  – Ventricular tachycardia
	  – Supraventricular tachycardia
	  – Atrial fibrillation and flutter
	  – Heart block
	  – Toxin-induced arrhythmias
	• Mechanical
	  – Valvular disease
	  – Ventricular septal defect

Hypovolemic	• Hemorrhagic
	  – Gastrointestinal bleeding
	  – Traumatic hemorrhage
	  – Retroperitoneal hemorrhage
	• Nonhemorrhagic
	  – Severe burns
	  – Dehydration can be secondary to vomiting and diarrhea
	  – Insensible losses perioperatively or during surgery

Obstructive	• Impaired diastolic filling due to mechanical obstruction
	  – Vena cava obstruction (clot or tumor)
	  – Tension pneumothorax
	  – Mechanical ventilation (breath stacking)
	  – Cardiac tamponade
	  – Constrictive pericarditis
	  – Restrictive cardiomyopathy
	• Impaired right ventricular systolic contraction
	  – Pulmonary embolism
	  – Pulmonary hypertension

may co-occur due to sepsis-induced cardiomyopathy. Hypovolemic shock can occur secondary to symptoms related to infection and increased insensible losses [52]. Sepsis may also lead to a hypercoagulable state, resulting in pulmonary embolism and obstructive shock [53].

Systemic inflammatory response syndrome (SIRS) can also result in distributive shock and is characterized by a robust inflammatory response to a major insult [54].

Causes include infection, pancreatitis, burns, major trauma, cardiac arrest, cardiopulmonary bypass, amniotic fluid embolism, and fat embolism.

Neurogenic shock is caused by a traumatic brain injury or spinal cord injury that results in the disruption of autonomic pathways, particularly of the sympathetic system. This typically results in decreased vascular resistance and increased parasympathetic tone, resulting in vasodilatory shock. Notably, there is often a component of cardiogenic shock from the resultant bradycardia. Severe trauma, however, often results in multiple injuries, and the diagnosis of neurogenic shock should only be made after excluding major hemorrhage.

Anaphylaxis is another common form of distributive shock. Anaphylaxis is caused by an IgE-mediated response to an allergen resulting in mast cell degranulation. In addition to systemic vasodilation, anaphylaxis will commonly cause rash (urticaria), bronchospasm, gastrointestinal symptoms, and mucosal swelling. Unlike many other causes of distributive shock, anaphylaxis is often rapidly reversible.

Adrenal crisis and decompensated hypothyroidism (myxedema coma) are two forms of shock caused by dysfunction of the endocrine system. Adrenal crisis may be due to primary adrenal insufficiency (Addisonian crisis) or secondary adrenal insufficiency.

14.4.2 Cardiogenic

Cardiogenic shock can be classified into three categories, which include cardiomyopathic, arrhythmic, and mechanical. Cardiogenic shock is primarily due to intrinsic cardiac pump failure, which may be due to many causes. Patients in cardiogenic shock may present in several ways. Classic cardiogenic shock can present with pulmonary edema, elevated JVP, and cold extremities. Patients, however, may also present without pulmonary edema, especially in the setting of right ventricular failure. Patients may also present with warm extremities in end-stage decompensated heart failure. Edema is another common finding in cardiogenic shock; however, it may not be present, especially in isolated acute left ventricular failure. Bedside ultrasound is a particularly useful tool available to clinicians to identify cardiac dysfunction at the bedside [55, 56]. Pulmonary ultrasound is useful in evaluating for pulmonary edema, which may be represented by B lines on lung ultrasound, as seen in Fig. 14.1 [58]. As discussed above, mixed venous or central venous oxygen saturation is classically low. Lactic acid may or may not be elevated, but an elevation in lactic acid is linked with mortality [14]. More invasive hemodynamic measurements obtained using devices like the PA catheter may show elevated pulmonary capillary wedge pressure, elevated central venous pressure, low cardiac output, and low cardiac index.

Cardiogenic shock can be classified into three categories, which include cardiomyopathic, arrhythmic, and mechanical.

Cardiomyopathic causes include acute ischemia, chronic ischemia, dilated cardiomyopathy, post-cardiac arrest myocardial stunning, myocarditis, takotsubo cardiomyopathy, sepsis-induced cardiomyopathy, and post-cardiopulmonary bypass.

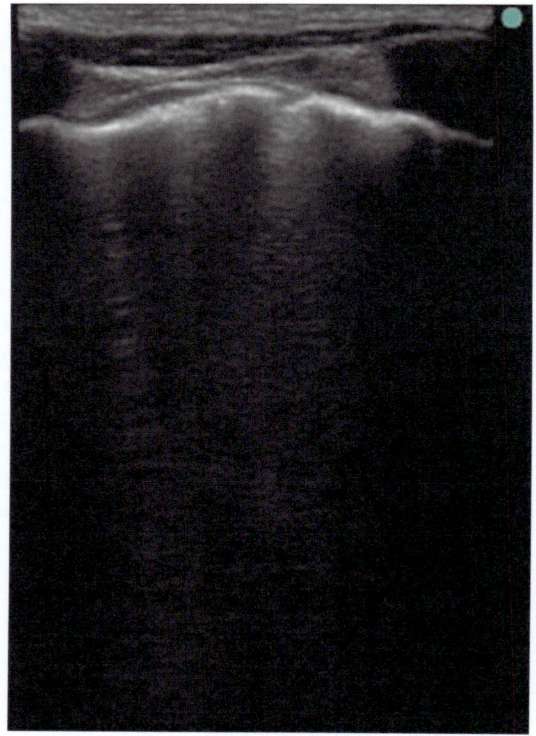

Fig. 14.1 Characteristics of B lines on lung ultrasound. Vertical echogenic wedge-shaped lines beginning at the pleura (bright line) and extending down the screen [57]

Both tachyarrhythmias and bradyarrhythmias may cause cardiogenic shock and may be of atrial or ventricular origin. Arrhythmias may be the primary etiology of shock or contribute to another shock state, such as atrial fibrillation with rapid ventricular response in a patient with septic shock.

Mechanical causes of cardiogenic shock include acute or acute on chronic valvular pathology, most commonly mitral or aortic. These may be stenotic or regurgitative lesions. Causes include chronic degeneration, masses, endocarditis, papillary muscle rupture, chordae tendineae rupture, retrograde aortic dissection into the aortic valve ring, and more. Another mechanical cause is cardiac masses such as atrial myxomas. Cardiac masses may impair outflow, cause valve incompetence, cause impaired contractility, or cause impaired cardiac compliance.

14.4.3 Hypovolemic

Hypovolemic shock is due to intravascular volume depletion. This results in decreased preload, decreased stroke volume, and decreased cardiac output. As a result, systemic vascular resistance is high. Lactic acid is often elevated. Mixed venous oxygen saturation is low, as discussed above. Clinically, patients exhibit tachycardia, narrow pulse pressure, weak pulses, low JVP, and cool skin.

Hypovolemic shock can broadly be categorized as hemorrhagic and nonhemorrhagic. The most common causes of hemorrhagic shock are gastrointestinal bleeding, trauma, and bleeding related to surgery. Nonhemorrhagic hypovolemic shock has many etiologies, which include major burns, vomiting, diarrhea, and insensible losses during surgery.

14.4.4   Obstructive

Obstructive shock is due to extracardiac causes that impair flow into or out of the heart. Often, these pathologies are associated with either right ventricular (RV) failure or impaired right ventricular and right atrial filling. Mixed venous oxygen saturation will typically be low. Hemodynamically, this typically manifests with narrow pulse pressure, elevated CVP, and elevated SVR. Cardiac output and cardiac index will be low. Lactic acid, as in other causes of shock, is often elevated. Physical exam findings are variable and based on the etiology of obstructive shock, which will be discussed below. Obstructive shock can best be broken down into two categories, which include pulmonary vascular obstruction and mechanical obstruction.

Pulmonary vascular causes of obstructive shock primarily include pulmonary embolism and pulmonary hypertension. Pulmonary embolism from venous thromboembolism causes acute right heart failure via several mechanisms. There is an acute increase in pulmonary vascular resistance from thrombus obstructing pulmonary arterial blood flow. In addition to this, there is the release of vasoactive mediators, which results in pulmonary vascular vasoconstriction. The RV subsequently cannot pump blood forward effectively. This results in decreased left ventricular preload and cardiac output. In addition to this, the RV will become dilated, which has several adverse effects. Significant right ventricular dilation will result in compression of the LV, further decreasing LV preload and cardiac output. In addition to this, RV dilation increases RV systolic and end-diastolic pressure, which decreases coronary perfusion in the RV and results in worsening RV dysfunction. The resultant decrease in LV preload and cardiac output contributes to hypotension, which further decreases RV coronary perfusion. This can result in rapid hemodynamic collapse. RV dysfunction may also be further exacerbated by hypoxemia, acidosis, and positive-pressure ventilation, as these all result in increased pulmonary vascular resistance [59]. Pulmonary hypertension is a less common cause of pulmonary vascular obstructive shock. Pulmonary hypertension may be due to primary pulmonary hypertension or a wide variety of other causes. The physiology of shock secondary to decompensated pulmonary hypertension is similar to that of pulmonary embolism [60]. Lastly, volume overload, sickle cell acute chest syndrome, and hypoxemic respiratory failure can also result in acute right ventricular failure and obstructive shock.

Mechanical causes of obstructive shock are somewhat broad, but most commonly include pericardial tamponade and tension pneumothorax. Pericardial tamponade can be acute (i.e., traumatic cardiac injury, aortic dissection, LV free wall rupture) or chronic (i.e., malignant effusion, uremia, infectious, inflammatory). Cardiac tamponade causes shock by compressing the cardiac chambers, which impairs their ability to fill as well as provide cardiac output. The rate at which tamponade causes hemodynamic collapse is related to the rate at which fluid accumulates. For example, in the case of LV free wall rupture, aortic dissection, and traumatic cardiac injuries, blood may accumulate rapidly, and the pericardium does not have time to stretch and accommodate pericardial fluid. This results in rapid compression of the cardiac chambers and hemodynamic collapse. Chronic effusions, however, build slowly over time, allowing the pericardium to stretch and accommodate more fluid. There is a point, however, where the pericardium cannot accommodate more fluid, and tamponade physiology ensues [61]. Pericardial tamponade is primarily a clinical diagnosis, though physical exam and diagnostic testing are essential for aiding in making the diagnosis. On exam, patients will typically have tachycardia, hypotension, and jugular venous pressure (JVP) elevation. Echocardiography is essential in diagnosing tamponade. Echocardiography helps determine the presence, location, and characteristics of an effusion; however, it also aids in assessing the hemodynamic significance of an effusion. Supportive findings on echocardiography include a dilated inferior vena cava, diastolic collapse of the right atrium or right ventricle, left-sided chamber collapse, and respiratory variations in volumes or flows [62]. Ultimately, the diagnosis of tamponade can only be confirmed through hemodynamic improvement after pericardial drainage.

Tension pneumothorax is another common mechanical cause of obstructive shock. When a large amount of air accumulates between the lung and chest wall, this may cause compression of the inferior vena cava (IVC), superior vena cava (SVC), and cardiac chambers. This will result in impaired cardiac filling. This may be exacerbated by positive-pressure ventilation, as pneumothorax on positive pressure is more likely to increase in size [63]. Large intrathoracic tumors may cause compression of the great veins, resulting in decreased cardiac filling (Fig. 14.2, Table 14.4).

Fig. 14.2 Echocardiography demonstrating a large pericardial effusion in a patient in tamponade [64]. *LV* left ventricle, *RV* right ventricle, *Ao* aorta, *LA* left atrium

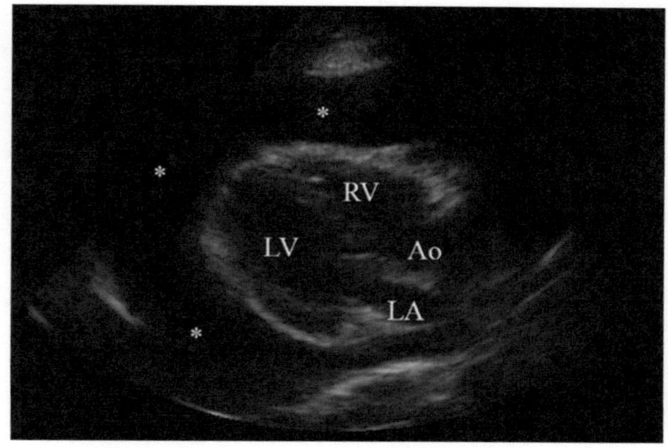

Table 14.4 Chart comparing clinical findings and hemodynamic variables among the several types of shock

	Distributive	Cardiogenic	Hypovolemic	Obstructive
Extremities Warm/cold	Warm	Cold	Cold	Cold
IVC size/ JVP	Normal/ normal	Enlarged/elevated	Small/decreased	Enlarged/ elevated
Pulse pressure	Wide/normal	Narrow	Narrow	Low
Cardiac output	High	Low	Low	Low
ScVO$_2$	Normal/high	Low	Low	Low
SVR	Low	High	High	High
PCWP	Normal/low	High	Low	Normal/low
Other	Fever	POCUS with LV, RV, or biventricular dysfunction Peripheral edema	Positive FAST exam Obvious hemorrhage Trauma	RV dilation on POCUS Pericardial effusion Absent lung sliding Pulsus paradoxus

14.5 Management

Any patient presenting with shock needs a detailed history and physical to evaluate the etiology of shock while simultaneously initiating resuscitation to improve survival. The steps in management are outlined in Flowchart 14.2. Early stabilization should include management of airway, breathing, and circulation in a critically ill patient. Adequate oxygenation should be maintained, and oxygen may be administered if oxygen saturation (sO$_2$) is less than 92%. If unable to treat hypoxia, patients may need endotracheal intubation and invasive mechanical ventilation.

Two peripheral wide-bore IV access should be established and fluid resuscitation initiated immediately. In many cases, central venous catheters may be necessary for infusing vasopressors and inotropes and also obtaining ScVO2 values. Crystalloids are preferred as the fluid of choice. Fluid boluses can be given with close monitoring for fluid overload with the use of POCUS or invasive monitoring. Early blood transfusion should be considered in cases of acute blood loss or if severe anemia is affecting oxygen delivery. The target of resuscitation is to maintain a mean arterial pressure (MAP) above or equal to 65 mmHg.

Studies have shown that longer duration of MAP less than 65 mmHg is an independent predictor of mortality in septic shock [65]. Research favors early administration of vasopressors, and it is recommended in septic shock, for improving perfusion, improving organ blood flow distribution, and decreasing the need for IV fluid and thus avoiding fluid overload [66]. Norepinephrine is the vasopressor of choice and may be started via a peripheral line in an emergency. Initiation of

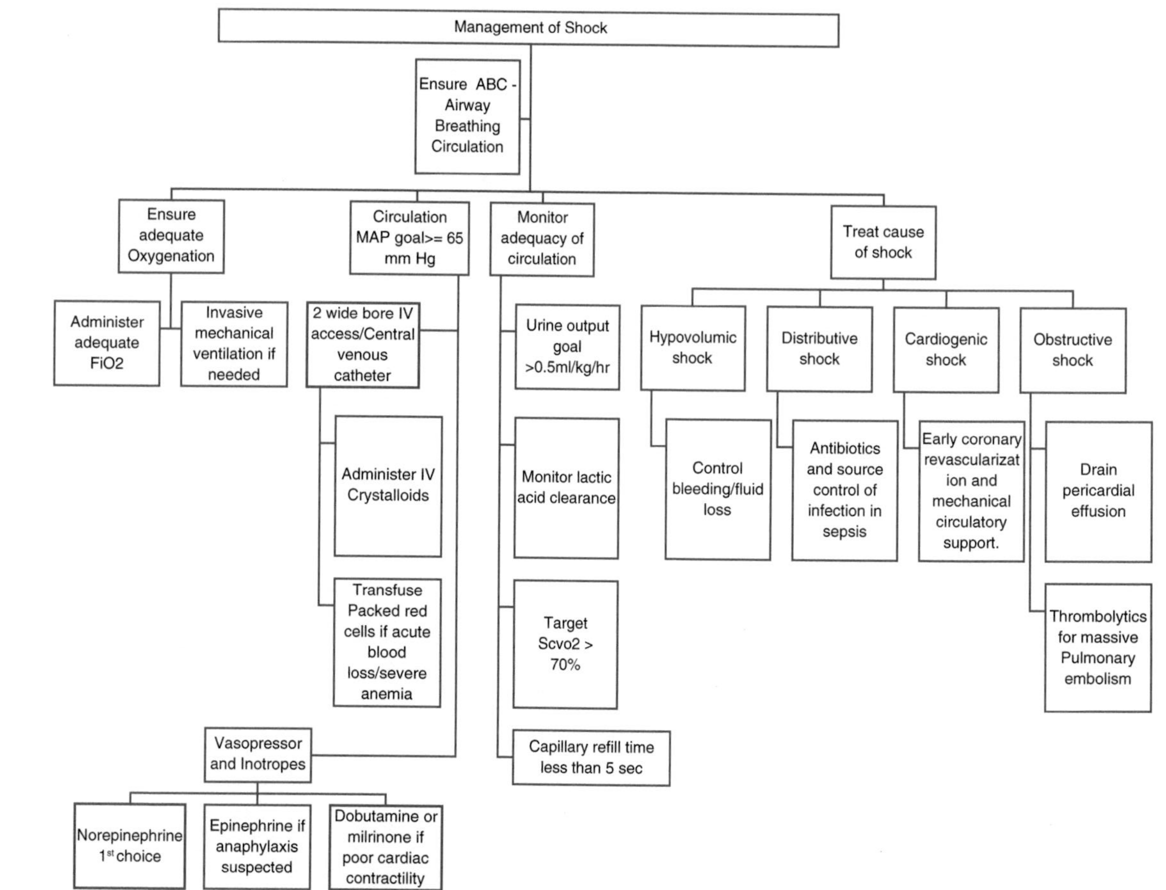

Flowchart 14.2 Management of shock

vasopressors should not be delayed till central venous access is established. Consider the use of inotropes (dobutamine or milrinone) if there is evidence of poor cardiac contractility/cardiogenic shock. Epinephrine is used as a drug of choice in anaphylactic shock.

Adequacy of resuscitation should be frequently assessed by the use of surrogate markers like urine output with a goal of at least 0.5 mL/kg/h or capillary refill time less than 5 s. Restoration of adequacy of tissue perfusion is assessed by lactate clearance and maintaining of $ScVO_2$ above 70%.

Concomitant treatment of the underlying etiology of shock is of paramount importance. In patients with hypovolemic shock, early efforts should be directed towards controlling the source of bleeding and fluid loss. If distributive shock is suspected to be secondary to sepsis, collect cultures, administer broad-spectrum antibiotics, and control the source of infection to correct septic shock. Coronary revascularization and mechanical circulatory support like extracorporeal membrane oxygenation (ECMO) or ventricular assist devices (VADs) should be considered when treating cardiogenic shock secondary to myocardial ischemia. When obstructive shock is diagnosed, pericardiocentesis should be done if evidence of cardiac tamponade and thrombolysis/pulmonary thrombectomy should be attempted if shock is secondary to massive pulmonary embolism. Chest tubes may be necessary to reverse pneumothorax.

14.6 Conclusion

Shock is a manifestation of poor organ perfusion and thus an imbalance of oxygen demand and supply to the tissues. Low blood pressure is not equivalent to shock. Prompt recognition and treatment have been shown to improve survival. Treatment includes rapid resuscitation to achieve hemodynamic stability and restore organ perfusion, along with treatment of the underlying cause of shock. If untreated, shock can lead to multiorgan failure and death.

Disclosure Authors report no conflict of interest.

References

1. Chaudry IH. Cellular mechanisms in shock and ischemia and their correction. Am J Phys. 1983;245(2):R117–34. https://doi.org/10.1152/ajpregu.1983.245.2.R117.
2. Chaudry IH, Ohkawa M, Clemens MG, Baue AE. Alterations in electron transport and cellular metabolism with shock and trauma. Prog Clin Biol Res. 1983;111:67–88.
3. Della Rocca Y, Fonticoli L, Rajan TS, Trubiani O, Caputi S, Diomede F, Pizzicannella J, Marconi GD. Hypoxia: molecular pathophysiological mechanisms in human diseases. J Physiol Biochem. 2022;78(4):739–52. https://doi.org/10.1007/s13105-022-00912-6.
4. Gorecki G, Cochior D, Moldovan C, Rusu E. Molecular mechanisms in septic shock (review). Exp Ther Med. 2021;22(4):1161. https://doi.org/10.3892/etm.2021.10595.

5. Nebout S, Pirracchio R. Should we monitor ScVO(2) in critically ill patients? Cardiol Res Pract. 2012;2012:370697. https://doi.org/10.1155/2012/370697.

6. Kushimoto S, Akaishi S, Sato T, Nomura R, Fujita M, Kudo D, Kawazoe Y, Yoshida Y, Miyagawa N. Lactate, a useful marker for disease mortality and severity but an unreliable marker of tissue hypoxia/hypoperfusion in critically ill patients. Acute Med Surg. 2016;3(4):293–7. https://doi.org/10.1002/ams2.207.

7. Pannu AK. Circulatory shock in adults in emergency department. Turk J Emerg Med. 2023;23(3):139–48. https://doi.org/10.4103/2452-2473.367400.

8. Vincent JL, Ince C, Bakker J. Clinical review: circulatory shock—an update: a tribute to Professor Max Harry Weil. Crit Care. 2012;16(6):239. https://doi.org/10.1186/cc11510.

9. Hernandez G, Ospina-Tascon GA, Damiani LP, Estenssoro E, Dubin A, Hurtado J, Friedman G, Castro R, Alegria L, Teboul JL, Cecconi M, Ferri G, Jibaja M, Pairumani R, Fernandez P, Barahona D, Granda-Luna V, Cavalcanti AB, Bakker J, The ASI, the Latin America Intensive Care N, Hernandez G, Ospina-Tascon G, Petri Damiani L, Estenssoro E, Dubin A, Hurtado J, Friedman G, Castro R, Alegria L, Teboul JL, Cecconi M, Cecconi M, Ferri G, Jibaja M, Pairumani R, Fernandez P, Barahona D, Cavalcanti AB, Bakker J, Hernandez G, Alegria L, Ferri G, Rodriguez N, Holger P, Soto N, Pozo M, Bakker J, Cook D, Vincent JL, Rhodes A, Kavanagh BP, Dellinger P, Rietdijk W, Carpio D, Pavez N, Henriquez E, Bravo S, Valenzuela ED, Vera M, Dreyse J, Oviedo V, Cid MA, Larroulet M, Petruska E, Sarabia C, Gallardo D, Sanchez JE, Gonzalez H, Arancibia JM, Munoz A, Ramirez G, Aravena F, Aquevedo A, Zambrano F, Bozinovic M, Valle F, Ramirez M, Rossel V, Munoz P, Ceballos C, Esveile C, Carmona C, Candia E, Mendoza D, Sanchez A, Ponce D, Ponce D, Lastra J, Nahuelpan B, Fasce F, Luengo C, Medel N, Cortes C, Campassi L, Rubatto P, Horna N, Furche M, Pendino JC, Bettini L, Lovesio C, Gonzalez MC, Rodruguez J, Canales H, Caminos F, Galletti C, Minoldo E, Aramburu MJ, Olmos D, Nin N, Tenzi J, Quiroga C, Lacuesta P, Gaudin A, Pais R, Silvestre A, Olivera G, Rieppi G, Berrutti D, Ochoa M, Cobos P, Vintimilla F, Ramirez V, Tobar M, Garcia F, Picoita F, Remache N, Granda V, Paredes F, Barzallo E, Garces P, Guerrero F, Salazar S, Torres G, Tana C, Calahorrano J, Solis F, Torres P, Herrera L, Ornes A, Perez V, Delgado G, Lopez A, Espinosa E, Moreira J, Salcedo B, Villacres I, Suing J, Lopez M, Gomez L, Toctaquiza G, Cadena Zapata M, Orazabal MA, Pardo Espejo R, Jimenez J, Calderon A, Paredes G, Barberan JL, Moya T, Atehortua H, Sabogal R, Ortiz G, Lara A, Sanchez F, Hernan Portilla A, Davila H, Mora JA, Calderon LE, Alvarez I, Escobar E, Bejarano A, Bustamante LA, Aldana JL. Effect of a resuscitation strategy targeting peripheral perfusion status vs serum lactate levels on 28-day mortality among patients with septic shock: the ANDROMEDA-SHOCK randomized clinical trial. JAMA. 2019;321(7):654–64. https://doi.org/10.1001/jama.2019.0071.

10. Levitt DG, Levitt JE, Levitt MD. Quantitative assessment of blood lactate in shock: measure of hypoxia or beneficial energy source. Biomed Res Int. 2020;2020:2608318. https://doi.org/10.1155/2020/2608318.

11. Chertoff J, Chisum M, Garcia B, Lascano J. Lactate kinetics in sepsis and septic shock: a review of the literature and rationale for further research. J Intensive Care. 2015;3:39. https://doi.org/10.1186/s40560-015-0105-4.

12. Suetrong B, Walley KR. Lactic acidosis in sepsis: It's not all anaerobic: implications for diagnosis and management. Chest. 2016;149(1):252–61. https://doi.org/10.1378/chest.15-1703.

13. Baxter J, Cranfield KR, Clark G, Harris T, Bloom B, Gray AJ. Do lactate levels in the emergency department predict outcome in adult trauma patients? A systematic review. J Trauma Acute Care Surg. 2016;81(3):555–66. https://doi.org/10.1097/TA.0000000000001156.

14. Jentzer JC, Schrage B, Patel PC, Kashani KB, Barsness GW, Holmes DR Jr, Blankenberg S, Kirchhof P, Westermann D. Association between the acidemia, lactic acidosis, and shock severity with outcomes in patients with cardiogenic shock. J Am Heart Assoc. 2022;11(9):e024932. https://doi.org/10.1161/JAHA.121.024932.

15. Alshiakh SM. Role of serum lactate as prognostic marker of mortality among emergency department patients with multiple conditions: a systematic review. SAGE Open Med. 2023;11:20503121221136401. https://doi.org/10.1177/20503121221136401.

16. Villar J, Short JH, Lighthall G. Lactate predicts both Short- and long-term mortality in patients with and without sepsis. Infect Dis (Auckl). 2019;12:1178633719862776. https://doi.org/10.1177/1178633719862776.

17. Wang Y, Feng Y, Yang X, Mao H. Prognostic role of elevated lactate in acute pulmonary embolism: a systematic review and meta-analysis. Phlebology. 2022;37(5):338–47. https://doi.org/10.1177/02683555221081818.

18. Gutierrez G. Central and mixed venous O(2) saturation. Turk J Anaesthesiol Reanim. 2020;48(1):2–10. https://doi.org/10.5152/TJAR.2019.140.

19. Mahajan RK, Peter JV, John G, Graham PL, Rao SV, Pinsky MR. Patterns of central venous oxygen saturation, lactate and veno-arterial CO2 difference in patients with septic shock. Indian J Crit Care Med. 2015;19(10):580–6. https://doi.org/10.4103/0972-5229.167035.

20. Textoris J, Fouche L, Wiramus S, Antonini F, Tho S, Martin C, Leone M. High central venous oxygen saturation in the latter stages of septic shock is associated with increased mortality. Crit Care. 2011;15(4):R176. https://doi.org/10.1186/cc10325.

21. van Beest P, Wietasch G, Scheeren T, Spronk P, Kuiper M. Clinical review: use of venous oxygen saturations as a goal—a yet unfinished puzzle. Crit Care. 2011;15(5):232. https://doi.org/10.1186/cc10351.

22. Walley KR. Use of central venous oxygen saturation to guide therapy. Am J Respir Crit Care Med. 2011;184(5):514–20. https://doi.org/10.1164/rccm.201010-1584CI.

23. Rimmer E, Garland A, Kumar A, Doucette S, Houston BL, Menard CE, Leeies M, Turgeon AF, Mahmud S, Houston DS, Zarychanski R. White blood cell count trajectory and mortality in septic shock: a historical cohort study. Can J Anaesth. 2022;69(10):1230–9. https://doi.org/10.1007/s12630-022-02282-5.

24. Vaz HA, Guimaraes RB, Dutra O. Challenges in high-sensitive troponin assay interpretation for intensive therapy. Rev Bras Ter Intensiva. 2019;31(1):93–105. https://doi.org/10.5935/0103-507X.20190001.

25. Berg I, Walpot K, Lamprecht H, Valois M, Lanctot JF, Srour N, van den Brand C. A systemic review on the diagnostic accuracy of point-of-care ultrasound in patients with undifferentiated shock in the emergency department. Cureus. 2022;14(3):e23188. https://doi.org/10.7759/cureus.23188.

26. Keikha M, Salehi-Marzijarani M, Soldoozi Nejat R, Sheikh Motahar Vahedi H, Mirrezaie SM. Diagnostic accuracy of rapid ultrasound in shock (RUSH) exam; a systematic review and meta-analysis. Bull Emerg Trauma. 2018;6(4):271–8. https://doi.org/10.29252/beat-060402.

27. Rahulkumar HH, Bhavin PR, Shreyas KP, Krunalkumar HP, Atulkumar S, Bansari C. Utility of point-of-care ultrasound in differentiating causes of shock in resource-limited setup. J Emerg Trauma Shock. 2019;12(1):10–7. https://doi.org/10.4103/JETS.JETS_61_18.

28. Yoshida T, Yoshida T, Noma H, Nomura T, Suzuki A, Mihara T. Diagnostic accuracy of point-of-care ultrasound for shock: a systematic review and meta-analysis. Crit Care. 2023;27(1):200. https://doi.org/10.1186/s13054-023-04495-6.

29. Gershengorn HB, Wunsch H, Scales DC, Zarychanski R, Rubenfeld G, Garland A. Association between arterial catheter use and hospital mortality in intensive care units. JAMA Intern Med. 2014;174(11):1746–54. https://doi.org/10.1001/jamainternmed.2014.3297.

30. Pinsky MR, Cecconi M, Chew MS, De Backer D, Douglas I, Edwards M, Hamzaoui O, Hernandez G, Martin G, Monnet X, Saugel B, Scheeren TWL, Teboul JL, Vincent JL. Effective hemodynamic monitoring. Crit Care. 2022;26(1):294. https://doi.org/10.1186/s13054-022-04173-z.

31. Binanay C, Califf RM, Hasselblad V, O'Connor CM, Shah MR, Sopko G, Stevenson LW, Francis GS, Leier CV, Miller LW, Investigators E, Coordinators ES. Evaluation study of congestive heart failure and pulmonary artery catheterization effectiveness: the ESCAPE trial. JAMA. 2005;294(13):1625–33. https://doi.org/10.1001/jama.294.13.1625.

32. Buhre W, Weyland A, Schorn B, Scholz M, Kazmaier S, Hoeft A, Sonntag H. Changes in central venous pressure and pulmonary capillary wedge pressure do not indicate changes in right and left heart volume in patients undergoing coronary artery bypass surgery. Eur J Anaesthesiol. 1999;16(1):11–7. https://doi.org/10.1046/j.1365-2346.1999.00406.x.

33. Connors AF Jr, Speroff T, Dawson NV, Thomas C, Harrell FE Jr, Wagner D, Desbiens N, Goldman L, Wu AW, Califf RM, Fulkerson WJ Jr, Vidaillet H, Broste S, Bellamy P, Lynn J, Knaus WA. The effectiveness of right heart catheterization in the initial care of critically ill patients. SUPPORT Investigators. JAMA. 1996;276(11):889–97. https://doi.org/10.1001/jama.276.11.889.

34. Friese RS, Shafi S, Gentilello LM. Pulmonary artery catheter use is associated with reduced mortality in severely injured patients: a National Trauma Data Bank analysis of 53,312 patients. Crit Care Med. 2006;34(6):1597–601. https://doi.org/10.1097/01.CCM.0000217918.03343.AA.

35. Harvey S, Harrison DA, Singer M, Ashcroft J, Jones CM, Elbourne D, Brampton W, Williams D, Young D, Rowan K, collaboration PA-Ms. Assessment of the clinical effectiveness of pulmonary artery catheters in management of patients in intensive care (PAC-Man): a randomised controlled trial. Lancet. 2005;366(9484):472–7. https://doi.org/10.1016/S0140-6736(05)67061-4.

36. Ivanov R, Allen J, Calvin JE. The incidence of major morbidity in critically ill patients managed with pulmonary artery catheters: a meta-analysis. Crit Care Med. 2000;28(3):615–9. https://doi.org/10.1097/00003246-200003000-00002.

37. National Heart L, Blood Institute Acute Respiratory Distress Syndrome Clinical Trials N, Wheeler AP, Bernard GR, Thompson BT, Schoenfeld D, Wiedemann HP, deBoisblanc B, Connors AF Jr, Hite RD, Harabin AL. Pulmonary-artery versus central venous catheter to guide treatment of acute lung injury. N Engl J Med. 2006;354(21):2213–24. https://doi.org/10.1056/NEJMoa061895.

38. Rhodes A, Cusack RJ, Newman PJ, Grounds RM, Bennett ED. A randomised, controlled trial of the pulmonary artery catheter in critically ill patients. Intensive Care Med. 2002;28(3):256–64. https://doi.org/10.1007/s00134-002-1206-9.

39. Richard C, Warszawski J, Anguel N, Deye N, Combes A, Barnoud D, Boulain T, Lefort Y, Fartoukh M, Baud F, Boyer A, Brochard L, Teboul JL, French Pulmonary Artery Catheter Study G. Early use of the pulmonary artery catheter and outcomes in patients with shock and acute respiratory distress syndrome: a randomized controlled trial. JAMA. 2003;290(20):2713–20. https://doi.org/10.1001/jama.290.20.2713.

40. Sandham JD, Hull RD, Brant RF, Knox L, Pineo GF, Doig CJ, Laporta DP, Viner S, Passerini L, Devitt H, Kirby A, Jacka M, Canadian Critical Care Clinical Trials G. A randomized, controlled trial of the use of pulmonary-artery catheters in high-risk surgical patients. N Engl J Med. 2003;348(1):5–14. https://doi.org/10.1056/NEJMoa021108.

41. Shah MR, Hasselblad V, Stevenson LW, Binanay C, O'Connor CM, Sopko G, Califf RM. Impact of the pulmonary artery catheter in critically ill patients: meta-analysis of randomized clinical trials. JAMA. 2005;294(13):1664–70. https://doi.org/10.1001/jama.294.13.1664.

42. Wiener RS, Welch HG. Trends in the use of the pulmonary artery catheter in the United States, 1993-2004. JAMA. 2007;298(4):423–9. https://doi.org/10.1001/jama.298.4.423.

43. Chiu C, Legrand M. Epidemiology of sepsis and septic shock. Curr Opin Anaesthesiol. 2021;34(2):71–6. https://doi.org/10.1097/ACO.0000000000000958.

44. Singer M, Deutschman CS, Seymour CW, Shankar-Hari M, Annane D, Bauer M, Bellomo R, Bernard GR, Chiche JD, Coopersmith CM, Hotchkiss RS, Levy MM, Marshall JC, Martin GS, Opal SM, Rubenfeld GD, van der Poll T, Vincent JL, Angus DC. The third international consensus definitions for sepsis and septic shock (Sepsis-3). JAMA. 2016;315(8):801–10. https://doi.org/10.1001/jama.2016.0287.

45. Eichenholz PW, Eichacker PQ, Hoffman WD, Banks SM, Parrillo JE, Danner RL, Natanson C. Tumor necrosis factor challenges in canines: patterns of cardiovascular dysfunction. Am J Phys. 1992;263(3 Pt 2):H668–75. https://doi.org/10.1152/ajpheart.1992.263.3.H668.

46. Hosenpud JD, Campbell SM, Mendelson DJ. Interleukin-1-induced myocardial depression in an isolated beating heart preparation. J Heart Transplant. 1989;8(6):460–4.

47. Kumar A, Krieger A, Symeoneides S, Kumar A, Parrillo JE. Myocardial dysfunction in septic shock: part II. Role of cytokines and nitric oxide. J Cardiothorac Vasc Anesth. 2001;15(4):485–511. https://doi.org/10.1053/jcan.2001.25003.

48. Parrillo JE. Pathogenetic mechanisms of septic shock. N Engl J Med. 1993;328(20):1471–7. https://doi.org/10.1056/NEJM199305203282008.

49. Pop-Began V, Paunescu V, Grigorean V, Pop-Began D, Popescu C. Molecular mechanisms in the pathogenesis of sepsis. J Med Life. 2014;7 Spec No. 2(Spec Iss 2):38–41.

50. Vincent JL, Bakker J, Marecaux G, Schandene L, Kahn RJ, Dupont E. Administration of anti-TNF antibody improves left ventricular function in septic shock patients. Results of a pilot study. Chest. 1992;101(3):810–5. https://doi.org/10.1378/chest.101.3.810.

51. Zhang YY, Ning BT. Signaling pathways and intervention therapies in sepsis. Signal Transduct Target Ther. 2021;6(1):407. https://doi.org/10.1038/s41392-021-00816-9.

52. Perner A, Cecconi M, Cronhjort M, Darmon M, Jakob SM, Pettila V, van der Horst ICC. Expert statement for the management of hypovolemia in sepsis. Intensive Care Med. 2018;44(6):791–8. https://doi.org/10.1007/s00134-018-5177-x.

53. Tsantes AG, Parastatidou S, Tsantes EA, Bonova E, Tsante KA, Mantzios PG, Vaiopoulos AG, Tsalas S, Konstantinidi A, Houhoula D, Iacovidou N, Piovani D, Nikolopoulos GK, Sokou R. Sepsis-induced coagulopathy: an update on pathophysiology, biomarkers, and current guidelines. Life (Basel). 2023;13(2):350. https://doi.org/10.3390/life13020350.

54. Balk RA. Systemic inflammatory response syndrome (SIRS): where did it come from and is it still relevant today? Virulence. 2014;5(1):20–6. https://doi.org/10.4161/viru.27135.

55. Polyzogopoulou E, Bezati S, Karamasis G, Boultadakis A, Parissis J. Early recognition and risk stratification in cardiogenic shock: well begun is half done. J Clin Med. 2023;12(7):2643. https://doi.org/10.3390/jcm12072643.

56. Ruben M, Molinas MS, Paladini H, Khalife W, Barbagelata A, Perrone S, Kaplinsky E. Emerging concepts in heart failure management and treatment: focus on point-of-care ultrasound in cardiogenic shock. Drugs Context. 2023;12:1. https://doi.org/10.7573/dic.2022-5-8.

57. Theerawit P, Touman N, Sutherasan Y, Kiatboonsri S. Transthoracic ultrasound assessment of B-lines for identifying the increment of extravascular lung water in shock patients requiring fluid resuscitation. Indian J Crit Care Med. 2014;18(4):195–9. https://doi.org/10.4103/0972-5229.130569.

58. Johannessen O, Claggett B, Lewis EF, Groarke JD, Swamy V, Lindner M, Solomon SD, Platz E. A-lines and B-lines in patients with acute heart failure. Eur Heart J Acute Cardiovasc Care. 2021;10(8):909–17. https://doi.org/10.1093/ehjacc/zuab046.

59. Shah IK, Merfeld JM, Chun J, Tak T. Pathophysiology and management of pulmonary embolism. Int J Angiol. 2022;31(3):143–9. https://doi.org/10.1055/s-0042-1756204.

60. Nowroozpoor A, Malekmohammad M, Seyyedi SR, Hashemian SM. Pulmonary hypertension in intensive care units: an updated review. Tanaffos. 2019;18(3):180–207.

61. Yuriditsky E, Horowitz JM. The physiology of cardiac tamponade and implications for patient management. J Crit Care. 2024;80:154512. https://doi.org/10.1016/j.jcrc.2023.154512.

62. McCanny P, Colreavy F. Echocardiographic approach to cardiac tamponade in critically ill patients. J Crit Care. 2017;39:271–7. https://doi.org/10.1016/j.jcrc.2016.12.008.

63. Thachuthara-George J. Pneumothorax in patients with respiratory failure in ICU. J Thorac Dis. 2021;13(8):5195–204. https://doi.org/10.21037/jtd-19-3752.

64. Doniger SJ, Ng N. Cardiac point-of-care ultrasound reveals unexpected, life-threatening findings in two children. Ultrasound J. 2020;12:4. https://doi.org/10.1186/s13089-020-0154-3.

65. Varpula M, Tallgren M, Saukkonen K, Voipio-Pulkki LM, Pettila V. Hemodynamic variables related to outcome in septic shock. Intensive Care Med. 2005;31(8):1066–71. https://doi.org/10.1007/s00134-005-2688-z.

66. Zhou HX, Yang CF, Wang HY, Teng Y, He HY. Should we initiate vasopressors earlier in patients with septic shock: a mini systemic review. World J Crit Care Med. 2023;12(4):204–16. https://doi.org/10.5492/wjccm.v12.i4.204.

Chapter 15
Cardiac Arrest

Alyson M. Esteves

15.1 Background

The incidence of adult in-hospital cardiac arrest (IHCA) is variable worldwide and likely influenced by many factors. Several countries maintain registries providing insight into the prevalence and outcomes associated with IHCA. IHCA incidence varies significantly across registries, with estimates of 1–17.5 IHCA per 1000 hospital admissions [1–4]. The American Heart Association (AHA) Get With The Guidelines® Resuscitation registry found the average annual incidence of adult IHCA in the United States to be ~292,000 and, when accounting for recurrent IHCA, ~357,900. It is worth noting that during the evaluated registry time period (2008–2017), there was a statistically significant increase in IHCA (incidence rate ratio, 1.03; 95% CI, 1.02–1.04; P = <0.001) [5]. More recent incidence data is limited, but trends are likely to continue increasing as the coronavirus disease 2019 (COVID-19) pandemic was associated with an increased incidence of IHCA [4].

Despite variable incidence, in comparison to out-of-hospital cardiac arrest (OHCA), IHCA has a more favorable survival to discharge rate (25.8 vs. 10.4%) and higher rates of good functional status (82 vs. 8.2%), albeit improvements in outcomes still exist and are continually emphasized through modifications to guideline recommendations [6]. COVID-19 data displayed worse morbidity and mortality outcomes associated with OHCA and IHCA; however, these trends are likely related to disease state-specific concerns, healthcare system strains, and other unmeasurable factors that will influence deviations from expected outcomes [4]. IHCA outcomes can be directly linked to early recognition and intervention, also referred to by the AHA as implementation of the Chain of Survival. The Chain of Survival for IHCA is broken down into six fundamental steps: early recognition and

A. M. Esteves (✉)
Dartmouth Hitchcock Medical Center, Lebanon, NH, USA
e-mail: alyson.m.esteves@hitchcock.org

Y. Alzaidi, M. A. Gebily (eds.), *The Pharmacist's Expanded Role in Critical Care Medicine*, https://doi.org/10.1007/978-3-031-77335-8_15

prevention, activation of emergency response, high-quality cardiopulmonary resuscitation (CPR), defibrillation, post-cardiac arrest care, and recovery [6]. Critical care pharmacists are effectively positioned to intervene in multiple phases during the Chain of Survival, which could directly improve IHCA patient outcomes.

15.2   Diagnosis

IHCA most commonly presents as a non-shockable rhythm, with the primary cause being a cardiac-inciting event [7]. Pharmacists should have a general understanding of cardiac rhythms that distinguish the AHA ACLS algorithms. These rhythms include asystole, pulseless electrical activity (PEA), ventricular fibrillation (VF), and pulseless ventricular tachycardia (pVT). Early identification of respiratory compromise, loss of pulse, and/or initial rhythm is pivotal in triaging an IHCA and deploying effective pharmacotherapy and defibrillation, as applicable. ACLS also includes noncardiac arrest algorithms; however, these will not be the focus of this chapter.

The primary causes of IHCA are either cardiac or respiratory in nature; however, there are numerous etiologies associated with cardiac arrest [7]. Reversible causes of cardiac arrest have been coined by the pneumonic "Hs and Ts." These causes include hypovolemia, hypoxia, hydrogen ion (acidosis), hypo/hyperkalemia, hypothermia, tension pneumothorax, cardiac tamponade, toxins, thrombosis pulmonary, and cardiac thrombosis [6]. A meta-analysis sought to confirm if this common pneumonic appropriately accounted for the most predominate underlying causes of IHCA. The most common causes of IHCA included hypoxia (26.46%), acute coronary syndrome (18.23%), arrhythmias (14.95%), hypovolemia (14.81%), infection (14.36%), and heart failure (12.64%). This study highlights the importance of considering a broader differential for IHCA causes beyond the common AHA-recognized etiologies [8].

15.3   Management

High-quality CPR is one of the most pivotal steps in the Chain of Survival and is essential regardless of the rhythm identified. CPR should be delivered at a rate of 100–120 compressions per minute, with a depth of 2 inches (5 cm), and allow for full chest recoil [6]. Compressors should be rotated every 2 min to align with rhythm checks to ensure that fatigue does not compromise compression quality [6]. Another key feature of high-quality CPR is the minimization of interruptions. Chest compression fraction (CCF) is a metric that has been derived to capture interruptions during ACLS. CCF is determined by the time spent providing active chest compressions divided by the total time of the code and represented as a percentage. The goal CCF according to the AHA is ≥60% [6]. Despite this value, CCF targets in clinical practice for IHCA are generally set at ≥80%. CCF targets have mostly been investigated in OHCA in mixed demographics of shockable and non-shockable rhythms. Outcome data has been mixed in publications; however, it is generally recognized that CCF remains an important target when determining high-quality CPR and has been linked to improving return of spontaneous circulation (ROSC) as well as survival in several studies [9–14]. IHCA code teams can improve CCF by ensuring that pauses for rhythm checks remain under 10 s, procedures are minimized that interrupt chest compressions, and, if applicable, the defibrillator is charging while compressions are ongoing [6].

After initiation of high-quality CPR, rhythm identification is the next essential step in IHCA management. The AHA provides a succinct algorithm outlining pathways for shockable (VF, pVT) and non-shockable (asystole/PEA) rhythms. Asystole is rapidly identifiable as a "flat line" on an electrocardiogram (ECG). In contrast, PEA is identifiable by an organized rhythm on the ECG, in the absence of a palpable pulse. VF (Fig. 15.1) is characterized by the absence of P waves, QRS complex, or T waves, in addition to varying amplitudes [15]. VT is a wide complex rhythm further classified into monomorphic VT or polymorphic VT. Monomorphic VT (Fig. 15.2) maintains relatively similar QRS complexes in comparison to polymorphic VT, which has variation in the QRS complex with each heartbeat [15]. An example of polymorphic VT is torsades de pointes. It is important for providers to quickly identify an initial rhythm, as early intervention has been linked to improvement in outcomes.

Non-shockable rhythms should have an emphasis on effective chest compressions and epinephrine administration. Epinephrine should be administered immediately after rhythm identification and then every 3–5 min for the duration of the code, despite changes in further rhythm development as the code progresses [6]. Epinephrine causes systemic vasoconstriction and provides additional increases in coronary perfusion pressure. Time to epinephrine administration is a pivotal

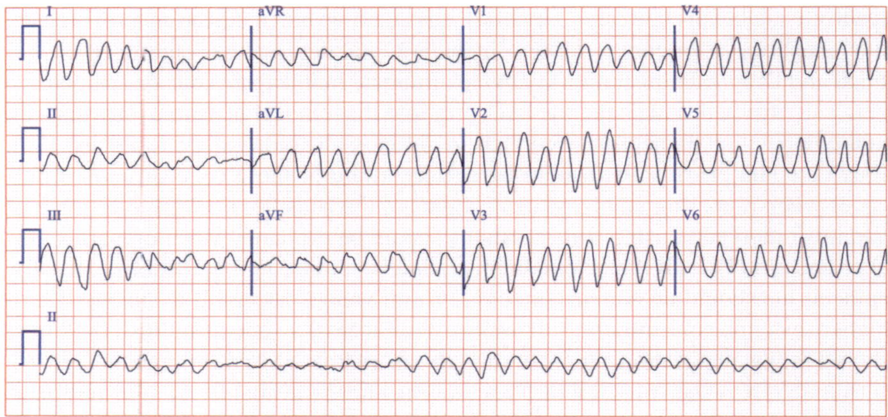

Fig. 15.1 An example of ventricular fibrillation cardiac arrest [15]

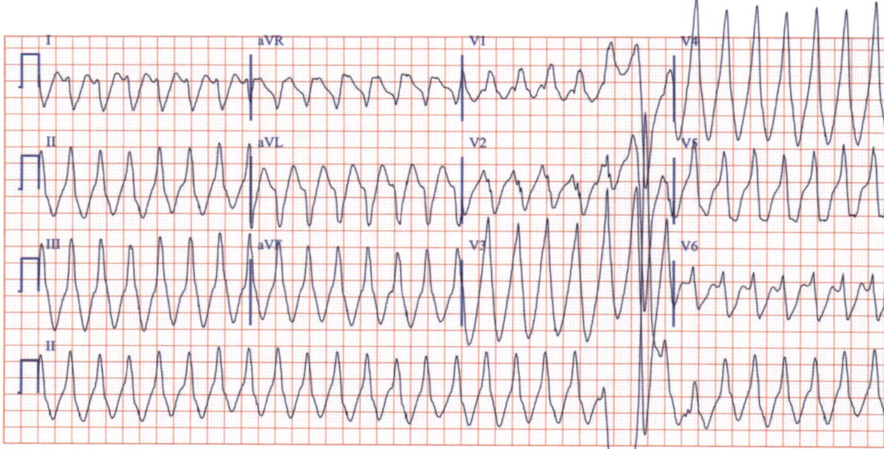

Fig. 15.2 Sustained monomorphic ventricular tachycardia [15]

intervention for an ICU pharmacist. Reductions in time to epinephrine administration in non-shockable rhythms have been linked to reduced time to ROSC, survival to hospital discharge, and improved neurologic outcomes [2, 15, 16]. Caution should be employed when evaluating epinephrine concentrations and dosages in the emergency setting, especially in light of medication and preparation shortages. Epinephrine should be administered via intravenous (IV) or intraosseous (IO) route of administration in a dose and concentration of 1 mg in 10 mL (0.1 mg/mL; 1:10,000). For ease of administration, prefilled luer-lock syringes are often available and should be the preferred stocked product to prevent medication safety errors from occurring. Epinephrine is also available in a 1 mg/mL concentration (1:1000) and must be diluted for administration in a code setting. This concentration is preferred for anaphylaxis emergencies or epinephrine infusion preparation and is often readily available in code carts. The ISMP has noted several medication errors related to epinephrine error concentrations, including fatalities, and has petitioned the US Food and Drug Administration (FDA) to eliminate ratio expressions of epinephrine [17, 18]. Over a decade later, the FDA required the removal of ratio expressions on non-combination epinephrine products to aid in medication safety awareness [19]. Providers and pharmacists should be acutely aware of these concentration differences when preparing emergent medications at the bedside. Furthermore, route of administration and dosing considerations should be evaluated when preparing epinephrine. The IV or IO route of administration is preferred for epinephrine. Ideally, epinephrine should be administered via central venous access, if available, due to higher systemic concentrations. Irrespective of access, an adequate flush (~10 mL) should follow medication administration to ensure full delivery through the line [6].

In rare IHCA scenarios, IV or IO access may not be available. Administration of epinephrine via an endotracheal tube (ETT) can be considered in these cases. Pharmacokinetics   and   pharmacodynamics   are   altered   via   this   route   of administration and have been linked to reduced serum concentrations, lower rates of ROSC, and reduced survival [6, 20]. The exact dose of ETT epinephrine is not known, but generally, it is recommended to administer 2–2.5 mg in 10 mL of normal saline [6, 20]. One important consideration to note is that chest compressions must be paused while ETT medications are being administered. Cessation of chest compressions is recommended to prevent aerosolization of the medication. After instillation, five manual ventilation breaths should be delivered to ensure disposition into the lung tissue to provide the most optimal chance at enhancing serum concentrations [21]. Given the importance of CCF as previously described, ETT administration of medications is likely more detrimental than beneficial, especially depending on initial rhythm identification (e.g., shockable rhythms).

In contrast to non-shockable rhythms, shockable rhythms rely on early defibrillation over medication administration. Understanding the importance and timing of defibrillation is essential to frame appropriate medication administration. Defibrillation quantity may vary per device; however, it is recommended to provide the maximum available dose, which is most commonly a monophasic defibrillation of 360 J [6]. Early defibrillation is a key step in the IHCA and OHCA chains of survival. Early defibrillation is defined as <3 min for IHCA [22]. Survival rates decrease rapidly when defibrillation is delayed, reducing to 50% after 5 min and <10% after 11 min [22]. Prior to defibrillation pad placement, pharmacists should recommend prompt removal of all transdermal medications in the locations of the pads. Patches may interfere with the efficacy of the delivered shock as well as cause burns [22].

Due to the essential role of defibrillation in terminating ventricular arrhythmias, medication administration is not considered until after the second defibrillation is delivered [6]. The first medication to be administered is epinephrine 1 mg in 10 mL IV (0.1 mg/mL; 1:10,000). Epinephrine should be administered every 3–5 min, and follow the same considerations described previously for non-shockable rhythms. It is essential to delay the initial administration of epinephrine. A prospective multi-center observational cohort study of IHCA evaluated the utilization of early epinephrine (within 2 min of the first defibrillation) vs. no epinephrine (>2 min or no administration) and associated outcomes. The cohort sizes were evenly divided, and the majority of patients in both arms received defibrillation <1 min after loss of pulse. Early epinephrine administration was found to reduce survival (OR 0.48, 95% CI 0.41–0.56; P = <0.001), reduce rates of ROSC (OR 0.55, 95% CI 0.46–0.95; P = <0.001), and reduce good functional outcome (OR 0.48, 95% CI 0.41–0.56; P = <0.001). It is unclear why early epinephrine administration was found to be harmful. Hypotheses include interference with other interventions, mechanisms of epinephrine in cardiac arrhythmias, and exposure to higher quantities of epinephrine throughout ACLS [23].

Antiarrhythmic therapy should be considered after the third unsuccessful defibrillation attempt. Antiarrhythmics alone do not have a role in successful conversion to a perfusing rhythm; however, they are considered to be an adjunct to defibrillation and may help in the reduction of recurrent arrhythmias [24]. Amiodarone has been a long-standing recommendation in the AHA guidelines for shock-refractory VF/

pVT. The first dose of amiodarone should be administered as an undiluted IV/IO bolus of 300 mg. A second dose of amiodarone may be administered if VF/pVT persists and should be administered as an undiluted IV/IO bolus of 150 mg. Limited data exists when considering the initiation of an amiodarone infusion in patients who achieve ROSC after amiodarone bolus administration. The AHA does not have any recommendations regarding amiodarone post-ROSC. A multicenter registry study evaluated amiodarone continuous infusions after ROSC in OHCA patients. Amiodarone was provided as a 1 mg/min continuous infusion for 6 h, followed by 0.5 mg/min for 18 h. The incidence of arrhythmia recurrence was 11.26% in the total cohort and 16.9% in the amiodarone cohort. After propensity matching, no difference was observed in arrhythmia recurrence reduction, survival to discharge, or neurologic recovery with the use of continuous infusion amiodarone [25]. Adverse effects of amiodarone infusions were not reported in this study but should be evaluated when considering initiation, most significantly hypotension and bradycardia in this patient population.

Lidocaine was a recent addition to the AHA ACLS algorithm for shockable rhythms. Lidocaine has been represented in prior iterations but was briefly removed. Lidocaine should be administered as an IV/IO bolos of 1–1.5 mg/kg followed by a second dose of 0.5–0.75 mg/kg if VF/pVT persists. Endotracheal administration of lidocaine can also be considered at 2–2.5 times the IV/IO dose. ETT administration considerations are the same as previously described for epinephrine. Literature surrounding the comparative efficacy of amiodarone vs. lidocaine is evolving and has mixed results. Lidocaine is efficacious and has benefits over placebo in refractory VF/pVT, specifically in ROSC achievement and survival to hospital arrival [26]. Two studies evaluating OHCA found no difference in mortality or neurologic outcomes with amiodarone vs. lidocaine [26, 27]. In contrast, a prospective interventional OHCA study found amiodarone to be associated with improved survival to hospital admission [28]. Furthermore, a Bayesian meta-analysis was conducted, which demonstrated that lidocaine may have superior survival to hospital discharge but no difference in survival to hospital admission, or ROSC [29]. The current AHA guidelines do not make a recommendation on which antiarrhythmic agent is preferred [6, 24]. Since the last guideline update in 2020, a retrospective cohort study evaluated IHCA amiodarone vs. lidocaine in refractory VF/pVT. This study showed that lidocaine was preferable to amiodarone and was associated with higher rates of ROSC, survival at various endpoints, and good neurologic outcome [30]. To date, the AHA has not made a statement on this data, but it suggests that lidocaine may be preferable in IHCA refractory VF/pVT. Initiation of lidocaine infusions post-ROSC is an additional area of controversy. A cohort study evaluated lidocaine-administered post-ROSC (dosing not specified) and found a reduction in VF/pVT recurrence but had no long-term outcome benefit [31]. The AHA states that there may be some consideration for utilization in patients where VF/pVT treatment may prove challenging, such as emergency medical service transport [24].

Adjunctive agents may play a role in ACLS management and are typically directed towards the correction of the inciting cardiac arrest etiology. In this chapter, we will cover the role of the most commonly used adjunctive agents in cardiac arrest. This list is not exhaustive, and additional adjuncts may be considered based on patient indication.

Magnesium sulfate is an adjunctive agent for patients experiencing polymorphic VT with a long QT interval (i.e., torsades de pointes) with or without hypomagnesemia [32]. In the setting of cardiac arrest, magnesium should be administered as an initial 2 g IV/IO bolus over 1–2 min [33]. Preparations of magnesium sulfate may vary. If using concentrated magnesium sulfate vials, doses should be diluted in 10 mL of dextrose 5% water [34]. Additional bolus doses should be considered until the cessation of torsades de pointes. Total dose recommendations vary, but 6 g is widely considered the maximum [34]. Serum magnesium levels are generally not followed in the cardiac arrest setting, but elevated serum concentrations (>3.5 mmol/L) may place patients at risk for toxicity [33]. After cessation of the inciting rhythm, magnesium and potassium should be replete appropriately to maintain normal serum levels. A medication administration record review should also be conducted by a pharmacist to ensure that the rhythm was not incited by a pharmacologic agent.

Hyperkalemia is a common etiology for cardiac arrest. Hyperkalemia can initially result in peaked T waves on an echocardiogram, progressing to loss of P waves, widening of the QRS complex, and ultimately resulting in asystole [35, 36]. A review of recent serum labs or labs available on an arterial blood gas should take place when considering the cause of the cardiac arrest. If hyperkalemia is present (>5.5 mEq/L), treatment should be initiated. Calcium should be immediately administered to stabilize the cardiac membrane and reduce the risk of ventricular fibrillation [35]. Calcium chloride 10% 1 g administered as an IV/IO bolus is the preferred modality. Calcium chloride is preferred as the elemental calcium content is approximately three times higher than calcium gluconate. If calcium chloride is unavailable, calcium gluconate can also be considered. Calcium gluconate 1–2 g IV/IO should be administered over 5–10 min [37]. Higher doses may be preferable due to the lower elemental calcium content. It is important to note that in the absence of a compelling indication (hyperkalemia or hypocalcemia), administration of calcium chloride had no benefit on ROSC achievement [38]. After administration of calcium, the focus should be on shifting potassium intracellularly. The most effective treatment modality is IV insulin. Insulin has a rapid onset of action (<15 min) and can reduce serum potassium by 0.6–1.2 mmol/L within 1 h [39, 40]. Insulin dosing strategies are variable. Historically, 10 units of regular insulin administered with 25 g of dextrose 50% (if serum blood glucose <250 mg/dL) was considered standard of care; however, this frequently resulted in hypoglycemic episodes, which have been correlated with increases in mortality [40]. Lower insulin dosing strategies have been evaluated to reduce the frequency of hypoglycemia. A single-center retrospective study evaluated 0.1 units/kg of insulin (maximum 10 units) in addition to dextrose administration. Rates of potassium reduction were similar (1.24 vs. 1.35 mmol/L) within 1 h, but hypoglycemic events were reduced (12 vs. 27%) [41]. A meta-analysis evaluated reduced insulin dosing strategies (5 units, 0.1 unit/kg, <10 units) in comparison to the standard 10 units for efficacy in potassium reduction and hypoglycemia rates. There was no difference seen in potassium reduction (mean difference −0.02 mmol/L, 95% CI, −0.11–0.07), but there was a reduction in hypoglycemia events (OR 0.55, 95% CI 0.43–0.69) and severe hypoglycemia (OR 0.41, 95% CI 0.27–0.64) [42]. A common prescribing/administration error with insulin for hyperkalemia is administration via the subcutaneous route. Insulin absorption and distribution are less predictable via this route and will impact the efficacy and rapid potassium reduction required for hyperkalemia correction. Lastly, potassium can be impacted by acidosis, causing more extracellular potassium to be present. In prolonged codes, acidosis is common. Sodium bicarbonate administration may be considered. It is estimated that potassium decreases by 0.3 mEq/L for every 0.1 unit increase in pH above normal [35]. Despite this knowledge, administration of sodium bicarbonate in this setting is controversial. Sodium bicarbonate administration resulting in hyperkalemia reduction has a long onset. The exact onset in the code setting is unknown. Furthermore, the most benefit in potassium reduction has been seen in patients with a pH <7.35, serum bicarbonate <17 mmol/L, serum potassium >6 mmol/L, and sodium bicarbonate doses >120 mEq [43]. The AHA only recommends sodium bicarbonate 50 mEq IV administered over 5 min, so the ultimate efficacy of this intervention remains unclear [35]. From an administration standpoint, pharmacists should avoid administration of sodium bicarbonate and calcium-containing products in the same line in the absence of significant flushing, as precipitation can occur [44].

Beyond hyperkalemia, administration of sodium bicarbonate is frequently considered and was recommended in prior AHA versions of the guidelines. The current AHA algorithm only recommends sodium bicarbonate in the setting of tricyclic antidepressant (TCA) overdoses [6]. Sodium bicarbonate provides a number of benefits in this overdose setting, which is beyond the scope of this chapter, but should be administered as an IV bolus of 8.4% 1–2 mEq/kg [45]. Sodium bicarbonate administration in the absence of hyperkalemia or overdose during cardiac arrest has not improved survival or neurologic outcomes as noted in numerous publications [46–48].

Although more prevalent in OHCA, opioid-induced/suspected cardiac arrest may prompt discussion of naloxone administration. One retrospective cohort study evaluated the use of naloxone in cardiac arrest patients with suspected opioid overdoses. Overall, the study size was small and lacked a comparator; however, it found that administration of naloxone had improved cardiac rhythms [49]. It is worth noting that the AHA comments that the cardiac rhythm improvement demonstrated in this study is not founded in enough data to support naloxone use during CPR [50]. With that being said, the AHA algorithm for opioid-associated emergencies for healthcare providers has a consideration for naloxone if administration will not impact other portions of ACLS [6]. Naloxone dosing in this setting is unclear but generally should be administered as an IV, IM, or subcutaneous bolus of 0.4–2 mg with the consideration for additional doses every 2–3 min [51]. Continuous infusions of naloxone are not likely to provide a clinical benefit in this setting but may play a role in post-resuscitative care to ensure that rebound hypoxia and somnolence do not occur in the setting of an opioid overdose. Pharmacists on the code team can help rule in or rule out the possibility of opioid-induced cardiac arrest based on patient presentation, urine drug screen evaluation, home medications, and/or inpatient medication administration. These data points can help supplement the discussion as to the value of naloxone in this clinical setting.

Thrombolytics may be used as adjunctive therapy in patients that have a suspected or confirmed pulmonary embolism (PE). The normal inciting rhythm during codes, secondary to massive pulmonary embolism, is PEA [6]. The AHA currently has a weak recommendation for the administration of thrombolytics in the setting of cardiac arrest secondary to a suspected/confirmed PE. Non-medication interventions also carry a weak recommendation [52]. Literature surrounding thrombolytic administration is limited, and many studies have conflicting results. To date, thrombolytics have not been found to favorably impact neurologic recovery or survival to hospital discharge [53–55]. There was some limited benefit seen in 30-day survival, ROSC achievement, and 24-h survival; however, conflicting studies exist for all of these outcomes [54–58]. Bleeding complications are more common in patients with thrombolysis; however, they were not found to be statistically significant, and administration is often a risk/benefit discussion [56]. Alteplase dosing is variable across literature and clinical practice for this indication. Described IV dosing regimens include 100 mg over 15 min, 50 mg over 2 min, divided bolus doses totaling 100 mg, or weight-based doses of 0.6–1 mg/kg (maximum 100 mg) [59]. Repeat doses up to 100 mg total are usually considered with lower initial bolus dosing strategies. A retrospective cohort review sought to characterize alteplase dosing and subsequent outcomes related to various dosing regimens. Alteplase 50 mg IV bolus was the most common dosing strategy. The review found that ROSC was associated with higher doses of alteplase (90.6 vs. 69.4 mg; $P = 0.03$) [59]. Tenecteplase may also be considered and may offer some advantages due to ease of admixture; however, dosing is more complex and weight based (Table 15.1) [60]. At this time, there are no head-to-head trials supporting the clinical safety and efficacy of one thrombolytic agent over another in this clinical setting.

Utilization of vasopressin, as an adjunctive agent or substitutive agent, has wavered in the AHA guidelines. Prior iterations of the guidelines recommended vasopressin 40 unit IV/IO bolus as a substitute for the first or second dose of epinephrine [61]. ETT administration can also be considered for vasopressin with previously described dosing considerations. Current iterations of the guidelines no longer recommend vasopressin as an alternative agent [6]. Vasopressin was removed from the guidelines due to lack of benefit in ROSC achievement, survival, or improvement in neurologic outcome [62]. One area of clinical controversy remains as to whether there is a benefit when vasopressin is combined with steroids and

Table 15.1 Tenecteplase dosing in pulmonary embolism [60]

Patient weight (kg)	Tenecteplase dose (mg)
<60	30
≥60 to <70	40
≥70 to <80	45
≥90	50

epinephrine. A number of trials have evaluated this combination of agents (vasopressin 20 units, methylprednisolone 40 mg, and epinephrine 1 mg) and have found benefit in ROSC achievement [63–65]. Data remains unclear of the benefit across shockable vs. non-shockable rhythms, survival to hospital discharge, long-term mortality outcomes, or improvement in neurologic function [63–65]. Due to the limited data with this combination, the AHA has not included this combination in the ACLS guideline [6]. It is important to note that no benefit has been seen with steroids alone in cardiac arrest [66, 67].

After ROSC attainment, pharmacists can play an additional role in the care provided. The AHA has an algorithm dedicated to post-resuscitative care, including airway management and corresponding respiratory goals, hemodynamic goals, pathways for consultative recommendations for targeted temperature management (TTM), or more in-depth cardiology workups [6]. The AHA recommends maintaining a systolic blood pressure >90 mmHg and a mean arterial pressure >65 mmHg, although exact clinical targets vary across ROSC trials [6]. In general, these hemodynamic parameters, or at minimum avoidance of hypotension, have been linked to improved neurologic recovery and reduced mortality [6, 68]. Pharmacists can aid in continuous infusion vasopressor initiation, agent selection, and titration, as appropriate, to meet these clinical targets. Appropriate agent selection should be based on patient-specific factors, including fluid responsiveness, underlying myocardial dysfunction, or need for inotropic support [69]. Agent consideration should include additional fluid support, norepinephrine, epinephrine, phenylephrine, dopamine, dobutamine, and/or milrinone. Furthermore, post-resuscitative sedation and analgesia should be evaluated. These considerations are also patient specific based on the timing of administration of paralytics for intubation, neurologic status after ROSC achievement, TTM and subsequent shivering considerations, presence of myoclonus, sources of pain including rib fractures, ventilator synchrony, and neuroprognostication concerns. According to the AHA, neuroprognostication should be in the setting of minimal sedation for a 72-h period [6]. Pharmacists can aid in agent selection and consideration of bolus vs. continuous infusion strategies for various agents. Additionally, pharmacists are poised to offer consultation on pharmacodynamics and pharmacokinetic considerations with various agents in the setting of subsequent hepatic failure, renal failure, or TTM initiation after ROSC.

15.4 Expanded Role of the Pharmacist

Critical care pharmacists are essential members of the code team. The role of the critical care pharmacist has evolved over time, and literature or survey responses can be found documenting pharmacist participation in virtually all primary code team roles. The Institute for Safe Medication Practices (ISMP) surveyed pharmacists regarding code response in 2022. At the time of the survey, 94% of respondents' organizations had pharmacists attending codes. Roles of pharmacists varied greatly in the survey and included medication preparation, medication consultation, chest compressions/ventilation, scribe, defibrillation, and intubation assistance [72]. Most commonly, pharmacists are positioned to run the code cart. Code cart leadership takes advantage of pharmacists' pharmacotherapy knowledge when considering various medication agents, timing, and determining anticipatory needs throughout the code. The ISMP survey was supported by a position paper on critical care pharmacy service offerings. The position paper has various levels of recommendations based on ICU structure (Table 15.2) for pharmacist participation in resuscitation events, attainment of the American Heart Association (AHA) Advanced Cardiac Life Support (ACLS) certification, and instructing ACLS courses [70, 71]. The position paper specifically emphasizes 24-h code coverage by a pharmacist [70]. It is important to note that this is an area of improvement for many institutions, as many survey respondents reported a lack of full-time coverage [72]. The position paper helps strengthen the role of the pharmacist as a leader in a code setting. Pharmacists are positioned as leaders in their ability to fill a number of code team roles, which is further strengthened by the "desirable" status for instructing ACLS courses [70].

Benefits of pharmacist presence at code events have been evaluated in a number of publications. Pharmacist presence and participation in various roles have been shown to contribute to ACLS guideline compliance [73–75]. Although guideline compliance does not have any specific long-term outcomes associated, it can be inferred that improvements in outcomes are likely made based upon the data supporting the series of proposed interventions. A retrospective review that demonstrated an improvement in guideline compliance also found an improvement in survival to hospital admission when emergency department (ED) pharmacists were included in code response. Although this survival trend did not persist to discharge, the preliminary influence supports that outcome improvements from pharmacist presence are likely [73]. Additionally, a Medicare database study found a significant reduction in mortality when pharmacists participated in cardiopulmonary resuscitation teams (12,880 reduced deaths, $P = 0.009$) [76]. Although not a correlator to patient outcomes but rather system improvements, pharmacist participation in code response has also been shown to reduce costs [73].

It is well established that emergency response scenarios are high-risk events and have an increased incidence of errors [77, 78]. The ISMP notes that the error incidence rate in code events is variable and has ranged from 1% to 15% in published literature [79]. A medication error database study highlighted that medication errors in this setting have a significantly higher likelihood of harm or death when compared to other medication error events [77]. Error types have been variable across

Table 15.2 Summary of critical care pharmacist roles by ICU level [70]

Role	ICU level 1*	ICU level 2*	ICU level 3*
Attendance at resuscitation events	Essential	Essential	Desirable
ACLS certification	Essential	Essential	Desirable
ACLS certification instructor	Desirable	Desirable	Desirable

*ICU levels are defined by critical care capabilities as outlined in prior publications [71]

studies and include incorrect medication selection, incorrect dose, improper preparation, and omissions [79]. The ISMP has recommended inclusion of pharmacists on code teams as a risk-reduction strategy to mitigate medication errors from occurring [79, 80].

Pharmacist training for code response is inconsistent across literature and survey results. One survey found that the most common training was basic life support (BLS) certification; however, comfort with code scenarios was correlated with BLS/ACLS certification and institution training programs [81]. The critical care position paper highlights the importance that pharmacists responding to codes should be ACLS certified [70]. Many of the fundamental pieces of ACLS go beyond traditional pharmacy didactic education, including ECG interpretation and other non-pharmacotherapy management portions of emergency resuscitation. A single-center review evaluated implementation of a pharmacist-centric code of blue education and found improvements in knowledge of various medication preparation questions, as well as perceived comfort. The training consisted of a 2-h didactic session, reference materials, and a hands-on skill portion [82]. Another single-center review evaluated training in addition to ACLS that focused on rhythm identification, ACLS pharmacology, and participation in multidisciplinary simulation ACLS scenarios. The addition of these supplemental experiences increased the confidence and comfort of the code responders [83].

References

1. Resuscitation Council UK [Internet]. [cited 2023 Jul 19]. Epidemiology of cardiac arrest Guidelines. https://www.resus.org.uk/library/2021-resuscitation-guidelines/epidemiology-cardiac-arrest-guidelines.
2. Perkins GD, Kenna C, Ji C, Deakin CD, Nolan JP, Quinn T, et al. The influence of time to adrenaline administration in the paramedic 2 randomised controlled trial. Intensive Care Med. 2020;46(3):426–36.
3. Shao F, Li CS, Liang LR, Qin J, Ding N, Fu Y, et al. Incidence and outcome of adult in-hospital cardiac arrest in Beijing, China. Resuscitation. 2016;102:51–6.
4. Bharmal M, DiGrande K, Patel A, Shavelle DM, Bosson N. Impact of coronavirus disease 2019 pandemic on cardiac arrest and emergency care. Cardiol Clin. 2022;40(3):355–64.
5. Holmberg MJ, Ross CE, Fitzmaurice GM, Chan PS, Duval-Arnould J, Grossestreuer AV, et al. Annual incidence of adult and pediatric in-hospital cardiac arrest in the United States. Circ Cardiovasc Qual Outcomes. 2019;12(7):e005580.
6. Panchal AR, Bartos JA, Cabañas JG, Donnino MW, Drennan IR, Hirsch KG, et al. Part 3: adult basic and advanced life support: 2020 American heart association guidelines for cardiopulmonary resuscitation and emergency cardiovascular care. Circulation. 2020;142(16_suppl_2):S366–468. https://doi.org/10.1161/CIR.0000000000000916.
7. Andersen LW, Holmberg MJ, Berg KM, Donnino MW, Granfeldt A. In-hospital cardiac arrest. JAMA. 2019;321(12):1200–10.
8. Allencherril J, Lee PYK, Khan K, Loya A, Pally A. Etiologies of in-hospital cardiac arrest: a systematic review and meta-analysis. Resuscitation. 2022;175:88–95.
9. Vaillancourt C, Petersen A, Meier EN, Christenson J, Menegazzi JJ, Aufderheide TP, et al. The impact of increased chest compression fraction on survival for out-of-hospital cardiac arrest patients with a non-shockable initial rhythm. Resuscitation. 2020;154:93–100.

10. Christenson J, Andrusiek D, Everson-Stewart S, Kudenchuk P, Hostler D, Powell J, et al. Chest compression fraction determines survival in patients with out-of-hospital ventricular fibrillation. Circulation. 2009;120(13):1241–7.
11. Vaillancourt C, Everson-Stewart S, Christenson J, Andrusiek D, Powell J, Nichol G, et al. The impact of increased chest compression fraction on return of spontaneous circulation for out-of-hospital cardiac arrest patients not in ventricular fibrillation. Resuscitation. 2011;82(12):1501–7.
12. Wik L, Olsen JA, Persse D, Sterz F, Lozano M, Brouwer MA, et al. Why do some studies find that CPR fraction is not a predictor of survival? Resuscitation. 2016;104:59–62.
13. Maddani S, Chaudhuri S, Krishna H, Rao S, Unnithan N, Ravindranath S. Evaluation of the quality of cardiopulmonary resuscitation provided by the emergency response team at a tertiary care hospital. Indian J Anaesth. 2022;66(2):126.
14. Vestergaard LD, Lauridsen KG, Krarup NHV, Kristensen JU, Andersen LK, Løfgren B. Quality of cardiopulmonary resuscitation and 5-year survival following in-hospital cardiac arrest. Open Access Emerg Med. 2021;13:553–60.
15. Nathanson LA, McClennen S, Safran C, Goldberger A. ECG Wave-Maven: Self-Assessment Program for Students and Clinicians [Internet]. [cited 2023 Oct 9]. http://ecg.bidmc.harvard.edu.
16. Hansen M, Schmicker RH, Newgard CD, Grunau B, Scheuermeyer F, Cheskes S, et al. Time to epinephrine administration and survival from nonshockable out-of-hospital cardiac arrest among children and adults. Circulation. 2018;137(19):2032–40.
17. Okubo M, Komukai S, Callaway CW, Izawa J. Association of timing of epinephrine administration with outcomes in adults with out-of-hospital cardiac arrest. JAMA Netw Open. 2021;4(8):e2120176.
18. Barnstein C. Institute for Safe Medication Practices. Petition for changes in labeling of epinephrine injection. 2004 [cited 2023 Sep 1]. https://www.ismp.org/sites/default/files/attachments/2018-04/USP%20Petition%20for%20Epinephrine%20labeling.pdf.
19. Institute for Safe Medication Practices [Internet]. It doesn't pay to play the percentages. 2002 [Cited 2023 Aug 25]. https://www.ismp.org/resources/it-doesnt-pay-play-percentages.
20. U.S. Food & Drug Administration [Internet]. Single entity injectable drug products. 2017. https://www.fda.gov/drugs/information-drug-class/single-entity-injectable-drug-products.
21. Niemann JT, Stratton SJ, Cruz B, Lewis RJ. Endotracheal drug administration during out-of-hospital resuscitation: where are the survivors? Resuscitation. 2002;53(2):153–7.
22. Easley RB, Schleien CL, Shaffner DH. Chapter 33—Pediatric cardiopulmonary resuscitation. In: Motoyama EK, Davis PJ, editors. Smith's anesthesia for infants and children. 7th ed. Philadelphia, PA: Mosby; 2006. p. 1110–54. https://www.sciencedirect.com/science/article/pii/B9780323026475500382.
23. Part 4: the automated external defibrillator: key Link in the chain of survival. Circulation. 2000;102(suppl_1) https://doi.org/10.1161/circ.102.suppl_1.I-60.
24. Andersen LW, Kurth T, Chase M, Berg KM, Cocchi MN, Callaway C, et al. Early administration of epinephrine (adrenaline) in patients with cardiac arrest with initial shockable rhythm in hospital: propensity score matched analysis. BMJ. 2016;353:i1577.
25. Panchal AR, Berg KM, Kudenchuk PJ, Del Rios M, Hirsch KG, Link MS, et al. 2018 American heart association focused update on advanced cardiovascular life support use of antiarrhythmic drugs during and immediately after cardiac arrest: an update to the American heart association guidelines for cardiopulmonary resuscitation and emergency cardiovascular care. Circulation. 2018;138(23). https://doi.org/10.1161/CIR.0000000000000613
26. Lee BK, Youn CS, Kim YJ, Ryoo SM, Lim KS, Nam GB, et al. Effect of prophylactic amiodarone infusion on the recurrence of ventricular arrhythmias in out-of-hospital cardiac arrest survivors: a propensity-matched analysis. J Clin Med. 2019;8(2):244.
27. Kudenchak PJ, Brown SP, Daya M, Rea T, Nichol G, Morrison LJ, et al. Amiodarone, lidocaine, or placebo in out-of-hospital cardiac arrest. N Engl J Med. 2016;374(18):1711–22.

28. Kishihara Y, Kashiura M, Amagasa S, Fukushima F, Yasuda H, Moriya T. Comparison of the effects of lidocaine and amiodarone for out-of-hospital cardiac arrest patients with shockable rhythms: a retrospective observational study from a multicenter registry. BMC Cardiovasc Disord. 2022;22(1):466.
29. Dorian P, Cass D, Schwartz B, Cooper R, Gelaznikas R, Barr A. Amiodarone as compared with lidocaine for shock-resistant ventricular fibrillation. N Engl J Med. 2002;346(12):884–90.
30. Khan SU, Winnicka L, Saleem MA, Rahman H, Rehman N. Amiodarone, lidocaine, magnesium or placebo in shock refractory ventricular arrhythmia: a Bayesian network meta-analysis. Heart Lung J Crit Care. 2017;46(6):417–24.
31. Wagner D, Kronick SL, Nawer H, Cranford JA, Bradley SM, Neumar RW. Comparative effectiveness of amiodarone and lidocaine for the treatment of in-hospital cardiac arrest. Chest. 2023;163(5):1109–19.
32. Kudenchuk PJ, Newell C, White L, Fahrenbruch C, Rea T, Eisenberg M. Prophylactic lidocaine for post resuscitation care of patients with out-of-hospital ventricular fibrillation cardiac arrest. Resuscitation. 2013;84(11):1512–8.
33. Zeppenfeld K, Tfelt-Hansen J, De Riva M, Winkel BG, Behr ER, Blom NA, et al. 2022 ESC guidelines for the management of patients with ventricular arrhythmias and the prevention of sudden cardiac death. Eur Heart J. 2022;43(40):3997–4126.
34. Thomas SHL, Behr ER. Pharmacological treatment of acquired QT prolongation and torsades de pointes: treatment of torsades de pointes. Br J Clin Pharmacol. 2016;81(3):420–7.
35. Magnesium Sulfate [Internet]. [cited 2023 Oct 9]. http://online.lexi.com.
36. Part 8: advanced challenges in resuscitation: section 1: life-threatening electrolyte abnormalities. Circulation. 2000;102(suppl_1):253–9. https://doi.org/10.1161/circ.102.suppl_1.I-217.
37. Simon LV, Hashmi MF, Farrell MW. Hyperkalemia. In: StatPearls [Internet]. Treasure Island, FL: StatPearls Publishing; 2023. [cited 2023 Aug 25]. http://www.ncbi.nlm.nih.gov/books/NBK470284/.
38. Calcium Gluconate [Internet]. [cited 2023 Oct 9]. http://online.lexi.com.
39. Vallentin MF, Granfeldt A, Meilandt C, Povlsen AL, Sindberg B, Holmberg MJ, et al. Effect of intravenous or intraosseous calcium vs saline on return of spontaneous circulation in adults with out-of-hospital cardiac arrest: a randomized clinical trial. JAMA. 2021;326(22):2268–76.
40. Weisberg LS. Management of severe hyperkalemia. Crit Care Med. 2008;36(12):3246.
41. Long B, Warix JR, Koyfman A. Controversies in management of hyperkalemia. J Emerg Med. 2018;55(2):192–205.
42. Wheeler DT, Schafers SJ, Horwedel TA, Deal EN, Tobin GS. Weight-based insulin dosing for acute hyperkalemia results in less hypoglycemia. J Hosp Med. 2016;11(5):355–7.
43. Moussavi K, Garcia J, Tellez-Corrales E, Fitter S. Reduced alternative insulin dosing in hyperkalemia: a meta-analysis of effects on hypoglycemia and potassium reduction. Pharmacother J Hum Pharmacol Drug Ther. 2021;41(7):598–607.
44. Abuelo JG. Treatment of severe hyperkalemia: confronting 4 fallacies. Kidney Int Rep. 2018;3(1):47–55.
45. Lexicomp Online [Internet]. [cited 2023 Oct 9]. Trissel's IV compatibility. https://online.lexi.com/lco/action/ivcompatibility/trissels.
46. Mirrakhimov AE, Ayach T, Barbaryan A, Talari G, Chadha R, Gray A. The role of sodium bicarbonate in the management of some toxic ingestions. Int J Nephrol. 2017;2017:1–8.
47. Ahn S, Kim YJ, Sohn CH, Seo DW, Lim KS, Donnino MW, et al. Sodium bicarbonate on severe metabolic acidosis during prolonged cardiopulmonary resuscitation: a double-blind, randomized, placebo-controlled pilot study. J Thorac Dis. 2018;10(4):2295–302.
48. Kawano T, Grunau B, Scheuermeyer FX, Gibo K, Dick W, Fordyce CB, et al. Prehospital sodium bicarbonate use could worsen long term survival with favorable neurological recovery among patients with out-of-hospital cardiac arrest. Resuscitation. 2017;119:63–9.
49. Vukmir RB, Katz L. Sodium bicarbonate improves outcome in prolonged prehospital cardiac arrest. Am J Emerg Med. 2006;24(2):156–61.

50. Saybolt MD, Alter SM, Dos Santos F, Calello DP, Rynn KO, Nelson DA, et al. Naloxone in cardiac arrest with suspected opioid overdoses. Resuscitation. 2010;81(1):42–6.
51. Dezfulian C, Orkin A, Maron B, Elmer J. Opioid-associated out-of-hospital cardiac arrest: distinctive clinical features and implications for health care and public responses: a scientific statement from the American heart association. Circulation. 2021;143(16):e836–70.
52. Naloxone [Internet]. [cited 2023 Oct 9]. http://online.lexi.com.
53. Berg KM, Soar J, Andersen LW, Böttiger BW, Cacciola S, Callaway CW, et al. Adult advanced life support: 2020 international consensus on cardiopulmonary resuscitation and emergency cardiovascular care science with treatment recommendations. Circulation. 2020;142(16_suppl_1):S92–S139. https://doi.org/10.1161/CIR.0000000000000893.
54. Böttiger BW, Arntz HR, Chamberlain DA, Bluhmki E, Belmans A, Danays T, et al. Thrombolysis during resuscitation for out-of-hospital cardiac arrest. N Engl J Med. 2008;359(25):2651–62.
55. Javaudin F, Lascarrou JB, Le Bastard Q, Bourry Q, Latour C, De Carvalho H, et al. Thrombolysis during resuscitation for out-of-hospital cardiac arrest caused by pulmonary embolism increases 30-day survival. Chest. 2019;156(6):1167–75.
56. Alshaya OA, Alshaya AI, Badreldin HA, Albalawi ST, Alghonaim ST, Al Yami MS. Thrombolytic therapy in cardiac arrest caused by cardiac etiologies or presumed pulmonary embolism: an updated systematic review and meta-analysis. Res Pract Thromb Haemost. 2022;6(4):e12745.
57. Janata K, Holzer M, Kürkciyan I, Losert H, Riedmüller E, Pikula B, et al. Major bleeding complications in cardiopulmonary resuscitation: the place of thrombolytic therapy in cardiac arrest due to massive pulmonary embolism. Resuscitation. 2003;57(1):49–55.
58. Sharifi M, Berger J, Beeston P, Bay C, Vajo Z, Javadpoor S. Pulseless electrical activity in pulmonary embolism treated with thrombolysis (from the "PEAPETT" study). Am J Emerg Med. 2016;34(10):1963–7.
59. De Paz D, Diez J, Ariza F, Scarpetta DF, Quintero JA, Carvajal SM. Emergency thrombolysis during cardiac arrest due to pulmonary thromboembolism: our experience over 6 years. Open Access Emerg Med. 2021;13:67–73.
60. Peppard SR, Parks AM, Zimmerman J. Characterization of alteplase therapy for presumed or confirmed pulmonary embolism during cardiac arrest. Am J Health Syst Pharm. 2018;75(12):870–5.
61. Tenecteplase [Internet]. [cited 2023 Oct 9]. http://online.lexi.com.
62. Neumar RW, Otto CW, Link MS, Kronick SL, Shuster M, Callaway CW, et al. Part 8: adult advanced cardiovascular life support: 2010 American heart association guidelines for cardiopulmonary resuscitation and emergency cardiovascular care. Circulation. 2010;122(18_suppl_3):S729–67. https://doi.org/10.1161/CIRCULATIONAHA.110.970988.
63. Yan W, Dong W, Song X, Zhou W, Chen Z. Therapeutic effects of vasopressin on cardiac arrest: a systematic review and meta-analysis. BMJ Open. 2023;13(4):e065061.
64. Mentzelopoulos SD, Zakynthinos SG, Tzoufi M, Katsios N, Papastylianou A, Gkisioti S, et al. Vasopressin, epinephrine, and corticosteroids for in-hospital cardiac arrest. Arch Intern Med. 2009;169(1):15–24.
65. Mentzelopoulos SD, Malachias S, Chamos C, Konstantopoulos D, Ntaidou T, Papastylianou A, et al. Vasopressin, steroids, and epinephrine and neurologically favorable survival after in-hospital cardiac arrest: a randomized clinical trial. JAMA. 2013;310(3):270–9.
66. Andersen LW, Isbye D, Kjærgaard J, Kristensen CM, Darling S, Zwisler ST, et al. Effect of vasopressin and methylprednisolone vs placebo on return of spontaneous circulation in patients with in-hospital cardiac arrest: a randomized clinical trial. JAMA. 2021;326(16):1586–94.
67. Shah K, Mitra AR. Use of corticosteroids in cardiac arrest-a systematic review and meta-analysis. Crit Care Med. 2021;49(6):e642–50.
68. Donnino MW, Andersen LW, Berg KM, Chase M, Sherwin R, Smithline H, et al. Corticosteroid therapy in refractory shock following cardiac arrest: a randomized, double-blind, placebo-controlled, trial. Crit Care Lond Engl. 2016;20:82.

69. Callaway CW, Donnino MW, Fink EL, Geocadin RG, Golan E, Kern KB, et al. Part 8: post–cardiac arrest care: 2015 American heart association guidelines update for cardiopulmonary resuscitation and emergency cardiovascular care. Circulation. 2015;132(18_suppl_2):S465–82. https://doi.org/10.1161/CIR.0000000000000262.

70. Jozwiak M, Bougouin W, Geri G, Grimaldi D, Cariou A. Post-resuscitation shock: recent advances in pathophysiology and treatment. Ann Intensive Care. 2020;10:170.

71. Institute for Safe Medication Practices [Internet]. Survey results from pharmacists provide support to enhance the organizational response to codes. 2022. https://www.ismp.org/resources/survey-results-pharmacists-provide-support-enhance-organizational-response-codes.

72. Lat I, Paciullo C, Daley MJ, MacLaren R, Bolesta S, McCann J, et al. Position paper on critical care pharmacy services (executive summary): 2020 update. Am J Health Syst Pharm. 2020;77(19):1619–24.

73. Haupt MT, Bekes CE, Brilli RJ, Carl LC, Gray AW, Jastremski MS, et al. Guidelines on critical care services and personnel: recommendations based on a system of categorization of three levels of care*. Crit Care Med. 2003;31(11):2677.

74. McAllister MW, Chestnutt JG. Improved outcomes and cost savings associated with pharmacist presence in the emergency department. Hosp Pharm. 2017;52(6):433–7.

75. Draper HM, Eppert JA. Association of pharmacist presence on compliance with advanced cardiac life support guidelines during in-hospital cardiac arrest. Ann Pharmacother. 2008;42(4):469–74.

76. Heavner MS, Rouse GE, Lemieux SM, Owusu KA, Pritchard D, Yazdi M, et al. Experience with integrating pharmacist documenters on cardiac arrest teams to improve quality. J Am Pharm Assoc. 2018;58(3):311–7.

77. Bond CA, Raehl CL. Clinical pharmacy services, pharmacy staffing, and hospital mortality rates. Pharmacotherapy. 2007;27(4):481–93.

78. Lipshutz AKM, Morlock LL, Shore AD, Hicks RW, Dy SM, Pronovost PJ, et al. Medication errors associated with code situations in U.S. hospitals: direct and collateral damage. Jt Comm J Qual Patient Saf. 2008;34(1):46–56.

79. Gokhman R, Seybert AL, Phrampus P, Darby J, Kane-Gill SL. Medication errors during medical emergencies in a large, tertiary care, academic medical center. Resuscitation. 2012;83(4):482–7.

80. Institute for Safe Medication Practices [Internet]. Preventing medication errors during codes. 2011. https://www.ismp.org/resources/preventing-medication-errors-during-codes.

81. Institute for Safe Medication Practices [Internet]. EPINEPHrine pre-filled syringe shortage. 2010. https://www.ismp.org/alerts/epinephrine-pre-filled-syringe-shortage.

82. Machado C, Barlows TG, Marsh WA, Coto-Depani Y, Dalin G. Pharmacists on the emergency cardiopulmonary resuscitation team: their responsibilities, training, and attitudes. Hosp Pharm. 2003;38(1):40–9.

83. Marlowe KF, Woods DD. Evaluating a training program for pharmacist code blue response. Hosp Pharm. 2005;40(1):49–54.

84. Bartel BJ. Impact of high-fidelity simulation and pharmacist-specific didactic lectures in addition to ACLS provider certification on pharmacy resident ACLS performance. J Pharm Pract. 2014;27(4):412–5.

Part IV
Neurocritical Care

Chapter 16
Traumatic Brain Injury

Lesly V. Jurado Hernández and Teresa A. Allison

16.1 Introduction

Traumatic brain injury (TBI) causes substantial challenges for public health systems, leading to long-term economic burdens to patients and health systems [1]. Globally, in 2019, there were 27.16 million new TBI cases [2]. These numbers are significantly underestimated, as they do not take into account TBIs treated in emergency departments and primary care or those that go untreated.

In addition to the acute care requirements, these patients often need long-term care and extensive rehabilitation. Many patients are young when injured and otherwise in good health; they can live for decades even if severely injured. It is thought that up to 15% of patients with even a "mild TBI" will experience a post-concussion syndrome (PCS), which consists of physical (fatigue, headaches), cognitive (difficulties with concentration and memory), and emotional (irritability, anxiety, depression) symptoms [3]. It can lead to disturbances in personal relationships as well as the ability to return to school or work weeks to months after injury [4]. The literature on PCS is limited due to difficulty studying this population. Symptoms are not specific to PCS and may overlap with other conditions. Additionally, it is questioned whether persistent symptoms are driven by neurological and/or other psychological factors and how premorbid conditions may influence these symptoms. The severity of PCS depends on many factors including the severity of TBI, multiple TBIs (as in contact sports),

L. V. Jurado Hernández
Department of Pharmacy, Novant Health New Hanover Regional Medical Center Wilmington, NC, USA

T. A. Allison (✉)
Department of Pharmacy, Memorial Hermann—Texas Medical Center, Houston, TX, USA
e-mail: Teresa.Allison@memorialhermann.org

Y. Alzaidi, M. A. Gebily (eds.), *The Pharmacist's Expanded Role in Critical Care Medicine*, https://doi.org/10.1007/978-3-031-77335-8_16

as well as neurological and psychological factors. Patients with moderate-to-severe TBI have been shown to be twice as likely to die as similar non-brain-injured people; their life expectancy is reduced by 7 years [5].

16.2 Classification of TBI

Traumatic brain injury can be described based on several different criteria. Injuries are classified as primary or secondary. The primary injury is the event causing the damage. It is immediate and not modifiable by treatment. Secondary injuries begin quickly after the primary injury and are thought to cause the majority of complications following a TBI. There are many causes of secondary injuries, with hypoxia ($PaO_2 < 60$ mmHg) and hypotension (SBP < 95 mmHg) considered to be the leading contributing factors. One incident of either hypoxia or hypotension has been shown to nearly double the mortality in severe TBI [6, 7].

There are two classical types of head injury: closed head injury (CHI) or penetrating TBI. CHI (also known as non-penetrating injury or blunt TBI) is caused by an external force strong enough to move the brain in the skull. This can be caused by falls, motor vehicle accidents, sports injuries, being struck with an object, or a blast injury. Penetrating TBI is caused when an object pierces the skull and enters the brain.

Traumatic brain injury can be classified based on the effects on the brain. Focal injuries occur at the site of the impact. The neurological deficits are predominantly confined to this area. Diffuse axonal injury is the shearing of axons in cerebral white matter, which leads to widespread damage. Hematomas are bleeds caused by a ruptured blood vessel and are further described based on the location of the hemorrhage. Intracerebral hemorrhage is when bleeding occurs into the brain tissue. Epidural hematomas occur in the area between the skull and the dura mater, the top layer of the meninges. Subdural hematomas occur in the area between the dura mater and arachnoid mater. Subarachnoid hemorrhages (SAHs) occur in the area between the arachnoid mater and pia mater. Traumatic SAHs are treated as a TBI per TBI guidelines, while aneurysmal SAH is considered a subset of stroke and is treated according to aneurysmal SAH guidelines [8]. Further discussion of aneurysmal SAH is outside the scope of this chapter. Contusions are a bruising or swelling when very small blood vessels bleed into the brain. Contusions are further classified as coup and contrecoup injuries. A coup injury occurs directly under the impact site, while the contrecoup injury occurs on the opposite side of the impact. Coup and contrecoup injuries often happen when the brain is bounced back and forth within the skull, such as in high-speed motor vehicle collisions or in shaken baby syndrome. Concussions are considered a mild TBI and a temporary injury. However, it can take the brain months to heal.

Traumatic brain injury is classified based on the severity of injury as mild, moderate, or severe. Table 16.1 describes the severity of injury.

Table 16.1 Classification of severity of traumatic brain injury [9, 10]

	Mild	Moderate	Severe
GCS	13–15	9–12	3–8
Loss of consciousness	<30 min	30 min–24 h	>24 h
Post-traumatic amnesia	0–1 days	>1–7 days	>7 days
Structural imaging	Normal	Normal or abnormal	Normal or abnormal
Interventions	No	Imaging and monitoring, possible treatment	Imaging, monitoring, and treatment

GCS Glasgow Coma Scale

16.3 Hemodynamics

The skull is a rigid compartment comprised of brain matter, blood, and cerebrospinal fluid (CSF). The Monro-Kellie hypothesis states that the sum of the volumes of brain tissue, intracranial blood, and CSF is constant. An increase in the volume of one component should cause a proportional decrease in one or both remaining components, or it will result in an increase in intracranial pressure (ICP) [11]. Intracranial blood (primarily venous) and CSF are the two components where the volume can adapt most easily to accommodate an increase in volume of intracranial contents. Once these compensatory mechanisms are exhausted, volume increases in any of the three components (e.g., hematoma, cerebral edema, space-occupying lesions, hemorrhage) will lead to increases in pressure, resulting in elevated ICP [11].

Intracranial pressure is the pressure within the cranial vault; the relationship between volume and pressure within the cranium is nonlinear. Cerebral perfusion pressure (CPP) is the mean arterial pressure (MAP) minus ICP and is used as a surrogate for cerebral blood flow (CBF). Mathematically, this is shown as CPP = MAP—ICP. Normally, CBF is maintained constant over a CPP range by cerebral autoregulation. Once autoregulation is impaired, changes in MAP or ICP can have direct effects on CBF [11].

The Brain Trauma Foundation Guidelines for the Management of Severe Traumatic Brain Injury fourth Edition (BTF Guidelines) recommend a CPP target between 60 and 70 mm Hg and ICP below 22 mm Hg, which has demonstrated to reduce 2-week mortality in traumatic brain injury [12, 13]. The goals of ICP management are to preserve adequate brain oxygen delivery, avoid secondary injury, and prevent herniation. Brain herniation syndrome results in an extreme elevation of ICP accompanied by Cushing's triad consisting of irregular respirations, bradycardia, and hypertension, followed by normalization of ICP [11]. Elevated ICP and cerebral herniation are life-threatening neurologic emergencies. Intracranial hypertension is defined as a sustained (>5 min) elevation of ICP to >22 mm Hg [13]. Additionally, the systolic blood pressure goal is >100 mm Hg for patients aged 50–69 years and >110 mm Hg for patients aged 15–49 and >70 years [13].

16.4   Neurological Evaluation and Imaging

Admission to a neurologic intensive care unit is associated with reduced morbidity and mortality in patients with TBI [14, 15]. After initial assessment in the emergency room, patients with severe TBI should be admitted to the ICU, a specialized neuro ICU if one is present. However, utilization of other services may be required depending on the extent of injuries.

In the acute phase of ICU management, hemodynamic and neurological assessments are performed on TBI patients every hour. As the patient's condition stabilizes, neurological assessment periods may be extended. Neurological evaluations are most commonly performed with a Glasgow Coma Scale (GCS), which objectively describes the extent of impaired consciousness [16]. The scale assesses three components of responsiveness, including eye-opening, verbal, and motor responses. The total score is a sum of each of these three components; see Table 16.2. A patient who is completely awake and intact will receive a score of 15, while patients in a coma will have a score of 8 or less. A completely unresponsive patient will receive a score of 3, which is the lowest possible score.

Neuroimaging with a non-contrast-enhanced computed tomography (CT) scan should be performed immediately in the emergency department in order to determine if neurosurgical interventions are possible [9]. If the injury is amenable to surgery, the patient should be taken to the operating room (OR) immediately. If the injury is not amenable to surgery, the patient should be taken immediately to the ICU.

The BTF Guidelines recommend monitoring ICP in all salvageable patients with a severe TBI and an abnormal CT scan with either hematomas, contusions, swelling, herniation, or compressed basal cisterns [13]. ICP monitoring is indicated in patients with severe TBI with a normal CT scan if two or more of the following features are noted at admission: age >40 years, unilateral or bilateral motor

Table 16.2 Glasgow Coma Scale [16]

	Response	Score
Eye opening	Spontaneous	4
	To speech	3
	To pain	2
	No response	1
Best verbal response	Oriented to person, place, and time	5
	Confused	4
	Inappropriate words	3
	Incomprehensible sounds	2
	No response	1
Best motor response	Obeys commands	6
	Moves to localized pain	5
	Flexion withdrawal from pain	4
	Abnormal flexion (decorticate)	3
	Abnormal extension (decerebrate)	2
	No response	1

posturing, or an SBP <90 mmHg. Typically, ICP and MAP are monitored, and CPP is calculated hourly in patients with an ICP monitor. There are two basic types of ICP monitors. The external ventricular drainage catheter is placed inside a ventricle; it can measure ICP and drain CSF. The ICP monitor known as a "bolt" is placed in the subarachnoid space, epidural space, or parenchyma. The bolt is only able to monitor the ICP.

Advanced cerebral monitoring techniques for blood flow and oxygen include transcranial Doppler (TCD)/duplex sonography, differences between arterial and arterio-jugular venous oxygen ($AVDO_2$), and measurements of local tissue oxygen. Arterio-jugular $AVDO_2$ globally measures cerebral oxygen extraction. Microdialysis measures brain metabolism, and electrocorticography determines cortical spreading depression. Currently, use of these monitoring techniques in clinical practice is limited due to insufficient evidence demonstrating a benefit as well as questions regarding how to use the data provided by these advanced cerebral monitors.

16.5 Pharmacological Management

Pharmacological management can be divided into management of CPP, management of ICP, and adjunct therapies. Management of CPP entails maintaining a MAP to balance the ICP. MAP is increased with fluids, blood products, and vasopressors. ICP is managed with pharmacological agents including hyperosmolar therapy, sedation and analgesia, and anesthetics. Nonpharmacological methods include decompressive craniectomy, prophylactic hypothermia, cerebrospinal fluid drainage, and ventilation strategies. Because fluids and vasopressors are covered elsewhere, the focus of this chapter will be the management of ICP.

16.5.1 Hyperosmolar Therapy

The administration of hyperosmolar agents is one of the principal strategies in treating cerebral edema and lowering elevated ICP. Hyperosmolar therapy primarily consists of mannitol and hypertonic saline (HTS). Current literature suggests that both agents are effective for managing acute intracranial hypertension in the setting of TBI; however, Class I evidence for this therapy is meager, and most evidence is derived from retrospective analyses or case series [13]. See Table 16.3 for comparisons of the two agents. The optimal agent, method of administration, and precise mechanism of action for this class continue to be examined.

Hyperosmolar agents have two main mechanisms of action. An immediate ICP reduction is observed through changes in blood fluid dynamics or rheology. The mechanisms underlying these rheological modifications include lowering of blood viscosity and increasing MAP, which lead to reduced cerebral blood volume and a compensatory cerebral vasoconstriction [17, 18]. Additionally,

Table 16.3 Comparison of mannitol and hypertonic saline [18, 20, 22, 23, 26, 27, 33, 37, 43, 46, 48–51, 55, 56]

	Mannitol	Hypertonic saline
Mechanism of action	Decreases blood viscosity and improves microcirculatory blood flow	Decreases blood viscosity and improves microcirculatory blood flow
Additional proposed benefits	Free radical scavenger and inhibits programed cell death	Anti-inflammatory processes
Onset of action	20 min	20 min
Duration of effect	90 min to 6 h	90 min to 4 h
Administration access	May be administered via peripheral line	Traditionally administered via central line; newer literature suggests that it is safe to administer via peripheral line. Institutional polices will dictate peripheral or central administration
Infusion	Infused via boluses	Infused via boluses or continuous infusion
Dose	Typically 20% solution at 0.5–1 g/kg	Dependent on sodium level, goal sodium level, and fluid status
Intravascular volume effects	Produces diuresis; beneficial in hypervolemic patients	Increases intravascular volume; beneficial in hypovolemic patients. However, can lead to hypervolemia and complications
Electrolyte disturbances	Risk of sodium and potassium abnormalities; hyper- or hypo- depending on the time of lab draw in relation to administration of mannitol	Risk of electrolyte abnormalities: Hypernatremia and hyperchloremia. Risk of metabolic acidosis due to hyperchloremia
Acute kidney injury	Risk of acute kidney injury (theoretically when osmolar gap >20 mOsm/kg)	Risk of acute kidney injury due to hypernatremia and hyperchloremia
Neurological complications	Administration of continuous infusions can lead to accumulation, worsening cerebral edema, and rebound ICP elevation	Risk of osmotic demyelination, especially in hyponatremic patients

ICP intracranial pressure

these agents have osmotic properties, which take effect in approximately 20 min after dosing. These osmotic properties produce a reduction in brain water content and a reduction in cerebrospinal fluid pressure. When administered in clinical doses, mannitol reduces brain water by approximately 2% [18]. Other features of mannitol that have been proposed to contribute to its therapeutic effects include that it is a free radical scavenger and it inhibits programmed cell death [19–21]. It has been proposed that hypertonic saline has additional vasoregulatory, immunomodulatory, and neurochemical effects that provide benefit in this patient population [22].

Both agents do appear to be effective at lowering ICP, but the literature has not demonstrated a superior agent. Additionally, neither agent has shown to improve neurological outcomes [23]. As such, guidelines have differing recommendations. The BTF Guidelines recommend mannitol at 0.25–1 g/kg, in one-time or as-needed doses.

Currently, there is insufficient evidence from comparative studies to support a formal recommendation regarding hypertonic saline [13]. However, the 2019 Seattle International Severe Traumatic Brain Injury Consensus Conference (SIBICC) recommends either hypertonic saline or mannitol boluses as initial (Tier 1) treatment for an elevated ICP and considers treatments within a tier to be equivalent [24]. The 2020 Neurocritical Care Society (NCS) Guidelines for the Acute Treatment of Cerebral Edema in Neurocritical Care Patients recommend hypertonic saline over mannitol for initial management of elevated ICP and cerebral edema in patients with TBI. The panel acknowledged that the quality of evidence was low; however, hypertonic saline was at least as safe and effective as mannitol. Additionally, the panel agreed that the purposed advantages of hypertonic saline over mannitol for fluid resuscitation and cerebral perfusion supported this recommendation [23]. The Western Trauma Association (WTA) management recommendations state that it is generally accepted that both agents are effective in reducing elevated ICP, though they suggest HTS in the polytrauma patient who requires vascular volume expansion in addition to lowering of the ICP [25].

Currently, the choice of agent is based on perceived advantages and disadvantages as well as pharmacokinetic and pharmacodynamic properties. Mannitol is a sugar alcohol that is excreted unchanged in the urine. The half-life is affected by glomerular filtration rate and averages 39–103 min [18, 26]. Mannitol is removed via hemodialysis and peritoneal dialysis [27]. The peak ICP-lowering effect occurs within 30–45 min and lasts around 6 h. Mannitol becomes less effective with repeated doses. Mannitol is most frequently administered as a 20% (1098 mOsm/L) or 25% (1375 mOsm/L) solution when given for ICP control. The dose can range from 0.25 to 2 g/kg, while most clinicians will use doses of 0.5–1 g/kg. Doses may be repeated every 4–6 h based on clinical need. Mannitol should be infused through an in-line ≤ 5 micron filter due to the risk of precipitation. The infusion length is typically 10–30 min, with the faster infusion rate of 10 min reserved for impending cerebral herniation.

The acute effect of mannitol on systemic arterial pressure is variable. A slight increase in pulse pressure and MAP is commonly observed. However, transient decreases in blood pressure secondary to decreases in systemic vascular resistance have been reported in the literature [28]. Hypotension is most likely to occur in patients who are relatively volume depleted. Acute mannitol-induced hypotension is rarely a serious problem. However, it can present a challenge when attempting to maintain CPP.

The potential complication of mannitol accumulating in damaged brain tissue and worsening fluid shifts appears to be more of an issue when the drug is not cleared from the blood between doses. A theoretical risk of mannitol is "rebound" intracranial pressure, which is most often attributed to continuous infusions or repeated high doses. In either case, it is proposed that prolonged therapy leads to penetration of osmotically active particles into brain tissue, especially in areas of a disrupted blood-brain barrier (BBB). Accumulation of mannitol leads to the creation of an osmotic gradient favoring water movement into the tissue, leading to edema [29]. Whether this actually occurs is unclear; several studies in animals and humans have reported no clinical evidence of rebound intracranial pressure [30–34]. Alternate proposed mechanisms include rapid volume depletion from administration of mannitol without adequate fluid administration as well as the administration of fluids that are hypotonic relative to the osmolarity of the patient combined with a rise in the number of intracellular osmotic particles induces movement of water back into regions with disrupted BBB and increased water permeability [20, 35]. Until the actual mechanism of rebound intracranial pressure can be determined, it is recommended not to administer mannitol as continuous infusions or more often than every 4–6 h.

Mannitol-induced acute kidney injury (AKI) has been extensively discussed in the literature; however, the mechanism remains unclear. Suggested mechanisms include renal vasoconstriction produced by a high dose/concentration of mannitol; profound diuresis and natriuresis, and osmotic nephropathy, which is isomeric tubular vacuolization or tubular cell swelling [36–38]. Furthermore, patients with preexisting risk factors including advanced age, underlying kidney disease, and concomitant use of nephrotoxic agents have been shown to be susceptible to the development of mannitol-induced AKI [36, 39, 40].

The risk of AKI is suggested to increase with a serum osmolality greater than 320 mOsm/kg [18]. Hence, many institutions continue to monitor serum osmolality when administering mannitol therapy with an upper allowable limit of 320 mOsm/kg [24]. While monitoring serum osmolality in patients who have received multiple doses of mannitol may be useful for associated toxicities, it does not predict mannitol concentrations [41]. The 2020 NCS Guidelines for the Acute Treatment of Cerebral Edema in Neurocritical Care Patients recommend using serum osmolar gap (measured serum osmolality—calculated osmolality) over serum osmolality to monitor for increased risk of AKI [23]. The osmolar gap has been shown to correlate better with mannitol serum concentrations than serum osmolality. Additionally, a normal osmolar gap concentration indicates that sufficient clearance of mannitol has occurred for additional dosing [42]. Retrospective analyses suggest that AKI with an osmolar gap <55 mOsm/kg is extremely rare and is more likely to occur once it exceeds 60–75 mOsm/kg [26, 43, 44]. The guidelines acknowledge that an upper limit of 20 mOsm/kg is often used as the threshold for AKI risk, although this number is not clearly supported by literature [23]. Mannitol-induced AKI is often reversible with cessation of the drug and will respond to hemodialysis, if required [44, 45].

It is important to closely monitor electrolytes while patients are receiving hyperosmolar therapy [23]. With mannitol, it is important to note the subacute phase in which electrolytes and the fluid status are being monitored. For example, hyponatremia may be observed immediately after the dose of mannitol secondary to dilution. However, hypernatremia may be observed in the diuresis period as it causes a net clearance of "free water." In addition to water and sodium chloride, abundant urine loss of potassium, phosphate, and magnesium can occur in patients receiving mannitol. Though exceedingly rare, mannitol can lead to volume overload with subsequent pulmonary edema or heart failure immediately following administration [26].

The ratio of urine diuresed to the volume of mannitol 25% solution administered can be as high as 5:1 [20]. For example, if 125 mL of mannitol is administered, the patient may diurese 625 mL. As such, patients can become severely dehydrated. Often, fluids and sodium will need to be replaced after a mannitol infusion using normal saline (0.9%), one-half normal saline (0.45%), or one-quarter normal saline (0.22%) depending on the sodium concentration. The volume replaced is dependent on the perceived volume status of the patient and may require ½ to 1 mL per mL diuresed.

A theoretical advantage of HTS to mannitol is that an intact BBB is less permeable to saline than to mannitol. The reflection coefficient, which is a measure of the ability of a membrane to prevent the passage of solutes, is 1 for sodium chloride vs. 0.9 for mannitol. Animal studies show that with an intact BBB, sodium administration increases CSF sodium concentrations but lags behind plasma levels by 1–4 h, creating an effective osmotic gradient.

Therapeutic HTS dosing regimens are more varied compared to mannitol. Regimens include concentrations ranging from 2% to 23.4%, which are administered as bolus doses or continuous infusions. There is no evidence to suggest that one regimen is superior to another. Currently, clear guidelines and specific sodium targets are lacking. Because of this, a 2011 survey of Neurocritical Care Society members showed that administration patterns varied considerably [46]. One-third of respondents used prophylactic continuous infusions, one-fourth reported using symptom-based bolus dosing, and one-fifth reported using a combination of the two strategies. Additionally, a small number reported using scheduled bolus dosing.

Traditionally, it has been recommended that concentrations of hypertonic saline solutions of 3% or greater be infused through a central catheter to avoid extravasation, thrombophlebitis, and tissue necrosis. It is thought that this recommendation was extrapolated from studies on peripheral administration of osmolar loads of total parenteral nutrition, which determined maximum osmolarity of peripherally infused solutions be limited to 900 mOsml/L. Currently, there is still concern for thrombophlebitis and extravasation; however, there is growing support in the literature for the peripheral administration of HTS [47–52]. Additionally, there are practical reasons for peripheral line administration. First, central venous access is not immediately available in the acute setting in all patients. This recommendation can lead to a delay in therapy and potentially worsen outcomes. Second, central catheters are associated with complications including infection, symptomatic thrombosis, and pneumothorax. Catheter-related complications are estimated to occur with up to 15–20% of catheters, depending on the site of placement [53]. Prior to a facility or ICU adopting peripheral administration of HTS, a protocol for administration and monitoring should be implemented. It should include the following: (a) infusing HTS only through large veins (18–20 gauge) in an upper extremity that are not in an area of flexion, (b) utilizing a dedicated line for infusion, (c) rotating the infusion site every 2–4 days for prolonged infusions, (d) scheduled monitoring of the line to ensure that it is functioning, and (e) scheduled monitoring of the sites for any changes in color, swelling, or tenderness.

There is no clear short-term benefit or documented evidence for long-term outcomes with the titration of continuous HTS infusions to a sodium goal. Currently, the primary advantage of utilizing a sodium goal is to reduce the risk of adverse events. The quality of evidence evaluating the risk of AKI associated with HTS is low. Due to the uncertain association, literature and guidelines recommend monitoring serum sodium and chloride concentrations while the patient is receiving HTS. The 2020 NCS Guidelines for the Acute Treatment of Cerebral Edema in Neurocritical Care Patients recommend an upper sodium limit of 150–160 mEq/L and an upper chloride limit of 110–115 mEq/L to limit the risk of AKI [23]. Furthermore, hypernatremia (above 150 mEq/L) has been associated with an increase in mortality in TBI patients [54–56]. This further suggests that HTS should only be administered for the treatment of elevated ICP and not to target a specific serum sodium level [57].

Large-volume administration of HTS can produce a metabolic acidosis due to hyperchloremia and volume expansion. It leads to volume expansion of the extracellular fluid and intravascular volume with bicarbonate-poor intracellular fluid, reducing the serum bicarbonate and resulting in a temporary decline in pH. Additionally, hyperchloremia is associated with AKI [58–61]. In order to alleviate the acid-base disturbances observed with a high-chloride load, buffered sodium solutions are used. Buffered sodium solutions can contain sodium acetate, sodium bicarbonate, or sodium lactate with or without sodium chloride. Buffered sodium solutions require compounding, and there is no standard formulation. This results in solutions with different concentrations and osmolarities, which has led to the recommendation that pharmacists formulate the admixture using milliequivalents of sodium rather than grams so that the osmolarity of the solution matches that of commercially available hypertonic sodium chloride solutions [62].

A significant concern with the use of HTS is overcorrection of the serum sodium concentration, leading to osmotic demyelination syndrome (ODS). ODS is most likely to occur in patients with extremely low serum sodium levels (<120 mEq/L) [63]. Osmotic demyelination syndrome has been reported in normonatremic (>135 mEq/L) patients, though not when being treated for cerebral edema. HTS should be administered cautiously, and serum sodium concentrations should be monitored.

16.5.2   Sedation and Analgesia

The use of sedation and analgesia has many purposes in ICU patients, including limiting the stress response to critical illness, providing anxiolysis, facilitating mechanical ventilator support and tolerance, and enabling ICU care. In the critically ill patient, pain arises from different sources and is subjective. TBI patients may experience moderate-to-severe pain at rest depending on the extent of their injuries, though they may also experience pain during routine care in the ICU. In patients who are able to self-report pain, the 0–10 numeric rating scale, administered either verbally or visually, is considered a valid and feasible pain scale. Validated pain scales, such as the behavioral pain scale (BPS) or the critical care pain observation tool (CPOT), allow clinicians to assess pain in patients that are unable to self-report it [64].

In the TBI patient, sedation and analgesia are used to provide adequate conditions that favor recovery of brain tissue and prevent secondary neuronal injury [65]. Because pain and agitation can lead to increases in ICP, intravenous sedation and analgesia are considered first-line therapy. Other neurological conditions TBI patients may experience, including status epilepticus and paroxysmal sympathetic hyperactivity (PSH), utilize sedation and analgesia as mainstays of therapy.

Sedation and analgesia are believed to be beneficial in managing elevated ICP through three mechanisms [66]. First, they decrease cerebral metabolic rate of oxygen ($CMRO_2$), subsequently leading to a reduction in CBF with a comparable decrease in cerebral blood volume. Based on the Monro-Kellie hypothesis, the reduction in cerebral blood volume will lead to a reduction in ICP. Second, sedation and analgesia reduce pain and agitation, which decreases the incidence of arterial hypertension and an associated increase in ICP. Third, analgesia reduces agitation and coughing associated with intolerance of the endotracheal tube. This reduces the intrathoracic pressure, leading to increased jugular venous outflow and decreased ICP. Table 16.4 gives a more complete summary of the physiologic effects of sedative and analgesic agents.

The neurological examination is the gold standard for monitoring TBI patients. Sedation and analgesia may impair the ability to get an accurate assessment of the patient's neurological status. It is often a balancing act between maintaining adequate sedation and analgesia as well as being able to assess the patient accurately. Additionally, agents may have side effects such as reducing CPP. The ideal agent for

Table 16.4 Systemic and cerebral physiologic effects of sedative and analgesic agents

	HR	CO	SVR	MAP	ICP	CPP	CBF	$CMRO_2$
Barbiturates	↑	↓	↑↓	↓↓	↓↓	↓	↓↓	↓↓
Benzodiazepines	↔□↑	↓↔□	↓↔□	↓	↓	↓	↓	↓
Dexmedetomidine	↓	↓	↔□↑	↓	↓?	↓?	↓↓	↔□
Etomidate	↔□	↔□	↔□	↔□	↓	↔□	↓	↓
Ketamine	↑	↑	↑	↑	↑	↔□	↑↑	↔□
Opioids	↓	↔□	↓↔□	↓	↓↔□	↓↔□	↔□	↓
Propofol	↔□	↓	↓↓	↓↓	↓↓	↓	↓↓	↓↓

↓, decrease; ↑, increase; ↔□ no change, *HR* heart rate, *CO* cardiac output, *SVR* systemic vascular resistance, *MAP* mean arterial pressure, *ICP* intracranial pressure, *CPP* cerebral perfusion pressure, *CBF* cerebral blood flow, *CMRO₂*, cerebral metabolic rate of oxygen
Adapted from Rhoney DH, Parker D. Use of sedative and analgesic agents in neurotrauma patients on cerebral physiology. Neurol Res 2001;23;237–59

a TBI patient would include (1) a quick onset and offset to allow for frequent neurological exams, (2) reduced ICP by cerebral blood volume reduction or cerebral vasoconstriction, (3) reduced CBF and $CMRO_2$ while maintaining coupling of the two, (4) maintained cerebral autoregulation, (5) allowing usual cerebral vascular reactivity to changes in $PaCO_2$, and (6) minimal cardiovascular depressant effects [65].

16.5.3 Barbiturate Coma

Barbiturates have been recommended to treat high and refractory ICP since the early 1980s [67, 68]. Barbiturates are thought to be neuroprotective through depression of cerebral metabolism and oxygen consumption. They may also lead to higher brain oxygenation with lower cerebral blood flow secondary to improving coupling of regional blood flow to metabolic demands. Additionally, this leads to decreased ICP from decreased cerebral blood volume. Other brain-protective mechanisms include inhibition of oxygen radical-mediated lipid peroxidation [69–71].

Despite the perceived benefits of barbiturates, the literature has not demonstrated a mortality benefit [72–74]. Furthermore, numerous complications occur with their use, including severe hypotension, decreased gastrointestinal motility, and increased incidence of infections. Currently, high-dose barbiturate administration is recommended to control elevated ICP refractory to maximum standard medical and surgical treatment [13]. However, hemodynamic stability is essential before and during barbiturate therapy. Due to the high incidence of hypotension, many patients will require a vasopressor and fluid support during barbiturate therapy.

16.6 Nonpharmacological Treatments

16.6.1 Body/Head Position

The standard posture for critically ill patients is a semi-recumbent position with head elevation at an angle of 30°. This position has been shown to reduce the frequency and risk of nosocomial pneumonia, especially in patients who receive enteral nutrition [75]. Several studies have demonstrated the benefits of elevating the head of the bed for lowering ICP in TBI patients [76–78]. One recent study showed that changing stable TBI patients from a head elevation of 30° to 15° and then to 0° resulted in a gradual increase in ICP. However, brain oxygenation and brain circulation were improved [79]. This study did not assess clinical outcomes resulting from these changes. Currently, there is limited evidence to recommend an ideal head position. Based on other perceived benefits, such as lowering the risk of nosocomial pneumonia, head elevation should be maintained at 30° and then individualized to the patient's needs.

16.6.2 Temperature Management

The United States Centers for Disease Control and Prevention defines fever in hospital-acquired infections as a measured temperature of greater than 38 °C. Similarly, the Society of Critical Care Medicine and Infectious Diseases Society of America define fever as a temperature equal to or greater than 38.3 °C [80]. Fever is observed in 20–50% of TBI patients, with nearly 90% having at least one episode within 7 days of hospitalization [81]. High fever (>39.0 °C) within 72 h of the injury has been associated with six times the mortality of afebrile patients, while even low-grade fever (38–39 °C) has been associated with increased mortality [82]. Fever burden, particularly early after TBI, is associated with poor prognosis [83]. Every 1 °C increase in temperature has been associated with a 2.2-fold increased risk of adverse outcomes. Further, a 0.5 °C rise in temperature can lead to a series of secondary injuries and neuron death [84].

While infection is the most common cause of fever, many causes in TBI patients exist including disruption of the hypothalamic set point by endogenous pyrogens released from injured neurons [85]. Through several complex mechanisms, fever can lead to cerebral edema and potentially a decrease in CPP [85, 86]. Fever increases the cerebral metabolic rate for oxygen and glucose, which can lead to an increase in CBF and eventually an increase in CBV and ICP [87]. Fever in TBI patients can lead to secondary injury including ischemic neuronal injury, mitochondrial dysfunction, reactive oxygen species, and thereby neuronal death.

Temperature in TBI patients should be maintained at normothermia (37.5 °C) to lessen the risk of secondary brain injury and elevated ICPs. First-line treatment of fever includes scheduled acetaminophen 650 mg every 4 h (4000 mg maximum in 24 h). Second-line therapy includes applying an external cooling blanket and ice packs to the axilla, groin, and neck if temperature remains >37.5 °C. Third-line therapy includes administration of cold IV fluids and 0.9% sodium chloride in 500–1000 mL if temperature remains elevated despite previous therapies. Fourth-line therapy, which includes intravascular or external cooling in non-intubated patients or esophageal cooling in intubated patients, is often reserved for those who cannot tolerate the additional volume. Once intravascular cooling is initiated, other external cooling methods can be [88] removed. The devices are regulated to a core body temperature that is measured by a bladder thermistor or esophageal temperature probe.

Aggressive fever control to maintain normothermia can lead to shivering. Shivering increases the patient's metabolic rate, which can have detrimental effects on oxygenation and ICP, making it challenging to achieve goal temperatures [88]. Shivering can be scored at the bedside by using the Bedside Shivering Assessment Scale (BSAS), with scores of 0 = no shivering, 1 = mild shivering localized to neck and/or thorax, 2 = moderate shivering with gross movement of upper extremities, and 3 = severe shivering that involves gross movements of the trunk and upper and lower extremities [88]. The goal BSAS is a score of ≤1. Medications to prevent shivering as well as counter warming during the cooling period have been protocolized to minimize shivering. Medications are given in a stepwise approach with the goal to maximize one agent prior to moving to the next; see Table 16.5.

16.6.3 Prophylactic Hypothermia

Prophylactic hypothermia is believed to be neuroprotective through several mechanisms including reduced ICP, reduced $CMRO_2$, reduced CBF, and maintenance of the BBB function. Additionally, it is thought to limit secondary brain injury by reducing the inflammatory response and biochemical cascade early after TBI [13, 89–91]. Nevertheless, there are significant risks associated with the use of prophylactic hypothermia including seizures and myoclonus and effects on the immune system leading to an increase in infections, predominantly pneumonia, coagulopathy, and ventricular ectopic beats [92]. Electrolyte disturbances, particularly hypokalemia and hyperkalemia, are common. Hypokalemia can lead to ventricular arrhythmias, cardiac arrest, and death. If prophylactic hypothermia is used, the pharmacist should participate in the development of an electrolyte protocol specific to the cooling and rewarming phases.

Prophylactic hypothermia for TBI has been studied since the 1990s in 14 randomized controlled trials with different TBI patient populations, outcomes, and cooling devices. Currently, the evidence is inconsistent and does not support improved morbidity and mortality. Prophylactic hypothermia is not recommended because of these findings as well as the increased risks associated with it [13].

Table 16.5 Medications used for management of shivering

Step	Intervention	Dose
1	Buspirone and magnesium sulfate infusion	Buspirone: 30 mg Q8 h 15 mg Q8 h if CrCl <50 mL/min Avoid use in CrCl <20 mL/min or ESRD Magnesium: Start at 0.5 mg/h; titrate by 0.25 g/h Q4 h, to goal magnesium level (3–3.5 mg/dL) Start at 0.25 mg/h if CrCl </=30 mL/min
2	Dexmedetomidine infusion or fentanyl infusion or meperidine	Dexmedetomidine: Initiate at 0.2 mcg/kg/h, titrate every 15 min to effect. Max dose 1.4 mcg/kg/h Fentanyl: Initiate at 25 mcg/h Meperidine: 12.5–75 mg IM or IV Q4 h as needed
3	Propofol infusion	Initiate at 20 mcg/kg/min; titrate to effect (max dose 75 mcg/kg/min); monitor patients for PRIS at higher doses
4	Vecuronium or rocuronium	Vecuronium: 0.1 mg/kg IV as needed based on BSAS score and TOF monitoring Rocuronium:1–1.2 mg/kg IV as needed based on BSAS score and TOF monitoring

BSAS bedside shivering assessment scale, *PRIS* propofol-related infusion syndrome, *TOF* train of four, *CrCl* creatinine clearance, ESRD end stage renal disease

Adapted from: Choi HA, Ko S-B, Presciutti M. Prevention of shivering during therapeutic temperature modulation: the Columbia anti-shivering protocol. Neurocrit Care. 2011;14:389–94

16.7 Adjunct Therapies

16.7.1 Seizure Prophylaxis

Patients with severe TBI have a high risk of seizures [13, 93]. Seizures usually occur in the area of the brain where scarring has developed secondary to the injury [94]. Post-traumatic seizures (PTSs) are classified as early (occurring within 7 days of injury) or late (occurring after 7 days of injury). Post-traumatic epilepsy (PTE) is defined as recurrent seizures more than 7 days following injury. Table 16.6 highlights risk factors for PTS and PTE. The rate of clinical PTS has been reported to be as high as 12–25%, including subclinical seizures detected on electroencephalography [95]. Early PTS is associated with higher mortality, longer hospital length of stay, and non-home discharge [96]. PTE doubles the rate of unfavorable outcomes at 2 years and increases the risk of unexpected death by a factor of 30 [5, 97, 98].

The BTF Guidelines recommend the use of anticonvulsants following TBI to prevent the occurrence of PTS. Phenytoin is recommended in the guidelines; however, the use of levetiracetam is increasing for this indication. Currently, there is a lack of comparative studies to recommend one agent over another. Table 16.7 compares the dosing and monitoring of the two agents.

Total phenytoin levels must be adjusted for hypoalbuminemia and renal dysfunction. The formula for dose adjustment that most accurately predicts adjustment based on albumin and renal dysfunction is the Winter-Tozer equation [101, 102]:

$$\text{Predicted free phenytoin} = \left[\left(\text{measured total PHT}\right) / \left(0.2 \times \text{albumin} + 0.10\right)\right] \times 0.1$$

Adverse events with phenytoin are predominantly concentration related. Adverse events associated with total concentrations less than 40 mcg/mL include nystagmus, blurred vision, diplopia, ataxia, slurred speech, and lethargy, while coma and death are associated with concentrations greater than 40 mcg/mL. Other concerns include cardiovascular collapse, extravasations and purple glove syndrome, Stevens-Johnson syndrome/toxic epidermal necrolysis, drug interactions, and enteral tube feed

Table 16.6 Risk factors for PTS and PTE after TBI [95, 99, 100]

PTS	PTE
Age ≤65 years	Acute intracerebral hematoma
Cortical contusion	Age >65 years
Chronic alcoholism	Cortical contusion
Epidural hematoma	Early PTS
Glasgow coma scale (GCS) score ≤10	History of depression
Intracerebral hemorrhage	Post-traumatic amnesia >24 h
Immediate seizures	Severe TBI
Linear or depressed skull fracture	
Penetrating head injury	
Post-traumatic amnesia >30 min	
Subdural hematoma	

Table 16.7 Comparison of phenytoin and levetiracetam for seizure prophylaxis [13, 110, 112, 114]

	Phenytoin	Levetiracetam
Loading dose	20 mg/kg IV × 1 (max 2000 mg)	NA
Maintenance dose	5 mg/kg/day or 100 mg IV/PO/GT every 8 h or 300 mg SR capsules PO daily	500–1000 mg every 12 h May be given IV/PO/GT
Duration	7 days	7 days
Monitoring	Total 10–20 mg/L Free 1–2 mg/L	NA

GT gastric tube, *IV* intravenous, *PO* oral, *SR* sustained release

interactions. Phenytoin can produce cardiovascular collapse when infused too quickly [103]. However, this is thought to be due to the diluent, which contains propylene glycol. Patients develop hypotension and bradyarrhythmias [104]. Phenytoin is a Vaughan-Williams class 1B antiarrhythmic. However, it has quick on-off kinetics at the sodium channel, making it less arrhythmogenic compared with agents with slow on-off kinetics, such as the class IC agents. Additionally, phenytoin can cause significant tissue damage when extravasation occurs. It leads to a purplish-black discoloration accompanied by edema and pain distal to the site of injection. On rare occasions, it may progress to necrosis, ischemia, vascular compression, or compartment syndrome requiring surgical interventions. It is termed purple glove syndrome (PGS) because of its appearance. The pathophysiology is not well understood, and several mechanisms have been proposed [105]. Phenytoin comes in a highly alkaline (pH = 12) solution, and it has been proposed that it may induce vasoconstriction resulting in leaking of the solution into surrounding interstitial soft tissue spaces. This is usually followed by damage to vascular endothelial integrity, promoting further leakage of phenytoin solution into adjacent interstitial soft tissue spaces. It has also been proposed that mixing of the highly alkaline solution with the more neutral pH of the blood may produce precipitation of phenytoin that may obstruct the vein and lead to phenytoin backup and leakage into soft tissue interstitial spaces and the development of PGS. Finally, IV phenytoin solution contains sodium hydroxide, propylene glycol, and ethanol, all of which are known tissue irritants that can cause damage in extravasations. In order to reduce the risk of extravasation, phenytoin should be administered through an 18-gauge peripheral IV catheter or larger or via a central line. Additionally, the nurse should check the patency of the line prior to infusion. Phenytoin should never be infused through lines in the hands or feet.

Fosphenytoin is a water-soluble prodrug of phenytoin. It has several advantages over phenytoin. It may be administered intravenously or intramuscularly. The maximum recommended infusion rate is 150 mg / min vs. 50 mg/min for phenytoin. The prodrug has an 8–15-min half-life of conversion to phenytoin. Due to this conversion time, the time to therapeutic levels is the same between agents [106–108]. It is often preferred over phenytoin due to better tolerance at the infusion site, lower risk of cardiac arrhythmias or hypotension, and lower risk of PGS [109]. However, fosphenytoin is converted to phenytoin and can cause similar electrocardiography (ECG) changes.

Additionally, it has been theorized to have direct effects on calcium equilibrium due to its metabolism to phenytoin and an inorganic phosphate. The inorganic phosphate binds with cations and leads to a reduction in both total and ionized calcium concentrations. The subsequent hypocalcemia has the potential to produce various cardiac arrhythmias. Continuous ECG monitoring, particularly during the loading dose, is recommended for both agents due to the potential for bradyarrhythmias.

Despite the knowledge that phenytoin interacts with enteral tube feeds for over 40 years, the mechanism of the interaction remains poorly understood. It is thought that phenytoin adheres to the plastic tubing or there is a physical incompatibility with the enteral feed. Regardless, phenytoin serum levels can be reduced by 50–75% when it is administered via the enteral feeding tube. Recommendations to overcome this issue include (1) flush tube before and after phenytoin administration and (2) hold tube feeds 1–2 h before and after each dose. Due to the complications of holding tube feeds and adjusting rates to ensure adequate nutrition, a reasonable option is to empirically increase the dose from 100 mg every 8 h to 200 mg every 12 h.

The use of levetiracetam for seizure prophylaxis is increasing due to a favorable adverse effect profile, more predictable pharmacokinetics making the need for therapeutic drug monitoring less burdensome, and similar clinical efficacy to phenytoin and valproic acid in status epilepticus. Currently, the ideal dose of levetiracetam for seizure prophylaxis is unknown. Recent evidence recommends lower doses due to the finding of no difference between higher and lower dosing regimens [110]. Intravenous levetiracetam is well tolerated when diluted in 100 mL of 0.9% sodium chloride and 5% dextrose and infused over 15–60 min. Recently, rapid IV push administration of undiluted drug at doses as high as 4500 mg has been shown to be safe and well tolerated [111, 112]. Administration of undiluted drugs can lead to a reduction in the time to administration secondary to delays in ordering and preparation and allowing for the drug to be stored on the unit in medication-dispensing units.

Adverse effects most often frequently observed with levetiracetam include psychiatric and behavioral symptoms [113]. Twenty to thirty-five percent of adults treated with levetiracetam for epilepsy experience behavioral adverse events. Specifically, patients experience greater irritability, aggression, depressive mood, and anxiety compared to other antiepileptics. Approximately 18% of patients will require cessation or dose reduction due to behavioral adverse effects. Additional adverse effects include psychotic symptoms, paranoid ideation, and hallucinations.

16.7.2 Venous Thromboembolism (VTE) Prophylaxis

The incidence of VTE in TBI patients is up to 54% in patients who do not receive prophylaxis and 25% in patients who are placed on sequential compression devices (SCDs) alone [115, 116]. The incidence of VTE increases with the severity of TBI. As such, surveillance protocols are recommended in high-risk patients to ensure early detection and intervention. Low-molecular-weight heparin (LMWH) or low-dose unfractionated heparin (UFH) may be used in combination with mechanical prophylaxis.

Low-molecular-weight heparin is the preferred agent in trauma patients with injury severity score (ISS) >10 per the Western Trauma Association (WTA) guidelines [117]. Enoxaparin 40 mg twice daily is considered the standard dose in most trauma patients, while the recommended dose for patients greater than 65 years old, with weight less than 50 kg, or who have a creatinine clearance (CrCl) of 30–60 mL/min is 30 mg subcutaneously (SC) twice daily. Additional enoxaparin weight-based dosing regimens exist. Anti-Xa levels should be monitored in patients on enoxaparin who are underweight, in females with less than 50 kg total body weight, in those with BMI greater than 40, in acute renal failure patients, in those at increased risk of bleeding, or in those who were initiated on weight-based doses. The recommended timing for anti-Xa levels is 4 h after the third dose. Most agree that the goal range for prophylaxis is 0.2–0.4 units/mL. Once in the goal range, anti-Xa levels should be rechecked if renal function declines.

Unfractionated heparin is recommended in patients with a CrCl less than 30 mg/dL or in renal failure. Dosing is 5000 units SC every 8 h if the body mass index (BMI) is less than 40 or 7500 units and SC Q8H if the BMI is greater than 40 and CrCl is less than 30 mL/min [13, 117, 118].

Pharmacological prophylaxis for VTE prophylaxis can be initiated safely 24 h after injury in most TBI patients with a stable head CT. However, there are several risk stratification scoring systems used to guide surveillance and prophylaxis in polytrauma and TBI patients. The risk for thromboembolism in trauma patients is assessed using the Greenfield Risk Assessment Profile. Risk factors are divided into categories: underlying conditions, iatrogenic factors, injury-related factors, and age. The maximum score is 14. A score of 5 or more has been shown to increase the DVT risk threefold; pharmacologic VTE prophylaxis should be initiated [119]. The Trauma Embolic Scoring System (TESS) is another VTE risk stratification scoring system for polytrauma patients determined by five clinical variables: age, Injury Severity Score (ISS), BMI, ventilator days, and presence of a lower extremity fracture [120]. A score of 0–2 indicates no risk, a score of 3–6 is low risk, and a score of 7–14 is considered moderate to high risk. This tool has been shown to be a useful clinical decision-making tool in predicting VTE in military trauma patients [121]. The Parkland Protocol is an algorithm for VTE prophylaxis specifically in TBI patients. It stratifies patients into categories for spontaneous progression of hemorrhage and provides recommendations on starting VTE prophylaxis [122]. In low-risk TBI patients, enoxaparin is started 24 h post-injury; in moderate-risk TBI patients, enoxaparin is initiated 72 h post-injury; and in high-risk TBI patients, a prophylactic inferior vena cava (IVC) filter is recommended.

16.7.3 Antibiotic Prophylaxis

The infection rate in patients with intracranial pressure monitors has been reported to be as high as 27% [123]. These infections are associated with high morbidity and mortality, longer intensive care unit and hospital stay, and increased healthcare costs [124–126].

Methods to prevent external ventricular drain (EVD) infections include disinfection of the skin, pre- and postoperative prophylaxis, shortening the duration of EVD use, antibiotic-impregnated shunts, prolonged prophylactic antibiotics, or combinations of these in protocols [126, 127]. Published protocols from some institutions have demonstrated rates as low as 0%. In patients with EVDs, systemic prophylactic antibiotics can prevent infection. The Neurocritical Care Society Consensus Statement on Insertion and Management of EVDs recommends to administer one dose of antimicrobials prior to EVD insertion and not continuing antibiotics for the duration of EVD placement [128].

For neurosurgery procedures, CSF-shunting procedures, the recommended regimen is cefazolin 2 g IV × 1 or 3 g IV × 1 for patients weighing ≥120 kg. Redosing of cefazolin if surgery continues longer than 4 h from the preoperative dose is recommended. Alternative agents for patients allergic to β-lactam antibiotics include vancomycin 15 mg/kg IV × 1 or clindamycin 900 mg IV × 1. Redosing of clindamycin if surgery continues longer than 6 h from the preoperative dose is recommended. The recommended duration of postoperative antimicrobials is a single dose or continuation for less than 24 h [129]. There is insufficient data to recommend continuation of antibiotics beyond 24 h postoperatively in patients with craniectomy or additional doses beyond the perioperative dose in patients with indwelling devices [123, 128, 130].

16.7.4 Stress Ulcer Prophylaxis (SUP)

Stress ulcers are superficial ulcers in the upper gastrointestinal (GI) tract that may develop during hospitalization and in the ICU setting [131, 132]. Stress ulcers develop because of either hypersecretion of acid or impaired mucosal protection secondary to GI tract hypoperfusion, mucosal ischemia, or disruption. Additionally, TBI patients are at an increased risk for developing gastric stress ulcers during their hospital stay because of increased ICP and overstimulation of the vagus nerve, which can lead to excess production of gastric acid as well as general hypoperfusion of the gut due to the stress of critical illness [133–135].

Stress ulcers in critically ill patients can be divided into four categories, including asymptomatic stress ulceration, stress ulceration with occult bleeding, stress ulceration with overt bleeding, and stress ulceration with clinically significant bleeding [131, 136, 137]. The incidence of asymptomatic stress ulceration in critically ill patients who do not receive prophylaxis may exceed 75%, while stress ulceration leading to clinically significant bleeding affects approximately 1–3% of patients in the ICU [138, 139]. Stress ulceration can lead to an increased length of stay as well as serious complications including perforation, hemorrhagic shock, and death. Stress ulcer management should focus on prevention.

Multiple risk factors have been linked to the risk of stress ulceration. Patients are considered to be at very high risk for developing a stress ulcer with clinically significant bleeding if they have either prolonged mechanical ventilation beyond 48 h or the presence of coagulopathy [140, 141]. Patients are at high risk if they have two of the following risk factors: GCS <10, head or spinal cord injury, high-dose corticosteroids (>250 mg/day of hydrocortisone or equivalent), history of GI bleeding within 1 year, hypotension, ICU admission >1 week, ileus, major surgery, multiple-organ failure, myocardial infarction, renal or hepatic failure, sepsis, severe burns (>35% body surface area), solid-organ transplant, and trauma [131, 137, 140–142].

The Surviving Sepsis Campaign guidelines recommend the use of a proton pump inhibitor (PPI) or histamine 2-receptor antagonist (H2RA) for stress ulcer prophylaxis [143]. Both medication classes lead to the inhibition of gastric acid secretion and an increase in gastric pH. Proton pump inhibitors block the hydrogen-potassium ATPase pump, while H2RAs bind to the histamine-2 receptor on parietal cells and inhibit the pathway histamine utilizes to stimulate proton pump activity. Sucralfate has also been used for SUP; however; it requires gastric access. The use of sucralfate is limited in the ICUs, as many have moved to jejunal nutrition to reduce aspiration. The choice of agent can vary per institution and patient population and should take into account administration, adverse effects, drug interactions, and cost. Many institutions will elect to administer pantoprazole orally or intravenously and lansoprazole enterally as a suspension. Compared to cimetidine and ranitidine, famotidine has a longer duration of action and fewer drug interactions involving the cytochrome P-450 hepatic enzyme system [144]. Combined with this and its general tolerability, famotidine is frequently the preferred H2RA. Table 16.8 highlights the dosing of agents used for stress ulcer prophylaxis.

Despite the benefits of these agents in preventing stress ulcers, concerns regarding the association between non-judicious acid suppression and increased risk of bacterial infections, particularly pneumonia and *Clostridioides difficile*, exist. The risk of infection is thought to be higher with the PPIs than the H2RAs. Additionally, both classes of agents have been associated with thrombocytopenia in case reports and case series. However, larger analyses were not able to confirm this concern. In most of the reports describing thrombocytopenia, patients had additional risk

Table 16.8 Stress ulcer prophylaxis agents [135, 137, 140, 144]

H 2-receptor antagonists		
Cimetidine	400 mg PO	Q6H
Famotidine	20 mg PO/NG/IV	Q12H Q24H (CrCl <50 mL/min)
Ranitidine	150 mg PO/IV	Q12H Q24H (CrCl <50 mL/min)
Proton pump inhibitors		
Esomeprazole	40 mg PO/IV	Q24H
Lansoprazole	30 mg NG	Q24H
Omeprazole	40 mg PO/NG	Q24H
Pantoprazole	40 mg PO/IV/NG	Q24H
Gastrointestinal protectant		
Sucralfate	1 g PO/NG	Q6H

IV intravenously, *NG* nasogastrically, *PO* orally

factors that could have caused or contributed to the development of thrombocytopenia. As such, the risks and benefits need to be considered. Therapy should be initiated and discontinued as applicable to the clinical situation. The pharmacist can play an important role in managing appropriate stress ulcer therapy.

16.7.5 Tranexamic Acid

Tranexamic acid (TXA) is a synthetic lysine analogue that competitively inhibits the conversion of plasminogen to plasmin. This reduces the proteolytic action of plasmin on fibrin clots, resulting in an inhibition of fibrinolysis [145, 146]. It has been shown to reduce surgical bleeding and decrease mortality in patients with extracranial bleeding [147, 148]. Intracranial bleeding starts at the moment of impact and can continue for several hours after injury [149, 150]. Increased fibrinolysis is often observed in TBI patients and predicts hemorrhagic expansion [151]. It has been proposed that early administration of TXA could prevent or decrease hemorrhagic expansion and therefore herniation and death.

The CRASH-3 trial concluded that the risk of death was reduced with early tranexamic acid use in patients with mild-to-moderate head injury. TXA should be administered as a loading dose of 1 g over 10 min, started within 3 h of injury, followed by a continuous infusion of 1 g over the next 8 h. However, the use of TXA in isolated TBI remains controversial due to several questions regarding the effect size, mortality only being observed in subgroups, quality of survival, mid-study protocol changes, safety, and other concerns about CRASH-3 and TXA use in general [152, 153]. A subsequent meta-analysis of 9 studies including CRASH-3 data concluded that in acute TBI patients, TXA may decrease hematoma expansion but probably has no effect on mortality or disability [154]. If TXA is to be considered, it is recommended to use it in moderate TBI patients with GCS 9–12 and preserved pupillary reactivity. What is likely to have more of an impact is limiting secondary brain injuries by preventing hypotension, hypoxemia, and pyrexia insults [7, 153, 155].

16.7.6 Glucose Targets

Acute hyperglycemia after TBI is common and has been associated with poor outcomes [156–158]. An early surge in sympathetic activity leads to an increase in systemic circulating catecholamines. The degree of sympathoadrenal response appears to increase linearly with the severity of the brain injury [159]. The catecholamine surge occurs within minutes of the insult and may be transient, while the circulating glucose surge that follows soon after is sustained. Studies indicate that hyperglycemia is harmful because it contributes to anaerobic metabolism in the brain, resulting in brain tissue lactic acidosis and secondary neuronal injury

[160–162]. However, data also suggests that moderate hyperglycemia may be necessary during acute TBI because glucose is the only energy source for the brain, and its utilization significantly increases to meet energy demands immediately following injury [163, 164]. It is unclear as to what level of hyperglycemia should be treated and if it will improve or worsen outcomes.

Tight glycemic control has been shown to increase global glucose uptake and increase cerebral metabolic distress after TBI [165]. Additionally, reduced CSF microdialysis levels of glucose after TBI have been demonstrated [166, 167]. Persistent low levels of glucose independently predict poor outcomes. Decreases in microdialysis glucose levels can be due to several causes, including brain ischemia, herniation, and seizures. Given that these processes could be occurring and that the brain has an increased need for glucose, it is reasonable to assume that a reduction in glucose supply would be harmful.

The BTF Guidelines do not provide a specific recommendation for glycemic control due to insufficient evidence. The 2024 Society of Critical Care Medicine Guidelines on Glycemic Control for Critically Ill Children and Adults state that "analysis from neurological ICUs yielded comparable findings, and these patients should be managed like unselected patients." The guidelines recommend treating persistent hyperglycemia greater than or equal to 180 mg/dL in critically ill adults. For the acute management of hyperglycemia, the guideline suggests using an IV insulin infusion vs. subcutaneous insulin. The recommended target glucose ranges are 140–200 mg/dL vs. 80–139 mg/dL in order to decrease the risk of hypoglycemia. While managing hyperglycemia with an IV insulin infusion, ≤ 1 h, continuous, or near-continuous glucose monitoring should occur.

16.7.7   Steroids

The only level 1 recommendation in the BTF Guidelines is against the use of steroids for improving outcomes or reducing ICP. In severe TBI, high-dose methylprednisolone was associated with increased mortality. Since the 1950s, glucocorticoids have been used to provide symptomatic relief to patients with brain tumors. A large portion of patients will experience symptomatic edema, which often produces a mass effect larger than the tumor [168]. This mass effect can lead to headaches and neurological deficits. Based on the benefits observed in patients with brain tumors in the perioperative phase, their use became common in other neurosurgical procedures and in the treatment of TBI. A systematic review in 1997 showed no benefit for improving outcomes in TBI patients; however, the authors recommended a larger trial to confirm these results [169].

The Corticosteroid Randomization After Significant Head Injury (CRASH) trial was an international, multicenter, randomized controlled trial of methylprednisolone in patients with TBI. The trial evaluated 10,008 adult hospitalized patients within 8 h of injury with a GCS <14. Patients received methylprednisolone 2 g IV followed by 0.4 mg/h for 48 h or placebo. The study was stopped early due to the increased risk of death in the steroid group [125, 167]. Six-month follow-up confirmed a higher risk of death.

16.8 Complications

16.8.1 Paroxysmal Sympathetic Hyperactivity

Paroxysmal sympathetic hyperactivity (PSH) is a syndrome that occurs in 8–10% of patients with TBI and is characterized by episodes of hypertension, tachypnea, hyperthermia, diaphoresis, and dystonic posturing [170, 171]. These episodes may last from minutes to hours and can occur several times a day or, in refractory cases, nearly continuously. It is associated with greater morbidity, increased healthcare costs, longer hospitalizations, and worse outcomes. Uncontrolled symptoms can lead to secondary brain injury from hypertension, hyperthermia, cardiac damage, and death [172]. Detailed descriptions of the time course of PSH are difficult to find in the literature. One study showed that the first episode occurred on average 5.9 ± 3.7 days after injury [173]. It may persist into the rehabilitation phase and may last for weeks to months after the injury. In severe cases, it may persist for more than 1 year [173, 174].

Significant risk factors for developing PSH after TBI include the severity of the initial brain injury, younger age, and male gender. Most agree that PSH is caused by a functional disconnection leading to unbalanced activation of brainstem systems controlling the autonomic nervous system. PSH can be caused by different mechanisms of injury in different locations, explaining the variability in symptoms and severity. Regardless of the lesion location, the final common pathway is an imbalance of adrenergic outflow.

Symptom-based findings are used for the early identification of PSH. As such, PSH is frequently only recognized once the patient begins to awaken. Diagnosis is often one of exclusion and recognition of a recurring pattern. An expert consensus group proposed the use of the PSH assessment measure (PSH-AM) tool shown in Table 16.9, which is a clinical scoring system used for probabilistic diagnosis [171]. There are two components in the PSH-AM tool; the clinical feature scale (CFS) assesses the severity of clinical features and motor activity, and the diagnosis likelihood tool (DLT) measures the presence of compatible features of PSH. Combined scores indicate the diagnostic likelihood of PSH as unlikely, possible, or probable. This assessment tool should be used on a daily basis in the ICU and through the rehabilitation phase.

Management of PSH requires a combination of pharmacological and nonpharmacological treatment modalities. The etiology of PSH is not well understood, which makes treatment difficult. Therapy focuses on the control of symptoms. A combination of medications from different classes is tried based on symptoms and

Table 16.9 PSH assessment measure tool

Clinical feature scale (CFS)					
	0	1	2	3	Score
Heart rate	<100	100–119	120–139	≥140	
Respiratory rate	<18	18–23	24–29	≥30	
Systolic blood pressure	<140	140–159	160–179	≥180	
Temperature	<37	37–37.9	38–38.9	≥39.0	
Sweating	Nil	Mild	Moderate	Severe	
Posturing during episodes	Nil	Mild	Moderate	Severe	
CFS subtotal					
Severity of clinical features					Nil 0 Mild 1–6 Moderate 7–12 Severe ≥13
Diagnosis likelihood tool (DLT): Score 1 point for each feature present					
Clinical features occur simultaneously					
Episodes are paroxysmal in nature					
Sympathetic over-reactivity to normally non-painful stimuli					
Features persist for ≥3 consecutive days					
Features persist for ≥2 weeks post-brain injury					
Features persist despite treatment of alternative differential diagnoses					
Medication administered to decrease sympathetic features					
≥2 episodes daily					
Absence of parasympathetic features during episode					
Absence of other presumed causes of features					
Antecedent acquired brain injury					
DLT subtotal					
CFS + DLT total					
PSH diagnostic likelihood					Unlikely <8 Possible 8–16 Probable >17

Adapted from Baguley IJ, Perkes IE, Fernandez-Ortega F. Paroxysmal sympathetic hyperactivity after acquired brain injury: consensus on conceptual definition, nomenclature, and diagnostic criteria. J Neurotrauma.2014;31:1515–1520

individualized to the patient. Pharmacological management of PSH focuses on symptom management, prevention of symptoms, and treatment of refractory issues. Optimizing outcomes with medications and minimizing side effects are important. A combination of short-acting medications for termination of symptoms should be used with long-acting agents to prevent symptoms. Intravenous medications and continuous infusions should be added for refractory symptoms. Table 16.10 highlights the commonly used medications used to treat PSH and the symptoms they treat via their proposed mechanism.

Symptoms are often triggered by minimal external stimuli from routine patient care. Because of this, patients can be placed on minimal stimulation protocols to reduce the number of times interventions are performed.

Table 16.10 Medications used for treatment of paroxysmal sympathetic hyperactivity [170, 172]

Medication	Symptoms treated	Proposed mechanism
Clonidine	Hypertension	α-Agonist
Dexmedetomidine	Hypertension, agitation, tachycardia	α-Agonist
Propranolol	Hypertension, tachycardia, fever	β-Blocker
Dantrolene	Muscle rigidity, posturing	Calcium ion blocker
Bromocriptine	Dystonia, fever, posturing	Dopamine agonist
Gabapentin	Spasticity, allodynic response	GABA agonist
Benzodiazepines	Agitation, hypertension, tachycardia, posturing	$GABA_A$ agonist
Baclofen (oral and intrathecal)	Pain, clonus, rigidity	$GABA_B$ agonist
Morphine	Tachycardia, peripheral vasodilation, allodynic response	μ-Opiate agonist

16.8.2 Infections in TBI Patients

Patients with TBI can be hospitalized for long periods, and they are exposed to nosocomial infections due to the need for mechanical ventilation and urinary catheters [175–177]. Nosocomial infections affect approximately 30% of patients in the ICU, while they affect up to 50% of TBI patients [178–180]. Infections can develop in severe TBI patients due to extracranial injuries; however, the TBI injury can contribute to infections due to its ability to cause immunosuppression [181, 182].

Infections of concern in TBI patients include those related to the EVD, ventriculitis, and meningitis. Reported ventriculostomy-related infection (VRI) rates are as high as 32%; however, rates of less than 10% are most often reported [128, 183, 184]. Empiric therapy for healthcare-associated ventriculitis and meningitis includes vancomycin plus an anti-pseudomonal β-lactam (cefepime, ceftazidime, or meropenem) per the 2017 IDSA guidelines [185]. In patients with allergies to β-lactams who are not able to tolerate meropenem or if it is contraindicated, ciprofloxacin or aztreonam is recommended. In patients with infections due to *Candida* species, liposomal amphotericin B combined with 5-flucytosine is recommended initially; once clinical improvement is demonstrated, therapy may be changed to fluconazole based on susceptibilities.

When treating infections in the neuro ICU, the possibility of neurotoxicity with β-lactams should be considered. Patients should be monitored for decreased levels of consciousness, nonconvulsive status epilepticus, myoclonus, and new-onset psychiatric disorders [186, 187]. Beta-lactams competitively inhibit the gamma-aminobutyric acid A ($GABA_A$) receptor, which could lead to the neurotoxicity [188–190]. However, higher serum concentrations of β-lactams have been associated with neurotoxicity, predominantly in the setting of renal failure [191]. Of the β-lactams, cefepime is most often associated with neurotoxicity [191–196]. Cefepime-induced neurotoxicity has been associated with supratherapeutic levels as well as total exposure, defined by duration of therapy [191]. Risk factors associated with β-lactam neurotoxicity include age, baseline cognitive dysfunction, inappropriate dosing, and kidney dysfunction [197]. Because of the risk of neurotoxicity with any of the β-lactam, appropriate dose adjustments should be made in patients with renal dysfunction. Additionally, patients should be monitored for signs of neurotoxicity.

16.8.3 Central Fever

Fever affects approximately 70% of critically ill patients at some point during their hospital admission. In neuro ICU patients, only 50% of fevers are associated with an infection [198]. Fever in brain injury patients leads to larger infarct size in ischemic stroke patients, poorer outcomes in the acute phase of brain injury, and increased mortality [199].

Central or neurogenic fever is a noninfectious source of fever in TBI patients. Studies have reported the incidence ranges from 4% to 37% in TBI survivors [200, 201]. It is likely the result of an injury to the hypothalamus leading to a disruption in the hypothalamic set point temperature and an abnormal increase in body temperature. It is often characterized by bradycardia, lack of perspiration, high temperatures, and a plateau-like temperature curve that persists for days to weeks [200, 202]. However, others report that it results in high temperatures, tachycardia, hyperhidrosis, hypertension, and sometimes seizures [200, 202–204].

There are several etiologies of fever in ICU patients, including infection, venous thromboembolism, medications, surgery, atelectasis, and PSH. Diagnosis of central fever is a diagnosis of exclusion. Antipyretic medications including acetaminophen and nonsteroidal anti-inflammatory drugs (NSAIDs) often do not provide adequate temperature control [205]. When these agents fail to control the temperature, external cooling devices or endovascular cooling catheters may be tried [198]. Case reports discuss the potential benefits of bromocriptine, propranolol, and baclofen for the treatment of central fever [201, 206–210]. However, further evaluation of these agents for this indication is needed.

16.8.4 Sodium and Water Disorders

Patients may experience one of the three sodium/water disorders after a TBI. Diabetes insipidus (DI) is on the opposite spectrum of syndrome of inappropriate antidiuretic hormone secretion (SIADH) with regard to renal handling of water. SIADH and cerebral salt wasting (CSW) syndrome appear clinically similar and are often misdiagnosed for the other. However, SIADH is a "water" issue, while CSW is a "sodium" issue.

16.8.4.1 Diabetes Insipidus

Diabetes insipidus (DI) is characterized by polyuria (>50 mL/kg per 24 h), hypotonic urine (<300 mOsm/kg), and polydipsia [211, 212]. Because patients are often unable to sense or respond to thirst, polydipsia is absent. Serum sodium levels are often elevated due to the lack of compensation with fluid intake. There are four etiologic categories of DI, including central (or neurogenic) DI, nephrogenic DI, primary polydipsia, and gestational DI. Primary polydipsia and gestational DI are outside the scope of this review.

Nephrogenic DI is due to a renal insensitivity to the antidiuretic effect of normal levels of antidiuretic hormone or arginine vasopressin (AVP). There are genetic causes; however, medications and electrolyte disturbances (hypercalcemia or hypokalemia) are the most common causes of nephrogenic DI in the ICU. Up to 20% of patients who take lithium long-term will develop nephrogenic DI. Other agents reported to cause DI include demeclocycline, ofloxacin, foscarnet, clozapine, and orlistat [211, 213].

Central DI, the most common etiology for DI in the ICU, is due to a loss of production of AVP. Several cerebral diseases, such as tumor, granulomatosis, or meningitis, can lead to a loss of ADH secretion. However, the most common cause is injury to the posterior pituitary or hypothalamic median eminence. This may be due to a TBI, pituitary surgery, or cerebral edema/herniation.

Treatment of DI primarily consists of (1) replacing AVP to prevent ongoing renal water loss and (2) replacing water loss to correct hypernatremia. In the case of medication-induced nephrogenic DI, the offending medication should be identified and immediately discontinued.

16.8.4.2 Syndrome of Inappropriate Antidiuretic Hormone Secretion (SIADH)

SIADH accounts for one-third of all hyponatremia cases [214]. It occurs when secretion of AVP continues inappropriately with normal or decreased plasma osmolality. SIADH is considered a euvolemic hypotonic hyponatremic state. Diagnostic criteria include (1) serum sodium level of <135 mEq/L, (2) urine osmolality >100 mOsm/kg, (3) urine sodium concentration >20–30 meq/L, (4) clinical euvolemia or hypervolemia, (5) absence of other potential causes, and (6) normal renal function and absence of diuretic use [215].

Treatment of SIADH most commonly includes fluid restriction, treatment of underlying pathology, hypertonic saline, loop diuretics, desmopressin, and vasopressin receptor antagonists or "vaptans." Previously, drugs that cause DI such as demeclocycline and lithium were used to manage SIADH. However, this is not recommended due to the adverse effects of these medications. Choice of treatment is determined by symptoms of hyponatremia and underlying conditions. Patients exhibiting mild-to-moderate symptoms may require fluid restriction and treatment of underlying pathology. Patients with severe symptoms such as seizures or severe somnolence will require hypertonic saline.

The speed at which the sodium is corrected depends on whether the hyponatremia is considered acute (<24–48 h) or chronic (>48 h). An increase of 4–6 mEq/L of the serum sodium is sufficient to reverse the serious manifestations of hyponatremia including brain herniation and neurological damage. If there is any question as to whether or not the hyponatremia is acute or chronic, chronic correction recommendations should be followed. Minimum correction of sodium should be no more than 4–8 mEq/L per day, and no more than 4–6 mEq/L per day if there is a concern for osmotic demyelination syndrome. Previously, it was recommended that the limit should not exceed 10–12 mEq/L per 24-h period [215]. However, many now advocate increasing the serum sodium to no more than 8 mEq/L in a 24-h period [216].

16.8.4.3 Cerebral Salt Wasting Syndrome

Cerebral salt wasting (CSW) syndrome is a loss of sodium and water in the urine leading to a decrease in intravascular volume and hyponatremia. It is often associated with neurological disorders including SAH, head injury, and neurosurgical procedures. Differentiating CSW from SIADH is almost impossible.

Volume restriction, which is commonly done in SIADH, can be detrimental in neurological conditions, particularly in SAH patients. For this reason, most neurological ICU patients with hyponatremia are managed with various concentrations of sodium chloride or balanced sodium solutions depending on the serum sodium level and perceived intravascular volume.

16.9 Conclusion

Traumatic brain injury is a potentially devastating disease that is complicated by secondary injuries. Complications lead to further increases in morbidity and mortality. Patients with TBI should be treated in a dedicated neuro ICU in order to improve outcomes.

References

1. Maas AIR, Stocchetti N, Bullock R. Moderate and severe traumatic brain injury in adults. Lancet Neurol. 2008;7(8):728–41. https://doi.org/10.1016/S1474-4422(08)70164-9.
2. Guan B, Anderson DB, Chen L, Feng S, Zhou H. Global, regional and national burden of traumatic brain injury and spinal cord injury, 1990-2019: a systematic analysis for the global burden of disease study 2019. BMJ Open. 2023;13(10):e075049. https://doi.org/10.1136/bmjopen-2023-075049.
3. Wood RL. Understanding the "miserable minority": a diasthesis-stress paradigm for post-concussional syndrome. Brain Inj. 2004;18(11):1135–53. https://doi.org/10.1080/02699050410001675906.

4. Ruff RM, Camenzuli L, Mueller J. Miserable minority: emotional risk factors that influence the outcome of a mild traumatic brain injury. Brain Inj. 1996;10(8):551–65. https://doi.org/10.1080/026990596124124.
5. Harrison-Felix C, Pretz C, Hammond FM, et al. Life expectancy after inpatient rehabilitation for traumatic brain injury in the United States. J Neurotrauma. 2015;32(23):1893–901. https://doi.org/10.1089/neu.2014.3353.
6. Chesnut RM, Marshall LF, Klauber MR, et al. The role of secondary brain injury in determining outcome from severe head injury. J Trauma. 1993;34(2):216–22. https://doi.org/10.1097/00005373-199302000-00006.
7. Miller JD, Becker DP. Secondary insults to the injured brain. J R Coll Surg Edinb. 1982;27(5):292–8.
8. Hoh BL, Ko NU, Amin-Hanjani S, et al. 2023 guideline for the management of patients with aneurysmal subarachnoid hemorrhage: a guideline from the American Heart Association/American Stroke Association. Stroke. 2023;54(7):e314–70. https://doi.org/10.1161/STR.0000000000000436.
9. Ling GSF, Marshall SA. Management of traumatic brain injury in the intensive care unit. Neurol Clin. 2008;26(2):409–26, viii. https://doi.org/10.1016/j.ncl.2008.02.001.
10. Heegaard W, Biros M. Traumatic brain injury. Emerg Med Clin North Am. 2007;25(3):655–78, viii. https://doi.org/10.1016/j.emc.2007.07.001.
11. Dunn LT. Raised intracranial pressure. J Neurol Neurosurg Psychiatry. 2002;73 Suppl 1(Suppl 1):i23–7. https://doi.org/10.1136/jnnp.73.suppl_1.i23.
12. Gerber LM, Chiu YL, Carney N, Härtl R, Ghajar J. Marked reduction in mortality in patients with severe traumatic brain injury. J Neurosurg. 2013;119(6):1583–90. https://doi.org/10.3171/2013.8.JNS13276.
13. Carney N, Totten AM, O'Reilly C, et al. Guidelines for the management of severe traumatic brain injury, fourth edition. Neurosurgery. 2017;80(1):6–15. https://doi.org/10.1227/NEU.0000000000001432.
14. Patel HC, Menon DK, Tebbs S, Hawker R, Hutchinson PJ, Kirkpatrick PJ. Specialist neurocritical care and outcome from head injury. Intensive Care Med. 2002;28(5):547–53. https://doi.org/10.1007/s00134-002-1235-4.
15. Elf K, Nilsson P, Enblad P. Outcome after traumatic brain injury improved by an organized secondary insult program and standardized neurointensive care. Crit Care Med. 2002;30(9):2129–34. https://doi.org/10.1097/00003246-200209000-00029.
16. Teasdale G, Jennett B. Assessment of coma and impaired consciousness. A practical scale. Lancet. 1974;2(7872):81–4. https://doi.org/10.1016/s0140-6736(74)91639-0.
17. Burke AM, Quest DO, Chien S, Cerri C. The effects of mannitol on blood viscosity. J Neurosurg. 1981;55(4):550–3. https://doi.org/10.3171/jns.1981.55.4.0550.
18. Diringer MN, Zazulia AR. Osmotic therapy: fact and fiction. Neurocrit Care. 2004;1(2):219–33. https://doi.org/10.1385/NCC:1:2:219.
19. Alvarez B, Ferrer-Sueta G, Radi R. Slowing of peroxynitrite decomposition in the presence of mannitol and ethanol. Free Radic Biol Med. 1998;24(7–8):1331–7. https://doi.org/10.1016/s0891-5849(98)00005-7.
20. Paczynski RP. Osmotherapy. Basic concepts and controversies. Crit Care Clin. 1997;13(1):105–29. https://doi.org/10.1016/s0749-0704(05)70298-0.
21. Korenkov AI, Pahnke J, Frei K, et al. Treatment with nimodipine or mannitol reduces programmed cell death and infarct size following focal cerebral ischemia. Neurosurg Rev. 2000;23(3):145–50. https://doi.org/10.1007/pl00011946.
22. Doyle JA, Davis DP, Hoyt DB. The use of hypertonic saline in the treatment of traumatic brain injury. J Trauma. 2001;50(2):367–83. https://doi.org/10.1097/00005373-200102000-00030.
23. Cook AM, Morgan Jones G, Hawryluk GWJ, et al. Guidelines for the acute treatment of cerebral edema in neurocritical care patients. Neurocrit Care. 2020;32(3):647–66. https://doi.org/10.1007/s12028-020-00959-7.

24. Hawryluk GWJ, Aguilera S, Buki A, et al. A management algorithm for patients with intracranial pressure monitoring: the Seattle international severe traumatic brain injury consensus conference (SIBICC). Intensive Care Med. 2019;45(12):1783–94. https://doi.org/10.1007/s00134-019-05805-9.
25. Alam HB, Vercruysse G, Martin M, et al. Western trauma association critical decisions in trauma: management of intracranial hypertension in patients with severe traumatic brain injuries. J Trauma Acute Care Surg. 2020;88(2):345–51. https://doi.org/10.1097/TA.0000000000002555.
26. Torre-Healy A, Marko NF, Weil RJ. Hyperosmolar therapy for intracranial hypertension. Neurocrit Care. 2012;17(1):117–30. https://doi.org/10.1007/s12028-011-9649-x.
27. Borges HF, Hocks J, Kjellstrand CM. Mannitol intoxication in patients with renal failure. Arch Intern Med. 1982;142(1):63–6.
28. Coté CJ, Greenhow DE, Marshall BE. The hypotensive response to rapid intravenous administration of hypertonic solutions in man and in the rabbit. Anesthesiology. 1979;50(1):30–5. https://doi.org/10.1097/00000542-197901000-00007.
29. Fishman RA. Brain edema. N Engl J Med. 1975;293(14):706–11. https://doi.org/10.1056/NEJM197510022931407.
30. Javid M, Gilboe D, Cesario T. The rebound phenomenon and hypertonic solutions. J Neurosurg. 1964;21:1059–66. https://doi.org/10.3171/jns.1964.21.12.1059.
31. Maioriello AV, Chaljub G, Nauta HJW, Lacroix M. Chemical shift imaging of mannitol in acute cerebral ischemia. Case report J Neurosurg. 2002;97(3):687–91. https://doi.org/10.3171/jns.2002.97.3.0687.
32. Anderson P, Boréus L, Gordon E, et al. Use of mannitol during neurosurgery: interpatient variability in the plasma and CSF levels. Eur J Clin Pharmacol. 1988;35(6):643–9. https://doi.org/10.1007/BF00637601.
33. Rudehill A, Gordon E, Ohman G, Lindqvist C, Andersson P. Pharmacokinetics and effects of mannitol on hemodynamics, blood and cerebrospinal fluid electrolytes, and osmolality during intracranial surgery. J Neurosurg Anesthesiol. 1993;5(1):4–12. https://doi.org/10.1097/00008506-199301000-00002.
34. James HE, Langfitt TW, Kumar VS, Ghostine SY. Treatment of intracranial hypertension. Analysis of 105 consecutive, continuous recordings of intracranial pressure. Acta Neurochir. 1977;36(3–4):189–200. https://doi.org/10.1007/BF01405391.
35. Ravussin P, Archer DP, Tyler JL, et al. Effects of rapid mannitol infusion on cerebral blood volume. A positron emission tomographic study in dogs and man. J Neurosurg. 1986;64(1):104–13. https://doi.org/10.3171/jns.1986.64.1.0104.
36. Lin SY, Tang SC, Tsai LK, et al. Incidence and risk factors for acute kidney injury following mannitol infusion in patients with acute stroke. Medicine (Baltimore). 2015;94(47):e2032. https://doi.org/10.1097/MD.0000000000002032.
37. Better OS, Rubinstein I, Winaver JM, Knochel JP. Mannitol therapy revisited (1940–1997). Kidney Int. 1997;52(4):886–94. https://doi.org/10.1038/ki.1997.409.
38. Pérez-Pérez AJ, Pazos B, Sobrado J, Gonzalez L, Gándara A. Acute renal failure following massive mannitol infusion. Am J Nephrol. 2002;22(5–6):573–5. https://doi.org/10.1159/000065279.
39. Dickenmann M, Oettl T, Mihatsch MJ. Osmotic nephrosis: acute kidney injury with accumulation of proximal tubular lysosomes due to administration of exogenous solutes. Am J Kidney Dis. 2008;51(3):491–503. https://doi.org/10.1053/j.ajkd.2007.10.044.
40. Bentley ML, Corwin HL, Dasta J. Drug-induced acute kidney injury in the critically ill adult: recognition and prevention strategies. Crit Care Med. 2010;38(6 Suppl):S169–74. https://doi.org/10.1097/CCM.0b013e3181de0c60.
41. Frank JI. Large hemispheric infarction, deterioration, and intracranial pressure. Neurology. 1995;45(7):1286–90. https://doi.org/10.1212/wnl.45.7.1286.
42. García-Morales EJ, Cariappa R, Parvin CA, Scott MG, Diringer MN. Osmole gap in neurologic-neurosurgical intensive care unit: its normal value, calculation, and relation-

ship with mannitol serum concentrations. Crit Care Med. 2004;32(4):986–91. https://doi.org/10.1097/01.ccm.0000120057.04528.60.

43. Dorman HR, Sondheimer JH, Cadnapaphornchai P. Mannitol-induced acute renal failure. Medicine (Baltimore). 1990;69(3):153–9. https://doi.org/10.1097/00005792-199005000-00003.

44. Gadallah MF, Lynn M, Work J. Case report: mannitol nephrotoxicity syndrome: role of hemodialysis and postulate of mechanisms. Am J Med Sci. 1995;309(4):219–22. https://doi.org/10.1097/00000441-199504000-00006.

45. Rabetoy GM, Fredericks MR, Hostettler CF. Where the kidney is concerned, how much mannitol is too much? Ann Pharmacother. 1993;27(1):25–8. https://doi.org/10.1177/106002809302700105.

46. Hays AN, Lazaridis C, Neyens R, Nicholas J, Gay S, Chalela JA. Osmotherapy: use among neurointensivists. Neurocrit Care. 2011;14(2):222–8. https://doi.org/10.1007/s12028-010-9477-4.

47. Erstad BL. Peripheral intravenous administration of 23.4% sodium chloride solution: a plea for caution. Am J Health Syst Pharm. 2023;80(15):1032–5. https://doi.org/10.1093/ajhp/zxad103.

48. Holden DN, Mucksavage JJ, Cokley JA, et al. Hypertonic saline use in neurocritical care for treating cerebral edema: a review of optimal formulation, dosing, safety, administration and storage. Am J Health Syst Pharm. 2023;80(6):331–42. https://doi.org/10.1093/ajhp/zxac368.

49. Perez CA, Figueroa SA. Complication rates of 3% hypertonic saline infusion through peripheral intravenous access. J Neurosci Nurs. 2017;49(3):191–5. https://doi.org/10.1097/JNN.0000000000000286.

50. Faiver L, Hensler D, Rush SC, Kashlan O, Williamson CA, Rajajee V. Safety and efficacy of 23.4% sodium chloride administered via peripheral venous access for the treatment of cerebral herniation and intracranial pressure elevation. Neurocrit Care. 2021;35(3):845–52. https://doi.org/10.1007/s12028-021-01248-7.

51. Jones GM, Bode L, Riha H, Erdman MJ. Safety of continuous peripheral infusion of 3% sodium chloride solution in neurocritical care patients. Am J Crit Care. 2016;26(1):37–42. https://doi.org/10.4037/ajcc2017439.

52. Mesghali E, Fitter S, Bahjri K, Moussavi K. Safety of peripheral line administration of 3% hypertonic saline and mannitol in the emergency department. J Emerg Med. 2019;56(4):431–6. https://doi.org/10.1016/j.jemermed.2018.12.046.

53. Merrer J, De Jonghe B, Golliot F, et al. Complications of femoral and subclavian venous catheterization in critically ill patients: a randomized controlled trial. JAMA. 2001;286(6):700–7. https://doi.org/10.1001/jama.286.6.700.

54. Vedantam A, Robertson CS, Gopinath SP. Morbidity and mortality associated with hypernatremia in patients with severe traumatic brain injury. Neurosurg Focus. 2017;43(5):E2. https://doi.org/10.3171/2017.7.FOCUS17418.

55. Aiyagari V, Deibert E, Diringer MN. Hypernatremia in the neurologic intensive care unit: how high is too high? J Crit Care. 2006;21(2):163–72. https://doi.org/10.1016/j.jcrc.2005.10.002.

56. Lee YI, Ahn J, Ryu JA. Clinical outcomes associated with degree of hypernatremia in neurocritically ill patients. J Korean Neurosurg Soc. 2023;66(1):95–104. https://doi.org/10.3340/jkns.2022.0161.

57. Hawryluk GWJ, Editorial. Sodium values and the use of hyperosmolar therapy following traumatic brain injury. Neurosurg Focus. 2017;43(5):E3. https://doi.org/10.3171/2017.8.FOCUS17506.

58. Nagami GT. Hyperchloremia—why and how. Nefrologia. 2016;36(4):347–53. https://doi.org/10.1016/j.nefro.2016.04.001.

59. Zhang Z, Xu X, Fan H, Li D, Deng H. Higher serum chloride concentrations are associated with acute kidney injury in unselected critically ill patients. BMC Nephrol. 2013;14:235. https://doi.org/10.1186/1471-2369-14-235.

60. Yunos NM, Bellomo R, Hegarty C, Story D, Ho L, Bailey M. Association between a chloride-liberal vs chloride-restrictive intravenous fluid administration strategy and kidney injury in critically ill adults. JAMA. 2012;308(15):1566–72. https://doi.org/10.1001/jama.2012.13356.

61. Semler MW, Self WH, Wanderer JP, et al. Balanced crystalloids versus saline in critically ill adults. N Engl J Med. 2018;378(9):829–39. https://doi.org/10.1056/NEJMoa1711584.

62. Cook AM, Cook TS, Rosen-Lamer A. Errors with extemporaneous compounding of buffered hypertonic saline. Am J Health Syst Pharm. 2020;77(19):1543–5. https://doi.org/10.1093/ajhp/zxaa226.

63. Aegisdottir H, Cooray C, Wirdefeldt K, Piehl F, Sveinsson O. Incidence of osmotic demyelination syndrome in Sweden: a nationwide study. Acta Neurol Scand. 2019;140(5):342–9. https://doi.org/10.1111/ane.13150.

64. Devlin JW, Skrobik Y, Gélinas C, et al. Clinical practice guidelines for the prevention and management of pain, agitation/sedation, delirium, immobility, and sleep disruption in adult patients in the ICU. Crit Care Med. 2018;46(9):e825–73. https://doi.org/10.1097/CCM.0000000000003299.

65. Rhoney DH, Parker D. Use of sedative and analgesic agents in neurotrauma patients: effects on cerebral physiology. Neurol Res. 2001;23(2–3):237–59. https://doi.org/10.1179/016164101101198398.

66. Oddo M, Crippa IA, Mehta S, et al. Optimizing sedation in patients with acute brain injury. Crit Care. 2016;20(1):128. https://doi.org/10.1186/s13054-016-1294-5.

67. Shapiro HM, Wyte SR, Loeser J. Barbiturate-augmented hypothermia for reduction of persistent intracranial hypertension. J Neurosurg. 1974;40(1):90–100. https://doi.org/10.3171/jns.1974.40.1.0090.

68. Bricolo AP, Glick RP. Barbiturate effects on acute experimental intracranial hypertension. J Neurosurg. 1981;55(3):397–406. https://doi.org/10.3171/jns.1981.55.3.0397.

69. Roberts I, Sydenham E. Barbiturates for acute traumatic brain injury. Cochrane Database Syst Rev. 2012;2012(12):CD000033. https://doi.org/10.1002/14651858.CD000033.pub2.

70. Roberts DJ, Hall RI, Kramer AH, Robertson HL, Gallagher CN, Zygun DA. Sedation for critically ill adults with severe traumatic brain injury: a systematic review of randomized controlled trials. Crit Care Med. 2011;39(12):2743–51. https://doi.org/10.1097/CCM.0b013e318228236f.

71. Bilotta F, Gelb AW, Stazi E, Titi L, Paoloni FP, Rosa G. Pharmacological perioperative brain neuroprotection: a qualitative review of randomized clinical trials. Br J Anaesth. 2013;110(Suppl 1):i113–20. https://doi.org/10.1093/bja/aet059.

72. Eisenberg HM, Frankowski RF, Contant CF, Marshall LF, Walker MD. High-dose barbiturate control of elevated intracranial pressure in patients with severe head injury. J Neurosurg. 1988;69(1):15–23. https://doi.org/10.3171/jns.1988.69.1.0015.

73. Schwartz ML, Tator CH, Rowed DW, Reid SR, Meguro K, Andrews DF. The University of Toronto head injury treatment study: a prospective, randomized comparison of pentobarbital and mannitol. Can J Neurol Sci. 1984;11(4):434–40. https://doi.org/10.1017/s0317167100045960.

74. Ward JD, Becker DP, Miller JD, et al. Failure of prophylactic barbiturate coma in the treatment of severe head injury. J Neurosurg. 1985;62(3):383–8. https://doi.org/10.3171/jns.1985.62.3.0383.

75. Drakulovic MB, Torres A, Bauer TT, Nicolas JM, Nogué S, Ferrer M. Supine body position as a risk factor for nosocomial pneumonia in mechanically ventilated patients: a randomised trial. Lancet. 1999;354(9193):1851–8. https://doi.org/10.1016/S0140-6736(98)12251-1.

76. Feldman Z, Kanter MJ, Robertson CS, et al. Effect of head elevation on intracranial pressure, cerebral perfusion pressure, and cerebral blood flow in head-injured patients. J Neurosurg. 1992;76(2):207–11. https://doi.org/10.3171/jns.1992.76.2.0207.

77. Kenning JA, Toutant SM, Saunders RL. Upright patient positioning in the management of intracranial hypertension. Surg Neurol. 1981;15(2):148–52. https://doi.org/10.1016/0090-3019(81)90037-9.

78. Ropper AH, O'Rourke D, Kennedy SK. Head position, intracranial pressure, and compliance. Neurology. 1982;32(11):1288–91. https://doi.org/10.1212/wnl.32.11.1288.
79. Burnol L, Payen JF, Francony G, et al. Impact of head-of-bed posture on brain oxygenation in patients with acute brain injury: a prospective cohort study. Neurocrit Care. 2021;35(3):662–8. https://doi.org/10.1007/s12028-021-01240-1.
80. O'Grady NP, Alexander E, Alhazzani W, et al. Society of critical care medicine and the infectious diseases society of America guidelines for evaluating new fever in adult patients in the ICU. Crit Care Med. 2023;51(11):1570–86. https://doi.org/10.1097/CCM.0000000000006022.
81. Marion DW. Controlled normothermia in neurologic intensive care. Crit Care Med. 2004;32(2 Suppl):S43–5. https://doi.org/10.1097/01.ccm.0000110731.69637.16.
82. Li J, Jiang J, yao. Chinese Head Trauma Data Bank: effect of hyperthermia on the outcome of acute head trauma patients. J Neurotrauma. 2012;29(1):96–100. https://doi.org/10.1089/neu.2011.1753.
83. Bao L, Chen D, Ding L, Ling W, Xu F. Fever burden is an independent predictor for prognosis of traumatic brain injury. PLoS One. 2014;9(3):e90956. https://doi.org/10.1371/journal.pone.0090956.
84. Puccio AM, Fischer MR, Jankowitz BT, Yonas H, Darby JM, Okonkwo DO. Induced normothermia attenuates intracranial hypertension and reduces fever burden after severe traumatic brain injury. Neurocrit Care. 2009;11(1):82–7. https://doi.org/10.1007/s12028-009-9213-0.
85. Greer DM, Funk SE, Reaven NL, Ouzounelli M, Uman GC. Impact of fever on outcome in patients with stroke and neurologic injury: a comprehensive meta-analysis. Stroke. 2008;39(11):3029–35. https://doi.org/10.1161/STROKEAHA.108.521583.
86. Stocchetti N, Protti A, Lattuada M, et al. Impact of pyrexia on neurochemistry and cerebral oxygenation after acute brain injury. J Neurol Neurosurg Psychiatry. 2005;76(8):1135–9. https://doi.org/10.1136/jnnp.2004.041269.
87. Cairns CJS, Andrews PJD. Management of hyperthermia in traumatic brain injury. Curr Opin Crit Care. 2002;8(2):106–10. https://doi.org/10.1097/00075198-200204000-00003.
88. Choi HA, Ko SB, Presciutti M, et al. Prevention of shivering during therapeutic temperature modulation: the Columbia anti-shivering protocol. Neurocrit Care. 2011;14(3):389–94. https://doi.org/10.1007/s12028-010-9474-7.
89. Lyeth BG, Jiang JY, Liu S. Behavioral protection by moderate hypothermia initiated after experimental traumatic brain injury. J Neurotrauma. 1993;10(1):57–64. https://doi.org/10.1089/neu.1993.10.57.
90. Polderman KH. Mechanisms of action, physiological effects, and complications of hypothermia. Crit Care Med. 2009;37(7 Suppl):S186–202. https://doi.org/10.1097/CCM.0b013e3181aa5241.
91. Sahuquillo J, Vilalta A. Cooling the injured brain: how does moderate hypothermia influence the pathophysiology of traumatic brain injury. Curr Pharm Des. 2007;13(22):2310–22. https://doi.org/10.2174/138161207781368756.
92. Wright S, Peralta S, Ranasinghe L. A review of adverse effects of targeted temperature management for post-cardiac arrest patients. AJBSR. 2020;9(1):043.
93. Uski J, Lamusuo S, Teperi S, Löyttyniemi E, Tenovuo O. Mortality after traumatic brain injury and the effect of posttraumatic epilepsy. Neurology. 2018;91(9):e878–83. https://doi.org/10.1212/WNL.0000000000006077.
94. Englander J, Cifu DX, Diaz-Arrastia R. Information/education page. Seizures and traumatic brain injury. Arch Phys Med Rehabil. 2014;95(6):1223–4. https://doi.org/10.1016/j.apmr.2013.06.002.
95. Torbic H, Forni AA, Anger KE, Degrado JR, Greenwood BC. Use of antiepileptics for seizure prophylaxis after traumatic brain injury. Am J Health Syst Pharm. 2013;70(9):759–66. https://doi.org/10.2146/ajhp120203.
96. Laing J, Gabbe B, Chen Z, Perucca P, Kwan P, O'Brien TJ. Risk factors and prognosis of early posttraumatic seizures in moderate to severe traumatic brain injury. JAMA Neurol. 2022;79(4):334–41. https://doi.org/10.1001/jamaneurol.2021.5420.

97. Pease M, Mallela AN, Elmer J, et al. Association of posttraumatic epilepsy with long-term functional outcomes in individuals with severe traumatic brain injury. Neurology. 2023;100(19):e1967–75. https://doi.org/10.1212/WNL.0000000000207183.

98. Pease M, Gonzalez-Martinez J, Puccio A, et al. Risk factors and incidence of epilepsy after severe traumatic brain injury. Ann Neurol. 2022;92(4):663–9. https://doi.org/10.1002/ana.26443.

99. Temkin NR. Risk factors for posttraumatic seizures in adults. Epilepsia. 2003;44(s10):18–20. https://doi.org/10.1046/j.1528-1157.44.s10.6.x.

100. Yablon SA. Posttraumatic seizures. Arch Phys Med Rehabil. 1993;74(9):983–1001.

101. Montgomery MC, Chou JW, McPharlin TO, Baird GS, Anderson GD. Predicting unbound phenytoin concentrations: effects of albumin concentration and kidney dysfunction. Pharmacotherapy. 2019;39(7):756–66. https://doi.org/10.1002/phar.2273.

102. Cheng W, Kiang TKL, Bring P, Ensom MHH. Predictive performance of the winter-Tozer and derivative equations for estimating free phenytoin concentration. Can J Hosp Pharm. 2016;69(4):269–79. https://doi.org/10.4212/cjhp.v69i4.1573.

103. Algren DA, Christian MR. Phenytoin toxicity unlikely to result in arrhythmias. JAMA Intern Med. 2014;174(1):167. https://doi.org/10.1001/jamainternmed.2013.11177.

104. Earnest MP, Marx JA, Drury LR. Complications of intravenous phenytoin for acute treatment of seizures. Recommendations for usage. JAMA. 1983;249(6):762–5.

105. Okogbaa JI, Onor IO, Arije OA, Harris MB, Lillis RA. Phenytoin-induced purple glove syndrome: a case report and review of the literature. Hosp Pharm. 2015;50(5):391–5. https://doi.org/10.1310/hpj5005-391.

106. Adams BD, Buckley NH, Kim JY, Tipps LB. Fosphenytoin may cause hemodynamically unstable bradydysrhythmias. J Emerg Med. 2006;30(1):75–9. https://doi.org/10.1016/j.jemermed.2005.01.034.

107. Thomson A. Fosphenytoin for the treatment of status epilepticus: an evidence-based assessment of its clinical and economic outcomes. Core Evid. 2005;1(1):65–75.

108. Swadron SP, Rudis MI, Azimian K, Beringer P, Fort D, Orlinsky M. A comparison of phenytoin-loading techniques in the emergency department. Acad Emerg Med. 2004;11(3):244–52. https://doi.org/10.1111/j.1553-2712.2004.tb02204.x.

109. Newman JW, Blunck JR, Fields RK, Croom JE. Fosphenytoin-induced purple glove syndrome: a case report. Clin Neurol Neurosurg. 2017;160:50–3. https://doi.org/10.1016/j.clineuro.2017.06.006.

110. Ohman K, Kram B, Schultheis J, et al. Evaluation of levetiracetam dosing strategies for seizure prophylaxis following traumatic brain injury. Neurocrit Care. 2023;38(2):345–55. https://doi.org/10.1007/s12028-022-01599-9.

111. Haller JT, Bonnin S, Radosevich J. Rapid administration of undiluted intravenous levetiracetam. Epilepsia. 2021;62(8):1865–70. https://doi.org/10.1111/epi.16961.

112. Morgan O, Medenwald B. Safety and tolerability of rapid administration undiluted levetiracetam. Neurocrit Care. 2020;32(1):131–4. https://doi.org/10.1007/s12028-019-00708-5.

113. Thelengana A, Shukla G, Srivastava A, et al. Cognitive, behavioural and sleep-related adverse effects on introduction of levetiracetam versus oxcarbazepine for epilepsy. Epilepsy Res. 2019;150:58–65. https://doi.org/10.1016/j.eplepsyres.2019.01.004.

114. Wu MF, Lim WH. Phenytoin: a guide to therapeutic drug monitoring. Proc Singapore Healthcare. 2013;22(3):198–202. https://doi.org/10.1177/201010581302200307.

115. Geerts WH, Code KI, Jay RM, Chen E, Szalai JP. A prospective study of venous thromboembolism after major trauma. N Engl J Med. 1994;331(24):1601–6. https://doi.org/10.1056/NEJM199412153312401.

116. Denson K, Morgan D, Cunningham R, et al. Incidence of venous thromboembolism in patients with traumatic brain injury. Am J Surg. 2007;193(3):380–3; discussion 383–384. https://doi.org/10.1016/j.amjsurg.2006.12.004.

117. Ley EJ, Brown CVR, Moore EE, et al. Updated guidelines to reduce venous thromboembolism in trauma patients: a Western trauma association critical decisions algorithm. J Trauma Acute Care Surg. 2020;89(5):971–81. https://doi.org/10.1097/TA.0000000000002830.

118. Vandiver JW, Ritz LI, Lalama JT. Chemical prophylaxis to prevent venous thromboembolism in morbid obesity: literature review and dosing recommendations. J Thromb Thrombolysis. 2016;41(3):475–81. https://doi.org/10.1007/s11239-015-1231-5.

119. Greenfield LJ, Proctor MC, Rodriguez JL, Luchette FA, Cipolle MD, Cho J. Posttrauma thromboembolism prophylaxis. J Trauma. 1997;42(1):100–3. https://doi.org/10.1097/00005373-199701000-00017.

120. Rogers FB, Shackford SR, Horst MA, et al. Determining venous thromboembolic risk assessment for patients with trauma: the trauma embolic scoring system. J Trauma Acute Care Surg. 2012;73(2):511–5. https://doi.org/10.1097/ta.0b013e3182588b54.

121. Walker PF, Schobel S, Caruso JD, et al. Trauma embolic scoring system in military trauma: a sensitive predictor of venous thromboembolism. Trauma Surg Acute Care Open. 2019;4(1):e000367. https://doi.org/10.1136/tsaco-2019-000367.

122. Phelan HA. Pharmacologic venous thromboembolism prophylaxis after traumatic brain injury: a critical literature review. J Neurotrauma. 2012;29(10):1821–8. https://doi.org/10.1089/neu.2012.2459.

123. Lozier AP, Sciacca RR, Romagnoli MF, Connolly ES. Ventriculostomy-related infections: a critical review of the literature. Neurosurgery. 2002;51(1):170–81; discussion 181–182. https://doi.org/10.1097/00006123-200207000-00024.

124. Hoefnagel D, Dammers R, Ter Laak-Poort MP, Avezaat CJJ. Risk factors for infections related to external ventricular drainage. Acta Neurochir. 2008;150(3):209–14; discussion 214. https://doi.org/10.1007/s00701-007-1458-9.

125. Edwards NC, Engelhart L, Casamento EMH, McGirt MJ. Cost-consequence analysis of antibiotic-impregnated shunts and external ventricular drains in hydrocephalus. J Neurosurg. 2015;122(1):139–47. https://doi.org/10.3171/2014.9.JNS131277.

126. Alleyne CH, Hassan M, Zabramski JM. The efficacy and cost of prophylactic and periprocedural antibiotics in patients with external ventricular drains. Neurosurgery. 2000;47(5):1124–7.; discussion 1127-1129. https://doi.org/10.1097/00006123-200011000-00020.

127. Edwards P, Arango M, Balica L, et al. Final results of MRC CRASH, a randomised placebo-controlled trial of intravenous corticosteroid in adults with head injury-outcomes at 6 months. Lancet. 2005;365(9475):1957–9. https://doi.org/10.1016/S0140-6736(05)66552-X.

128. Fried HI, Nathan BR, Rowe AS, et al. The insertion and management of external ventricular drains: an evidence-based consensus statement: a statement for healthcare professionals from the neurocritical care society. Neurocrit Care. 2016;24(1):61–81. https://doi.org/10.1007/s12028-015-0224-8.

129. Ratilal B, Costa J, Sampaio C. Antibiotic prophylaxis for surgical introduction of intracranial ventricular shunts: a systematic review. J Neurosurg Pediatr. 2008;1(1):48–56. https://doi.org/10.3171/PED-08/01/048.

130. Bratzler DW, Dellinger EP, Olsen KM, et al. Clinical practice guidelines for antimicrobial prophylaxis in surgery. Am J Health Syst Pharm. 2013;70(3):195–283. https://doi.org/10.2146/ajhp120568.

131. Quenot JP, Thiery N, Barbar S. When should stress ulcer prophylaxis be used in the ICU? Curr Opin Crit Care. 2009;15(2):139–43. https://doi.org/10.1097/MCC.0b013e32832978e0.

132. Moody FG, Cheung LY. Stress ulcers: their pathogenesis, diagnosis, and treatment. Surg Clin North Am. 1976;56(6):1469–78. https://doi.org/10.1016/s0039-6109(16)41099-6.

133. Kemp WJ, Bashir A, Dababneh H, Cohen-Gadol AA. Cushing's ulcer: further reflections. Asian J Neurosurg. 2015;10(2):87–94. https://doi.org/10.4103/1793-5482.154976.

134. Helmy A, Vizcaychipi M, Gupta AK. Traumatic brain injury: intensive care management. Br J Anaesth. 2007;99(1):32–42. https://doi.org/10.1093/bja/aem139.

135. Mohebbi L, Hesch K. Stress ulcer prophylaxis in the intensive care unit. Proc (Bayl Univ Med Cent). 2009;22(4):373–6. https://doi.org/10.1080/08998280.2009.11928562.

136. Cook D, Guyatt G. Prophylaxis against upper gastrointestinal bleeding in hospitalized patients. N Engl J Med. 2018;378(26):2506–16. https://doi.org/10.1056/NEJMra1605507.

137. Barletta JF, Bruno JJ, Buckley MS, Cook DJ. Stress ulcer prophylaxis. Crit Care Med. 2016;44(7):1395–405. https://doi.org/10.1097/CCM.0000000000001872.

138. Cook DJ, Griffith LE, Walter SD, et al. The attributable mortality and length of intensive care unit stay of clinically important gastrointestinal bleeding in critically ill patients. Crit Care. 2001;5(6):368–75. https://doi.org/10.1186/cc1071.

139. Tsiotos GG, Mullany CJ, Zietlow S, van Heerden JA. Abdominal complications following cardiac surgery. Am J Surg. 1994;167(6):553–7. https://doi.org/10.1016/0002-9610(94)90096-5.

140. ASHP Therapeutic Guidelines on Stress Ulcer Prophylaxis. ASHP commission on therapeutics and approved by the ASHP board of directors on November 14, 1998. Am J Health Syst Pharm. 1999;56(4):347–79. https://doi.org/10.1093/ajhp/56.4.347.

141. Spirt MJ. Stress-related mucosal disease: risk factors and prophylactic therapy. Clin Ther. 2004;26(2):197–213. https://doi.org/10.1016/s0149-2918(04)90019-7.

142. Cook DJ, Fuller HD, Guyatt GH, et al. Risk factors for gastrointestinal bleeding in critically ill patients. Canadian critical care trials group. N Engl J Med. 1994;330(6):377–81. https://doi.org/10.1056/NEJM199402103300601.

143. Rhodes A, Evans LE, Alhazzani W, et al. Surviving sepsis campaign: international guidelines for management of sepsis and septic shock: 2016. Crit Care Med. 2017;45(3):486–552. https://doi.org/10.1097/CCM.0000000000002255.

144. Schunack W. What are the differences between the H2-receptor antagonists? Aliment Pharmacol Ther. 1987;1(Suppl 1):493S–503S. https://doi.org/10.1111/j.1365-2036.1987.tb00658.x.

145. CRASH-3 trial collaborators. Effects of tranexamic acid on death, disability, vascular occlusive events and other morbidities in patients with acute traumatic brain injury (CRASH-3): a randomised, placebo-controlled trial. Lancet. 2019;394(10210):1713–23. https://doi.org/10.1016/S0140-6736(19)32233-0.

146. Lier H, Maegele M, Shander A. Tranexamic acid for acute hemorrhage: a narrative review of landmark studies and a critical reappraisal of its use over the last decade. Anesth Analg. 2019;129(6):1574–84. https://doi.org/10.1213/ANE.0000000000004389.

147. CRASH-2 Trial Collaborators, Shakur H, Roberts I, et al. Effects of tranexamic acid on death, vascular occlusive events, and blood transfusion in trauma patients with significant haemorrhage (CRASH-2): a randomised, placebo-controlled trial. Lancet. 2010;376(9734):23–32. https://doi.org/10.1016/S0140-6736(10)60835-5.

148. Kim C, Park SSH, Davey JR. Tranexamic acid for the prevention and management of orthopedic surgical hemorrhage: current evidence. J Blood Med. 2015;6:239–44. https://doi.org/10.2147/JBM.S61915.

149. Oertel M, Kelly DF, McArthur D, et al. Progressive hemorrhage after head trauma: predictors and consequences of the evolving injury. J Neurosurg. 2002;96(1):109–16. https://doi.org/10.3171/jns.2002.96.1.0109.

150. Narayan RK, Maas AIR, Servadei F, et al. Progression of traumatic intracerebral hemorrhage: a prospective observational study. J Neurotrauma. 2008;25(6):629–39. https://doi.org/10.1089/neu.2007.0385.

151. Zhang J, He M, Song Y, Xu J. Prognostic role of D-dimer level upon admission in patients with traumatic brain injury. Medicine (Baltimore). 2018;97(31):e11774. https://doi.org/10.1097/MD.0000000000011774.

152. Honeybul S, Ho KM, Rosenfeld JV. The role of tranexamic acid in traumatic brain injury. J Clin Neurosci. 2022;99:1–4. https://doi.org/10.1016/j.jocn.2022.02.029.

153. Taccone FS, Citerio G, Stocchetti N. Is tranexamic acid going to CRASH the management of traumatic brain injury? Intensive Care Med. 2020;46(6):1261–3. https://doi.org/10.1007/s00134-019-05879-5.

154. Lawati KA, Sharif S, Maqbali SA, et al. Efficacy and safety of tranexamic acid in acute traumatic brain injury: a systematic review and meta-analysis of randomized-controlled trials. Intensive Care Med. 2021;47(1):14–27. https://doi.org/10.1007/s00134-020-06279-w.

155. Jones PA, Andrews PJ, Midgley S, et al. Measuring the burden of secondary insults in head-injured patients during intensive care. J Neurosurg Anesthesiol. 1994;6(1):4–14.
156. Rovlias A, Kotsou S. The influence of hyperglycemia on neurological outcome in patients with severe head injury. Neurosurgery. 2000;46(2):335–42; discussion 342–343. https://doi.org/10.1097/00006123-200002000-00015.
157. Cochran A, Scaife ER, Hansen KW, Downey EC. Hyperglycemia and outcomes from pediatric traumatic brain injury. J Trauma. 2003;55(6):1035–8. https://doi.org/10.1097/01.TA.0000031175.96507.48.
158. De Salles AA, Muizelaar JP, Young HF. Hyperglycemia, cerebrospinal fluid lactic acidosis, and cerebral blood flow in severely head-injured patients. Neurosurgery. 1987;21(1):45–50. https://doi.org/10.1227/00006123-198707000-00009.
159. Rosner MJ, Newsome HH, Becker DP. Mechanical brain injury: the sympathoadrenal response. J Neurosurg. 1984;61(1):76–86. https://doi.org/10.3171/jns.1984.61.1.0076.
160. Welsh FA, Ginsberg MD, Rieder W, Budd WW. Deleterious effect of glucose pretreatment on recovery from diffuse cerebral ischemia in the cat. II Regional metabolite levels. Stroke. 1980;11(4):355–63. https://doi.org/10.1161/01.str.11.4.355.
161. Oddo M, Schmidt JM, Mayer SA, Chioléro RL. Glucose control after severe brain injury. Curr Opin Clin Nutr Metab Care. 2008;11(2):134–9. https://doi.org/10.1097/MCO.0b013e3282f37b43.
162. Zygun DA, Steiner LA, Johnston AJ, et al. Hyperglycemia and brain tissue pH after traumatic brain injury. Neurosurgery. 2004;55(4):877–81.; discussion 882. https://doi.org/10.1227/01.neu.0000137658.14906.e4.
163. Abi-Saab WM, Maggs DG, Jones T, et al. Striking differences in glucose and lactate levels between brain extracellular fluid and plasma in conscious human subjects: effects of hyperglycemia and hypoglycemia. J Cereb Blood Flow Metab. 2002;22(3):271–9. https://doi.org/10.1097/00004647-200203000-00004.
164. Parkin M, Hopwood S, Jones DA, et al. Dynamic changes in brain glucose and lactate in pericontusional areas of the human cerebral cortex, monitored with rapid sampling on-line microdialysis: relationship with depolarisation-like events. J Cereb Blood Flow Metab. 2005;25(3):402–13. https://doi.org/10.1038/sj.jcbfm.9600051.
165. Vespa P, McArthur DL, Stein N, et al. Tight glycemic control increases metabolic distress in traumatic brain injury: a randomized controlled within-subjects trial. Crit Care Med. 2012;40(6):1923–9. https://doi.org/10.1097/CCM.0b013e31824e0fcc.
166. Vespa P, Boonyaputthikul R, McArthur DL, et al. Intensive insulin therapy reduces microdialysis glucose values without altering glucose utilization or improving the lactate/pyruvate ratio after traumatic brain injury. Crit Care Med. 2006;34(3):850–6. https://doi.org/10.1097/01.CCM.0000201875.12245.6F.
167. Vespa PM, McArthur D, O'Phelan K, et al. Persistently low extracellular glucose correlates with poor outcome 6 months after human traumatic brain injury despite a lack of increased lactate: a microdialysis study. J Cereb Blood Flow Metab. 2003;23(7):865–77. https://doi.org/10.1097/01.WCB.0000076701.45782.EF.
168. Ryken TC, McDermott M, Robinson PD, et al. The role of steroids in the management of brain metastases: a systematic review and evidence-based clinical practice guideline. J Neuro-Oncol. 2010;96(1):103–14. https://doi.org/10.1007/s11060-009-0057-4.
169. Alderson P, Roberts I. Corticosteroids in acute traumatic brain injury: systematic review of randomised controlled trials. BMJ. 1997;314(7098):1855–9. https://doi.org/10.1136/bmj.314.7098.1855.
170. Samuel S, Allison TA, Lee K, Choi HA. Pharmacologic management of paroxysmal sympathetic hyperactivity after brain injury. J Neurosci Nurs. 2016;48(2):82–9. https://doi.org/10.1097/JNN.0000000000000207.
171. Baguley IJ, Perkes IE, Fernandez-Ortega JF, et al. Paroxysmal sympathetic hyperactivity after acquired brain injury: consensus on conceptual definition, nomenclature, and diagnostic criteria. J Neurotrauma. 2014;31(17):1515–20. https://doi.org/10.1089/neu.2013.3301.

172. Choi HA, Jeon SB, Samuel S, Allison T, Lee K. Paroxysmal sympathetic hyperactivity after acute brain injury. Curr Neurol Neurosci Rep. 2013;13(8):370. https://doi.org/10.1007/s11910-013-0370-3.
173. Fernandez-Ortega JF, Prieto-Palomino MA, Garcia-Caballero M, Galeas-Lopez JL, Quesada-Garcia G, Baguley IJ. Paroxysmal sympathetic hyperactivity after traumatic brain injury: clinical and prognostic implications. J Neurotrauma. 2012;29(7):1364–70. https://doi.org/10.1089/neu.2011.2033.
174. Baguley IJ, Heriseanu RE, Nott MT, Chapman J, Sandanam J. Dysautonomia after severe traumatic brain injury: evidence of persisting overresponsiveness to afferent stimuli. Am J Phys Med Rehabil. 2009;88(8):615–22. https://doi.org/10.1097/PHM.0b013e3181aeab96.
175. Sharma R, Shultz SR, Robinson MJ, et al. Infections after a traumatic brain injury: the complex interplay between the immune and neurological systems. Brain Behav Immun. 2019;79:63–74. https://doi.org/10.1016/j.bbi.2019.04.034.
176. Alharfi IM, Charyk Stewart T, Al Helali I, Daoud H, Fraser DD. Infection rates, fevers, and associated factors in pediatric severe traumatic brain injury. J Neurotrauma. 2014;31(5):452–8. https://doi.org/10.1089/neu.2013.2904.
177. Vincent JL, Bihari DJ, Suter PM, et al. The prevalence of nosocomial infection in intensive care units in Europe. Results of the European Prevalence of Infection in Intensive Care (EPIC) Study. EPIC International Advisory Committee. JAMA. 1995;274(8):639–44.
178. Dziedzic T, Slowik A, Szczudlik A. Nosocomial infections and immunity: lesson from brain-injured patients. Crit Care. 2004;8(4):266–70. https://doi.org/10.1186/cc2828.
179. Vincent JL. Nosocomial infections in adult intensive-care units. Lancet. 2003;361(9374):2068–77. https://doi.org/10.1016/S0140-6736(03)13644-6.
180. Kourbeti IS, Vakis AF, Papadakis JA, et al. Infections in traumatic brain injury patients. Clin Microbiol Infect. 2012;18(4):359–64. https://doi.org/10.1111/j.1469-0691.2011.03625.x.
181. Hazeldine J, Naumann DN, Toman E, et al. Prehospital immune responses and development of multiple organ dysfunction syndrome following traumatic injury: a prospective cohort study. PLoS Med. 2017;14(7):e1002338. https://doi.org/10.1371/journal.pmed.1002338.
182. Wolach B, Sazbon L, Gavrieli R, Broda A, Schlesinger M. Early immunological defects in comatose patients after acute brain injury. J Neurosurg. 2001;94(5):706–11. https://doi.org/10.3171/jns.2001.94.5.0706.
183. Chan KH, Mann KS. Prolonged therapeutic external ventricular drainage: a prospective study. Neurosurgery. 1988;23(4):436–8. https://doi.org/10.1227/00006123-198810000-00005.
184. Omar MA, Mohd Haspani MS. The risk factors of external ventricular drainage-related infection at Hospital Kuala Lumpur: an observational study. Malays J Med Sci. 2010;17(3):48–54.
185. Tunkel AR, Hasbun R, Bhimraj A, et al. 2017 Infectious Diseases Society of America's clinical practice guidelines for healthcare-associated ventriculitis and meningitis. Clin Infect Dis. 2017;64(6):e34–65. https://doi.org/10.1093/cid/ciw861.
186. Deshayes S, Coquerel A, Verdon R. Neurological adverse effects attributable to β-lactam antibiotics: a literature review. Drug Saf. 2017;40(12):1171–98. https://doi.org/10.1007/s40264-017-0578-2.
187. Bhattacharyya S, Darby RR, Raibagkar P, Gonzalez Castro LN, Berkowitz AL. Antibiotic-associated encephalopathy. Neurology. 2016;86(10):963–71. https://doi.org/10.1212/WNL.0000000000002455.
188. Sugimoto M, Uchida I, Mashimo T, et al. Evidence for the involvement of GABA(a) receptor blockade in convulsions induced by cephalosporins. Neuropharmacology. 2003;45(3):304–14. https://doi.org/10.1016/s0028-3908(03)00188-6.
189. Fujimoto M, Munakata M, Akaike N. Dual mechanisms of GABAA response inhibition by beta-lactam antibiotics in the pyramidal neurones of the rat cerebral cortex. Br J Pharmacol. 1995;116(7):3014–20. https://doi.org/10.1111/j.1476-5381.1995.tb15957.x.
190. Sugimoto M, Fukami S, Kayakiri H, et al. The beta-lactam antibiotics, penicillin-G and cefoselis have different mechanisms and sites of action at GABA(A) receptors. Br J Pharmacol. 2002;135(2):427–32. https://doi.org/10.1038/sj.bjp.0704496.

191. Barreto EF, Webb AJ, Pais GM, Rule AD, Jannetto PJ, Scheetz MH. Setting the beta-lactam therapeutic range for critically ill patients: is there a floor or even a ceiling? Crit Care Explor. 2021;3(6):e0446. https://doi.org/10.1097/CCE.0000000000000446.
192. Payne LE, Gagnon DJ, Riker RR, et al. Cefepime-induced neurotoxicity: a systematic review. Crit Care. 2017;21(1):276. https://doi.org/10.1186/s13054-017-1856-1.
193. Ojha N, Riaz S, Eranki A. Cefepime neurotoxicity in a patient with acute tubular necrosis. Cureus. 2020;12(8):e9911. https://doi.org/10.7759/cureus.9911.
194. Balderia PG, Chandorkar A, Kim Y, Patnaik S, Sloan J, Newman GC. Dosing cefepime for renal function does not completely prevent neurotoxicity in a patient with kidney transplant. J Patient Saf. 2018;14(2):e33–4. https://doi.org/10.1097/PTS.0000000000000225.
195. Tchapyjnikov D, Luedke MW. Cefepime-induced encephalopathy and nonconvulsive status epilepticus: dispelling an artificial dichotomy. Neurohospitalist. 2019;9(2):100–4. https://doi.org/10.1177/1941874418803225.
196. Maan G, Keitoku K, Kimura N, et al. Cefepime-induced neurotoxicity: systematic review. J Antimicrob Chemother. 2022;77(11):2908–21. https://doi.org/10.1093/jac/dkac271.
197. Chow KM, Hui AC, Szeto CC. Neurotoxicity induced by beta-lactam antibiotics: from bench to bedside. Eur J Clin Microbiol Infect Dis. 2005;24(10):649–53. https://doi.org/10.1007/s10096-005-0021-y.
198. Meier K, Lee K. Neurogenic Fever. J Intensive Care Med. 2017;32(2):124–9. https://doi.org/10.1177/0885066615625194.
199. Chatziparteli K, Alonso OF, Kraydieh S, Dietrich WD. Importance of posttraumatic hypothermia and hyperthermia on the inflammatory response after fluid percussion brain injury: biochemical and immunocytochemical studies. J Cereb Blood Flow Metab. 2000;20(3):531–42. https://doi.org/10.1097/00004647-200003000-00012.
200. Childers MK, Rupright J, Smith DW. Post-traumatic hyperthermia in acute brain injury rehabilitation. Brain Inj. 1994;8(4):335–43. https://doi.org/10.3109/02699059409150984.
201. Meythaler JM, Stinson AM. Fever of central origin in traumatic brain injury controlled with propranolol. Arch Phys Med Rehabil. 1994;75(7):816–8.
202. Segatore M. Fever after traumatic brain injury. J Neurosci Nurs. 1992;24(2):104–9. https://doi.org/10.1097/01376517-199204000-00010.
203. Cunha BA, Digamon-Beltran M, Gobbo PN. Implications of fever in the critical care setting. Heart Lung. 1984;13(5):460–5.
204. Powers JH, Scheld WM. Fever in neurologic diseases. Infect Dis Clin N Am. 1996;10(1):45–66. https://doi.org/10.1016/s0891-5520(05)70285-3.
205. Thompson HJ, Tkacs NC, Saatman KE, Raghupathi R, McIntosh TK. Hyperthermia following traumatic brain injury: a critical evaluation. Neurobiol Dis. 2003;12(3):163–73. https://doi.org/10.1016/s0969-9961(02)00030-x.
206. Kang SH, Kim MJ, Shin IY, Park DW, Sohn JW, Yoon YK. Bromocriptine for control of hyperthermia in a patient with mixed autonomic hyperactivity after neurosurgery: a case report. J Korean Med Sci. 2012;27(8):965–8. https://doi.org/10.3346/jkms.2012.27.8.965.
207. Yu KW, Huang YH, Lin CL, Hong CZ, Chou LW. Effectively managing intractable central hyperthermia in a stroke patient by bromocriptine: a case report. Neuropsychiatr Dis Treat. 2013;9:605–8. https://doi.org/10.2147/NDT.S44547.
208. Garg M, Garg K, Singh PK, et al. Neurogenic fever in severe traumatic brain injury treated with propranolol: a case report. Neurol India. 2019;67(4):1097–9. https://doi.org/10.4103/0028-3886.266258.
209. Huang YS, Hsiao MC, Lee M, Huang YC, Lee JD. Baclofen successfully abolished prolonged central hyperthermia in a patient with basilar artery occlusion. Acta Neurol Taiwanica. 2009;18(2):118–22.
210. Lee HC, Kim JM, Lim JK, Jo YS, Kim SK. Central hyperthermia treated with baclofen for patient with pontine hemorrhage. Ann Rehabil Med. 2014;38(2):269–72. https://doi.org/10.5535/arm.2014.38.2.269.

211. Harrois A, Anstey JR. Diabetes insipidus and syndrome of inappropriate antidiuretic hormone in critically ill patients. Crit Care Clin. 2019;35(2):187–200. https://doi.org/10.1016/j.ccc.2018.11.001.
212. Refardt J, Winzeler B, Christ-Crain M. Diabetes insipidus: an update. Endocrinol Metab Clin. 2020;49(3):517–31. https://doi.org/10.1016/j.ecl.2020.05.012.
213. Bendz H, Aurell M. Drug-induced diabetes insipidus: incidence, prevention and management. Drug Saf. 1999;21(6):449–56. https://doi.org/10.2165/00002018-199921060-00002.
214. Gross P. Clinical management of SIADH. Ther Adv Endocrinol Metab. 2012;3(2):61–73. https://doi.org/10.1177/2042018812437561.
215. Verbalis JG, Goldsmith SR, Greenberg A, et al. Diagnosis, evaluation, and treatment of hyponatremia: expert panel recommendations. Am J Med. 2013;126(10 Suppl 1):S1–42. https://doi.org/10.1016/j.amjmed.2013.07.006.
216. Sterns RH, Rondon-Berrios H, Adrogué HJ, et al. Treatment guidelines for hyponatremia: stay the course. Clin J Am Soc Nephrol. 2023;19(1):129–35. https://doi.org/10.2215/CJN.0000000000000244.

Chapter 17
Acute Ischemic Stroke

Brooke Barlow, Andrew J. Webb, and Karen Berger

17.1   Introductory Case

A 76-year-old man with a past medical history of hypertension, pancreatitis, and hyperlipidemia presents to the emergency department (ED) at 10:16 am via emergency medical service (EMS) with acute-onset right-sided hemiplegia. He was last seen well at 9:30 am that morning by his son, who was traveling with him to a family party. When the patient attempted to get out of the car, he was unable to stand and the son noted that he had a new right-sided facial droop and slurred speech. Concerned for the signs of a stroke, the son called 911.

In the ED, his initial blood pressure was 170/59 mm Hg, his heart rate was 85 beats per minute in normal sinus rhythm, and he had a respiratory rate of 18 with an SpO_2 of 100%. On initial exam, he was alert and oriented, followed commands, and had normal horizontal extraocular movements and intact visual fields. His motor exam was notable for mild right-sided facial droop, moderate right lower extremity drift, and mild-to-moderate dysarthria but normal left-sided movement and no loss of sensation, overall scoring 5 points on the National Institutes of Health Stroke Score (NIHSS). A non-contrast head computed tomography (CT) showed age-related parenchymal loss but no intracranial hemorrhage. The patient was diagnosed

B. Barlow
Memorial Hermann-The Woodlands Medical Center, Houston, TX, USA

A. J. Webb (✉)
Massachusetts General Hospital, Boston, MA, USA
e-mail: ajwebb@mgh.harvard.edu

K. Berger
Nova Southeastern University, Fort Lauderdale, FL, USA

Broward Health Medical Center, Fort Lauderdale, FL, USA

with an acute ischemic stroke and, after confirmation of eligibility and assent, received IV tenecteplase at 10:49 am.

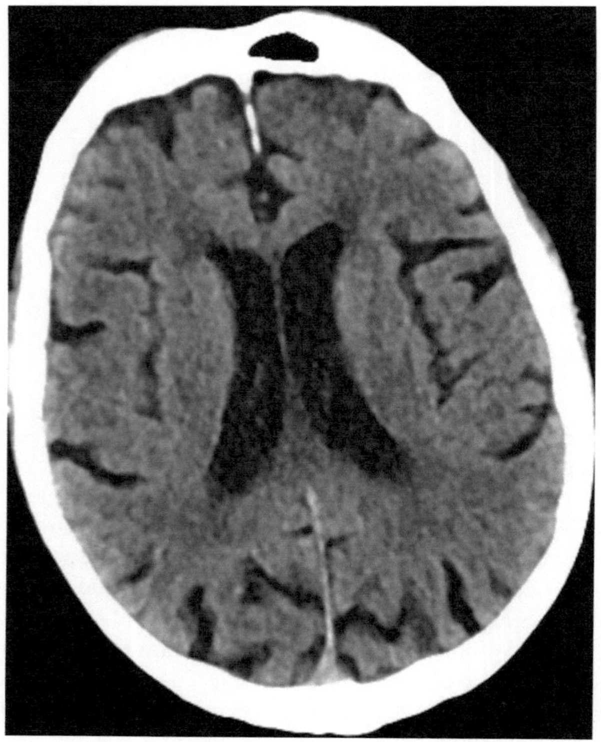

In this chapter, we will review the epidemiology, diagnosis, and management of acute ischemic stroke. Both acute and key secondary prevention therapies will be discussed, including potential complications and monitoring parameters key to the safe implementation of these therapies. A summary of the acute management of ischemic stroke is depicted in Fig. 17.1.

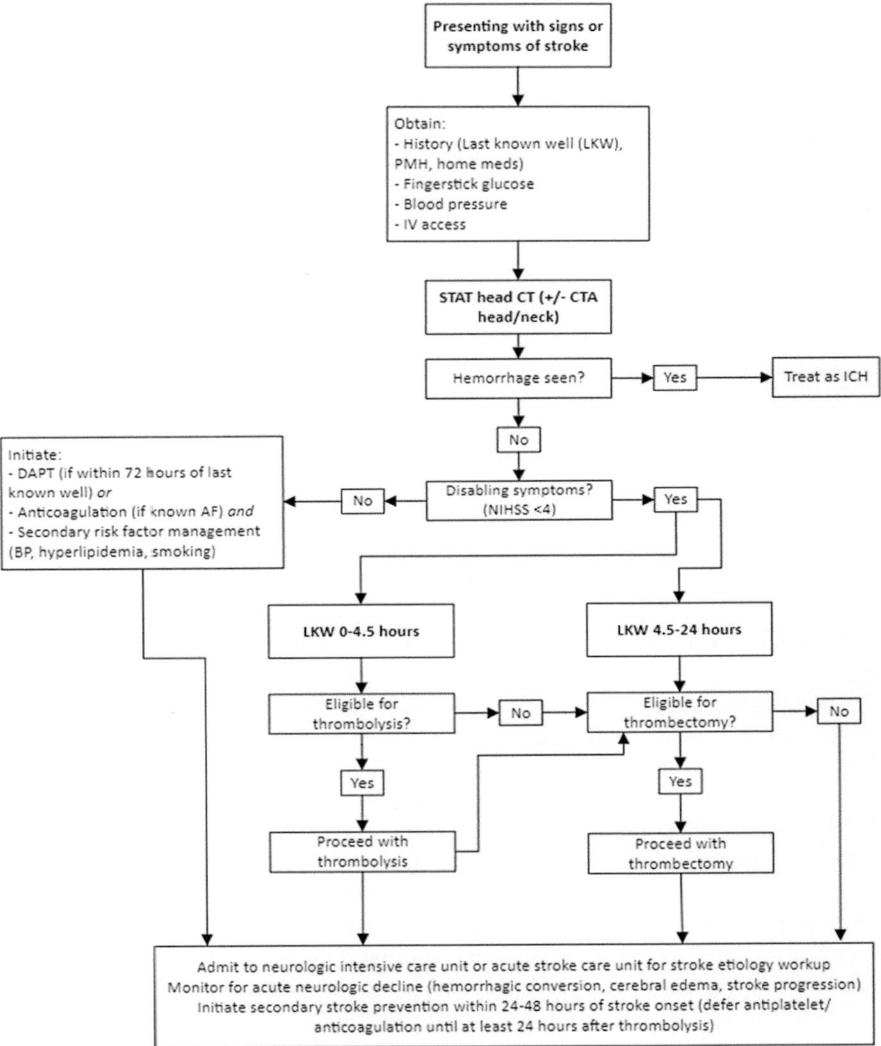

Fig. 17.1 Acute ischemic stroke treatment algorithm. Acute ischemic stroke must be managed rapidly and efficiently for optimal outcomes. Patients presenting with signs and symptoms of acute ischemic stroke should be rapidly assessed and triaged, and treatment should be initiated as soon as possible. Patients with non-disabling symptoms (generally defined as an NIHSS of 3 or less) can receive less emergent treatment but should still be closely monitored for neurologic worsening in which case they may become eligible for advanced therapies. Eligibility for thrombolysis and thrombectomy is discussed extensively throughout the chapter

17.2 Introduction

Stroke remains a global health burden and is a leading cause of death and disability worldwide. Approximately 795,000 people suffer from a stroke event annually, of which 75% account for first-time events, with the remaining experiencing a recurrent attack [1]. According to the American Heart Association's (AHA) Heart Disease and Stroke Statistics update, stroke accounts for 1 of every 21 deaths in the United States, with one stroke-related death occurring every 3 min and 17 s [1]. Of all strokes, acute ischemic stroke (AIS) is the most common, accounting for 87% of events, followed by intracranial hemorrhage (ICH) at 10% and subarachnoid hemorrhage at 3% [1]. Despite the marked advances in AIS management over the past decade, the prevalence of stroke is projected to increase by 20.5% in 2030 compared to 2012 [1]. This increase is proposed to be due to a near doubling in the rates of hypertension and diabetes, highlighting the importance of controlling modifiable risk factors for stroke prevention [2].

17.3 Symptoms and Presentation

Early, prompt recognition of stroke symptoms is of utmost importance in AIS to minimize the risk of potentially permanent, disabling long-term sequelae. Several screening tools have been developed to improve the general public's recognition of stroke symptoms and promote timely triage. Historically, FAST (face, arm, speech, time) was the most commonly used screening tool given its simple structure, ease of use, and high sensitivity (85%) for stroke detection [3]. However, in clinical trials, FAST failed to detect up to 40% of posterior circulation strokes, most notably due to the insensitivity of FAST to visual and gate disturbances [4]. In recognition of these shortcomings, the acronym was expanded to BEFAST (balance, eyes, face, arm, speech, time) to include the visual symptoms and limb ataxia experienced in posterior events to improve symptom recognition. This expansion was estimated to reduce the proportion of missed AIS events from 14% to 4.4% [5].

While these screening tools capture most stroke warning signs, symptomatology is highly dependent on the effected intracranial vascular territory. For example, an infarct in the left middle cerebral artery would manifest as contralateral hemiplegia, hemisensory loss, and expressive aphasia. In contrast, a patient with a basilar artery occlusion could present with depressed consciousness, hemi- or quadriparesis, and speech abnormalities accompanied by prodromal symptoms of nausea, vertigo, neck stiffness, and headache [6]. Attention should also be drawn to populations likely to present with atypical stroke symptoms, most notably amongst women and extremes of age [7, 8]. Women are two times more likely to present with atypical stroke symptoms, including loss of consciousness and nausea/vomiting, and have a lower likelihood of presenting with lower extremity paresis [8].

Table 17.1 National Institutes of Health Stroke Scale (NIHSS) interpretation [7]

0	No stroke symptoms
1–4	Minor stroke symptoms
5–15	Moderate stroke symptoms
16–20	Moderate–severe stroke symptoms
21–42	Severe stroke symptoms

Table 17.2 Modified Rankin scale (mRS)

0	No symptoms
1	No significant disability. Able to carry out all usual activities despite some symptoms
2	Slight disability. Able to look after own affairs without assistance but unable to carry out all previous activities
3	Moderate disability. Requires some help, but able to walk unassisted
4	Moderately severe disability. Unable to attend to own bodily needs without assistance, or unable to walk unassisted
5	Severe disability. Requires constant nursing care and attention, bedridden, incontinent
6	Dead

Determining stroke severity is important in the initial AIS assessment as it can aid in evaluating a patient's candidacy for certain treatment options and may predict the likelihood of an underlying large-vessel occlusion [9]. The National Institutes of Health Stroke Scale (NIHSS) is a 15-item neurologic examination scale used as a quantitative assessment tool to measure the degree of stroke-related neurologic deficits. The score ranges from 0 to 42, with higher scores indicating a higher stroke severity (Table 17.1) [7]. NIHSS is also used to follow changes in neurologic examination after treatment interventions such as thrombectomy or thrombolysis [7]. Higher scores on the NIHSS correlate with increasing severity of stroke, but it is important to note that the score may underestimate the severity of strokes occurring in the nondominant hemisphere or in the posterior circulation. The mRS is a 7-step ordinal scale which measures the degree of functional disability or dependence in those who experience a stroke (Table 17.2). Achieving an mRS of 0–1 at 90 days is traditionally considered to be an excellent outcome.

17.4 Pathophysiology

AIS is characterized by a mismatch of oxygen supply and demand in cortical tissue, leading to focal neurologic deficits. Insufficient arterial cerebral blood flow (CBF) to brain tissue leads to local ischemia as neurons receive insufficient oxygen to carry out normal cellular respiration, which inevitably leads to cell death if CBF cannot be restored [10]. While stroke was historically a purely clinical diagnosis, advances in magnetic resonance imaging (MRI) have allowed for identification of the hyperacute changes secondary to ischemia within minutes of CBF falling below the ischemic threshold of 10–20 mL/100 g/min [11]. Early hyperacute changes seen on

MRI are referred to as an ischemic core, and the vascular territory surrounding the core that is receiving suboptimal CBF and is at risk of ischemia is referred to as the penumbra. Core tissue is considered unsalvageable unless reperfusion occurs immediately, while penumbral tissue can be salvaged with acute therapies. Ischemic lesions tend to follow the vascular territory of the artery involved in the occlusion, apart from hypoperfusion strokes (also known as "watershed" strokes), which tend to cause damage at the border zones between vascular territories.

The cellular mechanisms underpinning cerebral ischemia have been the target of extensive research, both to understand the underlying pathways involved in neuronal cell death and to identify potential therapeutic targets to limit primary and secondary injury after AIS. Insufficient oxygen delivery to neurons leads to an incapacity to transport calcium across the cell membrane. Intracellular calcium accumulation paired with an inability to regulate extracellular glutamate concentrations leads to further alterations in cellular ion gradients, intracellular edema, and activation of apoptosis pathways. The accumulation of intracellular ions and excess water and the resulting production of reactive oxygen species lead to acidosis, DNA damage, and ultimately programmed cell death [10]. Pharmacotherapeutic agents targeting these pathways have been introduced in clinical trials but have yet to be demonstrated to be beneficial in humans.

The etiology of AIS can be broadly categorized into thromboembolic and hemodynamic categories. Thromboembolic strokes occur due to an abrupt cessation of CBF caused by either an embolus (such as a cardioembolism caused by atrial fibrillation) or a thrombosis (such as via stenosis caused by atherosclerosis). Hemodynamic strokes are less common and occur when blood supply to the brain is insufficient to meet cerebral demands. This can occur during prolonged hypotension because of increased cerebral metabolic demand or a mismatch in arterial blood flow between ischemic and nonischemic brain regions ("reversed Robin Hood syndrome"). Stroke etiologies are often further subdivided into the TOAST (Trial of Org 10172 in Acute Stroke Treatment Trial) criteria, categorizing strokes as caused by either large-artery atherosclerosis, cardioembolism, small-vessel disease, other determined etiology, or undetermined etiology (also referred to as cryptogenic or stroke of unknown source) [12]. While the acute management of AIS is largely similar across etiologies, determination of the cause of a stroke is critical to the selection of appropriate secondary stroke prevention therapy and is a core objective of index admission after AIS [13].

17.5 Acute Therapies

17.5.1 Thrombolytic Therapy

Intravenous thrombolysis is the cornerstone of acute therapy for patients with AIS. Thrombolytics catalyze the conversion of plasminogen to plasmin, a proteolytic enzyme responsible for breaking the cross-links between fibrin and destabilizing clot integrity. Dissolution of the fibrin-rich thrombus with thrombolytics restores blood flow and perfusion to ischemic areas and, if administered within a timely fashion, mitigates the risk of irreversible ischemic damage [14]. Alteplase (r-tPA) was the first FDA-approved thrombolytic for AIS based on the results of the 1995 NINDS trial, which demonstrated a 30% increased likelihood of a favorable functional outcome as measured on the modified Rankin scale (mRS) at 90 days compared to placebo [15]. The NINDS trial, in combination with the ECASS-III trial [16], established alteplase as the standard of care in eligible patients with AIS. The benefits of treatment are directly linked to the expediency of treatment initiation after last known well (LKW) [17]. When thrombolysis is initiated within 0–3 h of LKW, the number needed to treat (NNT) is estimated to be 10 for one patient to achieve an excellent functional outcome (mRS 0–1) at 90 days. The NNT increases to 19 when treatment is initiated within 3–4.5 h of LKW, emphasizing the critical importance of timely initiation in eligible patients. Thrombolysis significantly increases the risk of symptomatic intracranial hemorrhage (sICH) compared to placebo, but the long-term benefits of thrombolysis outweigh the risks in eligible patients.

Prolonged ischemic injury leads to capillary cell apoptosis, increased vascular permeability, inflammation, and oxidative stress, enhancing the risk of hemorrhagic transformation [18]. Thus, treatment initiation beyond 4.5 h is not recommended given the potential for higher rates of intracranial bleeding [7, 18]. However, advancements have been made in the subgroup of "wake-up" strokes, which were historically considered a contraindication to thrombolytic therapy given the unknown time of symptom onset and potential for a completed infarct. A series of trials evaluated the use of advanced imaging techniques using diffusion-weighted imaging MRI with fluid-attenuated inversion recovery (FLAIR) sequence or CT perfusion to identify the presence of a salvageable penumbra amenable for intervention with thrombolysis and/or thrombectomy [7, 19, 20]. A meta-analysis of three randomized trials evaluating the use of thrombolysis in patients with AIS presenting within 4.5–9 h of LKW who underwent advanced imaging to identify perfusion mismatches revealed that a higher proportion of patients achieved an excellent functional outcome with alteplase compared to placebo, demonstrating that careful patient selection could extend the window of eligibility [20].

Patients presenting with symptoms of AIS must be rapidly assessed for eligibility and contraindications to thrombolysis. Patients presenting within 4.5 h of LKW or within 9 h of LKW with perfusion mismatch on advanced imaging and who have disabling stroke symptoms (traditionally defined as an NIHSS >5) are considered potentially eligible for thrombolysis. The 2019 AHA/ASA Acute Stroke Guidelines provide a Level IA recommendation for thrombolysis within 3 h of LKW, Level IB-R for thrombolysis within 4.5 h of LKW, and Level IIa B-R for thrombolysis in the extended window for eligible patients [7]. Contraindications must be carefully evaluated prior to therapy, however, to ensure that the benefits outweigh the risk of such therapy. A full list of contraindications to thrombolytics is given in Table 17.3.

While alteplase has historically been the thrombolytic of choice for AIS, its complex dosing and long administration time have prompted investigation into alternative thrombolytics. Tenecteplase is a third-generation thrombolytic genetically

Table 17.3 Absolute and relative contraindications to thrombolysis in acute ischemic stroke [7]

Absolute contraindications	Relative contraindications
Presentation >4.5 h after onset (without the capability to determine extended-window eligibility)	Recent gastrointestinal or genitourinary bleeding more than 21 days prior to presentation
BP sustained >185/110 mm hg despite treatment	Major surgery or serious non-head trauma in previous 14 days
Current or history of intracranial hemorrhage or subarachnoid hemorrhage	Acute seizure at stroke onset
Intracranial or spinal surgery, serious head trauma, or previous stroke within 3 months	Pregnancy
Active internal bleeding	Acute pericarditis
Intracranial, gastric, or intra-axial intracranial neoplasm, arteriovenous malformation	Minor or rapidly improving symptoms
Bleeding diathesis (INR >1.7, aPTT >40 s, platelets <100,000/mm^3)	Recent myocardial infarction (<3 months)
Anticoagulation use—INR >1.7, DOAC use within 48 h, recipient of therapeutic-dose UFH or LMWH	Arterial puncture at noncompressible site within 7 days
Confirmed/suspected endocarditis or aortic arch dissection	Initial blood glucose <50 or >400 mg/dL
Recent gastrointestinal bleed (<21 days)	

Table 17.4 Comparison of alteplase and tenecteplase

	Alteplase (rt-PA)	Tenecteplase (TNK)
FDA approval	AIS (0–3 h), PE, acute myocardial infarction (MI)	Acute MI (off-label for AIS)
Product availability	50 mg, 100 mg vial	50 mg vial
Final concentration	1 mg/mL	5 mg/mL
Fibrin specificity	++	++++
Pharmacokinetics	PAI-1 resistance: Low Half-life: 5 min	PAI-1 resistance: High Half-life: 22 min
Stroke dosing	0.9 mg/kg (max 90 mg)	0.25 mg/kg (max 25 mg)
Administration	10% as IV bolus over 1 min, remainder as 60-min IV infusion	IV push over 5 s

modified to possess a 15-fold higher fibrin specificity and an 80-fold increased resistance to plasminogen activator inhibitor-1 (PAI-1), an enzyme responsible for the inactivation of tissue plasminogen activator [21]. The increased resistance to PAI-1 significantly prolongs the half-life of tenecteplase, allowing tenecteplase to be administered as an intravenous bolus compared to a bolus plus infusion [21]. Furthermore, the enhanced fibrin specificity prevents systemic fibrin degradation and may reduce the risk of bleeding (Table 17.4). The practical advantages of the simplified preparation and ease of administration with tenecteplase may translate to improved door-to-needle times and help expedite patient transfer to thrombectomy-capable centers [22].

Several studies have compared the safety and efficacy of tenecteplase to alteplase in doses ranging from 0.1 to 0.4 mg/kg. Initial studies were conducted in patients with large-vessel occlusions (LVOs) who were also eligible for mechanical thrombectomy. The EXTEND-IA TNK trial enrolled patients with LVO within a 4.5-h time window to 0.25 mg/kg of tenecteplase (maximum dose of 25 mg) vs. alteplase 0.9 mg/kg (maximum dose of 90 mg). The proportion of patients who achieved >50% reperfusion in the involved ischemic region was higher in the tenecteplase group at 22% compared to only 10% in those who received alteplase ($p = 0.002$). Tenecteplase also resulted in improved 90-day functional outcomes (median mRS 2 vs. 3, $p = 0.04$) with no differences in the rates of sICH. Several large RCTs conducted outside of the LVO cohort (AcT, TRACE-2, and others), have demonstrated non-inferiority in functional outcomes between alteplase and tenecteplase with no notable differences in bleeding events [23]. Notably, higher tenecteplase doses (0.4 mg/kg) have been shown to increase sICH rates and lead to worse functional outcomes [24]. Therefore, the recommended dosing for tenecteplase in AIS is 0.25 mg/kg (maximum of 25 mg) administered as a single intravenous bolus over 5 s. The 2019 AHA/ASA guidelines suggest that tenecteplase may be reasonable as an alternative to alteplase in those who are eligible for thrombolysis and who are also eligible to undergo mechanical thrombectomy [7]. These guidelines were however published before a majority of this research was conducted, and future renditions of the guidelines are likely to incorporate recommendations for tenecteplase that reflect the latest data. The 2023 European Stroke Organization (ESO) developed expedited expert consensus recommendations for the use of tenecteplase in AIS and provided a strong recommendation with moderate quality of evidence for use of tenecteplase as an alternative thrombolytic to alteplase in AIS for those who present within the 4.5-h time window [25].

17.5.2   Thrombectomy

Where thrombolytic therapy aims to pharmacologically dissolve culprit lesions causing ischemia, patients with visualized LVOs of the major cerebral vessels may also be eligible for endovascular thrombectomy to mechanically achieve reperfusion. Intra-arterial thrombectomy (IAT) has evolved dramatically over the last two decades and has been established as the most effective acute therapy for AIS in eligible patients. First-generation thrombectomy devices included either direct catheter aspiration or clot retrieval and were associated with increased rates of arterial reperfusion over intravenous thrombolytic administration alone, but the improved functional outcomes seen with second-generation stent retriever devices solidified IAT as the standard of care [26, 27]. Stent retrievers deploy a flexible stent into the target thrombus and expand the stent so that the thrombus becomes lodged within the stent, and the stent is then retracted. A patient-level meta-analysis of five international randomized controlled trials (MR CLEAN, ESCAPE, REVASCAT, SWIFT PRIME, and EXTEND IA) revealed that IAT was associated with a nearly three-times increased odds of good functional outcome at 3 months (adj. OR 2.71, 95% CI 2.07–3.55) and a number needed to treat to achieve an mRS of 0–2 at 90 days of 5. Rates of sICH were similar between arms (4.4 vs. 4.3%, $p = 0.81$), and mortality was similar in both arms (15.3 vs. 18.9%, $p = 0.15$) [26].

Initial trials enrolled patients within 6–12 h of LKW, but subsequent studies expanded eligibility to patients with appropriate clinical or imaging findings to treatment within 16–24 h of last known well [28, 29]. Patients with posterior circulation LVOs, particularly in the basilar artery, were also often excluded or under-represented in early trials of thrombectomy. Two trials, the BEST and BASICS trials, initially suggested that basilar artery thrombectomy did not improve functional outcomes in patients with basilar artery LVOs [30, 31]. Two follow-up trials, the BAOCHE and ATTENTION trials, enrolled a larger population of patients within basilar artery LVOs within 24 h of symptom onset and randomized them to undergo thrombectomy or receive standard of care. In both trials, thrombectomy was associated with significantly improved functional outcomes at 90 days with a favorable risk profile [32, 33], an effect confirmed after meta-analysis of all four trials (OR 1.54, 95% CI 1.16–2.06) [34].

The 2019 acute stroke guidelines provide a Level IA recommendation for IAT in patients presenting within 6–16 h of last known well and a level IIB recommendation for patients presenting within 24 h [7]. Traditional eligibility criteria include identification of an LVO in an anterior circulation vessel (ICA or M1 or M2 segment of MCA), low burden of early ischemic changes on CT as determined by an Alberta Stroke Programme Early CT Score (ASPECTS) of 6 or greater, good baseline functional status, and an NIHSS score of at least 6. Extended-window IAT (i.e., within 16–24 h of the last known well) should be considered in patients who have a mismatch between either clinical exam and ischemic core identified on perfusion imaging or sufficient "salvageable" tissue, defined as an ischemic core of less than 70 mL and a ratio of penumbra volume to core volume of greater than 1.8 identified via perfusion imaging. These criteria are based on the inclusion criteria of the major trials published at the time of the guideline's release; however, the benefit of IAT continues to be demonstrated in an expanded population of patients with LVOs. Thrombectomy has been shown to be beneficial in patients with posterior LVOs, large infarct cores [35, 36], baseline disability [37], and patients with low baseline NIHSS scores [38]. As evidence evolves, eligibility for IAT continues to expand, suggesting benefit in nearly all patients who present with an LVO within 24 h of last known well.

Reperfusion after IAT is graded on the Thrombolysis in Cerebral Infarction (TICI) score, which is a radiographic assessment of the success of revascularization. The modified TICI score (mTICI) ranges from a score of 0–3, with higher scores indicating higher degrees of reperfusion (Table 17.5) [39]. Successful reperfusion is considered to be attainment of a TICI score of 2B or greater, and reperfusion is obtained in approximately 70% of patients in the context of clinical trials [26] and in over 80% of patients in clinical practice [40]. Approximately 10–30% of patients

Table 17.5 Modified thrombolysis in cerebral infarction (mTICI) grades

mTICI score	Interpretation
0	No reperfusion obtained
1	Minimal reperfusion obtained
2A	Partial reperfusion of <50% of the affected territory
2B	Partial reperfusion of >50% of the affected territory
2C	Near-complete reperfusion of the affected territory except for slow flow in distal territory
3	Complete reperfusion

who receive a thrombolytic pre-procedure achieve spontaneous reperfusion, which is not included in the metrics of post-IAT reperfusion [41].

Failure to achieve successful reperfusion is associated with worse functional outcomes, and several strategies exist to rescue a failed IAT, including intra-arterial (IA) thrombolytic administration, rescue stenting, and antiplatelet infusions. Each hour of delay in time to reperfusion has been associated with a 6% lower likelihood of attaining a good outcome, and thus use of rescue therapies can be considered in the angiography suite to hasten time to reperfusion in difficult cases [42]. Adjunctive antiplatelet infusions including GIIb/IIIa inhibitors (eptifibatide, tirofiban) or P2Y12 inhibitors (cangrelor) can be used in isolation during mechanical thrombectomy, but their largest role is to prevent thrombosis of emergently placed neuroendovascular stents. The decision to place a carotid or intracranial stent is generally made during the index angiography, and thus pretreatment with oral antiplatelet agents may not be feasible or safe given recent administration of a thrombolytic. Infusions have the advantages of rapid onset, titratability (via platelet reactivity unit [PRU] testing for cangrelor), and ease of cessation in the setting of bleeding. All three agents can be used within the initial 24-h window after thrombolytic administration to prevent stent thrombosis. Suggested dosing of rescue agents and antiplatelet bridging strategies are summarized in Table 17.6.

17.5.3 Blood Pressure Management

An acute hypertensive response occurs in up to 75% of patients presenting with an AIS, which is thought to be an autoregulatory response to maintain cerebral perfusion [49]. Alterations in CBF are directly dependent on systemic blood pressure (BP); thus, any drastic change in BP can potentiate stroke progression or hemorrhagic transformation. An acute drop in SBP >30 mmHg or a cumulative decline >50 mmHg is associated with a decreased likelihood of a favorable outcome, with any drop >60 mmHg associated with an increased risk of death [50]. On the contrary, higher BP significantly increases the risk of hemorrhagic transformation, with a fourfold increased risk in those with an SBP >170 mmHg compared to 141–150 mmHg [51]. Despite the existing data, the ideal BP target in AIS remains

Table 17.6 Rescue adjunctive therapies in mechanical thrombectomy

Agent	Dosing	Notes
Fibrinolytics and thrombolytics		
Alteplase	Adjuvant use: Flat dose of 10 mg or 0.225 mg/kg (maximum 22.5 mg) infused IA over 15–30 min [43]	Doses vary, and adjuvant doses up to 40 mg have been reported [44]
Tenecteplase	1.5–10 mg as a bolus or infused IA at a rate of 0.4 mg/min [45, 46]	Given the high concentration of commercially available vial (5 mg/mL), may require further dilution for IA infusion
Antiplatelet agents		
Eptifibatide	180 mcg/kg IV/IA bolus (maximum 22.6 mg) followed by 0.75–2 mcg/kg/min (maximum 15 mg/h) for up to 24 h	Adjust doses for renal impairment. Administer antiplatelet agent 0–120 min before drip discontinuation
Tirofiban	0.4 mcg/kg IV bolus over 30 min followed by 0.1 mcg/kg/min for up to 48 h	Adjust doses for renal impairment. Administer antiplatelet agent 0–120 min before drip discontinuation. IA infusions have been reported using lower doses
Cangrelor	If used during stenting procedure: 30 mcg/kg IV bolus at least 10 min before stent deployment followed by 4 mcg/kg/min continuous infusion during procedure [47]. If used after stenting or post-thrombectomy: 0.75 mcg/kg/min IV continuous infusion	Doses can be titrated to a platelet reactivity unit (PRU) goal of 50–150 (higher values suggest more platelet reactivity and insufficient antiplatelet activity) [48]; ensure that samples are run immediately after drawing as cangrelor breaks down in serum and falsely high PRUs can be seen with delays to measurement. Some centers employ lower initial doses based on experience with supratherapeutic PRUs (i.e, PRU <50) using conventional doses. If starting clopidogrel: Administer loading dose at the time of infusion discontinuation and maintenance dose 24 h later. If starting ticagrelor: Administer loading dose 0–120 min before drip discontinuation and then maintenance dose 12 h later

poorly defined and requires a tailored approach based on factors such as preexisting comorbidities and eligibility for reperfusion therapies. Table 17.7 outlines the AHA/ASA guideline recommendations for blood pressure targets in those eligible or ineligible for reperfusion-based therapies and pharmacologic treatment options.

The current recommendations are based on the results of the ENCHANTED trial, which randomized 2196 patients who received thrombolysis with a baseline SBP ≥150 mmHg to intensive BP control (SBP 130–140 mmHg) vs. standard BP control (SBP <180 mmHg) [52]. The mean SBP was 144 mmHg in the intensive

Table 17.7 Recommendations for blood pressure control in acute ischemic stroke [7]

	Thrombolysis	Thrombectomy	No reperfusion therapy
Blood pressure target	Pre-thrombolytic: <185/110 mmHg Post-thrombolytic (× 24 h): <180/105 mmHg	Pre-thrombectomy <185/110 mmHg Post-thrombectomy (× 24 h): <180/105 mmHg	If present with BP ≥220/120 mmHg: Target 15% BP reduction during first 24 h
Monitoring	Monitor BP every 15 min × 2 h, then Q30 min × 6 h, then Q1 h × 16 h		Monitor BP hourly

Pharmacologic agents for acute blood pressure control

Drug	Dosing	Side effects
Labetalol	10–20 mg IVP, may repeat every 10 min (max 80 mg)	Bradycardia
Nicardipine	5 mg/h IV infusion, titrated by 2.5 mg/h every 5–15 min (max 15 mg/h)	Volume overload
Clevidipine	1–2 mg/h IV infusion, titrated by doubling dose every 2–5 min (max 32 mg/h)	Hypertriglyceridemia

control arm vs. 149 mmHg in the standard control arm. No difference was found in the primary outcome of mRS at 90 days, despite fewer intracranial hemorrhage events in the intensive control arm [52]. Excessive BP reduction can compromise cerebral perfusion, worsen the ischemic injury, and heighten the risk of acute kidney injury. After successful reperfusion (TICI2B-3) after IAT, aggressive BP control to an SBP <120 mmHg increases the risk of dependency (RR 1.23, CI 1.09–1.39) [53]. These findings were replicated in the OPTIMAL-BP trial with intensive BP control defined as <140 mmHg post-thrombectomy, leading to increased dependency compared to conventional targets (SBP 140–180 mmHg) [54]. High BP variability, defined as rapid fluctuations in BP, is also associated with early neurologic deterioration within 72 h in acute ischemic stroke [55]. Therefore, BP control after AIS requires a delicate balance of maintaining CBF through avoidance of hypo- and hypertension along with prevention of rapid variations in blood pressure to optimize patient outcomes.

Selection of the optimal antihypertensive for BP control in AIS requires a careful assessment of patient characteristics and comorbidities that may predict response (or nonresponse) to specific treatments. Labetalol is a mixed $\alpha 1$, $\beta 1$, and $\beta 2$ blocker, which induces vasodilation and negative chronotropic effects. Labetalol can be administered as an intravenous push (IVP) or by a continuous infusion. The primary dose-limiting side effect is bradycardia. Nicardipine is a dihydropyridine calcium channel blocker that is more selective towards inducing vasodilation and has minimal effects on myocardial calcium channels. A common approach may be to administer labetalol bolus in those who are otherwise candidates for thrombolysis but require BP reduction, given its rapid onset of action and ease of administration. In those who have persistent elevations in BP despite administration of bolus therapies, or if contraindications such as bradycardia prohibit labetalol administration, a continuous infusion of nicardipine is often considered. Comparative trials of labetalol and nicardipine are limited in their retrospective design but appear to suggest that an up-front approach with administration of nicardipine may result in improved time to target BP control and lower BP variability with no increased incidence of adverse effects [56–58]. Clevidipine is an alternative dihydropyridine calcium channel blocker with similar pharmacologic activity as nicardipine but differs in its formulation in a lipid emulsion and shorter half-life, which allows for more rapid titration. Head-to-head comparisons between clevidipine and nicardipine suggest similar efficacy in terms of blood pressure reduction but a lower overall volume administered with clevidipine, which may be advantageous in those at risk for volume overload [59, 60]. Hydralazine is a potent, direct-acting vasodilator that is frequently employed as an alternative to labetalol if an IVP agent is needed. However, hydralazine has been shown to increase intracranial pressure and decrease perfusion pressure, which can be deleterious in the setting of ischemia [61]. Furthermore, patient response to hydralazine is often unpredictable and its effects are prolonged, which can lead to precipitous drops in BP with a high degree of variability. The AHA/ASA guidelines suggest that hydralazine may be considered an alternative if other agents are unavailable or otherwise contraindicated [7]. Enalaprilat is the intravenous active metabolite of the angiotensin-converting enzyme inhibitor enalapril. Enalaprilat should be used with caution in AIS given its prolonged duration of action, which can prohibit titration and increase the risk of angioedema with ACE inhibitors when administered concomitantly with alteplase [62].

17.5.4 Acute Anticoagulation

Investigations into early initiation of anticoagulation in non-cardioembolic acute ischemic strokes have been performed under the hypothesis that anticoagulation could reduce thrombus propagation, decrease the volume of infarcted tissue, and thus reduce the degree of neurologic deficits. A systematic review including 28 trials of over 24,000 participants treated with unfractionated heparin, low-molecular-weight heparin, oral anticoagulants, or direct thrombin inhibitors failed to find any change in rates of disability or dependence (OR 0.98, 95% CI 0.92–1.03) [25]. While most of this data was based on initiation within the first 48 h from symptom onset, these findings remained consistent even when anticoagulation was initiated within 14 days. Although early anticoagulation reduced the rates of early recurrent strokes (0.75, 95% CI 0.65–0.88), this benefit was outweighed by the heightened risk of symptomatic intracranial (OR 2.47, 95% CI 1.90–3.21) and extracranial hemorrhagic events (OR 2.99, 95% CI 2.24–3.99) [63]. Thus, routine use of therapeutic anticoagulation outside of cardioembolic strokes is not recommended.

In patients presenting with a cardioembolic stroke, direct oral anticoagulants (DOACs) represent the preferred anticoagulation strategy, with evidence of reduced risk of ischemic stroke and bleeding compared to warfarin [64]. Timing of DOAC initiation remains a clinical challenge, as the risk of recurrent stroke and hemorrhagic transformation is highest within the first few days after stroke onset [65–67]. Stroke size and symptom severity are associated with an increased likelihood of hemorrhagic transformation; thus, a stratified approach based on these variables has been proposed. The European Society of Cardiology guidelines suggest the 1–3–6–12 rule, with initiation of DOAC therapy within 24 h for TIA, 3 days for mild stroke, 6 days for moderate stroke, and 12 days for severe strokes [68]. This recommendation was based on observational data; thus, more recent trials have aimed at defining the ideal timeframe in a randomized, prospective fashion. The Early vs. Later Anticoagulation for Stroke with Atrial Fibrillation (ELAN) trial was a prospective, open-label trial that randomized patients to receive DOAC therapy within 48 h after a minor or moderate stroke or on days 6–7 for a major stroke compared to later initiation at days 3–4 for minor strokes, 6–7 for moderate strokes, or 12–14 for major strokes. Of the 2013 participants enrolled, the proportions of minor (37%), moderate (40%), and major (23%) strokes were evenly distributed. The primary outcome, a composite of recurrent stroke, systemic embolism, or major bleeding within 30 days, occurred in 2.9% of the early treatment group compared to 4.1% of the later treatment group (95% CI −2.84 to 0.47) [69]. A meta-analysis including 12 trials (10 cohort studies, 2 RCT) involving 11,421 patients found that early initiation of DOAC therapy reduced the risk of recurrent ischemic events (OR 0.68, CI 0.55–0.84) with no significant difference in hemorrhagic events or all-cause mortality ($p = 0.20$). Cumulatively, these findings suggest that early initiation of anticoagulation in cardioembolic stroke may be safe and reduce the risk of recurrent ischemic events but requires a tailored approach based on stroke severity and patient-specific variables that would impact hemorrhage/stroke risk [70].

17.5.5 Antiplatelet Therapy

In patients ineligible or not indicated for thrombolytic or acute anticoagulation therapy, antiplatelets are the mainstay of treatment for AIS and form the backbone of most secondary prevention regimens. While not effective in providing immediate reperfusion of a thrombosed artery, antiplatelets can be effective in preventing early recurrent ischemic stroke and can help to stabilize atherosclerotic plaque. Early single antiplatelet therapy (SAPT) was demonstrated to be effective in the CAST trial, where over 21,000 patients were randomized to either aspirin 160 mg or placebo within 48 h of a suspected AIS. Aspirin led to a significant lower risk of recurrent ischemic stroke (1.6 vs. 2.1%, $p = 0.01$) and death (3.3 vs. 3.9%, $p = 0.04$) at 4 weeks. Rates of hemorrhagic stroke were similar between arms (1.1 vs. 0.9%, $p > 0.1$), but rates of extracranial bleeding were higher in the aspirin arm (0.8 vs. 0.6%, $p = 0.02$) [71]. Similar findings were reported in the IST trial [72], leading the initiation of aspirin within 24–48 h of stroke onset (but at least 24 h after thrombolytic administration, if applicable) to be a class IA recommendation in the 2019 acute ischemic stroke guidelines [7]. While the studied doses of aspirin in this context ranged from 160 to 300 mg, lower starting doses (i.e., 81 mg) are reasonable. In patients without enteral access, rectal aspirin 300 mg can be administered in the place of enteral aspirin.

Alternative SAPT regimens, including clopidogrel or ticagrelor, have been evaluated against aspirin in several international randomized controlled trials. The CAPRIE trial compared clopidogrel 75 mg daily to aspirin 325 mg daily as SAPT in patients with a history of stroke, myocardial infarction, or peripheral artery disease. While not specifically evaluating AIS (stroke onset had to be at least 1 week from randomization), rates of recurrent stroke were similar over a 36-month follow-up period in the stroke subgroup of patients (7.15 vs. 7.71%, $p = 0.26$). Rates of bleeding, including intracranial hemorrhage, were similar between groups. Ticagrelor was similarly evaluated against aspirin as SAPT in AIS in the SOCRATES trial [73]. Over 13,000 patients presenting with AIS within 24 h of symptom onset who were not eligible for thrombolysis because of minor stroke severity were randomized to ticagrelor (180 mg load followed by 90 mg twice daily) or aspirin (300 mg load followed by 100 mg daily). Rates of recurrent stroke, myocardial infarction, or death at 90 days were similar between arms (6.7 vs. 7.5%, $p = 0.07$) as were rates of major bleeding (0.5 vs. 0.6%, $p = 0.45$). Neither clopidogrel nor ticagrelor has notable advantages over the generally well-tolerated and inexpensive aspirin for acute SAPT, and thus aspirin remains first line for most patients. Given comparable safety profiles in both CAPRIE and SOCRATES, however, either could be reasonable in a patient who is allergic to or intolerant to aspirin.

Like in acute coronary syndrome, there has long been interest in whether dual-antiplatelet therapy (DAPT) may have a role in the treatment of AIS and prevention of recurrent events. Initial attempts to demonstrate the benefit of DAPT in stroke failed, however. The MATCH trial randomized 7599 patients who had a stroke or transient ischemic attack within the previous 3 months and risk factors for recurrent stroke to clopidogrel 75 mg daily with aspirin 75 mg daily or clopidogrel 75 mg daily alone [74]. The mean time to randomization was 26.5 days after the index stroke. After 18 months of follow-up, rates of recurrent stroke were similar between arms (8 vs. 9%, $p = 0.353$), but rates of life-threatening bleeding were significantly higher in the DAPT arm (3 vs. 1%, $p < 0.0001$).

While MATCH was interpreted as a negative trial, the positive signal from other trials including CHARISMA [75], ACTIVE-A [76], CARESS [77], FASTER [78], and CLAIR [79] suggested that identifying an enriched population that would be most likely to benefit from DAPT was still worthwhile. Because the risk of recurrent stroke rapidly increases over the first 7 days from stroke onset (11.5% at 7 days) and plateaus over time (15% at 1 month and 18.5% at 3 months) [80], initial negative results from the MATCH trial may have been driven by missing the window of time when patients would be most likely to benefit from the intensity of DAPT. Early DAPT after minor stroke or major TIA has subsequently been evaluated in five large international randomized controlled trials with consistent results, and thus the initiation of clopidogrel-based DAPT in patients presenting with non-cardioembolic minor stroke (presenting NIHSS <4) or major TIA (ABCD2 score >3) within 24 h of symptom onset has a class IA recommendation in the 2019 acute stroke guidelines [7]. Each of the major trials (CHANCE [81], POINT [82], THALES [73], CHANCE2 [83], and INSPIRES [84]) has minor differences and is summarized in Table 17.8. Two trials (THALES and CHANCE2) have evaluated ticagrelor instead of clopidogrel as the backbone of DAPT; ticagrelor produces a similar effect size to clopidogrel with more bleeding, except in the case of CYP2C19 loss of function, where ticagrelor has been demonstrated to be superior to clopidogrel for recurrent stroke prevention. In addition to minor stroke and major TIA, DAPT with full-dose aspirin (325 mg) is also recommended in the case of documented intracranial atherosclerosis as the etiology of stroke based on the results of the Stenting and Aggressive Medical Management for Preventing Recurrent Stroke in Intracranial Stenosis (SAMMPRIS) trial [85].

While the benefits of DAPT have consistently been demonstrated in select populations, caution should be employed in over-applying the results of trials to additional populations as the therapy is not without risk. Nearly a third of patients who

Table 17.8 Dual-antiplatelet therapy trials in acute ischemic stroke

Trial	Population	Treatment	Ischemic outcome	Hemorrhagic outcome
CHANCE (2013) [81]	Minor ischemic stroke (NIHSS <4) or major TIA (ABCD2 ≥4) within 24 h of symptom onset Patients with baseline disability (mRS >2), a clear indication for anticoagulation, who received a thrombolytic were excluded All centers in China	Arm 1: Clopidogrel 300 mg ×1 followed by 75 mg daily with aspirin 75 mg daily for 21 days followed by clopidogrel 75 mg monotherapy until day 90 Arm 2: Aspirin 75 mg daily monotherapy until day 90	Recurrent stroke by day 90: 8.2% (DAPT) vs. 11.7% (SAPT), $p < 0.001$	Moderate-to-severe bleeding: 0.3% (DAPT) vs. 0.3% (SAPT), $p = 0.73$
POINT (2018) [82]	Minor ischemic stroke (NIHSS <4) or major TIA (ABCD2 ≥ 4) within 12 h of symptom onset Patients with a clear indication for anticoagulation, who were eligible for endovascular therapy, or who received a thrombolytic were excluded Centers in North America, Europe, Australia, and New Zealand	Arm 1: Clopidogrel 600 mg ×1 followed by 75 mg daily with aspirin 50–325 mg daily for 90 days Arm 2: Aspirin 50–325 mg daily for 90 days	Composite of stroke, MI, or vascular death by 90 days: 5% (DAPT) vs. 6.5% (SAPT), $p = 0.02$	Major hemorrhage: 0.9% (DAPT) vs. 0.4%, $p = 0.02$

(continued)

Table 17.8 (continued)

Trial	Population	Treatment	Ischemic outcome	Hemorrhagic outcome
THALES (2020) [73]	Ischemic stroke (NIHSS <6) or major TIA (ABCD2 ≥6) or symptomatic extracranial or intracranial stenosis within 24 h of symptom onset Patients with a clear indication for anticoagulation, who were eligible for endovascular therapy or who received a thrombolytic, were excluded	Arm 1: Ticagrelor 180 mg ×1 followed by 90 mg twice daily with aspirin 300 mg loading dose followed by 75–100 mg daily for 30 days followed by aspirin 75–100 mg monotherapy until day 90 Arm 2: Aspirin 300 mg loading dose followed by 75–100 mg daily monotherapy until day 90	Stroke or death at 90 days: 5.5% (DAPT) vs. 6.5% (SAPT), $p = 0.02$	Severe bleeding: 0.5% (DAPT) vs. 0.1% (SAPT), $p = 0.001$ ICH or fatal bleeding: 0.4% (DAPT) vs. 0.1% (SAPT), $p = 0.005$
CHANCE2 (2021) [83]	Minor ischemic stroke (NIHSS <4) or major TIA (ABCD2 ≥4) within 24 h of symptom onset and CYP2C19 loss-of-function genotype Patients with baseline disability (mRS >2), a clear indication for anticoagulation, who received a thrombolytic were excluded All centers in China	Arm 1: Clopidogrel 300 mg ×1 followed by 75 mg daily with aspirin 75 mg daily for 21 days followed by clopidogrel 75 mg monotherapy until day 90 Arm 2: Ticagrelor 180 mg ×1 followed by 90 mg twice daily with aspirin 75 mg daily until day 21 and then ticagrelor 90 mg twice-daily monotherapy until day 90	Recurrent stroke by day 90: 6.0% (ticagrelor) vs. 7.6% (clopidogrel), $p = 0.008$	Moderate or severe bleeding: 0.3% (ticagrelor) vs. 0.3% (clopidogrel), $p = 0.66$
INSPIRES (2023) [84]	Ischemic stroke (NIHSS <6) or high risk TIA (ABCD2 ≥4) within 24–72 h of symptom onset and >50% stenosis if a major intracranial or extracranial artery or stroke of presumed atherosclerotic origin Patients with baseline disability (mRS >2), a clear indication for anticoagulation, who received a thrombolytic were excluded All centers in China	Arm 1: Clopidogrel 300 mg ×1 followed by 75 mg daily with aspirin 100 mg daily for 21 days followed by clopidogrel 75 mg monotherapy until day 90 Arm 2: Aspirin 100 mg daily monotherapy until day 90	Recurrent stroke within 90 days: 7.3% (DAPT) vs. 9.2% (SAPT), $p = 0.008$	Moderate-to-severe bleeding: 0.9% (DAPT) vs. 0.4% (SAPT), $p = 0.03$

started on DAPT for secondary stroke prevention in a cohort of Italian patients did not meet the inclusion criteria of the major trials [86]. While time to initiation of up to 72 h has now been demonstrated to be effective (INSPIRES trial), initiation of DAPT after receipt of a thrombolytic or thrombectomy and in more severe strokes has limited supporting evidence. The Antiplatelet vs. R-tPA for Acute Mild Ischemic Stroke (ARAMIS) trial randomized 760 patients presenting with mild stroke within 4.5 h of symptom onset to either clopidogrel-based DAPT or alteplase 0.9 mg/kg and demonstrated similar rates of excellent functional outcomes at 90 days (RR 1.36, 95% CI 0.80–2.30) or recurrent stroke at 90 days (0.3 vs. 0.6%, $p = 0.45$), suggesting that intravenous thrombolysis provides equivalent benefit to DAPT in patients with minor stroke, and the safety of initiating DAPT after thrombolysis has yet to be systematically analyzed [87].

17.6 Early Complications

17.6.1 Hemorrhagic Conversion

Ischemic tissue is at high risk of hemorrhagic conversion given the friable nature of the vascular bed around the stroke. Hemorrhagic conversion is variably defined but occurs in up to 40% of patients with ischemic stroke on a varied scale of severity [88]. Hemorrhagic conversion is graded as either hemorrhagic infarction (HI) or parenchymal hematoma (PH), with each having further classifications as either grade 1 (less severe) or grade 2 (more severe) [89]. Conversion can further be classified as either symptomatic (associated with worsening or decompensating neurologic status) or asymptomatic (identified on routine head imagining without associated symptoms). Conversion classification is associated with clinical status and is not universally associated with worse outcomes. The presence of HI (in contrast to PH) may represent successful reperfusion of at-risk tissue and has been associated with significant improvements in ischemic symptoms compared to both PH and no hemorrhagic conversion at all [90].

Several factors contribute to the risk of hemorrhagic transformation after stroke. Older age, higher baseline NIHSS score, higher baseline serum glucose, mass effect present on pretreatment imaging, and hypofibrinogenemia (<150 mg/dL) after treatment with alteplase are commonly cited risk factors associated with conversion [91]. Importantly, while treatment with thrombolytic agents significantly increases the risk of hemorrhagic conversion, spontaneous symptomatic hemorrhagic conversion still occurs in at least 1.3% of patients not treated with thrombolytics, and thus avoidance of thrombolytics in otherwise eligible patients does not entirely negate the risk of sICH [17]. Incidence also varies by definition; differences in the description of "symptomatic" and time, the course in which conversion occurs, can change the reported incidence in clinical trials and cohort studies. sICH as defined by the National Institute of Neurological Diseases and Stroke (NINDS) trial defined any clinical suspicion for decline in neurologic status with any degree of hemorrhage on head CT within 36 h of stroke onset as sICH [15], while the European Cooperative Acute Stroke Study (ECASS) and Safe Implementation of Thrombolysis in Stroke: Monitoring Study (SITS-MOST) provide more stringent criteria of a worsening of at least 4 points in the NIHSS score associated with hemorrhage within 36 h of stroke onset [16, 92].

Regardless of definition, any acute change in neurologic status should prompt clinical evaluation and consideration for emergent repeat head imaging to assess for bleeding. Patients typically undergo scheduled hourly or every other hour neurologic exams in the first 24 h after stroke to rapidly identify new deficits and prompt further evaluation. The NINDS trial protocol mandated a routine 24-h head CT to screen for hemorrhagic conversion, and while this practice has been questioned [93], it provides a "cap" to the 24-h monitoring window when patients are most likely to experience hemorrhagic conversion.

Treatment of hemorrhagic conversion should involve an assessment of the time from thrombolysis administration (if administered) and if other factors that could contribute to conversion (i.e., coagulopathy, antithrombotic therapy) are present. The 2019 acute stroke guidelines and 2017 AHA/ASA scientific statement on hemorrhagic transformation after alteplase provide treatment recommendations for patients who experience conversion [7, 91]. First, patients who experience minor, asymptomatic hemorrhagic conversion (such as HI1 per the Heidelberg criteria) may not require alterations in management. Patients with petechial hemorrhagic conversion generally tolerate the initiation of antiplatelet agents, and petechial hemorrhage was not an exclusion criterion for the ELAN trial, which evaluated early initiation of DOACs in stroke patients [69, 94]. In patients with sICH, deciding whether to provide hemostatic therapy ("thrombolytic reversal") should be based primarily on the timing of thrombolytic administration. While the alteplase and tenecteplase are terminally eliminated after 6 and 12 h, respectively, the effect of plasminogen activation persists for longer than the medications are present in circulation. Alteplase and tenecteplase exhibit both their intended pharmacologic action and their potential toxicities (bleeding) indirectly (i.e., through activation of plasminogen to plasmin, where plasmin then dissolves fibrin into fibrin degradation products); therefore, reversal should take into account both the pharmacokinetic properties of the parent agents and the pharmacodynamic relationship between the thrombolytic and the endogenous coagulation system. Fibrinogen, plasminogen, and D-dimer concentrations have been used as surrogates for this relationship and remain altered up to 24 h after thrombolytic administration [94, 95]. Therefore, treating sICH that occurs within 24 h of thrombolytic administration with hemostatic therapy may be reasonable to prevent hemorrhagic expansion.

Specific agents to consider when treating thrombolytic-associated sICH are summarized in Table 17.9. Notably, none are direct reversal agents for the thrombolytic agent itself per se but rather work to counteract the pharmacodynamic effect of plasminogen activation. Additionally, dosing, monitoring, and considerations are largely based on expert opinion, and no randomized controlled trials exist to guide the selection of agents. Adjunctive agents, including prothrombin complex concentrate, vitamin K, fresh frozen plasma (FFP), platelet transfusion, or recombinant

Table 17.9 Hemostatic therapy for sICH after thrombolysis administration [16, 56]

Agent	Dosing	Notes
Cryoprecipitate IV	10 units	10 units are expected to increase serum fibrinogen by 50 mg/dL Consider repeating until serum fibrinogen $\geq$150 mg/dL. **Note:** tenecteplase does not significantly affect serum fibrinogen concentrations
Fibrinogen concentrate (RiaSTAP, Fibryga) IV	40–70 mg/kg If baseline fibrinogen is known, can calculate dose: Dose in mg/kg = (150 measured fibrinogen [mg/dL])/1.7	Dosing extrapolated from recommendations for congenital fibrinogen deficiency
Tranexamic acid IV	10 mg/kg (consider empiric dosing of 1000 mg)	
Aminocaproic acid IV	4 g infusion over 1 h followed by 1 g/h for 8 h or until stable on repeat imaging	

factor VIIa, can be considered in specific circumstances but generally do not have a role in therapy for bleeding associated with thrombolytics. Despite this, treatment with adjunct agents is common—in a multicenter cohort study of 128 patients who experienced thrombolytic-associated sICH, 28.9% received a platelet transfusion, 20.3% received FFP, and 10.1% received vitamin K, PCC, or rFVIIa. None were protective for in-hospital mortality or hematoma expansion, and platelet transfusion was found to be associated with a higher rate of hematoma expansion (45.8 vs. 18.9%, $p = 0.01$) [96]. Lack of treatment with any product was common (38.2% received no therapy), which may suggest confounding by indication, where more severely ill patients received a higher intensity of therapy.

The role of cryoprecipitate or fibrinogen concentrate is to correct hypofibrinogenemia, which is both a consequence of thrombolytic administration and a potential mediator of hemorrhagic conversion. Treatment typically targets a serum fibrinogen concentration of $\geq$150 mg/dL, but it is reasonable to treat even if fibrinogen concentrations are above this at baseline. Tenecteplase does not significantly affect serum fibrinogen concentrations, and thus repeat dosing to a target fibrinogen concentration in patients who received tenecteplase may not be feasible [95]. Blood banks often release pools of cryoprecipitate in batches of 10 units, which is the basis for the empiric dosing recommendation, but this may vary by institution. A cohort study of 19 patients who received cryoprecipitate for thrombolysis-associated sICH reported that the median dose was 5 units, likely because this was the size of the pool released by the institution's blood blank. In this cohort, the median time to administration was 6.9 h after alteplase administration, 74% of patients received concurrent alternative blood products, and rates of thrombosis were low (5%). Hemostasis, defined as stable ICH size on repeat head imaging within 24 h of hemostatic therapy administration, was observed in 4 of the 14 (29%) patients who had imaging available for evaluation [97]. A similar cohort of 24 patients who received fibrinogen concentrate for thrombolysis-associated sICH received a median dose of fibrinogen concentrate of 2215 mg (mg/kg dose not reported) and reported a thrombosis rate of 12.5%. In this cohort, a higher rate of hemostasis was observed (77.2%) [98].

Support for the use of antifibrinolytic agents to supplement treatment in thrombolytic-associated sICH is mostly limited to case reports and series. Three case reports describe effective hemostasis with tranexamic acid after thrombolysis-associated sICH, with doses ranging from 1000 to 1670 mg [99–101]. TXA was selected either because of patient preference not to receive blood products, hyperfibrinolysis was identified on rotational thromboelastometry (ROTEM), or the patient experienced a transfusion reaction to cryoprecipitate. Outcomes associated with aminocaproic acid have been described in two case series by the same author group. The first is a cohort of 16 patients who received aminocaproic acid for thrombolysis-associated hemorrhage, of which 10 had received alteplase for stroke. Dosing varied, but the median bolus dose was 4 g, and the median infusion dose was 1 g/h for 5 h. Half of the included patients only received a single bolus. Of the included patients who received alteplase for stroke and experienced sICH (7/10), 50% of patients with evaluable repeat imaging (2/4) achieved hemostasis [102]. In a follow-up series by the same authors evaluating cryoprecipitate (discussed above), receipt of both cryoprecipitate and aminocaproic acid was associated with a 67% rate of hemostasis compared to 8% for cryoprecipitate alone [97].

Other aspects of managing hemorrhagic conversion follow similar principles to spontaneous ICH. It is reasonable to acutely control blood pressure and maintain SBP less than 140 mm Hg, avoid fever, avoid hyperglycemia, and reverse other potential coagulopathies. While secondary causes of ICH were excluded from key trials evaluating these interventions in ICH [103], the principles likely apply to hemorrhagic conversion as well.

17.6.2 Angioedema

An additional acute complication of acute ischemic stroke in patients treated with intravenous thrombolysis is contralateral orolingual angioedema. Angioedema is rare following thrombolysis, occurring in approximately 1–5% of treated patients, but it can be life threatening if not identified early and managed appropriately [62]. The endogenous fibrinolytic system is directly involved in the activation and upregulation of the kallikrein-bradykinin system and has been implicated in the pathophysiology of hereditary angioedema (HAE) [104]. The introduction of recombinant tissue plasminogen activator to serum thus accelerates the generation of bradykinin and increases the risk of angioedema, as has been seen with alteplase and tenecteplase treatment in patients with stroke [105, 106].

Several factors notably increase the risk of angioedema in patients treated with intravenous thrombolysis. Strokes localized to the right insulo-opercular area have been associated with angioedema [106, 107], as has pre-stroke treatment with ACE inhibitors [108]. A meta-analysis of 12 observational cohort studies identified that patients on ACE inhibitors had more than a five-times greater risk of developing angioedema compared to patients not on ACE inhibitors (crude prevalence of 12.58 vs. 1.97%). This effect was distinct to ACE inhibitors, as rates of angioedema were similar in patients taking angiotensin receptor blockers, beta-blockers, diuretics, and calcium channel blockers [108]. Rates of angioedema appear to be similar between alteplase and tenecteplase, although evidence evaluating this endpoint is limited [109].

While angioedema following thrombolysis can be mild and self-limiting, the need for urgent intubation and ultimately tracheostomy because of persistent angio-edema has been reported [110]. Angioedema onset is typically rapid, within 1–2 h of thrombolysis administration in most cases [111]. If angioedema develops during alteplase infusion, the infusion should be discontinued immediately.

The 2019 AHA/ASA guidelines for the management of acute ischemic stroke provide a class 1B statement recommending preparedness for potential emergent adverse events to thrombolysis, of which angioedema is specifically listed [7]. Guideline-recommended management of thrombolysis-associated angioedema is largely based on expert opinion and includes definitive securement of the airway if needed, discontinuation of alteplase if infusion is still running, cessation of angiotensin-converting enzyme (ACE) inhibitor therapy if currently ordered, and treatment with intravenous corticosteroids, antihistamines (diphenhydramine and famotidine), and nebulizers if needed. Therapies approved for HAE, such as icati-bant or plasma-derived C1 esterase, are suggested, but it is unclear if these will be effective in this population. Other therapies for angioedema, including fresh frozen plasma (FFP), tranexamic acid (TXA), or ecallantide, are not mentioned and only have case report-level evidence supporting their use for this indication. Therapy recommendations are summarized in Table 17.10.

17.6.3 Malignant Cerebral Edema

As neurons die after ischemic insult, they lose their ability to regulate electron gra-dients across cell membranes as the energy required to maintain sodium-potassium ATP-ase pumps is no longer produced. Without electron gradients, water flows pas-sively into neurons, causing progressive swelling and cytotoxic cerebral edema. While some cerebral edema is present in nearly 25% of all strokes, "malignant" cerebral edema (characterized by edema leading to mass effect and/or midline shift) is less common, occurring in approximately 5% of patients and most commonly in hemispheric MCA territory strokes [119]. Cerebral edema generally begins to develop 24–48 h after stroke onset, with incidence peaking at 3–5 days [120], and patients should be closely monitored for clinical signs of cerebral edema during this

Table 17.10 Therapies for thrombolysis-associated angioedema

Agent	Dose	Notes
First-line therapy		
Methylprednisolone IV	125 mg	Can be scheduled every 6 h if response is not immediate
Diphenhydramine IV	50 mg	Generally only needed once but can be scheduled every 6–12 h
Famotidine IV	20 mg	Generally only needed once but can be scheduled every 12 h
Second-line and rescue therapies		
Epinephrine SC	0.3 mg	**Generally avoided because of risk of posttreatment hypertension,** but considered if not responding to steroids and antihistamines
Icatibant SC	30 mg	Approved for hereditary angioedema treatment; dose can be repeated in 6 h if insufficient response is noted. Improvements have been observed in three case reports and no response in one [112–115]
Plasma-derived C1 esterase inhibitor IV (Ruconest, Berinert)	20 IU/ kg	Approved for hereditary angioedema treatment. Improvements have been observed in one case report [116]
Ecallantide SC	30 mg	Approved for hereditary angioedema treatment. No published reports support its role for thrombolysis-associated angioedema
Tranexamic acid IV	1000 mg	Theoretically beneficial (inhibits bradykinin production). No published reports support its role for thrombolysis-associated angioedema, but cohort studies support its role in ACEi-associated angioedema [117, 118]. **Caution** that TXA may partially reverse the thrombolytic effect of thrombolysis

time period. Outcomes in the absence of surgical decompression are dismal; 78% of patients in an early cohort of 55 patients who experienced malignant cerebral edema died as a result of poststroke herniation [120]. Several factors, including younger age, female sex, higher baseline NIHSS, early signs of ischemia and hyperdense vessel sign on baseline head CT, and a history of diabetes, hypertension, atrial fibrillation, or heart failure, have been associated with increased odds of developing malignant edema [119].

The management of patients who develop malignant cerebral edema after stroke is summarized in a 2014 scientific statement from the American Heart Association and the American Stroke Association and involves medical management of increased intracranial pressure and considerations for decompressive hemicraniectomy [121]. Strokes involving the MCA territory and cerebellar hemispheres are at the highest risk of causing herniation and thus warrant the most aggressive management. Because of the low quality of evidence with some signal for harm, both the 2014 malignant cerebral edema recommendations and 2020 NCS cerebral edema guidelines recommend against the use of prophylactic hyperosmolar agents in patients at risk of cerebral edema [121, 122].

Hyperosmolar therapy does have a role in patients who develop clinical or radiographic signs of mass effect with or without clinical herniation, however. If patients develop worsening levels of consciousness, signs of Cushing's triad (bradycardia, widening pulse pressure, irregular respirations), or changes in brainstem reflexes, urgent imaging should be obtained to assess for the development of edema and hyperosmolar therapy should be considered. Bolus hyperosmolar therapy (sodium chloride 3 or 23.4% or mannitol 20 or 25%) is preferable to continuous infusion in the setting of acute increases in intracranial pressure, as boluses have been reported to reverse clinical herniation [123]. There is insufficient evidence to support whether hypertonic solutions should be given on an "as-needed" basis for clinical events or if scheduled hyperosmolar therapy is ideal.

In cases of severe hemispheric cerebral edema, medical management with hyperosmolar therapy is insufficient to adequately treat increased intracranial pressure. Hypertonic solutions establish an osmotic gradient across a healthy blood-brain barrier to cause a shift in water content out of brain tissue and out of the cranial vault and also improve the rheological properties of red blood cells to improve perfusion to at-risk tissue. Because the blood-brain barrier is damaged in ischemic tissue, hypertonic solutions mainly shrink the volume of non-infarcted tissue and may not impact the volume of edema in the stroke bed. In one study of seven patients with hemispheric strokes with midline shift who were administered 1.5 g/kg of mannitol, brain volume overall decreased by an average of 8.1 mL (0.62%). The decrease was primarily in the non-infarcted hemisphere, however, with an average decrease of 0.82% in the non-infarcted hemisphere vs. 0.0% in the infarcted hemisphere ($p < 0.05$) [124].

If edema progresses, the definitive management involves decompressive hemicraniectomy. Decompressive hemicraniectomy has been evaluated in nine randomized controlled trials and has uniformly been found to be a lifesaving procedure in patients with malignant cerebral edema. Trials generally randomized patients without substantial premorbid disability who presented with strokes occupying 50–66% of the MCA or cerebellar vascular territory within 24–48 h of symptom onset associated with high baseline NIHSS scores and alterations in levels of consciousness to surgical decompression or medical management [125]. Across 526 randomized patients, surgical decompression was associated with a significant reduction in the risk of death at 6–12 months (OR 0.18, 95% CI 0.12–0.27) as well as death or disability (mRS >3) at 6–12 months (OR 0.34, 95% CI 0.22–0.52), but rates of severe disability (mRS 5) were similar between arms (OR 0.73, 95% CI 0.36–1.44). While the number of patients who experienced severe disability is higher in those who underwent decompression, this is counterbalanced by the number of patients who survive and are able to recover to lower levels of disability. Mortality is common in patients managed with medical therapy alone (68.3%). Positive effects of decompression are consistent between younger (<60 years) and older (>60 years) patients and whether decompression occurred before or after 48 h from symptom onset, although a trend towards improved outcomes with earlier decompression was noted [126]. While additional trials have been published since the AHA/ASA recommendation, the 2014 recommendation provides a class I LOE B recommendation for decompressive hemicraniectomy in patients <60 years of age with hemispheric infarctions who experience neurologic deterioration and a class IIb LOE C recommendation for patients >60 years of age.

Post-decompression, it is unclear what the role of hypertonic therapy is, as the restrictive effect of the skull has been removed from the mass lesion. It may be reasonable to continue therapy post-decompression to prevent rebound edema. Additional medical management considerations post-decompressive hemicraniectomy include seizure prophylaxis, as seizures occur in 25–36% of patients within a week of decompression [127–129]. Prophylaxis with levetiracetam 500–1000 mg twice daily may be reasonable for 1 week post-decompression, although evidence supporting this is limited to retrospective observational data. It may also be reasonable to withhold antithrombotic secondary stroke prevention therapy for 2–7 days postoperatively, but it is unknown when the ideal time to resume antiplatelet or anticoagulant therapy is after a hemicraniectomy.

17.7 Secondary Prevention

The risk of stroke recurrence is highest within the first 30 days post-event, a risk which can be mitigated with appropriate secondary preventive measures. Secondary prevention of stroke includes a comprehensive approach to risk factor modification, stroke prevention, diet and lifestyle adjustment, and prevention of complications. A simplified acronym to remember the key factors of secondary stroke prevention includes the "ABCDEFGs." A stands for antithrombotic therapy, either antiplatelet or anticoagulant, which should be prescribed during the hospital stay. Patients with atrial fibrillation should have an appropriate prescription for an oral anticoagulant, with counseling provided to ensure that patients are aware of the signs and symptoms of recurrent stroke or bleeding events. As mentioned in the previous section on antiplatelet therapy, candidates for DAPT should be sure that they are informed of the appropriate duration of therapy (21 vs. 90 days) to minimize the risk of adverse sequelae from prolonged treatment. B stands for blood pressure control. Patients with hypertension poststroke should be prescribed guideline-based antihypertensives, including an ACEi, ARB, or thiazide diuretic, which have been shown to effectively lower BP and risk of recurrent stroke [13, 130]. The optimal blood pressure target for long-term management is <130/80 mmHg [13]. C stands for smoking cessation and cholesterol management with high-intensity statin therapy. Smoking cessation is a critical factor in reducing the risk of stroke recurrence, as persistent smoking after an initial event increased the risk of recurrent stroke 1.68-fold with 10–20 cigarettes a day which increases to 2.72 in those who smoke more than 40 cigarettes daily [131]. Smoking cessation strategies can include nicotine replacement therapies (patch, gum, lozenges) or use of prescription-based treatments such as varenicline or bupropion [132]. A meta-analysis of 11 randomized trials and 12 observational studies found that statins reduced the risk of recurrent stroke by 20–33% [133]. Patients should be discharged on a high-intensity statin (atorvastatin 40–80 mg, rosuvastatin 20–40 mg) with a target LDL <70 mg/dL [13]. Diet, exercise, flu vaccination, and glucose control complete the DEFGs of secondary stroke prevention management, all of which are important educational points for patients upon discharge. Addressing barriers to adherence for medications and lifestyle should also be addressed to ensure the best possible outcomes for patients.

References

1. Tsao CW, Aday AW, Almarzooq ZI, et al. Heart disease and stroke statistics-2023 update: a report from the American Heart Association. Circulation. 2023;147(8):e93–e621. https://doi.org/10.1161/CIR.0000000000001123.
2. Pu L, Wang L, Zhang R, Zhao T, Jiang Y, Han L. Projected global trends in ischemic stroke incidence, deaths and disability-adjusted life years from 2020 to 2030. Stroke. 2023;54(5):1330–9. https://doi.org/10.1161/STROKEAHA.122.040073.
3. Zhao H, Pesavento L, Coote S, et al. Ambulance clinical triage for acute stroke treatment. Stroke. 2018;49(4):945–51. https://doi.org/10.1161/STROKEAHA.117.019307.
4. Huwez F, Casswell EJ. FAST-AV or FAST-AB tool improves the sensitivity of FAST screening for detection of posterior circulation strokes. Int J Stroke. 2013;8(3):E3. https://doi.org/10.1111/ijs.12008.
5. Aroor S, Singh R, Goldstein LB. BE-FAST (balance, eyes, face, arm, speech, time): reducing the proportion of strokes missed using the FAST mnemonic. Stroke. 2017;48(2):479–81. https://doi.org/10.1161/STROKEAHA.116.015169.
6. Demel SL, Broderick JP. Basilar occlusion syndromes. Neurohospitalist. 2015;5(3):142–50. https://doi.org/10.1177/1941874415583847.
7. Powers WJ, Rabinstein AA, Ackerson T, et al. Guidelines for the early management of patients with acute ischemic stroke: 2019 update to the 2018 guidelines for the early management of acute ischemic stroke a guideline for healthcare professionals from the American Heart Association/American Stroke A. Stroke. 2019;50(49):e344–418. https://doi.org/10.1161/STR.0000000000000211.
8. Eddelien HS, Butt JH, Christensen T, Danielsen AK, Kruuse C. Sex and age differences in patient-reported acute stroke symptoms. Front Neurol. 2022;13:846690. https://doi.org/10.3389/fneur.2022.846690.
9. Nicholls JK, Ince J, Minhas JS, Chung EML. Emerging detection techniques for large vessel occlusion stroke: a scoping review. Front Neurol. 2022;12:780324. https://doi.org/10.3389/fneur.2021.780324.
10. Jovin TG, Demchuk AM, Gupta R. Pathophysiology of acute ischemic stroke. Continuum Lifelong Learning Neurol. 2008;14(6):28. https://doi.org/10.1212/01.CON.0000275639.07451.e7.
11. Allen LM, Hasso AN, Handwerker J, Farid H. Sequence-specific MR Imaging findings that are useful in dating ischemic stroke. Radiographics. 2012;32(5):1285–97; discussion 1297-9. https://doi.org/10.1148/rg.325115760.
12. Adams HP, Bendixen BH, Kappelle LJ, et al. Classification of subtype of acute ischemic stroke. Definitions for use in a multicenter clinical trial. TOAST. Trial of Org 10172 in Acute Stroke Treatment. Stroke. 1993;24(1):35–41. https://doi.org/10.1161/01.str.24.1.35.
13. Kleindorfer DO, Towfighi A, Chaturvedi S, et al. 2021 guideline for the prevention of stroke in patients with stroke and transient ischemic attack: a guideline from the American Heart Association/American Stroke Association. Stroke. 2021;52(7):e364–467. https://doi.org/10.1161/STR.0000000000000375.
14. Tsivgoulis G, Katsanos AH, Sandset EC, et al. Thrombolysis for acute ischaemic stroke: current status and future perspectives. Lancet Neurol. 2023;22(5):418–29. https://doi.org/10.1016/S1474-4422(22)00519-1.

15. The National Institute of Neurological Disorders and Stroke rt-PA Stroke Study Group. Tissue plasminogen activator for acute ischemic stroke. N Engl J Med. 1995;333(24):1581–8. https://doi.org/10.1056/NEJM199512143332401.

16. Hacke W, Kaste M, Bluhmki E, et al. Thrombolysis with alteplase 3 to 4.5 hours after acute ischemic stroke. N Engl J Med. 2008;359(13):1317–29. https://doi.org/10.1056/NEJMoa0804656.

17. Emberson J, Lees KR, Lyden P, et al. Effect of treatment delay, age, and stroke severity on the effects of intravenous thrombolysis with alteplase for acute ischaemic stroke: a meta-analysis of individual patient data from randomised trials. Lancet. 2014;384(9958):1929–35. https://doi.org/10.1016/S0140-6736(14)60584-5.

18. Charbonnier G, Bonnet L, Biondi A, Moulin T. Intracranial bleeding after reperfusion therapy in acute ischemic stroke. Front Neurol. 2021;11:11. https://doi.org/10.3389/fneur.2020.629920.

19. Thomalla G, Simonsen CZ, Boutitie F, et al. MRI-guided thrombolysis for stroke with unknown time of onset. N Engl J Med. 2018;379(7):611–22. https://doi.org/10.1056/NEJMoa1804355.

20. Campbell BCV, Ma H, Ringleb PA, et al. Extending thrombolysis to 4·5-9 h and wake-up stroke using perfusion imaging: a systematic review and meta-analysis of individual patient data. Lancet. 2019;394(10193):139–47. https://doi.org/10.1016/S0140-6736(19)31053-0.

21. Menon BK, Singh N, Sylaja PN. Tenecteplase use in patients with acute ischaemic stroke. Lancet. 2023;401(10377):618–9. https://doi.org/10.1016/S0140-6736(22)02633-2.

22. Hall J, Thon JM, Heslin M, et al. Tenecteplase improves door-to-needle time in real-world acute stroke treatment. Stroke. 2021;1(1):e000102. https://doi.org/10.1161/SVIN.121.000102.

23. Kobeissi H, Ghozy S, Turfe B, et al. Tenecteplase vs. alteplase for treatment of acute ischemic stroke: a systematic review and meta-analysis of randomized trials. Front Neurol. 2023;14:1102463. https://doi.org/10.3389/fneur.2023.1102463.

24. Kvistad CE, Næss H, Helleberg BH, et al. Tenecteplase versus alteplase for the management of acute ischaemic stroke in Norway (NOR-TEST 2, part a): a phase 3, randomised, open-label, blinded endpoint, non-inferiority trial. Lancet Neurol. 2022;21(6):511–9. https://doi.org/10.1016/S1474-4422(22)00124-7.

25. Alamowitch S, Turc G, Palaiodimou L, et al. European Stroke Organisation (ESO) expedited recommendation on tenecteplase for acute ischaemic stroke. Eur Stroke J. 2023;8(1):8–54. https://doi.org/10.1177/23969873221150022.

26. Goyal M, Menon BK, van Zwam WH, et al. Endovascular thrombectomy after large-vessel ischaemic stroke: a meta-analysis of individual patient data from five randomised trials. Lancet. 2016;387(10029):1723–31. https://doi.org/10.1016/S0140-6736(16)00163-X.

27. Nogueira RG, Lutsep HL, Gupta R, et al. Trevo versus merci retrievers for thrombectomy revascularisation of large vessel occlusions in acute ischaemic stroke (TREVO 2): a randomised trial. Lancet. 2012;380(9849):1231–40. https://doi.org/10.1016/S0140-6736(12)61299-9.

28. Nogueira RG, Jadhav AP, Haussen DC, et al. Thrombectomy 6 to 24 hours after stroke with a mismatch between deficit and infarct. N Engl J Med. 2018;378(1):11–21. https://doi.org/10.1056/NEJMoa1706442.

29. Albers GW, Marks MP, Kemp S, et al. Thrombectomy for stroke at 6 to 16 hours with selection by perfusion imaging. N Engl J Med. 2018;378(8):708–18. https://doi.org/10.1056/NEJMoa1713973.

30. Liu X, Dai Q, Ye R, et al. Endovascular treatment versus standard medical treatment for vertebrobasilar artery occlusion (BEST): an open-label, randomised controlled trial. Lancet Neurol. 2020;19(2):115–22. https://doi.org/10.1016/S1474-4422(19)30395-3.

31. Langezaal LCM, van der Hoeven EJRJ, Mont'Alverne FJA, et al. Endovascular therapy for stroke due to basilar-artery occlusion. N Engl J Med. 2021;384(20):1910–20. https://doi.org/10.1056/NEJMoa2030297.

32. Tao C, Nogueira RG, Zhu Y, et al. Trial of endovascular treatment of acute basilar-artery occlusion. N Engl J Med. 2022;387(15):1361–72. https://doi.org/10.1056/NEJMoa2206317.

33. Jovin TG, Li C, Wu L, et al. Trial of thrombectomy 6 to 24 hours after stroke due to basilar-artery occlusion. N Engl J Med. 2022;387(15):1373–84. https://doi.org/10.1056/NEJMoa2207576.

34. Malik A, Drumm B, D'Anna L, et al. Mechanical thrombectomy in acute basilar artery stroke: a systematic review and meta-analysis of randomized controlled trials. BMC Neurol. 2022;22(1):415. https://doi.org/10.1186/s12883-022-02953-2.

35. Bendszus M, Fiehler J, Subtil F, et al. Endovascular thrombectomy for acute ischaemic stroke with established large infarct: multicentre, open-label, randomised trial. Lancet. 2023;402(10414):1753–63. https://doi.org/10.1016/S0140-6736(23)02032-9.

36. Yoshimura S, Sakai N, Yamagami H, et al. Endovascular therapy for acute stroke with a large ischemic region. N Engl J Med. 2022;386(14):1303–13. https://doi.org/10.1056/NEJMoa2118191.

37. Siegler JE, Qureshi MM, Nogueira RG, et al. Endovascular vs medical management for late anterior large vessel occlusion with prestroke disability. Neurology. 2023;100(7):e751–63. https://doi.org/10.1212/WNL.0000000000201543.

38. Patel K, Taneja K, Shu L, et al. Anterior circulation thrombectomy in patients with low national institutes of health stroke scale score: analysis of the national inpatient sample. Stroke 2023 4(2):e000998. https://doi.org/10.1161/SVIN.123.000998.

39. Tung EL, McTaggart RA, Baird GL, et al. Rethinking thrombolysis in cerebral infarction 2b. Stroke. 2017;48(9):2488–93. https://doi.org/10.1161/STROKEAHA.117.017182.

40. Wollenweber FA, Tiedt S, Alegiani A, et al. Functional outcome following stroke Thrombectomy in clinical practice. Stroke. 2019;50(9):2500–6. https://doi.org/10.1161/STROKEAHA.119.026005.

41. Yogendrakumar V, Churilov L, Guha P, et al. Tenecteplase treatment and thrombus characteristics associated with early reperfusion: an EXTEND-IA TNK trials analysis. Stroke. 2023;54(3):706–14. https://doi.org/10.1161/STROKEAHA.122.041061.

42. Fransen PSS, Berkhemer OA, Lingsma HF, et al. Time to reperfusion and treatment effect for acute ischemic stroke: a randomized clinical trial. JAMA Neurol. 2016;73(2):190–6. https://doi.org/10.1001/jamaneurol.2015.3886.

43. Renú A, Millán M, San Román L, et al. Effect of intra-arterial alteplase vs placebo following successful thrombectomy on functional outcomes in patients with large vessel occlusion acute ischemic stroke: the CHOICE randomized clinical trial. JAMA. 2022;327(9):826–35. https://doi.org/10.1001/jama.2022.1645.

44. Qureshi AI, Suri MF, Shatla AA, et al. Intra-arterial recombinant tissue plasminogen activator for ischemic stroke: an accelerating dosing regimen. Neurosurgery. 2000;47(2):473–6. discussion 477–9

45. Georgiadis AL, Memon MZ, Shah QA, et al. Intra-arterial tenecteplase for treatment of acute ischemic stroke: feasibility and comparative outcomes. J Neuroimaging. 2012;22(3):249–54. https://doi.org/10.1111/j.1552-6569.2011.00628.x.

46. Zhao ZA, Qiu J, Wang L, et al. Intra-arterial tenecteplase is safe and may improve the first-pass recanalization for acute ischemic stroke with large-artery atherosclerosis: the BRETIS-TNK trial. Front Neurol. 2023;14:1155269. https://doi.org/10.3389/fneur.2023.1155269.

47. Elhorany M, Lenck S, Degos V, et al. Cangrelor and stenting in acute ischemic stroke: monocentric case series. Clin Neuroradiol. 2021;31(2):439–48. https://doi.org/10.1007/s00062-020-00907-0.

48. Holden DN, Entezami P, Bush MC, et al. Characterization of antiplatelet response to low-dose cangrelor utilizing platelet function testing in neuroendovascular patients. Pharmacotherapy. 2021;41(10):811–9. https://doi.org/10.1002/phar.2619.

49. Qureshi AI, Ezzeddine MA, Nasar A, et al. Prevalence of elevated blood pressure in 563,704 adult patients presenting to the emergency department with stroke in the United States. Am J Emerg Med. 2007;25(1):32–8. https://doi.org/10.1016/j.ajem.2006.07.008.

50. Silver B, Lu M, Morris DC, Mitsias PD, Lewandowski C, Chopp M. Blood pressure declines and less favorable outcomes in the NINDS tPA stroke study. J Neurol Sci. 2008;271(1–2):61–7. https://doi.org/10.1016/j.jns.2008.03.012.

51. Ahmed N, Wahlgren N, Brainin M, et al. Relationship of blood pressure, antihypertensive therapy, and outcome in ischemic stroke treated with intravenous thrombolysis: retrospective analysis from safe implementation of thrombolysis in stroke-international stroke thrombolysis register (SITS-ISTR). Stroke. 2009;40(7):2442–9. https://doi.org/10.1161/STROKEAHA.109.548602.

52. Anderson CS, Huang Y, Lindley RI, et al. Intensive blood pressure reduction with intravenous thrombolysis therapy for acute ischaemic stroke (ENCHANTED): an international, randomised, open-label, blinded-endpoint, phase 3 trial. Lancet. 2019;393(10174):877–88. https://doi.org/10.1016/S0140-6736(19)30038-8.

53. Zaki HA, Lloyd SA, Elmoheen A, et al. Antihypertensive interventions in acute ischemic stroke: a systematic review and meta-analysis evaluating clinical outcomes through an emergency medicine paradigm. Cureus. 2023;15(10):e47729. https://doi.org/10.7759/cureus.47729.

54. Nam HS, Kim YD, Heo J, et al. Intensive vs conventional blood pressure lowering after endovascular thrombectomy in acute ischemic stroke: the OPTIMAL-BP randomized clinical trial. JAMA. 2023;330(9):832–42. https://doi.org/10.1001/jama.2023.14590.

55. Todo K. Blood pressure variability in acute ischemic stroke. Hypertens Res. 2024;4:1–2. https://doi.org/10.1038/s41440-023-01556-9.

56. Hao F, Yin S, Tang L, Zhang X, Zhang S. Nicardipine versus labetalol for hypertension during acute stroke: a systematic review and meta-analysis. Neurol India. 2022;70(5):1793–9. https://doi.org/10.4103/0028-3886.359214.

57. Liu-DeRyke X, Levy PD, Parker D, Coplin W, Rhoney DH. A prospective evaluation of labetalol versus nicardipine for blood pressure management in patients with acute stroke. Neurocrit Care. 2013;19(1):41–7. https://doi.org/10.1007/s12028-013-9863-9.

58. Poyant JO, Kuper PJ, Mara KC, et al. Nicardipine reduces blood pressure variability after spontaneous intracerebral hemorrhage. Neurocrit Care. 2019;30(1):118–25. https://doi.org/10.1007/s12028-018-0582-0.

59. Rosenfeldt Z, Conklen K, Jones B, Ferrill D, Deshpande M, Siddiqui FM. Comparison of nicardipine with clevidipine in the management of hypertension in acute cerebrovascular diseases. J Stroke Cerebrovasc Dis. 2018;27(8):2067–73. https://doi.org/10.1016/j.jstrokecerebrovasdis.2018.03.001.

60. Finger JR, Kurczewski LM, Brophy GM. Clevidipine versus nicardipine for acute blood pressure reduction in a neuroscience intensive care population. Neurocrit Care. 2017;26(2):167–73. https://doi.org/10.1007/s12028-016-0349-4.

61. Overgaard J, Skinhøj E. A paradoxical cerebral hemodynamic effect of hydralazine. Stroke. 1975;6(4):402–4. https://doi.org/10.1161/01.STR.6.4.402.

62. Fröhlich K, Macha K, Gerner ST, et al. Angioedema in stroke patients with thrombolysis. Stroke. 2019;50(7):1682–7. https://doi.org/10.1161/STROKEAHA.119.025260.

63. Wang X, Ouyang M, Yang J, Song L, Yang M, Anderson CS. Anticoagulants for acute ischaemic stroke. Cochrane Database Syst Rev. 2021;2021(10):CD000024. https://doi.org/10.1002/14651858.CD000024.pub5.

64. Ruff CT, Giugliano RP, Braunwald E, et al. Comparison of the efficacy and safety of new oral anticoagulants with warfarin in patients with atrial fibrillation: a meta-analysis of randomised trials. Lancet. 2014;383(9921):955–62. https://doi.org/10.1016/S0140-6736(13)62343-0.

65. Seiffge DJ, Traenka C, Polymeris A, et al. Early start of DOAC after ischemic stroke: risk of intracranial hemorrhage and recurrent events. Neurology. 2016;87(18):1856–62. https://doi.org/10.1212/WNL.0000000000003283.

66. Abdul-Rahim AH, Fulton RL, Frank B, et al. Association of improved outcome in acute ischaemic stroke patients with atrial fibrillation who receive early antithrombotic therapy: analysis from VISTA. Eur J Neurol. 2015;22(7):1048–55. https://doi.org/10.1111/ene.12577.

67. Marchis GMD, Seiffge DJ, Schaedelin S, et al. Early versus late start of direct oral anticoagulants after acute ischaemic stroke linked to atrial fibrillation: an observational study and

individual patient data pooled analysis. J Neurol Neurosurg Psychiatry. 2022;93(2):119–25. https://doi.org/10.1136/jnnp-2021-327236.

68. Heidbuchel H, Verhamme P, Alings M, et al. EHRA practical guide on the use of new oral anticoagulants in patients with non-valvular atrial fibrillation: executive summary. Eur Heart J. 2013;34(27):2094–106. https://doi.org/10.1093/eurheartj/eht134.

69. Fischer U, Koga M, Strbian D, et al. Early versus later anticoagulation for stroke with atrial fibrillation. N Engl J Med. 2023;388(26):2411–21. https://doi.org/10.1056/NEJMoa2303048.

70. Jiang M, Wang C, Zhang Y. Comparison of early and delayed anticoagulation therapy after ischemic stroke in patients with atrial fibrillation: a systematic review and meta-analysis. J Thromb Thrombolysis. 2023;56(4):603–13. https://doi.org/10.1007/s11239-023-02872-0.

71. Chen ZM. CAST: randomised placebo-controlled trial of early aspirin use in 20 000 patients with acute ischaemic stroke. Lancet. 1997;349(9066):1641–9. https://doi.org/10.1016/S0140-6736(97)04010-5.

72. The international stroke trial (IST): a randomised trial of aspirin, subcutaneous heparin, both, or neither among 19 435 patients with acute ischaemic stroke. Lancet. 1997;349(9065):1569–81. https://doi.org/10.1016/S0140-6736(97)04011-7.

73. Johnston SC, Amarenco P, Denison H, et al. Ticagrelor and aspirin or aspirin alone in acute ischemic stroke or TIA. N Engl J Med. 2020;383(3):207–17. https://doi.org/10.1056/NEJMoa1916870.

74. Diener HC. Bogousslavsky J, Brass LM, et al. Aspirin and clopidogrel compared with clopidogrel alone after recent ischaemic stroke or transient ischaemic attack in high-risk patients (MATCH): randomised, double-blind, placebo-controlled trial. Lancet. 2004;364(9431):331–7. https://doi.org/10.1016/S0140-6736(04)16721-4.

75. Bhatt DL, Fox KAA, Hacke W, et al. Clopidogrel and aspirin versus aspirin alone for the prevention of atherothrombotic events. N Engl J Med. 2006;354(16):1706–17. https://doi.org/10.1056/NEJMoa060989.

76. Effect of clopidogrel added to aspirin in patients with atrial fibrillation. N Engl J Med. 2009;360(20):2066–78. https://doi.org/10.1056/NEJMoa0901301.

77. Markus HS, Droste DW, Kaps M, et al. Dual antiplatelet therapy with clopidogrel and aspirin in symptomatic carotid stenosis evaluated using doppler embolic signal detection: the clopidogrel and aspirin for reduction of emboli in symptomatic carotid stenosis (CARESS) trial. Circulation. 2005;111(17):2233–40. https://doi.org/10.1161/01.CIR.0000163561.90680.1C.

78. Kennedy J, Hill MD, Ryckborst KJ, Eliasziw M, Demchuk AM, Buchan AM. Fast assessment of stroke and transient ischaemic attack to prevent early recurrence (FASTER): a randomised controlled pilot trial. Lancet Neurol. 2007;6(11):961–9. https://doi.org/10.1016/S1474-4422(07)70250-8.

79. Wong KSL, Chen C, Fu J, et al. Clopidogrel plus aspirin versus aspirin alone for reducing embolisation in patients with acute symptomatic cerebral or carotid artery stenosis (CLAIR study): a randomised, open-label, blinded-endpoint trial. Lancet Neurol. 2010;9(5):489–97. https://doi.org/10.1016/S1474-4422(10)70060-0.

80. Amarenco P, Lavallée PC, Labreuche J, et al. One-year risk of stroke after transient ischemic attack or minor stroke. N Engl J Med. 2016;374(16):1533–42. https://doi.org/10.1056/NEJMoa1412981.

81. Wang Y, Wang Y, Zhao X, et al. Clopidogrel with aspirin in acute minor stroke or transient ischemic attack. N Engl J Med. 2013;369(1):11–9. https://doi.org/10.1056/NEJMoa1215340.

82. Johnston SC, Easton JD, Farrant M, et al. Clopidogrel and aspirin in acute ischemic stroke and high-risk TIA. N Engl J Med. 2018;379(3):215–25. https://doi.org/10.1056/NEJMoa1800410.

83. Wang Y, Meng X, Wang A, et al. Ticagrelor versus clopidogrel in CYP2C19 loss-of-function carriers with stroke or TIA. N Engl J Med. 2021;385(27):2520–30. https://doi.org/10.1056/NEJMoa2111749.

84. Gao Y, Chen W, Pan Y, et al. Dual antiplatelet treatment up to 72 hours after ischemic stroke. N Engl J Med. 2023;389(26):2413–24. https://doi.org/10.1056/NEJMoa2309137.

85. Chimowitz MI, Lynn MJ, Derdeyn CP, et al. Stenting versus aggressive medical therapy for intracranial arterial stenosis. N Engl J Med. 2011;365(11):993–1003. https://doi.org/10.1056/NEJMoa1105335.
86. De Matteis E, De Santis F, Ornello R, et al. Divergence between clinical trial evidence and actual practice in use of dual antiplatelet therapy after transient ischemic attack and minor stroke. Stroke. 2023;54(5):1172–81. https://doi.org/10.1161/STROKEAHA.122.041660.
87. Chen HS, Cui Y, Zhou ZH, et al. Dual antiplatelet therapy vs alteplase for patients with minor nondisabling acute ischemic stroke: the ARAMIS randomized clinical trial. JAMA. 2023;329(24):2135–44. https://doi.org/10.1001/jama.2023.7827.
88. Larrue V, von Kummer R, del Zoppo G, Bluhmki E. Hemorrhagic transformation in acute ischemic stroke. Stroke. 1997;28(5):957–60. https://doi.org/10.1161/01.STR.28.5.957.
89. von Kummer R, Broderick JP, Campbell BCV, et al. The Heidelberg bleeding classification. Stroke. 2015;46(10):2981–6. https://doi.org/10.1161/STROKEAHA.115.010049.
90. Molina CA, Alvarez-Sabín J, Montaner J, et al. Thrombolysis-related hemorrhagic infarction: a marker of early reperfusion, reduced infarct size, and improved outcome in patients with proximal middle cerebral artery occlusion. Stroke. 2002;33(6):1551–6. https://doi.org/10.1161/01.STR.0000016323.13456.E5.
91. Yaghi S, Willey JZ, Cucchiara B, et al. Treatment and outcome of hemorrhagic transformation after intravenous alteplase in acute ischemic stroke: a scientific statement for healthcare professionals from the American Heart Association/American Stroke Association. Stroke. 2017;48(12):e343–61. https://doi.org/10.1161/STR.0000000000000152.
92. Wahlgren N, Ahmed N, Dávalos A, et al. Thrombolysis with alteplase for acute ischaemic stroke in the safe implementation of thrombolysis in stroke-monitoring study (SITS-MOST): an observational study. Lancet. 2007;369(9558):275–82. https://doi.org/10.1016/S0140-6736(07)60149-4.
93. Guhwe M, Utley-Smith Q, Blessing R, Goldstein LB. Routine 24-hour computed tomography brain scan is not useful in stable patients post intravenous tissue plasminogen activator. J Stroke Cerebrovasc Dis. 2016;25(3):540–2. https://doi.org/10.1016/j.jstrokecerebrovasdis.2015.11.006.
94. Tanswell P, Seifried E, Su PCAF, Feuerer W, Rijken DC. Pharmacokinetics and systemic effects of tissue-type plasminogen activator in normal subjects. Clin Pharmacol Therap. 1989;46(2):155–62. https://doi.org/10.1038/clpt.1989.120.
95. Cannon CP, Gibson CM, McCabe CH, et al. TNK–tissue plasminogen activator compared with front-loaded alteplase in acute myocardial infarction. Circulation. 1998;98(25):2805–14. https://doi.org/10.1161/01.CIR.98.25.2805.
96. Yaghi S, Boehme AK, Dibu J, et al. Treatment and outcome of thrombolysis-related hemorrhage: a multicenter retrospective study. JAMA Neurol. 2015;72(12):1451–7. https://doi.org/10.1001/jamaneurol.2015.2371.
97. Verkerk BS, Lesch C, Cham S, Berger K. Cryoprecipitate for alteplase-related hemorrhagic conversion of acute ischemic stroke. J Pharm Pract. 2023;36(5):1253–9. https://doi.org/10.1177/08971900221102116.
98. Barra ME, Feske SK, Sylvester KW, et al. Fibrinogen concentrate for the treatment of thrombolysis-associated hemorrhage in adult ischemic stroke patients. Clin Appl Thromb Hemost. 2020;26:1076029620951867. https://doi.org/10.1177/1076029620951867.
99. French KF, White J, Hoesch RE. Treatment of intracerebral hemorrhage with tranexamic acid after thrombolysis with tissue plasminogen activator. Neurocrit Care. 2012;17(1):107–11. https://doi.org/10.1007/s12028-012-9681-5.
100. Rosafio F, Vandelli L, Bigliardi G, et al. Usefulness of thromboelastography in the detection and management of tissue plasminogen activator-associated hyperfibrinolysis. J Stroke Cerebrovasc Dis. 2017;26(2):e29–31. https://doi.org/10.1016/j.jstrokecerebrovasdis.2016.10.039.
101. Hailu K, Ragoonanan D, Davis H. Tranexamic acid for treatment of symptomatic hemorrhagic conversion following administration of tenecteplase for acute ischemic stroke. Am J Emerg Med. 2022;59:216.e1–5. https://doi.org/10.1016/j.ajem.2022.06.022.

102. Verkerk BS, Berger K, Lesch CA. Aminocaproic acid for the reversal of alteplase: a case series. J Pharm Pract. 2020;33(6):919–25. https://doi.org/10.1177/0897190019840095.
103. Ma L, Hu X, Song L, et al. The third intensive care bundle with blood pressure reduction in acute cerebral haemorrhage trial (INTERACT3): an international, stepped wedge cluster randomised controlled trial. Lancet. 2023;402(10395):27–40. https://doi.org/10.1016/S0140-6736(23)00806-1.
104. Nilsson T, Bäck O. Elevated plasmin-alpha 2-antiplasmin complex levels in hereditary angioedema: evidence for the in vivo efficiency of the intrinsic fibrinolytic system. Thromb Res. 1985;40(6):817–21. https://doi.org/10.1016/0049-3848(85)90318-4.
105. Molinaro G, Gervais N, Adam A. Biochemical basis of angioedema associated with recombinant tissue plasminogen activator treatment: an in vitro experimental approach. Stroke. 2002;33(6):1712–6. https://doi.org/10.1161/01.str.0000017284.77838.87.
106. Fugate JE, Kalimullah EA, Wijdicks EFM. Angioedema after tPA: what neurointensivists should know. Neurocrit Care. 2012;16(3):440–3. https://doi.org/10.1007/s12028-012-9678-0.
107. Werner R, Keller M, Woehrle JC. Facial angioedema and stroke. Cerebrovasc Dis. 2014;38(2):101–6. https://doi.org/10.1159/000365205.
108. Mas-Serrano M, García-Pastor A, Iglesias-Mohedano AM, et al. Related factors with orolingual angioedema after intravenous alteplase in acute ischemic stroke: results from a single-center cohort and meta-analysis. Neurol Sci. 2022;43(1):441–52. https://doi.org/10.1007/s10072-021-05279-y.
109. Flint AC, Eaton A, Melles RB, et al. Comparative safety of tenecteplase vs alteplase for acute ischemic stroke. J Stroke Cerebrovasc Dis. 2023;33(1):107468. https://doi.org/10.1016/j.jstrokecerebrovasdis.2023.107468.
110. Lekoubou A, Philippeau F, Derex L, et al. Audit report and systematic review of orolingual angioedema in post-acute stroke thrombolysis. Neurol Res. 2014;36(7):687–94. https://doi.org/10.1179/1743132813Y.0000000302.
111. Vigneron C, Lécluse A, Ronzière T, et al. Angioedema associated with thrombolysis for ischemic stroke: analysis of a case-control study. J Intern Med. 2019;286(6):702–10. https://doi.org/10.1111/joim.12962.
112. Benoit C, Cantier M, Rodriguez-Régent C, Gout O, Obadia M. Orolingual and abdominal angioedema post thrombolysis and thrombectomy. Neurology. 2018;90(3):140–1. https://doi.org/10.1212/WNL.0000000000004834.
113. Brown E, Campana C, Zimmerman J, Brooks S. Icatibant for the treatment of orolingual angioedema following the administration of tissue plasminogen activator. Am J Emerg Med. 2018;36(6):1125.e1–2. https://doi.org/10.1016/j.ajem.2018.03.018.
114. Cheong E, Dodd L, Smith W, Kleinig T. Icatibant as a potential treatment of life-threatening alteplase-induced angioedema. J Stroke Cerebrovasc Dis. 2018;27(2):e36–7. https://doi.org/10.1016/j.jstrokecerebrovasdis.2017.09.039.
115. Wollmach AD, Zehnder D, Schwendinger M, Tarnutzer AA. Unilateral orolingual angioedema in a patient with sarcoidosis after intravenous thrombolysis due to acute stroke without improvement after treatment with icatibant. BMJ Case Rep. 2020;13(12):e236643. https://doi.org/10.1136/bcr-2020-236643.
116. Pahs L, Droege C, Kneale H, Pancioli A. A novel approach to the treatment of orolingual angioedema after tissue plasminogen activator administration. Ann Emerg Med. 2016;68(3):345–8. https://doi.org/10.1016/j.annemergmed.2016.02.019.
117. Martinez Manzano JM, Lo KB, Patarroyo-Aponte G, Azmaiparashvili Z. The use of intravenous tranexamic acid for patients with angiotensin-converting enzyme inhibitor–induced angioedema: a case series. Ann Allergy Asthma Immunol. 2021;126(6):725–6. https://doi.org/10.1016/j.anai.2021.02.011.
118. Hasara S, Wilson K, Amatea J, Anderson J. Tranexamic acid for the emergency treatment of angiotensin-converting enzyme inhibitor-induced angioedema. Cureus. 2021;13(9):e18116. https://doi.org/10.7759/cureus.18116.

119. Thorén M, Azevedo E, Dawson J, et al. Predictors for cerebral edema in acute ischemic stroke treated with intravenous thrombolysis. Stroke. 2017;48(9):2464–71. https://doi.org/10.1161/STROKEAHA.117.018223.
120. Hacke W, Schwab S, Horn M, Spranger M, De Georgia M, von Kummer R. "Malignant" middle cerebral artery territory infarction: clinical course and prognostic signs. Arch Neurol. 1996;53(4):309–15. https://doi.org/10.1001/archneur.1996.00550040037012.
121. Wijdicks EFM, Sheth KN, Carter BS, et al. Recommendations for the management of cerebral and cerebellar infarction with swelling. Stroke. 2014;45(4):1222–38. https://doi.org/10.1161/01.str.0000441965.15164.d6.
122. Cook AM, Morgan Jones G, Hawryluk GWJ, et al. Guidelines for the acute treatment of cerebral edema in neurocritical care patients. Neurocrit Care. 2020;32(3):647–66. https://doi.org/10.1007/s12028-020-00959-7.
123. Koenig MA, Bryan M, Lewin JL, Mirski MA, Geocadin RG, Stevens RD. Reversal of transtentorial herniation with hypertonic saline. Neurology. 2008;70(13):1023–9. https://doi.org/10.1212/01.wnl.0000304042.05557.60.
124. Videen TO, Zazulia AR, Manno EM, et al. Mannitol bolus preferentially shrinks non-infarcted brain in patients with ischemic stroke. Neurology. 2001;57(11):2120–2. https://doi.org/10.1212/WNL.57.11.2120.
125. Reinink H, Jüttler E, Hacke W, et al. Surgical decompression for space-occupying hemispheric infarction: a systematic review and individual patient meta-analysis of randomized clinical trials. JAMA Neurol. 2021;78(2):208–16. https://doi.org/10.1001/jamaneurol.2020.3745.
126. Dower A, Mulcahy M, Maharaj M, et al. Surgical decompression for malignant cerebral oedema after ischaemic stroke. Cochrane Database Syst Rev. 2022;11 https://doi.org/10.1002/14651858.CD014989.pub2.
127. Brondani R, Garcia de Almeida A, Abrahim Cherubini P, et al. High risk of seizures and epilepsy after decompressive hemicraniectomy for malignant middle cerebral artery stroke. Cerebrovasc Dis Extra. 2017;7(1):51–61. https://doi.org/10.1159/000458730.
128. Yeap MC, Chen CC, Liu ZH, et al. Postcranioplasty seizures following decompressive craniectomy and seizure prophylaxis: a retrospective analysis at a single institution. J Neurosurg. 2018;131(3):936–40. https://doi.org/10.3171/2018.4.JNS172519.
129. Franco AC, Fernandes T, Peralta AR, et al. Frequency of epileptic seizures in patients undergoing decompressive craniectomy after ischemic stroke. Seizure. 2022;101:60–6. https://doi.org/10.1016/j.seizure.2022.07.011.
130. Hankey GJ. Angiotensin-converting enzyme inhibitors for stroke prevention. Stroke. 2003;34(2):354–6. https://doi.org/10.1161/01.STR.0000054261.97525.4B.
131. Chen J, Li S, Zheng K, et al. Impact of smoking status on stroke recurrence. J Am Heart Assoc. 2019;8(8):e011696. https://doi.org/10.1161/JAHA.118.011696.
132. Parikh NS, Omran SS, Kamel H, Elkind MSV, Willey J. Smoking-cessation pharmacotherapy for patients with stroke and TIA: systematic review. J Clin Neurosci. 2020;78:236–41. https://doi.org/10.1016/j.jocn.2020.04.026.
133. Yin Y, Zhang L, Marshall I, Wolfe C, Wang Y. Statin therapy for preventing recurrent stroke in patients with ischemic stroke: a systematic review and meta-analysis of randomized controlled trials and observational cohort studies. Neuroepidemiology. 2022;56(4):240–9. https://doi.org/10.1159/000525672.

Chapter 18
Status Epilepticus and Refractory Status Epilepticus

Morgan Trammel, Cina Sasannejad, Beverly Tomita, and Cherylee W. J. Chang

18.1 Introduction

In neurocritical care, a critical care pharmacist brings added expertise when well versed in cerebral pathophysiology, nuances of neuropathology, updated or newly established guidelines, and emerging neuro-pharmacotherapeutics [1, 2]. This specialty-specific knowledge includes strategies for prophylaxis or management of seizures or status epilepticus (SE). SE was redefined by the International League Against Epilepsy (ILAE) in 2015 as "a condition resulting either from the failure of the mechanisms responsible for seizure termination or from the initiation of mechanisms which lead to abnormally prolonged seizures (after time point t1)." It is a condition that can have long-term consequences (after time point t2), including neuronal death, neuronal injury, and alteration of neuronal networks, depending on the type and duration of seizures [3]. The intent is to utilize the operational time points to determine when treatment should be considered or started (time point t1, which the ILAE defined as 5 min) and to utilize time point t2 (defined as 30 min) to determine the aggressiveness

M. Trammel
Department of Pharmacy, Duke University Hospital, Durham, USA

C. Sasannejad
Department of Neurology, Duke University School of Medicine, Durham, NC, USA

B. Tomita
Carle Illinois College of Medicine, University of Illinois, Urbana, IL, USA

C. W. J. Chang (✉)
Department of Neurology, Duke University School of Medicine, Durham, NC, USA

Department of Neurosurgery, Duke University School of Medicine, Durham, NC, USA

Department of Medicine Division of Pulmonary, Allergy and Critical Care, Duke University School of Medicine, Durham, NC, USA
e-mail: Cherylee.Chang@duke.edu

Y. Alzaidi, M. A. Gebily (eds.), *The Pharmacist's Expanded Role in Critical Care Medicine*, https://doi.org/10.1007/978-3-031-77335-8_18

471

of treatment to prevent long-term consequences, e.g., neuronal injury or death. Refractory status epilepticus (RSE) is defined as intractable seizures unresponsive to a first-line anti-seizure medication (ASM), i.e., initial benzodiazepine (BZP), and an adequate second-line ASM, e.g., a full loading dose of an intravenous (IV) ASM. Super-refractory SE (SRSE) is defined as RSE that continues or recurs 24 h or longer despite the initiation of IV anesthetic agents [4, 5]. Even more recently, consensus definitions to standardize terminology to facilitate communication for clinical care and research include (1) new-onset RSE (NORSE), which is a clinical presentation in a patient without known epilepsy or preexisting relevant neurological disorder or clear structural, toxic, or metabolic etiology; (2) febrile infection-related epilepsy syndrome (FIRES) as a subcategory of NORSE that requires a prior febrile infection between 24 h and 2 weeks prior to the onset of RSE; (3) prolonged RSE (PRSE), which is RSE that lasts for at least 7 days despite appropriate management, but without the use of anesthetics; and (4) prolonged SRSE (PSRSE), which is SRSE that persists for at least 7 days including the ongoing need for anesthetics [6] (Table 18.1).

Table 18.1 Nomenclature and definitions of status epilepticus [3, 4, 6]

	Definition	Time course	IV anesthetic use	Potential for secondary injury
Status epilepticus (SE)	Abnormally prolonged seizures that can have long-term consequences if not treated depending on seizure type and duration	5–30+ min	May be required	Variable
Nonconvulsive SE (NCSE)	Electrographic seizures without overt symptomatology other than decreased LOC	5–30+ min	May be required	Variable
Refractory SE (RSE)	Intractable seizures unresponsive to a first-line ASM	30 min–24 h with anesthetics; 30 min–7 days without anesthetics	May be required	Moderate
Prolonged RSE (PRSE)	RSE lasting 7+ days despite appropriate management without the use of anesthetics	7+ days	No	High
Super refractory SE (SRSE)	RSE continuing or recurring 24 h+ despite the initiation of IV anesthetic agents	24+ h	Yes	High
Prolonged SRSE (PSRSE)	SRSE persisting 7+ days including ongoing need for IV anesthetic agents	7+ days	Yes	High
NORSE	New-onset RSE in a patient without known epilepsy or preexisting relevant neurological disorder or clear structural, toxic, or metabolic etiology	Variable	May be required	High
FIRES	NORSE with febrile infection 24 h to 2 weeks prior to onset of RSE	Variable	May be required	High

In a patient, the clinical signs and symptoms or semiology of the seizures may change over time in SE; however, it has been established that nonconvulsive seizures (NCSz) and NCSE, i.e., electrographic ictal activity without overt motor symptomatology except a decreased level of consciousness (LOC), can cause secondary neuronal injury [7]. Electroencephalography (EEG) is an important tool to detect occult NCSz and NCSE in the ICU since patients are frequently mechanically ventilated and sedated without obvious convulsive activity [8].

Depending on the cohort, SE has been associated with 30-day mortality varying between 8.5% and 31% [9, 10]. In the United States, a nationwide cohort of 33,814 patients showed a higher 30-day mortality in adults (10.2%) than in children (1.8%). The combined 1-year mortality was 25.1% (30.3% in adults and 4.6% in children); however, neurologic disability was highest in children aged 5–9 years (21.3%) [9]. In this cohort, prognostic factors for both 30-day and 1-year mortality included older age, no active (recent) history of epilepsy, presence of an acute etiology, and refractoriness of SE. Other studies also found that older age, duration, and NCSE were associated with new neurological deficits, which predicted worse 2-year survival [11]. In one German cohort of 2585 patients with SE, discharge mortality increased from 9.6% in non-refractory SE to 15.0% ($p < 0.001$) in RSE and 39.9% ($p < 0.001$) in SRSE [12]. These factors highlight the importance of terminating SE as quickly as possible.

After reviewing the cellular pathophysiology of SE, which informs the basis for pharmacotherapeutic modalities, this chapter provides a compendium of the most recent and commonly utilized ASM in SE and caveats and indications of use and explores novel methods for treatment.

18.2 Cellular Pathophysiology of Status Epilepticus

Typically fueled by an underlying etiology, when seizures persist, *N*-methyl-D-aspartate (NMDA) receptors accumulate in the synapse [13]. Subsequent enhanced glutaminergic excitotoxicity coincides with the internalization of γ-aminobutyric acid (GABA)$_A$ receptors, producing a functional decrease in the synaptic inhibitory GABAergic activity. The loss of inhibition, coupled with synaptic excitation, decreases not only the likelihood of spontaneous termination but also the likelihood that GABAergic medications such as BZPs and barbiturates will be effective to terminate seizures in SE and may explain the therapeutic efficacy of NMDA antagonists in SE [14, 15]. Increased NMDA receptor activity results in excessive intraneuronal calcium entry with activation of nitric oxide synthase, calpains, and NADPH oxidase with reactive oxygen species causing oxidative stress. This results in widespread damage to DNA, proteins, and lipids followed by neuroinflammation and neuronal death. Increased calcium accumulation results in mitochondrial failure due to changes in the membrane potential with opening of the mitochondrial permeability transition pore, followed by decrease in ATP production, mitochondrial swelling, and apoptosis [5, 16].

Understanding the mechanistic changes to receptors, the effect on neurotransmitters, and the cascade of injury may help tailor appropriate and timely therapy to prevent neuronal injury, death, and cognitive decline after SE (Figs. 18.1 and 18.2).

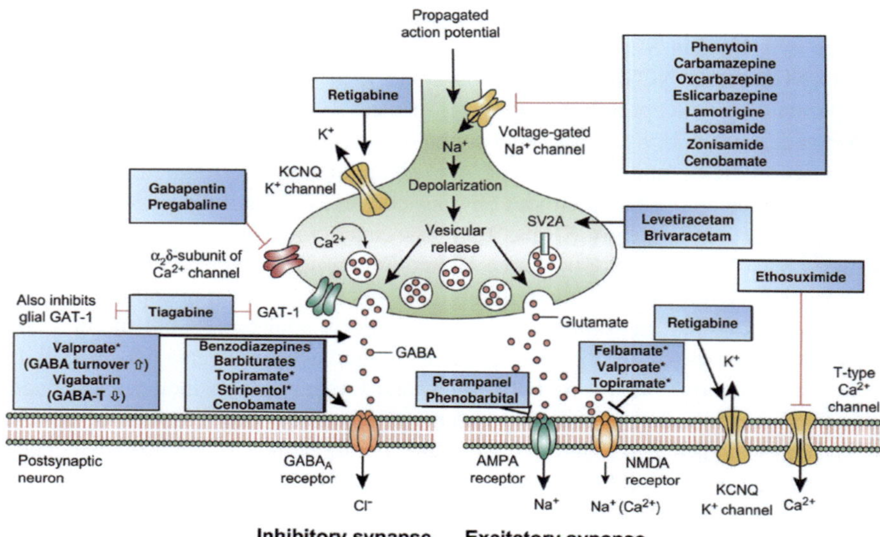

Fig. 18.1 Location of the mechanism of action of anti-seizure medications (Reproduced with permission from Löscher W, Klein P. The Pharmacology and Clinical Efficacy of Anti-seizure Medications: From Bromide Salts to Cenobamate and Beyond. CNS Drugs 2021;35:935–63 [17]). Asterisks indicate multiple mechanisms of action (MOA), although only the primary MOA is shown in the figure. *AMPA* α-amino-3-hydroxy-5-methyl-4-isoxazolepropionic acid, *Ca²⁺* calcium, *Cl⁻* chloride, *GABA* γ-aminobutyric acid, *GABA-T* GABA aminotransferase, *GAT-1* GABA transporter 1, *K⁺* potassium, *KCNQ Kv7* potassium channel family, *Na⁺* sodium, *NMDA* N-methyl-D-aspartate, *SV2A* synaptic vesicle protein 2A

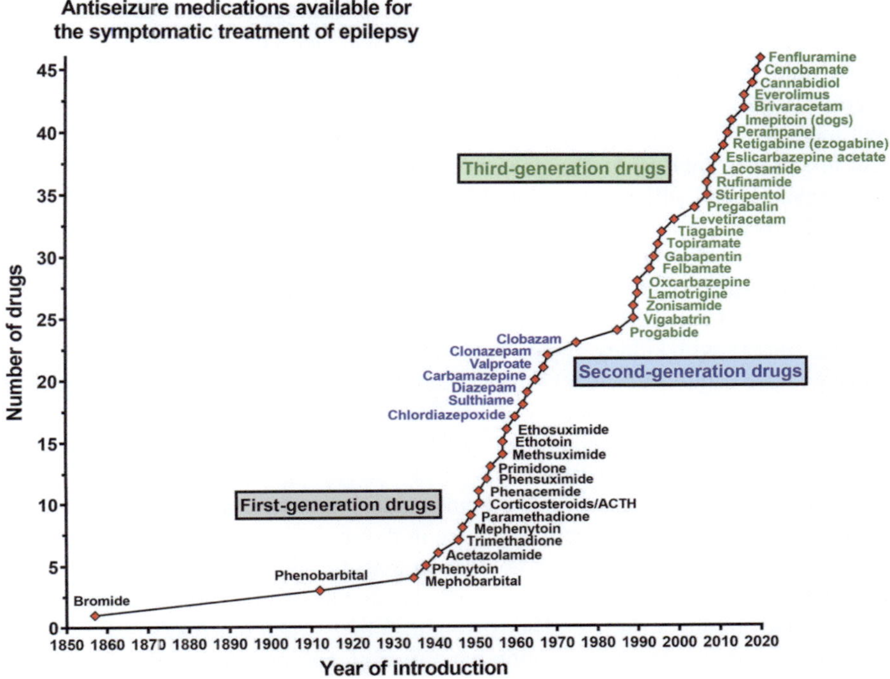

Fig. 18.2 The timeline of available anti-seizure medications (Reproduced with permission from Löscher W, Klein P. The Pharmacology and Clinical Efficacy of Anti-seizure Medications: From Bromide Salts to Cenobamate and Beyond. CNS Drugs 2021;35:935–63 [17])

18.3 Pharmacokinetics and Drug-Drug Interactions

A distinctive role for the pharmacist in the management of patients with SE involves understanding key principles of absorption and lipo- or hydrophilicity, which affect the volume of distribution (Vd), central nervous system (CNS) penetration, metabolism, and elimination of each ASM. Especially salient are (1) protein-binding properties that result in competition for binding sites on albumin and (2) induction or inhibition of hepatic enzymes. These properties can result in significant drug-drug interactions (DDIs) [18]. Careful consideration should also be given when contemplating initiation, increase, decrease, or discontinuation of a medication that is a known inducer or inhibitor of enzymes. Similarly, adding a medication to known inducers or inhibitors should be carefully evaluated. It is beyond the scope of this chapter to review all DDIs; however, there are many electronic databases and online applications that are readily available to assess these interactions.

Most ASMs are metabolized by the cytochrome P450 system in the liver by hydroxylation or conjugation, with metabolites being excreted by the kidneys [19]. Cytochrome P450 enzymes have broad substrate specificity; therefore, a single drug may be a substrate for multiple enzymes, such as CYP3A4, 2CP9, and 2C19.

Additionally, metabolism can occur by hepatic conjugation and mitochondrial β-oxidation. Common inducers that increase clearance and decrease steady-state concentrations include phenobarbital (PHB), phenytoin (PHT), primidone, carbamazepine (CBZ), and topiramate (TPM). Inhibitors of metabolism that slow clearance and increase the steady-state concentrations of ASMs include valproic acid (VPA) and non-ASMs such as omeprazole, verapamil, macrolide antibiotics, paroxetine, ketoconazole, and sulfamethoxazole [20]. Of ASMs, levetiracetam (LEV) has the fewest DDIs.

ASM elimination, expressed as the biological half-life, is the time required for the drug's serum concentration to decrease by 50% after absorption and distribution. Half-life is commonly most affected by renal function, and dose adjustment is often necessary with kidney impairment and renal replacement therapy. Metabolism and clearance can be dependent on concomitant medications, hepatic function, and, as is the case of PHT, nonlinearity at baseline.

Additionally, there are patient factors that may play a role in the pharmacokinetics of medications. The pharmacist considers several patient-specific issues when choosing medications, routes of administration, and clearance. These include changes in drug metabolism and clearance in the setting of preexisting or evolving kidney injury or hepatic failure, shock, hypotension, hyperthermia, or pregnancy; gastrointestinal absorption and gut motility; and changes in nutritional status (e.g., albumin and protein intake), total body weight, or body water that may impact the Vd.

Other key concepts when treating patients with SE include tapering of ASMs, especially in the setting of an infusion that has been administered at anesthetic doses. Both BZPs and barbiturates can have withdrawal symptoms of anxiety, restlessness, insomnia, irritability, confusion, nausea, vomiting, tremor, muscle stiffness, seizure, psychosis, and autonomic changes such as hypertension, tachycardia, and diaphoresis.

18.4 Therapeutic Drug Monitoring

Although some providers titrate an ASM to medication effect (i.e., termination of seizures, which requires continuous electroencephalography unless the patient awakens to baseline state), a best practice guideline was established for therapeutic drug monitoring (TDM) of ASM levels for key reasons: (1) to identify a target therapeutic concentration after titrating to clinical effectiveness since the cause of a change in drug response in the future may be identified by a level that varies from this target; (2) to evaluate for medication toxicity, especially when the therapeutic index (TI), i.e., the margin between the therapeutic dose and toxic dose, is narrow; (3) to assess compliance, especially in patients with uncontrolled or breakthrough seizures; (4) to guide dosage adjustment when pharmacokinetics may vary (e.g., metabolic changes, concomitant medications, pregnancy); and (5) to guide dose adjustment with medications with dose-dependent pharmacokinetics, e.g., PHT [21].

TI is defined as ED50/TD50, or the ratio of the drug concentration at which the drug is therapeutic or effective for 50% of patients (ED50) to the concentration that is toxic to 50% of patients (TD50) [22]. Older-generation ASMs such as PHT have a narrow TI with complicated pharmacokinetics and a high potential for DDIs. Although newer ASMs are less likely to have these concerns, TDM of newer ASMs in a real-world study showed clinical benefit in seizure reduction and decreases in side effects [23].

Since albumin levels may fluctuate widely during the hospital course of a critically ill patient, TDM is especially helpful when ASMs are significantly protein bound, e.g., PHT and VPA. In this situation, free levels might be helpful, although unless obtained on-site; delays in results can render the information less relevant in an ICU setting. When concomitant medications are administered, TDM can potentially assist the clinician in atypical dosing that may be necessary, although reference ranges can be misleading. The references are based on statistics of when the majority of patients experienced optimal response and may not be relevant to the index patient.

The optimal timing to draw a medication level is when the ASM has reached a steady state, typically 4–5 half-lives after starting treatment or a dose adjustment. ASMs with long half-lives do not require a trough level; however, ASMs with mid- or short half-lives (<12 h) may experience more fluctuation with inconsistent anti-seizure efficacy, and a trough obtained just before a "steady-state" dosage administration might be useful (e.g., LEV, VPA, or TPM) (Table 18.2).

Table 18.2 Target therapeutic index (TI) for selected ASMs

Drug	Established target TI
Carbamazepine[a] (CBZ)	4–11 µg/mL
Clobazam[a] (CLO)	0.03–0.3 µg/mL
Phenobarbital[a] (PHB)	10–40 µg/mL
Phenytoin[a] (PHT)	Total: 10–20 µg/mL Free: 1–2 µg/mL
Valproic acid[a] (VPA)	50–100 µg/mL
Drug	**Potential or suggested TI**
Levetiracetam[b] (LEV)	10–40 µg/mL
Brivaracetam[b] (BRV)	0.2–2 µg/mL
Ganaxolone[c] (GX)	85–250 ng/mL
Lacosamide[b] (LCM)	3–10 µg/mL
Lamotrigine[b] (LTG)	3–13 µg/mL
Perampanel[b] (PMP)	0.1–1 µg/mL
Topiramate[b] (TPM)	2–10 µg/mL

[a] [21]
[b] [24]
[c] [25]

18.5 Adverse Drug Effects

Consideration of adverse drug effects (ADEs) includes (1) acute dose-related effects that are typically rapidly reversible, e.g., sedation, fatigue, sodium levels, platelets, and transaminases; (2) idiosyncratic ADEs that are less common but serious and often dose dependent, such as Stevens-Johnson syndrome and toxic epidermal necrolysis; and (3) cumulative toxicity, which is less likely a concern in SE when initiating ASM, as this typically requires a prolonged exposure over several months to years.

18.6 Management Strategies for Termination of SE

In a study of patients with generalized convulsive status, successful termination with first-line treatment with GABAergic medications such as lorazepam, PHB, or diazepam (DZP) with PHT varied between 64.9%, 58.2%, and 55%, respectively; however, the response rates for a second-line agent were 7.0% and 2.3% for third-line agents [26]. Thus, 35–45% of patients with SE fail first-line therapy, and rapid escalation may help prevent RSE and improve outcomes [27].

When considering termination of SE, two major strategies include (1) enhancement of inhibitory processes and (2) opposition of excitatory processes. Initial immediate termination focuses on a fast-acting BZP to activate the $GABA_A$ receptor that allows negatively charged chloride cellular influx with neuronal inhibition. Subsequent second- and third-line therapy continues to attempt to leverage GABAergic inhibition through GABA receptors, GABA transaminase, or GABA-synthesizing enzyme glutamate decarboxylase. Additional strategies include (1) modulation of excitatory processes through decreases in the glutaminergic excitatory activity (i.e., NMDA or AMPA glutamate receptors); (2) modulation of synaptic vesicles, i.e., synaptic vesicle glycoprotein 2A (SV2A); and (3) direct or indirect action on voltage-gated sodium, calcium, or potassium ion channels by modification of the synthesis, metabolism, or function of neurotransmitters and receptors. SE termination often requires multiple mediations utilizing different targets of action.

18.6.1 Guidelines for SE Termination

Various guidelines have been created to address strategies for the termination of SE [28, 29]. The guidelines universally discuss the initial use of a fast-acting BZP, followed by second-line parenteral medications. The Established Status Epilepticus Treatment Trial (ESETT) of 384 patients with SE refractory to BZP showed equivalent efficacy of seizure termination in patients randomized to an infusion over

10 min of (1) LEV 60 mg/kg, maximum dose of 4500 mg; (2) valproate 40 mg/kg, maximum dose of 3000 mg; or (3) fosphenytoin 20 mg/kg, maximum dose of 1500 mg [30]. There were no significant differences in hypotension, intubation, or death. As such, these agents are the most frequently utilized second-line ASMs in SE. The primary outcome of cessation of SE and improvement in the level of consciousness at 60 min occurred in 47% of patients treated with LEV, 46% with VPA, and 45% with fosphenytoin. However, 10.7–11.2% of patients had recurrent seizures or RSE.

The most recent SE guideline published in 2020 addresses refractory convulsive SE and evaluates the strength of evidence for the efficacy of eight parenteral ASMs as a third-line treatment [27]. For RSE, administration of parenteral medications often requires anesthetic/sedating doses that require endotracheal intubation. While administering parenteral agents to terminate seizures, enteral agents are often added with the eventual goal to wean parenteral medications but with adequate anti-seizure effect to prevent seizure/SE recurrence.

18.7　Anti-seizure Medications

18.7.1　Available Parenteral Preparations

18.7.1.1　Benzodiazepines: $GABA_A$ Receptor Activation

BZPs are positive allosteric modulators of postsynaptic $GABA_A$ receptors, which are ligand-gated chloride channels. BZPs bind to the $\alpha+/\gamma-$ subunit interface of the $GABA_A$ receptor, increasing the affinity of GABA binding to receptors. This increases the frequency of opening of the chloride channels, leading to membrane hyperpolarization with subsequent inhibition of neuronal activity. Other positive modulators that bind to different sites on the $GABA_A$ receptor include barbiturates, alcohol, propofol (PRO), etomidate, and volatile anesthetics such as isoflurane [31–33].

The lipophilic property of each of the BZPs often drives the bedside therapeutic choice. DZP, the most lipophilic, has fast CNS penetration but rapid redistribution, causing a short-acting anti-seizure effect. DZP may therefore be the ideal agent in a patient undergoing epilepsy monitoring in preparation for potential resection of an epileptogenic focus, as it can terminate a seizure to prevent SE but allow another seizure to occur, facilitating the localization of the nidus for resection. However, in most patients with SE, a longer-acting agent, such as lorazepam, is preferable to allow secondary administration of a longer-acting ASM to prevent further seizures when the BZP effect clears.

The SE guidelines universally address the essential initial step in the acute setting to terminate seizures as quickly as possible given the synaptic changes and the loss of GABAergic responsiveness following prolonged seizures. Rectal DZP is useful in an outpatient setting but with less ease of use and rapidity than an intramuscular (IM) or IV route. As noted above, DZP is less utilized as an IV first-line therapy due to its lipophilic properties conferring a shorter effective half-life for seizure termination compared to lorazepam. The RAMPART trial in the pre-hospital setting demonstrated that administration of IV lorazepam had faster termination of seizures than IM midazolam (MDZ) when IV access is already established. However, when IV access is not yet obtained, the time to effective cessation of seizures is faster with IM MDZ when compared with IV lorazepam [28, 29, 34].

Secondary effects of BZPs and other GABAergic agents such as PRO and barbiturates include a decrease in cerebral metabolic rate and cerebral blood flow [35]. Systemic effects include hypotension and respiratory depression influenced by dosage, rate of administration, and concomitant medications. Acute reversal with flumazenil, a 1,4-imidazobenzodiazepine competitive antagonist at the BZP-binding site on the $GABA_A$ receptor, is not recommended in patients with SE, as seizures may be further potentiated [36]. Instead, hemodynamic and mechanical ventilatory support should be initiated accordingly if cardiac or respiratory ADEs occur.

Infusion/Anesthetic Dosing of BZP as a Third-Line Therapy

When seizures persist despite the administration of both first-line GABAergic treatment and a second-line therapy (e.g., LEV, VPA, and/or fosphenytoin), i.e., RSE, the guidelines recommend a third-line strategy of a parenteral infusion of an ASM with anesthetic properties to terminate seizures. Continuous EEG monitoring to detect NCSz/NCSE is essential. Current guidelines target seizure cessation, or alternatively, a burst-suppression pattern [27, 28], although anecdotally, achieving a burst suppression pattern does not necessarily prevent break-through ictal activity (i.e. seizures) and close continuous EEG monitoring is essential.

Lorazepam, while an excellent first-line IV ASM, is not an ideal option for a continuous infusion due to a diluent, propylene glycol (1,2-propanediol). Propylene glycol is metabolized by alcohol dehydrogenase in the liver to lactaldehyde and then by aldehyde dehydrogenase to lactate, acetate, and pyruvate, causing both a severe anion gap metabolic acidosis and an osmolar gap [37]. Missing the diagnosis of an unexplained anion gap acidosis, typically associated with an osmolar gap, may lead to progressive hypotension and acute kidney injury due to acute tubular necrosis [38]. Propylene toxicity can also occur when administering high-dose injections or infusions of diazepam or pentobarbital (PTB).

MDZ is water soluble at lower pH and does not require propylene glycol to maintain stability as an infusion. MDZ infusions are well tolerated and require higher doses on average to reach therapeutic efficacy for seizure cessation when compared to doses needed for sedative effects. MDZ has excellent CNS penetration due to its lipophilicity and is 94–98% protein bound. Agents, e.g., aspirin, that compete for the site where MDZ binds to albumin may enhance the action of MDZ [39]. The therapeutic effect of MDZ is complex due to metabolism by hepatic and intestinal CYP3A4 to its active metabolite, 1′-hydroxymidazolam, followed by glucuronidation and renal excretion. As expected, inhibitors of CYP3A4 activity such as erythromycin, diltiazem, verapamil, and azole antifungals can prolong the effect of MDZ. Although prolonged use of MDZ infusions induces hepatic CYP3A activity, the half-life of MDZ can increase due to a rise in its Vd and an increase in its free fraction [40]. Importantly, for patients with SE, other ASMs are often co-administered and can affect the action of MDZ.

It is essential to recall the potential for withdrawal complications when an MDZ infusion is used for a prolonged period and at high doses. Adding a long-acting enteral BZP such as clonazepam or clobazam may increase the safety of weaning a parenteral infusion (Table 18.3).

18.7.1.2 Other GABAergic Therapies

In addition to MDZ, other parenteral medications, such as barbiturates and PRO, can be utilized to terminate seizures.

Barbiturates: GABAergic

First used in 1912, phenobarbital (PHB) was predated by the first documented ASM, potassium bromide, which was isolated from the Mediterranean Sea in 1826 [43]. Barbiturates bind to the β-subunit of the $GABA_A$ receptor to increase the duration of the opening of the chloride channel without altering the channel conductance or opening frequency. This increase in the mean open duration results in neuronal hyperpolarization and inhibition. However, at higher plasma concentrations (>50 μM), such as those achieved with PTB infusions, barbiturates directly open $GABA_A$ receptors in the absence of GABA [44]. Barbiturates also reduce AMPA/kainate receptor-mediated signals resulting in decreasing glutamate excitatory post-synaptic currents [45]. Studies show that barbiturates decrease cerebral metabolic rate and cerebral blood flow in animals and brain-injured humans, which can also decrease intracranial hypertension in a low cerebral compliance state [46, 47].

Table 18.3 Benzodiazepines for seizure termination [27, 41, 42]

Drug	Pros	Cons
Lorazepam	Optimal choice for IV bolus administration	Dilute 1:1 with saline due to high viscosity. IV product contains propylene glycol. Not recommended for infusion
Midazolam	Optimal choice agent for IM administration and IV infusion at anesthetic dosages	Rapid redistribution (short duration of action), renal and hepatic dysfunction can result in accumulation of active metabolites. IV product contains propylene glycol, but infusion does not
Diazepam	Rectal route available	Rapid redistribution with a short duration of action. IV product contains propylene glycol

IV intravenous, *IM* intramuscular

Phenobarbital

Phenobarbital (PHB), albeit the oldest ASM still in use, is no longer a treatment of choice for seizures because of sedation and significant DDIs but may be considered as a bridge to weaning from a long-term PTB infusion. PHB is approximately 50% protein bound with an estimated Vd of 0.6 L/kg [48]. It is metabolized in the liver primarily by CYP2C9, with minor metabolism by CYP2C19 and CYP2E1, and approximately 25% is excreted unchanged in the urine. It has a long half-life of 100–160 h in adults. In children, metabolism is increased with a reported half-life of 103 h in term infants and 67 h in infants 4 weeks of age [49].

PHB is a potent inducer of hepatic enzymes and can speed the metabolism of other hepatically cleared medications, thereby decreasing their efficacy [50]. However, the metabolism and clearance of PHB can be inhibited with subsequent PHB accumulation by felbamate, oxcarbazepine, PHT, and VPA [51–53]. PHB ADEs are similar to all barbiturates: lethargy and somnolence are major complaints.

Infusion/Anesthetic Dosing of Barbiturates as a Third-Line Therapy

Pentobarbital Infusion

Pentobarbital (PTB) is 45–75% protein-bound, metabolized by hydroxylation to an inactive metabolite with urinary excretions after glucuronidation. PTB is a potent inducer of hepatic enzymes such as CYP2A6. It is moderately lipophilic and readily crosses the blood-brain barrier. The IV solution has a pH of 9.5 and requires a propylene glycol diluent, which makes it incompatible with many other IV medications and requires monitoring for osmolar or anion gap acidosis at higher doses. Given its lipophilicity and hepatic metabolism, elimination is biphasic. The first phase is about 4 h and may require additional loading boluses to reach a steady-state plasma concentration; the second phase is 35–50 h and can be longer depending on drug accumulation in adipose and muscle [54].

PTB ADEs frequently include hypotension due to peripheral and splanchnic blood vessel dilation [55] and are accentuated with rapid administration. More complicated ADEs typically appear with high doses of PTB. Effects on the brainstem include cardiorespiratory depression [56], progressive loss of cough reflex, shivering response, corneal reflexes, and eventually pupillary dilation. Systemically, higher levels of PTB can correspond to loss of tracheal epithelium ciliary motility [57], ileus [58], and suppression of the immunological response to infection by inhibiting lymphocytic activation and inhibiting phagocytosis by leukocytes [59].

Thiopental Infusion

Thiopental (THP) is less frequently utilized than PTB for SE. Although it is typically considered a short-acting anesthetic, it is more lipophilic than PTB, and as a result, it rapidly redistributes to the muscle and fat with an initial half-time of

15 min. The secondary half-life of THP is approximately 7 h due to a high Vd secondary to its lipophilicity [60]; thus, long-term thiopental infusions can result in elimination half-lives ranging from 18 to 36 h [61], and its use can be complicated by prolonged emergence from sedation once an infusion is stopped.

Propofol Infusion: GABAergic

Propofol (PRO) is an alkylphenol that acts as a $GABA_A$ receptor agonist that activates the β-1 subunit of the chloride channel in the receptor increasing the duration of channel opening. PRO also influences presynaptic GABAergic transmission through GABA uptake and GABA release [62]. When utilized for SE cessation, weaning of PRO has been associated with seizure recurrence; therefore, additional ASM therapies may be necessary before decreasing or stopping the PRO infusion [63].

PRO is highly lipid-soluble with poor water solubility and is formulated in a lipid emulsion of 10% soybean oil, 2.25% glycerol, and 1.2% lecithin from purified egg phosphatide. It must be used with caution in patients with egg yolk allergies or patients with disorders of fat metabolism. The risk for infection is high; therefore, vials and tubing must be changed every 12 h. PRO is more than 95% protein-bound and highly lipophilic with a quick onset of action. It is primarily metabolized to inactive metabolites through hepatic glucuronidation and excreted in urine, although extrahepatic sites such as the lungs are responsible for the biotransformation of PRO to an inactive metabolite [64].

Like other GABAergic anesthetics, PRO decreases cerebral metabolic rate and cerebral blood flow. PRO can be associated with profound hypotension due to a decrease in cardiac β-adrenoceptor responsiveness [65] and peripheral vasodilation due to inhibition of sympathetic vasoconstriction [66] with decreased cerebral perfusion pressure unless caution is taken during administration. PRO is classically associated with respiratory depression and hypertriglyceridemia; therefore, adjustment of enteral or parenteral nutrition may be necessary to avoid overfeeding the patient when administered at high dosages [67]. A rare but potentially life-threatening complication of PRO includes propofol-related infusion syndrome (PRIS). PRIS is characterized by opisthotonos, muscle rigidity, choreoathetoid movements, myoclonus, seizures, hyperthermia, hyperkalemia, and metabolic and lactic acidosis due to direct mitochondrial respiratory chain inhibition or impaired mitochondrial fatty acid metabolism. When untreated, patients can progress to rhabdomyolysis, acute kidney injury, transaminitis, hypotension, and arrhythmias, including ventricular tachycardia and fibrillation, or bradycardia leading to asystole/cardiac failure. First reported in children, it has also been found in adults, typically with higher dose (>5 mg/kg/h) infusions lasting more than 48 h [68].

18.7.1.3 Second-Line Non-anesthetic ASMs

Phenytoin and Fosphenytoin: Sodium Channel Blocker

Phenytoin (PHT), synthesized as a barbiturate derivative in 1908 and first used as an ASM in 1937, is the second oldest ASM still in clinical use. Fosphenytoin (fosPHT) is a phosphorylated ester prodrug of PHT that was first approved in 1996. The IV solution of PHT has poor water solubility, and its diluents include propylene glycol and alcohol adjusted to a pH of 12. FosPHT has a pH of 8.6–9.0 that enhances the solubility and safety if an infusion extravasates and in the hemodynamic tolerance to rapid infusion. FosPHT is more frequently utilized in clinical practice due to its safety profile and is rapidly metabolized to PHT by red blood cell and liver phosphatases in a 1:1 conversion to PHT.

PHT binds to the neuronal inner cytoplasmic membrane at the inner vestibule of the pore of the voltage-gated sodium channel in its inactive state. This action prolongs the neuronal refractory period and stabilizes the neuronal membrane [69, 70]. PHT may also inhibit postsynaptic voltage-gated calcium channels [71, 72]. PHT is 90–95% protein bound, and active free levels are increased by hypoalbuminemia or displacement by other medications, such as VPA. Its Vd increases with the dose from 0.52 to 0.78 L/kg. PHT is metabolized primarily hepatically via CYP2C9 and CYP2C19 enzymes to an active metabolite that is excreted in the urine. The metabolite is saturable, which results in a nonlinear dose-serum concentration relation. PHT demonstrates first-order kinetics at low plasma levels, but at therapeutic levels and saturable hepatic metabolism, it shifts to zero-order kinetics with large changes in plasma levels with small dose adjustments. It reaches peak plasma concentration in about 30 min.

PHT significantly induces hepatic enzymes and affects levels of PHB, CBZ, felbamate, oxcarbazepine, TPM, omeprazole, MDZ, fluoxetine, amiodarone, digoxin, cyclosporine, estrogens, progestogens, voriconazole, fluconazole, and itraconazole [73].

Short-term toxic side effects include nystagmus, loss of smooth extraocular pursuit, diplopia, ataxia, skin rash, or fever. Long-term use can be complicated by gingival hyperplasia, calvarial hyperostosis, hirsutism, peripheral neuropathy, cerebellar atrophy, and vitamin D and B12 deficiency [74].

When transitioning from parenteral dosing to enteral administration, it is important to recognize that only the PHT sodium salt extended-release oral formulation can be given once a day, while other formulations in suspension, chewable tablets, or IV should be dosed at least twice or three times per day.

Valproic Acid: GABAergic, Sodium, and Calcium Channel Activity

Valproic acid (VPA) is a simple 8-carbon branched-chain fatty (carboxylic) acid derived from valeric acid that is different from most ASMs that are heterocyclic nitrogen-containing compounds. VPA is typically well-tolerated as a rapid infusion, although it does have significant DDIs [53, 75]. VPA has multiple mechanisms of action, including attenuation of voltage-gated sodium ion channels by blocking the neuronal entry of sodium; inhibition of GABA transaminase, which blocks GABA degradation; increasing GABA synthesis by increasing the expression and activity of glutamic acid decarboxylase; modulation of calcium channels and NMDA receptors; and inhibition of histone deacetylase, which affects gene regulation associated with synaptic transmission, neurogenesis, inflammation, and neuronal plasticity [76].

VPA is 90% protein-bound, with saturable binding at higher therapeutic levels resulting in higher free VPA levels. The Vd of VPA is 0.15–0.22 L/kg. VPA undergoes extensive hepatic biotransformation by mitochondrial β-oxidation, microsomal hydroxylation, glucuronidation, and other conjugation reactions with excretion of its multiple metabolites in the urine. Less than 3% is excreted unchanged in the urine. As a fatty acid, VPA is a substrate for fatty acid β-oxidation, which takes place primarily in mitochondria. VPA-induced impairment of mitochondrial function and fatty acid metabolism is likely the cause of its significant ADEs [77]. VPA has a well-identified risk for hyperammonemia due to the interference of the conversion of ammonia to urea and is contraindicated in children and adults with known or suspected mitochondrial disorders or disorders of fatty acid metabolism or risk for hyperammonemia. Given the effect of VPA on the carnitine shuttle that results in the depletion of carnitine stores during long-term or high-dose therapy, co-administration of L-carnitine may prevent VPA hepatotoxicity and hyperammonemia [78]. VPA has a black box warning for hepatotoxicity, pancreatitis, and teratogenicity due to the 1–2% risk for neural tube defects, e.g., spina bifida, if used during the first trimester of pregnancy. Other side effects include tremor, somnolence, weight-gain, nausea, vomiting, and thrombocytopenia [79].

The co-administration of ASMs that induce hepatic enzymes such as CBZ, barbiturates, or PHT will accelerate VPA metabolism and require an increase in dosages. Conversely, VPA competes with PHT and BZPs for serum protein-binding sites, and concomitant administration raises the free concentration of VPA [80]. Free levels of VPA may be helpful when ASM co-administration is necessary; however, results are often delayed and not clinically relevant in an emergent setting due to off-site testing.

Unlike most ASMs that induce hepatic enzymes, increasing clearance and decreasing plasma levels, VPA is well known to inhibit enzymatic metabolism and increase plasma levels of ASMs such as PHB, PHT, CBZ, and lamotrigine (LTG) [19, 81]. Thus, the unpredictable relationship between VPA and other medications often makes it a challenging medication in complicated patients.

Levetiracetam: Synaptic Vesicle Protein 2A Binding

Levetiracetam (LEV) is a pyrrolidinone that was first approved in 1999, and the IV preparation in 2006. Unlike most ASMs, its primary mechanism of action is not through inhibitory or excitatory neurotransmitter receptor activity but a novel presynaptic mechanism of regulating the release of neurotransmitters through interaction with the synaptic vesicle protein 2A (SV2A), a transmembrane glycoprotein and galactose transporter [82]. LEV decreases the synchronization of bursts through the downstream effects on GABA as well as glutamate through AMPA and NMDA receptors (which also affects calcium homeostasis) to decrease neuronal excitability, seizures, and neuronal death [83]. It has a wide TI and is well tolerated and neither causes nor is impacted by DDIs. Given that it is available in both parenteral and enteral preparations, it has become widely used, often as a first-line medication, and as noted above, guidelines recommend its use in SE as a second-line treatment.

LEV has few serious ADEs on other organs. Side effects are typically neurologic, including irritability, aggression, anxiety, hyperactivity, depression, somnolence, fatigue, dizziness, and, rarely, psychosis and suicidal thoughts [84]. Other rare effects include thrombocytopenia, eosinophilia, pancytopenia, pharyngitis, nasopharyngitis, vomiting, nausea, and anorexia. Hypotension (0–5%) and respiratory depression (0–12%) have been reported in neonates [85] but are not common complications in adults.

LEV is less than 10% protein bound; therefore, LEV does not compete with other drugs for binding sites. The Vd ranges from 0.5 to 0.7 L/kg in adults and 0.6 to 0.9 L/kg in premature infants and children [86]. It is not metabolized by the liver but is primarily excreted unchanged in the urine, with 24% enzymatically hydrolyzed in the blood to an inactive metabolite [87]. The lack of dependence on cytochrome P450 metabolism and its lack of protein binding make it useful in patients with liver dysfunction and decrease DDIs. LEV reaches a steady state within 24–48 h, and the half-life is reported between 6 and 9 h [83, 87].

Brivaracetam: Voltage-Gated Sodium Channels and SV2a Receptors

Brivaracetam (BRV) is a 4-n-propyl analog of LEV that has a 15- to 30-fold higher affinity for SV2A than LEV [88]. Approved by the FDA in 2016, it is highly lipid soluble which increases the crossing of the blood-brain barrier. Unlike LEV, it also appears to inhibit voltage-gated sodium channels, thereby prolonging the refractory period of cortical neurons [89]; however, further studies suggest that its primary action is through its select high-affinity binding to presynaptic SV2a receptors [90]. BRV has a time-to-peak serum concentration within 1 h with a steady state reached in less than 48 h. It has less than 20% of protein binding with a Vd slightly less than water and a half-life of about 9 h [87]. BRV is extensively metabolized primarily by amidase hydrolysis to a carboxylic metabolic that is hydroxylated by CYP2C9. Additionally, the propyl side chain undergoes β-oxidation by CYP2C19 to three inactive metabolites. Greater than 95% of BRV is eliminated by the urine with 8.6% excreted unchanged. Dissimilar to LEV, P450-inducing medications increase clearance of BRV, and hepatic dysfunction increases BRV exposure necessitating dose reduction. Although affected by other medications, BRV does not significantly affect CYP450 or levels of other hepatically cleared medications such as ASMs. The exception is an elevation of the active metabolite of CBZ, carbamazepine epoxide (CE), due to BRV-mediated inhibition of epoxide hydrolase, the enzyme that hydrolyzes CE [91].

Similar to LEV, BRV is associated with somnolence, dizziness, and, predominantly, neurological/psychiatric ADEs such as irritability, insomnia, anxiety, and depression, but is typically well tolerated. In a retrospective evaluation and real-world experience, BRV has been used for successful SE resolution [92, 93].

Lacosamide: Voltage-Gated Sodium Channels

Lacosamide (LCM), like PHT and CBZ, is an ASM that acts on voltage-gated sodium channels. However, its action is novel by selectively enhancing the slow inactivation of voltage-gated sodium channels rather than acting on the fast synaptic transmission targeted by most ASMs. Through this mechanism, LCM affects excitatory and inhibitory ligand-gated ion channels and AMPA, NMDA, and $GABA_A$ receptors, thereby stabilizing hyperexcitable neuronal membranes and reducing long-term ion channel availability without impairing physiologic function [94]. LCM is a "functionalized" amino acid with a chiral center allowing the synthesis of an (R)-enantiomer that confers anti-seizure properties [95]. Interestingly, one study in rats with SE treated with LCM showed a dose-dependent neuroprotective effect with a reduction in neuronal cell loss in the hippocampus CA1 region and piriform cortex [96].

First approved in 2008, LCM is typically well tolerated, although side effects include dizziness, vertigo, fatigue, nausea and headache, vomiting, dyspepsia, and somnolence [97]. Its most life-threatening complications include its effect on the cardiac conduction system. Previously, the most common arrhythmias included first- and second-degree atrioventricular block and sinus node dysfunction [94]. A more recent systematic review showed ventricular tachycardia (29.4%) to be the most frequent arrhythmia, and in descending order: new-onset atrial fibrillation (17.6%), complete heart block (17.6%), Mobitz type 1 atrioventricular block (11.8%), sinus pauses (11.8%), pulseless electrical activity (5.9%), and widening QRS complex (5.9%) [98]. When initiating LCM or escalating the dose, a patient should first be evaluated for cardiac conduction delays, severe cardiac disease, known cardiac sodium channelopathies, and concomitant medications that prolong the QTc interval.

LCM is minimally protein bound, less than 15%, with a Vd of 0.7 L/kg fixed to total body water due to its hydrophilicity. Forty percent of a dose is eliminated unchanged in the urine, with the remainder hepatically metabolized to inactive metabolites by demethylation, primarily by CY2C19, and to a lesser extent by CYP3A4 and CYP2C9. These metabolites are renally excreted. No adjustment is needed in mild-to-moderate kidney injury, but with severe kidney impairment, the maximum dose should be adjusted [94]. LCM does not induce P450 enzymes. Its terminal half-life is 13 h in young patients and 14–16 h in the elderly.

Ketamine: NMDA Antagonist

Inhibition of glutamate receptors can interrupt the excitatory cascade that occurs with SE.

Ketamine (KET) is a noncompetitive NMDA glutamate receptor antagonist that is found to be effective, especially in RSE [99]. An animal study of SE demonstrated that PHB administered 15 min after seizure initiation controlled seizures in 66% of the animals; however, if seizures persisted, at 60 min, only 25% of seizures were controlled. Conversely, if KET was administered 15 min after seizure initiation, it had no effect, but at 60 min, KET at a dose of 100 mg/kg effectively controlled seizures in all animals [100]. This study demonstrated a dose effect, since 25 mg/kg was not effective at any time point, and underscores the concept that responsiveness to $GABA_A$ receptor-mediated inhibition wanes during SE.

KET is most effective when the NMDA channel was previously opened by glutamate binding and has other binding sites such as the mu, delta, and kappa opioid receptors. KET causes a hyperadrenergic state by inhibiting norepinephrine uptake and interacting with serotonin transporters to inhibit both dopamine and serotonin uptake. KET also directly inhibits nicotinic and muscarinic receptors and antagonizes sodium and potassium channels. These many properties explain the hypnotic, analgesic, and dissociative/hallucinogenic effects of KET with the preservation of hemodynamics [101].

Eighty percent of KET is demethylated by hepatic microsomal enzymes to an active metabolite, norketamine, which is hydrolyzed and eventually excreted in bile and urine after glucuronide conjugation. Small amounts of KET are also hydrolyzed in the kidneys, intestine, and lungs. KET has low protein binding (10–30%) but is lipid soluble with a high Vd of 2.3 L/kg. KET clearance is highly dependent on hepatic blood flow with a half-life of 2–3 h. It is also cleared 20% faster in females than males. Norketamine has analgesic properties and can accumulate when KET is administered as a continuous infusion. Prolonged ketamine exposure may result in up- and downregulation of regulatory neuronal proteins and has been associated with impairment of cognitive function and memory [102].

Ganaxolone: Neurosteroid, GABA Receptor

Neurosteroids present a novel treatment for SE. As noted previously, following excessive neuronal excitation and synchronization, persistent seizures result in brain inflammation with subsequent astrogliosis, microgliosis, receptor loss, and cell death. Ganaxolone (GX) was approved by the FDA in 2022 for use in children with cyclin-dependent kinase-like 5 (CDKL5) deficient epilepsy, and IV GX has been in clinical trials for RSE [103]. GX is a synthetic 3β-methyl analog of the naturally occurring neurosteroid allopregnanolone (also known as brexanolone). Neurosteroids are synthesized in the brain and inhibit neuronal excitability by directly opening chloride channels through allosteric modulation of the synaptic and extra-synaptic $GABA_A$ receptors at a receptor site separate from the BZP-binding site. GX is highly protein bound (99%) with a large Vd and a short half-life of 4 h after a single oral dose but a terminal half-life of 34 h. It undergoes hydroxylation to a weakly active metabolite, followed by stereoselective reduction of the ketone and sulfation in the liver. It is primarily excreted in the feces (80%) and urine (20%). Cytochrome P450 inducers (CYP2C19, CYP3A4, CYP2B6) will decrease GX levels.

Except for CNS side effects of somnolence, dizziness, fatigue, and headache, GX has no demonstrable organ or system ADEs. Unlike other steroids, neurosteroids have no systemic steroidal action. Given its GABAergic actions, there is a risk for withdrawal symptoms with abrupt discontinuation and should be tapered slowly after continued use [104]. In 2024, preliminary information from the first Phase III trial of IV GX in RSE showed a statistically significant increase in those achieving seizure termination within 30 min but did not impact the progression to IV anesthesia for 36 h after GX [105]. Despite these initial results, neurosteroids represent a promising agent for RSE and SRSE.

18.7.2 Enteral Agents

Adjunctive therapy is sometimes necessary to assist in the termination of status epilepticus. Choosing an ASM with different mechanisms of action can include less traditional medications that do not have a parenteral formulation.

18.7.2.1 Clobazam: GABA Receptor and GABA Transporter

Clobazam (CLO) and clonazepam (CLZ) are less conventional BZPs, as they have no parenteral preparation but may be useful adjunctive therapy, especially when transitioning from a parenteral infusion. CLO is an oral 1,5 BZP that activates the $GABA_A$ receptor and increases the production of the GABA transporter. CLO has less sedative effect than other BZPs due to its greater selectivity for α_2-subunits rather than α_1-subunits of the $GABA_A$ receptor. It takes 1–4 h to reach peak concentration, and due to its lipophilicity, it acts quickly and is evenly distributed with a half-life of 18 h. It is 85% protein-bound and rapidly hepatically metabolized to an active metabolite, N-desmethylclobazam, through the cytochrome P450 enzymes, CYP3A4 and CYP2C19. The metabolite has a long half-life of 50 h [106]. CLO also has anxiolytic properties and sedative effects. Tolerance can occur like with other BZPs, and abruptly stopping the medication can result in withdrawal symptoms. CLO is typically titrated to drug effect, although TDM is occasionally utilized for both CLO and its active metabolite.

18.7.2.2 Clonazepam: Serotonin agonist and GABA Receptor

Clonazepam (CLZ), unlike CLO, has the traditional 1–4 structure like other BDZs; however, it also has serotonergic effects, which appear to imbue anti-myoclonic efficacy. It has been utilized for SE [107]. It is metabolized by hepatic CYP3A, which is excreted in the urine. CLZ has a half-life of 20–80 h.

18.7.2.3 Topiramate: Sodium and Calcium Channel, GABA Receptor, Glutamate Receptors

Topiramate (TPM), first approved in Germany in 1998, is a sulfamate derivative of fructose with several mechanisms of action including (1) reduction of the frequency of activation of voltage-sensitive, use-dependent sodium channels; (2) potentiation of GABA inhibition by activity on the $GABA_A$ receptor-independent from the BZP-binding site; (3) inhibition of glutamate through antagonism of the AMPA and NMDA receptors; (4) reduction of the amplitude of voltage-gated L-type calcium channels; and (5) inhibition of type II and type IV carbonic anhydrase, which modulates pH-dependent activation of voltage- and receptor-activated ion channels [108].

TPM has low protein binding (~15%) and is minimally metabolized in the liver, as 75–80% is excreted unchanged in the urine. The Vd is 0.6–0.8 L/kg, suggesting that it is distributed into the volume of total body water with linear elimination kinetics and a long half-life of 18–23 h [109]. The half-life is reduced by inducing ASMs such as PHT, PB, and CBZ despite their extensive renal clearance. TPM is not a strong inducer of hepatic enzymes and has little clinically significant effect on LTG and PHT but does increase the clearance of digoxin and oral ethinylestradiol, which may affect contraceptive efficacy [110]. Side effects include fatigue, cognitive slowing, word-finding difficulty, amnesia, nausea, and anorexia. Additionally, a hyperchloremic non-anion gap metabolic acidosis can occur due to inhibition of carbonic anhydrase and may also contribute to nephrolithiasis, paresthesias, and somnolence [111–113].

18.7.2.4 Perampanel: AMPA Receptor Antagonist

Perampanel (PMP) was first approved for ages greater than 12 years by the FDA as an oral preparation in 2012 for partial-onset seizures, with expanded approval in 2015 for generalized tonic-clonic seizures. It is a novel noncompetitive selective antagonist of the postsynaptic AMPA glutamate receptors. PMP was approved in 2024 as a parenteral formulation in Japan but is only available as an oral agent in the United States. It is highly protein bound (~95%) and metabolized by CYP3A4/5, CYP1A2, and CYP2B6 and excreted in urine and feces as oxidative and conjugated metabolites. The peak plasma concentration occurs within 15 min to 2 h, with a terminal half-life of 105 h, which is shortened by enzyme-inducing concomitant medications. Steady state is not reached for 2–3 weeks. One group evaluated the efficacy and safety at doses of 4 mg in 12 patients and showed clinical and electrographic improvement in only 2 patients with no adverse events [114]. The enteral formulation of PMP and its slow time to steady state may limit its use and utility for rapid effect in terminating active seizures. The same group performed a retrospective analysis with a higher initial dose of up to 24 mg and showed seizure termination with PMP in 17% of 30 patients with RSE and SRSE. Another study of PMP in SRSE utilized 6 mg and suggested that loading doses higher than 6 mg or dose intervals shorter than 24 h might be more effective [115]; however, there are no robust safety data regarding this practice.

There is a black box warning regarding serious or life-threatening psychiatric and behavioral ADEs that include irritability, aggression, belligerence, hostility, and homicidal ideation in up to 20% of patients at higher doses. Less severe ADEs include dizziness, somnolence, fatigue, and headache [116]. In the acute setting of RSE and SRSE, these symptoms will not be apparent, but when the emergence of wakefulness occurs, it will be helpful to know that the frequency of these behaviors is dose dependent.

18.7.2.5 Carbamazepine and Lamotrigine: Voltage-Gated Sodium and Calcium Channels

Other oral agents that might be considered for the treatment of seizures are carbamazepine (CBZ) and lamotrigine (LTG). CBZ modulates voltage-gated sodium and calcium channels and can cause agranulocytosis, aplastic anemia, hepatic and renal injury, and hyponatremia.

LTG was first approved in 1994 and appears to bind and inhibit voltage-gated sodium channels to stabilize presynaptic neuronal membranes and inhibit presynaptic glutamate and aspartate release. It may also act on the voltage-gated calcium channels [117]. LTG has been associated with skin rash, headaches, nausea, dizziness, and ataxia. More life-threatening ADEs include Stevens-Johnson syndrome and hemophagocytic lymphohistiocytosis (HLH) [118]. HLH is an uncontrolled response by the immune system with symptoms of persistent fever, hepatosplenomegaly with liver dysfunction, cytopenias, hypertriglyceridemia, and coagulopathy with hypofibrinogenemia [119].

Both CBZ and LTG have been reported to exacerbate seizures, SE or NCSE, mostly in children with severe myoclonic epilepsy [120–123]. In one cohort of patients 2–18 years of age, LTG resulted in a greater than 50% increase in convulsive seizures in 8 (40%) of 20 patients, and myoclonic seizures worsened in 6 (33%) of 18 patients [124]. Both CBZ and LTG should be used with caution in patients with SE.

18.8 Less Conventional Methods of SE Cessation

18.8.1 Immunomodulation

When seizures persist, inflammatory mediators may not only generate seizures but also play a role in facilitating epileptic networks to fuel ongoing epileptogenesis [125]. Additionally, the underlying etiology of the SRSE may be an inflammatory disease such as autoimmune or viral encephalitis that may be responsive to immunomodulatory therapy [126]. Adrenocorticotropic hormone (ACTH) has been useful for infantile spasms; however, a meta-analysis evaluating corticosteroids, including ACTH, showed a lack of efficacy for childhood seizures other than spasms [127]. Corticosteroids (IV dexamethasone and methylprednisolone) have been utilized successfully in case reports and case series of SRSE [128–130].

No data shows that IV immunoglobulin (IVIg) is efficacious in terminating seizures independent of its effect on the underlying inflammatory etiology. A literature review regarding IVIg in RSE included 24 original studies published prior to 2017. This review showed an unclear impact on seizure freedom [131]. A Cochrane systematic review in 2019 found only one study that randomized patients to IVIg as an add-on therapy and showed no significant difference compared to an add-on placebo [132].

18.8.2 Ketogenic Diet

A high-fat, moderate-protein, low-carbohydrate diet in a 3:1 or 4:1 ratio of fat to protein induces ketosis to mimic a fasting state. It was first introduced as a treatment for epilepsy in 1921 [133]. More recently, a ketogenic diet (KD) has been shown to achieve seizure freedom in 13% of adult patients with drug-resistant epilepsy and can reduce seizure frequency by up to 50% [134]. Although the mechanism is not fully understood, various changes in dopamine, serotonin metabolites, orexigenic neuropeptide galanin, GABA, or kynurenic acid have been reported. Alterations in neurotransmitters, ion channels, oxidative stress, and brain energy metabolism increase the seizure threshold to prevent seizures [135]. KD appears to modulate inflammation through mechanisms that might include decreases in leptin levels, binding of ketone bodies to hydroxycarboxylic acid receptors, changes in glucagon and cyclic AMP, or modulation of adenosine. A meta-analysis of multiple studies showed that a KD reduces the inflammatory markers of tumor necrosis factor-α and interleukin-6. This effect on inflammation may make KD particularly useful in patients with SRSE due to an inflammatory condition [136].

Due to the difficulties in implementation especially in an intensive care setting, a KD is typically only considered after patients fail therapeutic coma with anesthetic dosing of medications as described earlier. In a survey of professional societies that included 156 respondents, of whom 80% were physicians and 18% nonphysicians, up to 25.7% cited the lack of pharmacist support as the most important missing resource in implementing this strategy for seizure termination. A dietician who is experienced in managing this unique source of calories is also essential [137].

Important monitoring includes frequent assessments of serum basic metabolic panel, including acid-base status, magnesium, phosphorus, liver function tests, complete blood cell count, lipid profile, calcium, vitamin D levels, urine ketones, and free carnitine. When unable to attain ketosis, it is necessary to undertake a careful assessment of concomitant medications such as elixirs that contain sorbitol, xylitol, or other alcoholic sugars or sources of carbohydrates. Steroids have antiketogenic properties and may inhibit ketosis; however, KD may increase the synthesis of neuroactive steroids, which can enhance levels of GABA and modulate $GABA_A$ receptors, thereby decreasing seizures [138].

Contraindications to KD include pregnancy, disorders related to fatty acid transport or oxidation, and metabolic conditions that require a high-carbohydrate diet, such as pyruvate carboxylase deficiency and porphyria [139]. In the critical care setting, severe hemodynamic instability is a contraindication, as acidosis may worsen hypotension and decrease the effectiveness of vasopressors [140]. Medications to avoid with a KD include carbonic anhydrase inhibitors such as zonisamide and TPM, which can worsen metabolic acidosis and nephrolithiasis. Most importantly, the induction of a KD with concurrent PRO infusion has resulted in PRIS with fatal arrhythmias and should be avoided. This may be due to the finding that PRO impairs fatty acid metabolism, and energy metabolism becomes impaired in the setting of a KD where lipids are the primary source of energy [139, 141].

18.8.3   *Hypothermia*

In animal models, hyperthermia with seizures for 20-min duration results in neocortical neuronal damage and necrosis at 45 min at temperatures of 39.5 °C and hippocampal injury at 41 °C. Conversely, hypothermia by a decrease of 5 °C reduced neocortical injury [142].

Hypothermia decreases the release of excitatory amino acids such as glutamate; inhibits accumulation of intracellular calcium; decreases free radical production, lipid peroxidation, cytokines, and inflammatory cascade; and prevents DNA damage and mitochondrial dysfunction. Furthermore, hypothermia decreases cerebral metabolic rate and may stabilize the blood-brain barrier and decrease cerebral edema [143]. There has been extensive work in animal models and human clinical trials evaluating hypothermia as a neuroprotectant in the setting of focal and global ischemia, i.e., acute ischemic stroke [144] and cardiac arrest [145] as well as traumatic brain injury [146]. Similarly, hypothermia has been utilized for RSE and SRSE [143]. Current guidelines, and suggested treatment approaches, recommend hypothermia as a potential adjuvant therapy for RSE and SRSE [4, 28]; however, some investigators have demonstrated seizure suppression with hypothermia induction but seizure recurrence when the patient is returned to normothermia [147].

For the pharmacist, the importance of hypothermia is the slowing of the systemic metabolic rate, changes in protein binding, hepatic and renal blood flow, renal tubular secretion, and enzymatic processes which will alter the pharmacokinetics and pharmacodynamics of different medications variably and result in drug toxicity or therapeutic failure. Dosage adjustment may be necessary [148, 149].

18.8.4 Magnesium

IV magnesium sulfate ($MgSO_4$) has been utilized for eclamptic seizures; however, it has also been utilized in non-eclamptic RSE and SRSE [150]. $MgSO_4$ inhibits NMDA-glutamate receptors and may also block calcium channels to decrease cell excitability [151]. ADEs associated with $MgSO_4$ include vasodilation, flushing, hypotension, and constipation, although at high dosages, weakness and heart block have been reported [150, 152]. $MgSO_4$ has few significant DDI. A systematic review evaluating 19 original articles of 28 patients with SE or RSE showed seizure reduction of up to 50%, but similar to hypothermia, seizures recur when the $MgSO_4$ infusion was discontinued [150]. The strategies of hypothermia and magnesium may best be employed while titrating other ASM agents that have a slow onset of action.

18.9 Novel Approaches

When conventional pharmacological modalities fail with SRSE, electroconvulsive therapy (ECT) [153, 154] and surgical options such as temporal lobectomy [155] may be considered but are beyond the scope of this chapter. Of great interest are novel, promising technological alternatives that will require pharmacological expertise. Nano-strategies have been proposed to enhance the efficacy of ASM. The challenge is to cross the blood-brain barrier protected by membrane lipophilicity and tight junctions, prevent enzymatic degradation of the active drug, and target the specific brain cells. Strategies include encapsulation of the drug as a pharmaceutical nanocarrier by micelles, liposomes, polymeric nanoparticles (NP), solid-lipid NP, nanoemulsions, and dendrimers [156, 157].

There are clinically available FDA-approved nanoformulated drugs. Many are targeted for oncological conditions, iron deficiency, and infection, e.g., liposomal preparations of vincristine and irinotecan, iron dextran, and liposomal amphotericin B. Neurologically targeted agents include glatiramer acetate and pegylated interferon β-1a for multiple sclerosis that uses polymer nanoparticle (NP) technology and tizanidine HCl, a muscle relaxant, and dexmethylphenidate HCl, a psychostimulant. These last two medications employ a nanocrystal NP strategy to promote high drug loading and bioavailability. Nanoengineering is ongoing for Alzheimer disease, Parkinson disease, Huntington disease, brain tumors, and stroke. For epilepsy, CBZ-loaded to solid lipid NP or poly lactic-glycolic acid NP has been developed to enhance their anti-seizure effect [158]. More recently, NPs have been developed to target voltage-gated calcium channels. Targeted binding can block the flow of ions but also induce conformational changes that alter ion fluxes. Carbon-based nanomaterials, including single-walled carbon nanotubes, reversibly block potassium channels and appear to decrease oxidative stress [159, 160]. This novel technology may expand the options for treatment and revolutionize the efficacy of pharmacotherapy for SE, RSE, and SRSE [158].

18.10   Summary

Critical care pharmacists play an essential role in the management of patients with RSE and SRSE. While guidelines direct the first steps in terminating seizures in SE, multiple ASMs and a deeper depth of sedation to anesthetic levels may be necessary when seizures persist. Less conventional but more complex strategies may sometimes be needed. The multiprofessional team approach of incorporating a pharmacist brings the added expertise of assessing DDIs, changes in metabolism/clearance of medications, and risk of ADEs to the bedside. In the future, the pharmacist will be able to leverage new formulations that utilize advanced technologies to enhance the CNS penetration of ASMs, their targets, and ASM efficacy to improve the care of the patient with SE (Tables 18.4 and 18.5).

Table 18.4 Key aspects of common anti-seizure medications

Drug	Mechanism of action	Dosing	Administration notes	Bioavailability	Vd	Protein binding	Metabolism	Elimination
Midazolam [27, 40, 161]	Positive allosteric modulator of GABA$_A$ receptors in the CNS, increasing permeability to chloride ions leading to hyperpolarization leads to increased frequency of channel opening	IM: 0.2 mg/kg, up to 10 mg Infusion: 0.05–2 mg/kg/h, may bolus 0.1–0.2 mg/kg and titrate by 0.05–0.1 mg/kg/h every 3–4 h with EEG	Administer IM doses as a deep injection into a large muscle mass	IM: >90%	1–3.1 L/kg	97%	Hepatic: CYP3A4; metabolism is induced with prolonged use increasing clearance 5–10×	Renal: 45–57% as conjugated drug; $T_{1/2}$ 3–4.2 h, prolonged in obesity, heart failure (2× increase), hepatic impairment (2.5× increase), renal failure (>25 h)
Propofol [27, 62, 63, 162]	GABA$_A$ receptor agonist	Infusion: 5–200 µg/kg/min, 1–2 mg/kg bolus may be given for breakthrough SE and rate titrated by 5–10 µg/kg/min every 5 min	IV product and tubing must be changed every 12 h; formulated in a lipid emulsion		2–10 L/kg, increasing with length of therapy	>95%	Hepatic: CYP2B6	Renal: 90%; $T_{1/2}$ 3–12 h (biphasic)
Ketamine [27, 101, 102]	Noncompetitive NMDA glutamate receptor antagonist	Loading: 1–2.5 mg/kg IV, followed by 1–10 mg/kg/h	Consider administering loading/bolus doses over 2–3 min; consider administering with a BZP		2.1–3.1 L/kg	10–30%	Primary: CYP3A; secondary: 2B6 and 2C9	Renal: 91%; $T_{1/2}$ 2.5 h (beta phase)

Drug	Mechanism of action	Dose	Administration	Bioavailability	V_d	Protein binding	Metabolism	Elimination/half-life
Pentobarbital [27, 54]	Binds synaptic and extrasynaptic GABA$_A$ receptors to enhance neuronal chloride channel opening and inhibition of cortical function; also inhibits AMPA receptors, resulting in suppression of glutaminergic neurotransmission	Infusion: 5–20 mg/kg bolus followed by 0.5–5 mg/kg/h with EEG; 5 mg/kg bolus doses may be given for breakthrough SE and rate titrated by 0.5–1 mg/kg/h every 12 h	Administer IV bolus doses no faster than 50 mg/min		1.06–1.1 L/kg	45–70%	Hepatic: hydroxylation and glucuronidation	$T_{1/2}$ 15–50 h
Lorazepam [41]	Positive allosteric modulator of GABA$_A$ receptors in the CNS, increasing permeability to chloride ions leading to hyperpolarization = increased frequency of channel opening	IV: 0.1 mg/kg, up to 4 mg per dose, may repeat in 3–5 min	IV: dilute 1:1 with sterile water for injection, NS, or D5W and mix gently prior to administration; do not exceed 2 mg/min	IM: 83–100%, PO: 90–93%	1.3 L/kg	85–91%	Hepatic: conjugation, rapid and extensive enterohepatic recirculation	Renal: 88%; $T_{1/2}$ 12–14 h, ≥25% prolonged in renal impairment
Diazepam [42]	Positive allosteric modulator of GABA$_A$ receptors in the CNS, increasing permeability to chloride ions leading to hyperpolarization → increased frequency of channel opening	IV: 0.15–0.2 mg/kg, max 10 mg per dose, may repeat dose in 3–5 min (90 mg/day)	Administer IV doses no faster than 5 mg/min	PO, IM: 94%	0.8–1 L/kg	95–99.3%	Hepatic: CYP3A4 and 2C19	Renal: primarily as metabolites; $T_{1/2}$ 20–100 h, prolonged in cirrhosis (2–5× increase) and older age
Clonazepam [21, 163]	Increases frequency of GABA-mediated chloride channel openings	PO/tube: 0.5–1 mg/day in 1–3 divided doses		PO: 90%	1.5–6.4 L/kg	85%	Hepatic: CYP3A4	$T_{1/2}$ 17–60 h

(continued)

Table 18.4 (continued)

Drug	Mechanism of action	Dosing	Administration notes	Bioavailability	Vd	Protein binding	Metabolism	Elimination
Phenobarbital [21, 27, 48, 49, 164]	Prolongs GABA-mediated chloride channel openings, some additional blockade of voltage-dependent sodium channels	IV loading: 15–20 mg/kg administered at 50–100 mg/min, may give additional 5–10 mg/kg 10 min after loading dose; maintenance dose 1–3 mg/kg/day in divided doses		PO: 90%	0.54–0.73 L/kg	20–45%	Hepatic: primarily CYP 2C9, some CYP2C19, CYP 2E1, N-glycosylation	Renal: 25%; $T_{1/2}$ 53–140 h
Valproate sodium [21, 27, 75, 76]	Enhances GABA transmission in specific circuits, some additional blockade of voltage-dependent sodium channels	IV loading: 20–40 mg/kg (max 3000 mg/dose) administered at 3–6 mg/kg/min, may give additional 20 mg/kg 10 min after loading dose; maintenance dosing: 10–15 mg/kg/day in divided doses		PO: ~90% (ER tabs)	0.15–0.22 L/kg	80–90%	Hepatic: glucuronidation, CYP2C9	Renal: 30–50%; $T_{1/2}$ 9–19 h
Phenytoin [21, 70, 73, 164]	Blocks voltage-dependent sodium channels at high firing frequencies	IV loading: 20 mg/kg, may give an additional 5–10 mg/kg 10 min after loading dose; maintenance dose 4–6 mg/kg/day in divided doses	Administer IV doses no faster than 50 mg/min, ideally through a large peripheral or central vein	PO: 80%, absorption is highly dependent on enteral formulation	0.52–0.78 L/kg	90–95%	Hepatic: CYP2C9, CYP2C19; first-order to zero-order kinetics	Renal: primarily as inactive metabolites; $T_{1/2}$ 12–36 h

Drug	Mechanism	Dose	Administration		Vd	Protein binding	Metabolism	Elimination
Fosphenytoin [165]	Blocks voltage-dependent sodium channels at high firing frequencies	IV loading: 20 mg PE/kg (max 1500 mg PE/dose), may give additional 5 mg PE/kg 10 min after loading dose; IV maintenance dosing: 4–6 mg PE/kg/day	Administer IV doses no faster than 150 mg PE/min (US boxed warning)		4.3–10.8 L	95–99%	See Phenytoin	See Phenytoin
Lacosamide [27, 94, 97, 166]	Enhances slow inactivation voltage-gated sodium channels, affects AMPA, NMDA, GABA$_A$ receptors	IV loading: 200–400 mg; maintenance dose 100–200 mg BID	Loading dose can be given IV push	PO: 100%	0.6–0.67 L/kg	<15%	Hepatic: CYP 3A4, 2C9, 2C19	Renal: 95%; $T_{1/2}$ 13 h
Topiramate [21, 109, 167]	Blocks voltage-dependent sodium channels at high firing frequencies, increases frequency at which GABA opens chloride channels (separate site from BZP action), antagonizes glutamate action at AMPA, inhibition of carbonic anhydrase	PO loading: 200–400 mg PO/via tube; maintenance: 300–1600 mg/day in divided doses		PO: 80%	0.6–0.8 L/kg	15–40% (inversely related to plasma concentrations)	Minimal metabolism; hepatic: hydroxylation, hydrolysis, and glucuronidation; renal: renal tubular reabsorption	Renal: 70%; $T_{1/2}$ 21 h (will vary depending on concomitant DDI and/or degree of renal failure)
Levetiracetam [21, 27, 86, 168, 169]	Proposed to bind SV2A proteins and AMPA receptors and to inhibit high voltage-activated calcium channels	IV loading: 40–60 mg/kg (max 4500 mg); maintenance 1000–1500 mg BID	Administer loading doses over 5–15 min, or consider IV push	PO: 100%	0.5–0.7 L/kg	<10%	Minimal metabolism, enzymatic hydrolysis primarily in the blood	Renal: 66%; $T_{1/2}$ 6–8 h
Brivaracetam [27, 170, 171]	Binds SV2A presynaptically with high affinity	IV loading: dose not well established; maintenance: 100 mg BID	Administer over 2–15 min, may give undiluted or diluted	PO: >90%	0.5 L/kg	<20%	Hepatic: CYP3A4, 2C9, 2C19	Renal: >95%; T_f 9 h

CNS central nervous system, D5W 5% dextrose in water, DDI drug-drug interactions, EEG electroencephalogram, IM intramuscular, IV intravenous, NA sodium, NS normal saline, PO oral, Vd volume of distribution

Table 18.5 Drug-drug interactions and notable adverse events

Drug	Drug-drug interactions	Notable adverse drug events
Midazolam [27, 40, 62]	Increased CNS depression seen with other medications that produce sedation and/or CNS depression; increased exposure to midazolam with major CYP3A4 inhibitors; reduced exposure to midazolam with CYP3A4 inducers	Respiratory depression, hypotension, delirium, withdrawal ± seizure recurrence with abrupt discontinuation, accumulation of active metabolite in renal and hepatic dysfunction, IV push products contain propylene glycol—IV infusion does not contain propylene glycol
Propofol [27, 62, 63, 162]	Increased CNS depression seen with other medications that produce sedation and/or CNS depression; risk of respiratory depression, hypotension, and bradycardia when combined with opioids or other sedatives	Allergy to egg/soy, hypotension, respiratory depression, hypertriglyceridemia, propofol-related infusion syndrome, green discoloration of urine, seizure recurrence with abrupt discontinuation
Ketamine [27, 101, 102]	Hypertension, tachycardia, increased cardiac output, respiratory depression, emergency reactions, withdrawal syndrome	Dissociative psychosis, excessive sympathomimetic stimulation, reports of increased intracranial pressure
Pentobarbital [27, 54]	Major enzyme inducer producing DDIs	Vasodilation with rapid administration, hypotension, cardiac depression, ileus, respiratory depression, propylene glycol toxicity, withdrawal ± seizures with abrupt discontinuation; rare: Stevens-Johnson syndrome, megaloblastic anemia
Lorazepam [37, 41]	Increased CNS depression seen with other medications that produce sedation and/or CNS depression	Respiratory depression, hypotension, delirium, withdrawal ± seizure recurrence with abrupt discontinuation, propylene glycol toxicity
Diazepam [42]	Increased CNS depression seen with other medications that produce sedation and/or CNS depression	Respiratory depression, hypotension, delirium, withdrawal ± seizure recurrence with abrupt discontinuation, propylene glycol toxicity
Clonazepam [163]	Increased CNS depression seen with other medications that produce sedation and/or CNS depression	Respiratory depression, hypotension, delirium, withdrawal ± seizure recurrence with abrupt discontinuation, propylene glycol toxicity
Phenobarbital [21, 27, 48, 49, 164]	Major enzyme inducer producing DDIs	Sedation, hypotension, respiratory depression; rare: rash and hepatitis; contains propylene glycol
Valproate sodium [21, 27, 75, 76, 79]	Major enzyme inhibitor producing DDIs; highly bound to plasma proteins and may be involved in the displacement of other protein-bound drugs; carbapenem antibiotics reduce serum concentrations of VPA	Hyperammonemia, pancreatitis, thrombocytopenia, nausea, dizziness, tremor; black box warning for hepatotoxicity

(continued)

Table 18.5 (continued)

Drug	Drug-drug interactions	Notable adverse drug events
Phenytoin [21, 70, 73, 164]	Major enzyme inducer producing DDIs; highly bound to plasma proteins and may be involved in the displacement of other protein-bound drugs	Arrhythmias, bradycardia, GI distress, purple glove syndrome; rare: rash, hepatitis, nystagmus; contains propylene glycol
Fosphenytoin	See Phenytoin	See Phenytoin
Lacosamide [27, 94, 97, 98, 166]	Minimal	Prolongation of PR interval, bradycardia, hypotension, heart block, rash, dizziness, nausea
Topiramate [21, 109, 167]	Increased CNS depression seen with other medications that produce sedation and/or CNS depression; risk of metabolic acidosis when combined with other carbonic anhydrase inhibitors	Somnolence, paresthesias, acute myopia, metabolic acidosis, nephrolithiasis
Levetiracetam [21, 27, 86, 168, 169]	Minimal	Sedation, fatigue, dizziness; rare: psychiatric disturbances and leukopenia
Brivaracetam [27, 170, 171]	BRV increases serum concentrations of PHT and carbamazepine epoxide	Accumulation in renal failure, bronchospasm, angioedema

References

1. Mucksavage JJ, Tesoro EP. The role of pharmacy in neurocritical care. Curr Treat Options Neurol. 2023;25:469–76.
2. Bourne RS, Dorward BJ. Clinical pharmacist interventions on a UK neurosurgical critical care unit: a 2-week service evaluation. Int J Clin Pharm. 2011;33:755–8.
3. Trinka E, Cock H, Hesdorffer D, et al. A definition and classification of status epilepticus—report of the ILAE Task Force on Classification of Status Epilepticus. Epilepsia. 2015;56:1515–23.
4. Shorvon S. Super-refractory status epilepticus: an approach to therapy in this difficult clinical situation. Epilepsia. 2011;52:53–6.
5. Shorvon SD, Ferlisi M. The treatment of super-refractory status epilepticus: a critical review of available therapies and a clinical treatment protocol. Brain. 2011;134:2802–18.
6. Hirsch LJ, Gaspard N, van Baalen A, et al. Proposed consensus definitions for new-onset refractory status epilepticus (NORSE), febrile infection-related epilepsy syndrome (FIRES), and related conditions. Epilepsia. 2018;59:739–44.
7. Lothman E. The biochemical basis and pathophysiology of status epilepticus. Neurology. 1990;40(Suppl 2):13–23.
8. Claassen J, Mayer SA, Kowalski RG, et al. Detection of electrographic seizures with continuous EEG monitoring in critically ill patients. Neurology. 2004;62:1743–8.
9. Choi SA, Lee H, Kim K, et al. Mortality, disability, and prognostic factors of status epilepticus: a nationwide population-based retrospective cohort study. Neurology. 2022;99:e1393–401.
10. Lu M, Faure M, Bergamasco A, et al. Epidemiology of status epilepticus in the United States: a systematic review. Epilepsy Behav. 2020;112:107459. https://doi.org/10.1016/j.yebeh.2020.107459.

11. Roberg LE, Monsson O, Kristensen SB, et al. Prediction of long-term survival after status epilepticus using the ACD Score. JAMA Neurol. 2022;79:604–13.

12. Strzelczyk A, Ansorge S, Hapfelmeier J, et al. Costs, length of stay, and mortality of super-refractory status epilepticus: a population-based study from Germany. Epilepsia. 2017;58:1533–41.

13. Naylor DE, Liu H, Niquet J, et al. Rapid surface accumulation of NMDA receptors increase glutamatergic excitation during status epilepticus. Neurobiol Dis. 2013;54:225–38.

14. Naylor DE, Liu H, Wasterlain CG. Trafficking of GABA(A) receptors, loss of inhibition, and a mechanism for pharmacoresistance in status epilepticus. J Neurosci. 2005;25:7724–33.

15. Wasterlain CG, Naylor DE, Liu H, et al. Trafficking of NMDA receptors during status epilepticus: therapeutic implications. Epilepsia. 2013;54(Suppl 6):78–80.

16. Walker MC. Pathophysiology of status epilepticus. Neurosci Lett. 2018;667:84–91.

17. Löscher W, Klein P. The pharmacology and clinical efficacy of antiseizure medications: from bromide salts to cenobamate and beyond. CNS Drugs. 2021;35:935–63.

18. Perucca E. Clinically relevant drug interactions with antiepileptic drugs. Br J Clin Pharmacol. 2006;61:246–55.

19. Johannessen SI, Landmark CJ. Antiepileptic drug interactions—principles and clinical implications. Curr Neuropharmacol. 2010;8:254–67.

20. Deodhar M, Al Rihani SB, Arwood MJ, et al. Mechanisms of CYP450 inhibition: understanding drug-drug interactions due to mechanism-based inhibition in clinical practice. Pharmaceutics. 2020; https://doi.org/10.3390/pharmaceutics12090846.

21. Patsalos PN, Berry DJ, Bourgeois BF, et al. Antiepileptic drugs—best practice guidelines for therapeutic drug monitoring: a position paper by the subcommission on therapeutic drug monitoring, ILAE Commission on Therapeutic Strategies. Epilepsia. 2008;49:1239–76.

22. Canadian Society of Pharmacology and Therapeutics. Glossary of pharmacology: therapeutic index. 2020. https://pharmacologycanada.org/Therapeutic-Index. Accessed 1 Jun 2024.

23. Lim SN, Wu T, Chang CW, et al. Clinical impact of therapeutic drug monitoring for newer anti-seizure medications in patients with epilepsy: a real-world observation study. Biom J. 2023;47:100680. https://doi.org/10.1016/j.bj.2023.100680.

24. Reimers A, Berg JA, Burns ML, et al. Reference ranges for antiepileptic drugs revisited: a practical approach to establish national guidelines. Drug Des Devel Ther. 2018;12:271–80.

25. Gasior M, Husain A, Barra ME, et al. Intravenous ganaxolone: pharmacokinetics, pharmacodynamics, safety, and tolerability in healthy adults. Clin Pharmacol Drug Dev. 2024;13:248–58.

26. Treiman DM, Meyers PD, Walton NY, et al. A comparison of four treatments for generalized convulsive status epilepticus. Veterans Affairs Status Epilepticus Cooperative Study Group. N Engl J Med. 1998;339:792–8.

27. Vossler DG, Bainbridge JL, Boggs JG, et al. Treatment of refractory convulsive status epilepticus: a comprehensive review by the American Epilepsy Society Treatments Committee. Epilepsy Curr. 2020;20:245–64.

28. Brophy GM, Bell R, Claassen J, et al., Neurocritical Care Society Status Epilepticus Guideline Writing Committee. Guidelines for the evaluation and management of status epilepticus. Neurocrit Care. 2012;17:3–23.

29. Glauser T, Shinnar S, Gloss D, et al. Evidence-based guideline: treatment of convulsive status epilepticus in children and adults: report of the Guideline Committee of the American Epilepsy Society. Epilepsy Curr. 2016;16:48–61.

30. Kapur J, Elm J, Chamberlain JM, et al. Randomized trial of three anticonvulsant medications for status epilepticus. N Engl J Med. 2019;381:2103–13.

31. Ghit A, Assal D, Al-Shami AS, et al. GABA$_A$ receptors: structure, function, pharmacology, and related disorders. J Genet Eng Biotechnol. 2021; https://doi.org/10.1186/s43141-021-00224-0.

32. Olsen RW, Li GD. GABA(A) receptors as molecular targets of general anesthetics: identification of binding sites provides clues to allosteric modulation. Can J Anaesth. 2011;58:206–15.

33. Baur R, Sigel E. Benzodiazepines affect channel opening of GABA A receptors induced by either agonist binding site. Mol Pharmacol. 2005;67:1005–8.

34. Silbergleit R, Durkalski V, Lowenstein D, et al. Intramuscular versus intravenous therapy for prehospital status epilepticus. N Engl J Med. 2012;366:591–600.
35. Slupe AM, Kirsch JR. Effects of anesthesia on cerebral blood flow, metabolism, and neuroprotection. J Cereb Blood Flow Metab. 2018;38:2192–208.
36. Haverkos GP, DiSalvo RP, Imhoff TE. Fatal seizures after flumazenil administration in a patient with mixed overdose. Ann Pharmacother. 1994;28:1347–9.
37. Wilson KC, Reardon C, Theodore AC, et al. Propylene glycol toxicity: a severe iatrogenic illness in ICU patients receiving IV benzodiazepines: a case series and prospective, observational pilot study. Chest. 2005;128:1674–81.
38. Zar T, Graeber C, Perazella MA. Recognition, treatment, and prevention of propylene glycol toxicity. Semin Dial. 2007;20:217–9.
39. Halliday NJ, Dundee JW, Collier PS, et al. Influence of plasma proteins on the onset of hypnotic action of intravenous midazolam. Anaesthesia. 1985;40:763–6.
40. Bodmer M, Link B, Grignaschi N, et al. Pharmacokinetics of midazolam and metabolites in a patient with refractory status epilepticus treated with extraordinary doses of midazolam. Ther Drug Monit. 2008;30:120–4.
41. National Center for Biotechnology Information. PubChem compound summary for CID 3958, Lorazepam. 2024. https://pubchem.ncbi.nlm.nih.gov/compound/Lorazepam. Accessed 15 Jul 2024.
42. National Center for Biotechnology Information. PubChem compound summary for CID 3016, Diazepam. 2024. https://pubchem.ncbi.nlm.nih.gov/compound/Diazepam. Accessed 15 Jul 2024.
43. Safdari F, Rabbani M, Hosseini-Sharifabad A. Effect of acute and long term potassium bromide administration on spatial working memory in rat. Res Pharm Sci. 2017;12:154–9.
44. Sieghart W. Structure and pharmacology of gamma-aminobutyric acid A receptor subtypes. Pharmacol Rev. 1995;47:182–234.
45. Nardou R, Yamamoto S, Bhar A, et al. Phenobarbital but not diazepam reduces AMPA/kainate receptor mediated currents and exerts opposite actions on initial seizures in the neonatal rat hippocampus. Front Cell Neurosci. 2011; https://doi.org/10.3389/fncel.2011.00016.
46. Baughman VL, Hoffman WE, Miletich DJ, et al. Effects of phenobarbital on cerebral blood flow and metabolism in young and aged rats. Anesthesiology. 1986;65:500–5.
47. Nordström CH, Messeter K, Sundbärg G, et al. Cerebral blood flow, vasoreactivity, and oxygen consumption during barbiturate therapy in severe traumatic brain lesions. J Neurosurg. 1988;68:424–31.
48. Nelson E, Powell JR, Conrad K, et al. Phenobarbital pharmacokinetics and bioavailability in adults. J Clin Pharmacol. 1982;22:141–8.
49. Pacifici GM. Clinical pharmacology of phenobarbital in neonates: effects, metabolism and pharmacokinetics. Curr Pediatr Rev. 2016;12:48–54.
50. Gupte S. Phenobarbital and metabolism of metronidazole. N Engl J Med. 1983;308:529.
51. Reidenberg P, Glue P, Banfield CR, et al. Effects of felbamate on the pharmacokinetics of phenobarbital. Clin Pharmacol Ther. 1995;58:279–87.
52. Flesch G. Overview of the clinical pharmacokinetics of oxcarbazepine. Clin Drug Investig. 2004;24:185–203.
53. Keys PA. Valproic acid: interactions with phenytoin and phenobarbital. Drug Intell Clin Pharm. 1982;16:737–9.
54. National Center for Biotechnology Information. PubChem compound summary for CID 4737, Pentobarbital. 2004. https://pubchem.ncbi.nlm.nih.gov/compound/Pentobarbital. Accessed 4 Jun 2024.
55. Kawaue Y, Iriuchijima J. Changes in cardiac output and peripheral flows on pentobarbital anesthesia in the rat. Jpn J Physiol. 1984;34:283–94.
56. Yamada KA, Moerschbaecher JM, Hamosh P, et al. Pentobarbital causes cardiorespiratory depression by interacting with a GABAergic system at the ventral surface of the medulla. J Pharmacol Exp Ther. 1983;226:349–55.
57. Iida H, Matsuura S, Shirakami G, et al. Differential effects of intravenous anesthetics on ciliary motility in cultured rat tracheal epithelial cells. Can J Anaesth. 2006;53:242–9.

58. Newey CR, Wisco D, Nattanmai P, et al. Observed medical and surgical complications of prolonged barbiturate coma for refractory status epilepticus. Ther Adv Drug Saf. 2016;7:195–203.
59. Neuwelt EA, Kikuchi K, Hill SA, et al. Barbiturate inhibition of lymphocyte function. Differing effects of various barbiturates used to induce coma. J Neurosurg. 1982;56:254–9.
60. Brandon RA, Baggot JD. The pharmacokinetics of thiopentone. J Vet Pharmacol Ther. 1981;4:79–85.
61. Turcant A, Delhumeau A, Premel-Cabic A, et al. Thiopental pharmacokinetics under conditions of long-term infusion. Anesthesiology. 1985;63:50–4.
62. Trapani G, Altomare C, Liso G, et al. Propofol in anesthesia. Mechanism of action, structure-activity relationships, and drug delivery. Curr Med Chem. 2000;7:249–71.
63. Stecker MM, Kramer TH, Raps EC, et al. Treatment of refractory status epilepticus with propofol: clinical and pharmacokinetic findings. Epilepsia. 1998;39:18–26.
64. Dawidowicz AL, Fornal E, Mardarowicz M, et al. The role of human lungs in the biotransformation of propofol. Anesthesiology. 2000;93:992–7.
65. Zhou W, Fontenot HJ, Wang SN, et al. Propofol-induced alterations in myocardial β-adrenoceptor binding and responsiveness. Anesth Analg. 1999;89:604–8.
66. Robinson BJ, Ebert TJ, O'Brien TJ, et al. Mechanisms whereby propofol mediates peripheral vasodilation in humans. Sympathoinhibition or direct vascular relaxation? Anesthesiology. 1997;86:64–72.
67. Dickerson RN, Buckley CT. Impact of propofol sedation upon caloric overfeeding and protein inadequacy in critically ill patients receiving nutrition support. Pharmacy. 2021; https:// doi.org/10.3390/pharmacy9030121.
68. Hemphill S, McMenamin L, Bellamy MC, et al. Propofol infusion syndrome: a structured literature review and analysis of published case reports. Br J Anaesth. 2019;122:448–59.
69. Keppel Hesselink JM. Phenytoin: repurposing an old molecule and patent strategies for neuropathic pain. J Clin Trials Pat. 2018;3(1):3.
70. Keppel Hesselink JM, Kopsky DJ. Phenytoin: 80 years young, from epilepsy to breast cancer, a remarkable molecule with multiple modes of action. J Neurol. 2017;264:1617–21.
71. Yaari Y, Selzer ME, Pincus JH. Phenytoin: mechanisms of its anticonvulsant action. Ann Neurol. 1986;20:171–84.
72. Schumacher TB, Beck H, Steinhäuser C, et al. Effects of phenytoin, carbamazepine, and gabapentin on calcium channels in hippocampal granule cells from patients with temporal lobe epilepsy. Epilepsia. 1998;39:355–63.
73. Rodriguez-Vera L, Yin X, Almoslem M, et al. Comprehensive physiologically based pharmacokinetic model to assess drug-drug interactions of phenytoin. Pharmaceutics. 2023; https:// doi.org/10.3390/pharmaceutics15102486.
74. LoPinto-Khoury C. Long-term effects of antiseizure medications. Semin Neurol. 2022;42:583–93.
75. Ghodke-Puranik Y, Thorn CF, Lamba JK, et al. Valproic acid pathway: pharmacokinetics and pharmacodynamics. Pharmacogenet Genomics. 2013;23:236–41.
76. Romoli M, Mazzocchetti P, D'Alonzo R, et al. Valproic acid and epilepsy: from molecular mechanisms to clinical evidences. Curr Neuropharmacol. 2019;17:926–46.
77. Silva MF, Aires CC, Luis PB, et al. Valproic acid metabolism and its effects on mitochondrial fatty acid oxidation: a review. J Inherit Metab Dis. 2008;31:205–16.
78. Bohan TP, Helton E, Mc Donald I, et al. Effect of L-carnitine treatment for valproate-induced hepatotoxicity. Neurology. 2001;56:1405–9.
79. Dreifuss FE, Langer DH. Side effects of valproate. Am J Med. 1988;84(Suppl 1A):34–41.
80. Bourgeois BF. Pharmacologic interactions between valproate and other drugs. Am J Med. 1988;84(Suppl 1A):29–33.
81. Bruni J, Gallo JM, Lee CS, et al. Interactions of valproic acid with phenytoin. Neurology. 1980;30:1233–6.
82. Rossi R, Arjmand S, Bærentzen SL, et al. Synaptic vesicle glycoprotein 2A: features and functions. Front Neurosci. 2022; https://doi.org/10.3389/fnins.2022.864514.

83. Contreras-García IJ, Cárdenas-Rodríguez N, Romo-Mancillas A, et al. Levetiracetam mechanisms of action: from molecules to systems. Pharmaceuticals (Basel). 2022; https://doi.org/10.3390/ph15040475.
84. Cramer JA, De Rue K, Devinsky O, et al. A systematic review of the behavioral effects of levetiracetam in adults with epilepsy, cognitive disorders, or an anxiety disorder during clinical trials. Epilepsy Behav. 2003;4:124–32.
85. Qiao MY, Cui HT, Zhao LZ, et al. Efficacy and safety of levetiracetam vs. phenobarbital for neonatal seizures: a systematic review and meta-analysis. Front Neurol. 2021; https://doi.org/10.3389/fneur.2021.747745.
86. Wright C, Downing J, Mungall D, et al. Clinical pharmacology and pharmacokinetics of levetiracetam. Front Neurol. 2013; https://doi.org/10.3389/fneur.2013.00192.
87. Steinhoff BJ, Staack AM. Levetiracetam and brivaracetam: a review of evidence from clinical trials and clinical experience. Ther Adv Neurol Disord. 2019; https://doi.org/10.1177/1756286419873518.
88. Gillard M, Fuks B, Leclercq K, et al. Binding characteristics of brivaracetam, a selective, high affinity SV2A ligand in rat, mouse and human brain: relationship to anti-convulsant properties. Eur J Pharmacol. 2011;664:36–44.
89. Zona C, Pieri M, Carunchio I, et al. Brivaracetam (ucb 34714) inhibits Na(+) current in rat cortical neurons in culture. Epilepsia. 2010;88:46–54.
90. Niespodziany I, André VM, Leclère N, et al. Brivaracetam differentially affects voltage-gated sodium currents without impairing sustained repetitive firing in neurons. CNS Neurosci Ther. 2015;21:241–51.
91. Klein P, Diaz A, Gasalla T, Whitesides J. A review of the pharmacology and clinical efficacy of brivaracetam. Clin Pharmacol. 2018;10:1–22.
92. Orlandi N, Bartolini E, Audenino D, et al. Intravenous brivaracetam in status epilepticus: a multicentric retrospective study in Italy. Seizure. 2021;86:70–6.
93. Martellino C, Laganà A, Atanasio G, et al. The real-world effectiveness of intravenous brivaracetam as a second-line treatment in status epilepticus. Epilepsy Behav. 2023;148:109464. https://doi.org/10.1016/j.yebeh.2023.109464.
94. Cawello W. Clinical pharmacokinetic and pharmacodynamic profile of lacosamide. Clin Pharmacokinet. 2015;54:901–14.
95. Rogawski MA, Tofighy A, White HS, et al. Current understanding of the mechanism of action of the antiepileptic drug lacosamide. Epilepsy Res. 2015;110:189–205.
96. Licko T, Seeger N, Zellinger C, et al. Lacosamide treatment following status epilepticus attenuates neuronal cell loss and alterations in hippocampal neurogenesis in a rate electrical status epilepticus model. Epilepsia. 2013;54:1176–85.
97. Beydoun A, D'Souza J, Hebert D, et al. Lacosamide: pharmacology, mechanisms of action and pooled efficacy and safety data in partial-onset seizures. Expert Rev Neurother. 2009;9:33–42.
98. Yadav R, Schrem E, Yadav V, et al. Lacosamide-related arrhythmias: a systematic analysis and review of the literature. Cureus. 2021;13:e20736. https://doi.org/10.7759/cureus.20736.
99. Alkhachroum A, Der-Nigoghossian CA, Mathews E, et al. Ketamine to treat super-refractory status epilepticus. Neurology. 2020;95:e2286–94.
100. Borris DJ, Bertram EH, Kapur J. Ketamine controls prolonged status epilepticus. Epilepsy Res. 2000;42:117–22.
101. Mion G, Villevieille T. Ketamine pharmacology: an update (pharmacodynamics and molecular aspects, recent findings). CNS Neurosci Ther. 2013;19:370–80.
102. Strous JFM, Weeland CJ, van der Draai FA, et al. Brain changes associated with long-term ketamine abuse, a systematic review. Front Neuroanat. 2022; https://doi.org/10.3389/fnana.2022.795231.
103. Vaitkevicius H, Ramsay RE, Swisher CB, et al. Intravenous ganaxolone for the treatment of refractory status epilepticus: results from an open-label, dose-finding, phase 2 trial. Epilepsia. 2022;63:2381–91.

104. Reddy DS. Neurosteroids as novel anticonvulsants for refractory status epilepticus and medical countermeasures for nerve agents: a 15-year journey to bring ganaxolone from bench to clinic. J Pharmacol Exp Ther. 2024;388:273–300.

105. Marinus Pharmaceuticals. Marinus Pharmaceuticals announces topline results from Phase 3 RAISE trial of IV ganaxolone in refractory status epilepticus. 2024. https://ir.marinuspharma. com/news/news-details/2024/Marinus-Pharmaceuticals-Announces-Topline-Results-from-Phase-3-RAISE-Trial-of-IV-Ganaxolone-in-Refractory-Status-Epilepticus/default.aspx. Accessed 19 Jun 2024.

106. Gauthier AC, Mattson RH. Clobazam: a safe, efficacious, and newly rediscovered therapeutic for epilepsy. CNS Neurosci Ther. 2015;21:543–8.

107. D'Anto J, Beuchat I, Rossetti AO, et al. Clonazepam loading dose in status epilepticus: is more always better? CNS Drugs. 2023;37:523–9.

108. Mula M, Cavanna AE, Monaco F. Psychopharmacology of topiramate: from epilepsy to bipolar disorder. Neuropsychiatr Dis Treat. 2006;2:475–88.

109. Bourgeois BF. Pharmacokinetics and metabolism of topiramate. Drugs Today (Barc). 1999;35:43–8.

110. Bialer M, Doose DR, Murthy B, et al. Pharmacokinetic interactions of topiramate. Clin Pharmacokinet. 2004;43:763–80.

111. Mirza N, Marson AG, Pirmohamed M. Effect of topiramate on acid-base balance: extent, mechanism and effects. Br J Clin Pharmacol. 2009;68:655–61.

112. Karim N, Sheikh AA. A rare, unreported cognitive side effect of topiramate: do we know it all yet? Cureus. 2020;12:e11342. https://doi.org/10.7759/cureus.11342.

113. Fechner A, Hubert K, Jahnke K, et al. Treatment of refractory and superrefractory status epilepticus with topiramate: a cohort study of 106 patients and a review of the literature. Epilepsia. 2019;60:2448–58.

114. Rohracher A, Höfler J, Kalss G, et al. Perampanel in patients with refractory and super-refractory status epilepticus in a neurological intensive care unit. Epilepsy Behav. 2015;49:354–8.

115. Redecker J, Wittstock M, Benecke R, et al. Efficacy of perampanel in refractory nonconvulsive status epilepticus and simple partial status epilepticus. Epilepsy Behav. 2015;45:176–9.

116. Greenwood J, Valdes J. Perampanel (Fycompa): a review of clinical efficacy and safety in epilepsy. P T. 2016;41:683–98.

117. Costa B, Vale N. Understanding lamotrigine's role in the CNS and possible future evolution. Int J Mol Sci. 2023; https://doi.org/10.3390/ijms24076050.

118. FDA Drug Safety Communication. FDA warns of serious immune system reaction with seizure and mental health medicine lamotrigine (Lamictal). 2018. https://www.fda.gov/drugs/drug-safety-and-availability/fda-drug-safety-communication-fda-warns-serious-immune-system-reaction-seizure-and-mental-health. Accessed 25 Jun 2024.

119. Henter JI, Horne A, Aricó M, et al. HLH-2004: diagnostic and therapeutic guidelines for hemophagocytic lymphohistiocytosis. Pediatr Blood Cancer. 2007;48:124–31.

120. Marini C, Parmeggiani L, Masi G, et al. Nonconvulsive status epilepticus precipitated by carbamazepine presenting as dissociative and affective disorders in adolescents. J Child Neurol. 2005;20:693–6.

121. Prasad AN, Stefanelli M, Nagarajan L. Seizure exacerbation and developmental regression with carbamazepine. Can J Neurol Sci. 1998;25:287–94.

122. Guerrini R, Belmonte A, Parmeggiani L, et al. Myoclonic status epilepticus following high-dosage lamotrigine therapy. Brain Dev. 1999;21:420–4.

123. Dinnerstein E, Jobst BC, Williamson PD. Lamotrigine intoxication provoking status epilepticus in an adult with localization-related epilepsy. Arch Neurol. 2007;64:1344–6.

124. Guerrini R, Dravet C, Genton P, et al. Lamotrigine and seizure aggravation in severe myoclonic epilepsy. Epilepsia. 1998;39:508–12.

125. Rana A, Musto AE. The role of inflammation in the development of epilepsy. J Neuroinflammation. 2018; https://doi.org/10.1186/s12974-018-1192-7.

126. Abboud H, Probasco JC, Irani S, et al., Autoimmune Encephalitis Alliance Clinicians Network. Autoimmune encephalitis: proposed best practice recommendations for diagnosis and acute management. J Neurol Neurosurg Psychiatry. 2021;92:757–68.

127. Mehta V, Ferrie CD, Cross JH, et al. Corticosteroids including ACTH for childhood epilepsy other than epileptic spasms. Cochrane Database Syst Rev. 2015;2015:CD005222. https://doi.org/10.1002/14651858.CD005222.pub3.

128. Kimizu T, Takahashi Y, Oboshi T, et al. Methylprednisolone pulse therapy in 31 patients with refractory epilepsy: a single center retrospective analysis. Epilepsy Behav. 2020;109:107116. https://doi.org/10.1016/j.yebeh.2020.107116.

129. Pantazou V, Novy J, Rossetti AO. Intravenous corticosteroids as an adjunctive treatment for refractory and super-refractory status epilepticus: an observational cohort study. CNS Drugs. 2019;33:187–92.

130. Ramos AB, Cruz RA, Villemarette-Pittman NR, et al. Dexamethasone as abortive treatment for refractory seizures or status epilepticus in the inpatient setting. J Investig Med High Impact Case Rep. 2019; https://doi.org/10.1177/2324709619848816.

131. Zeiler FA, Matuszczak M, Teitelbaum J, et al. Intravenous immunoglobulins for refractory status epilepticus, Part I: A scoping systematic review of the adult literature. Seizure. 2017;45:172–80.

132. Geng J, Dong J, Li Y, et al. Intravenous immunoglobulins for epilepsy. Cochrane Database Syst Rev. 2019;2019:CD008557. https://doi.org/10.1002/14651858.CD008557.pub4.

133. Wilder RM. The effect on ketonemia on the course of epilepsy. Mayo Clin Bull. 1921;2:307.

134. Williams TJ, Cervenka MC. The role for ketogenic diets in epilepsy and status epilepticus in adults. Clin Neurophysiol Pract. 2017;2:154–60.

135. Zhu H, Bi D, Zhang Y, et al. Ketogenic diet for human disease: the underlying mechanisms and potential for clinical implementations. Signal Transduct Target Ther. 2022; https://doi.org/10.1038/s41392-021-00831-w.

136. Ji J, Fotros D, Sohouli MH, et al. The effect of a ketogenic diet on inflammation-related markers: a systematic review and meta-analysis of randomized controlled trials. Nutr Rev. 2024;83:40. https://doi.org/10.1093/nutrit/nuad175.

137. Teixeira FJP, Shannon J, Busl KM, et al. Utilization of the ketogenic diet for adults with status epilepticus. Epilepsy Behav. 2023;144:109279. https://doi.org/10.1016/j.yebeh.2023.109279.

138. Rhodes ME, Talluri J, Harney JP, et al. Ketogenic diet decreases circulating concentrations of neuroactive steroids of female rats. Epilepsy Behav. 2005;7:231–9.

139. Kaul N, Laing J, Nicolo JP, et al. Practical considerations for ketogenic diet in adults with super-refractory status epilepticus. Neurol Clin Pract. 2021;11:438–44.

140. Kimmoun A, Novy E, Auchet T, et al. Hemodynamic consequences of severe lactic acidosis in shock states: from bench to bedside. Crit Care. 2015. https://doi.org/10.1186/s13054-015-0896-7. Erratum in: Crit Care. 2017 Feb 21;21(1):40.

141. Baumeister FA, Oberhoffer R, Liebhaber GM, et al. Fatal propofol infusion syndrome in association with ketogenic diet. Neuropediatrics. 2004;35:250–2.

142. Lundgren J, Smith ML, Blennow G, et al. Hyperthermia aggravates and hypothermia ameliorates epileptic brain damage. Exp Brain Res. 1994;99:43–55.

143. Legriel S. Hypothermia as a treatment in status epilepticus: a narrative review. Epilepsy Behav. 2019;101:106298. https://doi.org/10.1016/j.yebeh.2019.04.051.

144. You JS, Kim JY, Yenari MA. Therapeutic hypothermia for stroke: unique challenges at the bedside. Front Neurol. 2022; https://doi.org/10.3389/fneur.2022.951586.

145. Behringer W, Böttiger BW, Biasucci DG, et al. Temperature control after successful resuscitation from cardiac arrest in adults: a joint statement from the European Society for Emergency Medicine and the European Society of Anaesthesiology and Intensive Care. Eur J Anaesthesiol. 2024;41:278–81.

146. Trieu C, Rajagopalan S, Kofke WA, et al. Overview of hypothermia, its role in neuroprotection, and the application of prophylactic hypothermia in traumatic brain injury. Anesth Analg. 2023;137:953–62.

147. Corry JJ, Dhar R, Murphy T, et al. Hypothermia for refractory status epilepticus. Neurocrit Care. 2008;9:189–97.
148. van den Broek MP, Groenendaal F, Egberts AC, et al. Effects of hypothermia on pharmacokinetics and pharmacodynamics: a systematic review of preclinical and clinical studies. Clin Pharmacokinet. 2010;49:277–94.
149. Zhou J, Poloyac SM. The effect of therapeutic hypothermia on drug metabolism and response: cellular mechanisms to organ function. Expert Opin Drug Metab Toxicol. 2011;7:803–16.
150. Zeiler FA, Matuszczak M, Teitelbaum J, et al. Magnesium sulfate for non-eclamptic status epilepticus. Seizure. 2015;32:100–8.
151. Abdelmalik PA, Politzer N, Carlen PL. Magnesium as an effective adjunct therapy for drug resistant seizures. Can J Neurol Sci. 2012;39:323–7.
152. Jhang WK, Lee YJ, Kim YA, et al. Severe hypermagnesemia presenting with abnormal electrocardiographic findings similar to those of hyperkalemia in a child undergoing peritoneal dialysis. Korean J Pediatr. 2013;56:308–11.
153. Woodward MR, Doddi S, Marano C, et al. Evaluating salvage electroconvulsive therapy for the treatment of prolonged super refractory status epilepticus: a case series. Epilepsy Behav. 2023;144:109286. https://doi.org/10.1016/j.yebeh.2023.109286.
154. Ong MJY, Lee VLL, Teo SL, et al. Electroconvulsive therapy in refractory and super-refractory status epilepticus in adults: a scoping review. Neurocrit Care. 2024;41:681. https://doi.org/10.1007/s12028-024-02003-4.
155. Weimer T, Boling W, Pryputniewicz D, et al. Temporal lobectomy for refractory status epilepticus in a case of limbic encephalitis. J Neurosurg. 2008;109:742–5.
156. Bennewitz MF, Saltzman WM. Nanotechnology for delivery of drugs to the brain for epilepsy. Neurotherapeutics. 2009;6:323–36.
157. Zhou Y, Peng Z, Seven ES, et al. Crossing the blood-brain barrier with nanoparticles. J Control Release. 2018;270:290–303.
158. Naqvi S, Panghal A, Flora SJS. Nanotechnology: a promising approach for delivery of neuroprotective drugs. Front Neurosci. 2020; https://doi.org/10.3389/fnins.2020.00494.
159. Movahedpour A, Taghvaeefar R, Asadi-Pooya AA, et al. Nano-delivery systems as a promising therapeutic potential for epilepsy: current status and future perspectives. CNS Neurosci Ther. 2023;29:3150–9.
160. Pedrero SG, Staedler D, Gerber-Lemaire S. Recent developments on the use of nanomaterials for the treatment of epilepsy. Mini Rev Med Chem. 2022;22:1460–75.
161. National Center for Biotechnology Information. PubChem compound summary for CID 4192, Midazolam. 2024. https://pubchem.ncbi.nlm.nih.gov/compound/Midazolam. Accessed 15 Jul 2024.
162. National Center for Biotechnology Information. PubChem compound summary for CID 4943, Propofol. 2024. https://pubchem.ncbi.nlm.nih.gov/compound/Propofol. Accessed 15 Jul 2024.
163. National Center for Biotechnology Information. PubChem compound summary for CID 2802, Clonazepam. 2024. https://pubchem.ncbi.nlm.nih.gov/compound/Clonazepam. Accessed 15 Jul 2024.
164. National Center for Biotechnology Information. PubChem compound summary for CID 1775, Phenytoin. 2024. https://pubchem.ncbi.nlm.nih.gov/compound/Phenytoin. Accessed 15 Jul 2024.
165. National Center for Biotechnology Information. PubChem compound summary for CID 56339, Fosphenytoin. 2024. https://pubchem.ncbi.nlm.nih.gov/compound/Fosphenytoin. Accessed 15 Jul 2024.
166. National Center for Biotechnology Information. PubChem compound summary for CID 219078, Lacosamide. 2024. https://pubchem.ncbi.nlm.nih.gov/compound/Lacosamide. Accessed 15 Jul 2024.
167. National Center for Biotechnology Information. PubChem compound summary for CID 5284627, Topiramate. 2024. https://pubchem.ncbi.nlm.nih.gov/compound/Topiramate. Accessed 15 Jul 2024.

168. Haller JT. Rapid administration of undiluted intravenous levetiracetam. Epilepsia. 2021;62:1865–70.
169. National Center for Biotechnology Information. PubChem compound summary for CID 5284583, Levetiracetam. 2024. https://pubchem.ncbi.nlm.nih.gov/compound/Levetiracetam. Accessed 15 Jul 2024.
170. National Center for Biotechnology Information. PubChem compound summary for CID 9837243, Brivaracetam. 2024. https://pubchem.ncbi.nlm.nih.gov/compound/Brivaracetam. Accessed 15 Jul 2024.
171. Rolan P, Sargentini-Maier ML, Pigeolet E, Stockis A. The pharmacokinetics, CNS pharmacodynamics and adverse event profile of brivaracetam after multiple increasing oral doses in healthy men. Br J Clin Pharmacol. 2008;66:71–5.

Further Reading

National Center for Biotechnology Information. PubChem compound summary for CID 4763, Phenobarbital. 2024. https://pubchem.ncbi.nlm.nih.gov/compound/Phenobarbital. Accessed 15 Jul 2024.

Chapter 19
Delirium in the ICU: Pathophysiology, Diagnosis and Management

Neil Glassford, Robert Olver, and Yahya Shehabi

19.1 Delirium in Perspective

Whether arising from the Latin deliro-delirare (to go out of the furrow, to deviate from a straight line, to be deranged) [1], or the Greek leros (silly talk, nonsense) [2], delirium has been described in one form or another in medical literature since antiquity [3]. However, the first clear clinical definitions of this acute and fluctuant

N. Glassford (✉)
Department of Intensive Care Medicine, Victorian Heart Hospital, Monash Health, Clayton, VIC, Australia

Department of Intensive Care Medicine, Monash Medical Centre, Monash Health, Clayton, VIC, Australia

Division of Acute and Critical Care, School of Public Health and Preventive Medicine, Monash University, Monash Health, Melbourne, VIC, Australia

School of Clinical Sciences, Monash University, Clayton, VIC, Australia
e-mail: Neil.Glassford2@monashhealth.org

R. Olver
Department of Intensive Care Medicine, Victorian Heart Hospital, Monash Health, Clayton, VIC, Australia

Department of Intensive Care Medicine, Monash Medical Centre, Monash Health, Clayton, VIC, Australia

Y. Shehabi
Department of Intensive Care Medicine, Victorian Heart Hospital, Monash Health, Clayton, VIC, Australia

School of Clinical Sciences, Monash University, Clayton, VIC, Australia

Prince of Wales Clinical School of Medicine, University of New South Wales, Randwick, Sydney, NSW, Australia

© The Author(s), under exclusive license to Springer Nature Switzerland AG 2025
Y. Alzaidi, M. A. Gebily (eds.), *The Pharmacist's Expanded Role in Critical Care Medicine*, https://doi.org/10.1007/978-3-031-77335-8_19

neuropsychiatric syndrome were only provided in the 1990s (Table 19.1). This framework has evolved over the last four decades, as has our understanding of the pathophysiological basis of this syndromic expression of a final common pathway of multiple insults resulting from acute illness and comorbid conditions resulting in impaired brain function. Delirium causes profound distress to patients, their families and those providing their care [4]. Moreover, it is associated with increased intensive care unit morbidity and mortality, as well as a range of other patient-orientated adverse outcomes and healthcare costs [5]. With more than 50% of critically ill patients estimated to experience delirium during their intensive care unit (ICU) admission [6], the burden of delirium in this setting is a global public health priority, yet effective therapies to prevent and treat delirium have proven elusive [7].

19.1.1 Motoric Subtypes

For almost as long as delirium has been recognised, the different presentations of acute confusional states have been described by clinicians [8]. These are typically identified as the hyperactive, hypoactive and mixed subtypes, on the basis of their motoric symptoms (Table 19.1) [9]. These may differ not only in symptomatology, but also in epidemiology, pathophysiology and potential response to therapy. This has important implications for study design, and while these subtypes have long been recognised, relatively few studies account for these potential differences. Hypoactive delirium can be particularly difficult to identify, given the confounding interventions such as paralysis and sedation in the ICU environment and the difficulty distinguishing it from other neuropsychiatric conditions [10].

19.1.2 Subsyndromal Delirium

Subsyndromal delirium, or "attenuated delirium syndrome", is a more recently described construct that may represent a milder condition or an early stage in the development of delirium (Table 19.1). While not universally recognised or well characterised, even patients not meeting full diagnostic criteria for delirium have longer hospital stays, though the impact on mortality and the benefits of pharmacotherapy, if any, remain unproven [11].

Table 19.1 Definitions and diagnostic criteria for delirium

DSM-V diagnostic criteria

Criteria	Description
A	Disturbance in attention + reduced awareness
B	Acute and fluctuant deviation from baseline
C	An additional disturbance in cognition including language, memory, pertception, etc.
D	A and C are not due to an existing neurocognitive disorder and do not occur in the context of coma
E	Occurs due to another medical condition, substance exposure, intoxication, or withdrawal

*Must fulfill all of the criteria listed above for a diagnosis of delirium to be made

Motor subtype definitions

Hyperactive	Hyperactive psychomotor activity ± mood lability ± agitation ± refusal to cooperate with medical care
Hypoactive	Hypoactive psychomotor activity ± sluggishness ± lethargy ± stupor
Mixed	Normal psychomotor activity Disturbed attention and awareness or Rapid cycling between hypoactive and hyperactive states

Additional definitions and refinements

Subsyndromal	Condition meeting some but not all of the criteria for delirium Typically, less severe cognitive impairment Considered with an ICDSC score of 1–3/8 Considered with a CAM score of 2/4
Acute	Lasts hours–days
Persistent	Lasts weeks–months

Adapted from Refs. [11, 53, 54, 103]

DSM-V Diagnostic and Statistical Manual of Mental Disorders, 5th Edition; *ICDSC* Intensive Care Delirium Screening Checklist; *CAM* Confusion Assessment Method

19.2   Pathophysiology

The pathophysiology of delirium is complex and nebulous. Multiple theories are proposed, but a common pathophysiological pathway has yet to be defined. Delirium involves an underlying predisposition followed by a variety of different inciting events or acute stressors [12]. The multiple aetiologies of delirium suggest that there may be discreet neurophysiological pathways or multifactorial mechanisms from a given precipitant that converge to the clinical phenotype of delirium [13]. The most common predisposing factors and pathophysiological mechanisms will be discussed here.

19.2.1 Ageing, Cognitive Decline and Frailty

Delirium is a marker of underlying brain vulnerability and hence is substantially more common in elderly populations and those with pre-existing cognitive decline and frailty [14]. The risk of delirium increases progressively with age, with patients over the age of 75 up to 10× more likely to experience delirium than younger patients [15]. Rates of delirium are 3–4 times higher in those with pre-existing cognitive decline or dementia and 2–3 times higher in those with pre-existing frailty [16–18].

While delirium, frailty and cognitive decline are all unique and complex processes, they all share a generalised reduction in functional capacity and reduced resilience to tolerate acute stressors [18]. Additionally, episodes of delirium are associated with long-term reductions in independence and new diagnoses of cognitive decline [19]. These diseases share common pathophysiologic mechanisms, which may explain their association, including increases in systemic and neuronal inflammation, alterations in vascular permeability and brain perfusion and changes in brain connectivity [20].

19.2.2 Drugs and Neurotransmitters

Multiple classes of medications have been implicated in the pathogenesis and pathophysiology of delirium. The most common are opiates, benzodiazepines, antipsychotics and drugs with antihistamine or anti-cholinergic effects [21]. The evidence for these effects and the proposed pathophysiological mechanisms are based on alterations in neurotransmitter balance, particularly decreases in cholinergic transmission, hyperdopaminergic states and alterations in the levels of GABA and noradrenaline; however, the quality of evidence is inconsistent [22]. Studies that have examined CSF levels of various neurotransmitters during delirium have found inconsistent results [23].

An extensive meta-analysis of frequently implicated drugs found strong evidence that benzodiazepines increased the risk of delirium in ICU settings, but that this was not as clearly demonstrated in non-ICU settings [22]. The same meta-analysis suggested that opiates may increase delirium risk in a dose-dependent fashion; however, it is worth noting that poorly controlled pain is also a risk factor [24]. Anti-cholinergic agents were associated with a threefold increase in the risk of delirium, but the evidence supporting this was graded as low to very low quality. Regarding anti-psychotics, there was moderate- to high-quality evidence that the antipsychotics haloperidol and olanzapine did not increase the risk of delirium. Anti-psychotic drugs are frequently used to treat hyperactive delirium in clinical practice despite multiple large trials failing to demonstrate any significant preventative or treatment effect on delirium [25, 26]. The absence of demonstrable benefit calls into question hyperdopaminergic theories of delirium, at least as a stand-alone mechanism. A novel methodology big data trial from a New Zealand registry demonstrated that in addition to stand-alone agents, drug combinations may be a significant contributor to delirium, consistent with previous descriptions of polypharmacy as a risk factor [27].

While various classes of drugs have been implicated in the pathogenesis and incitement of delirium over time, gaps in the evidence suggest that more research as to their role in the pathophysiology of delirium is necessary. Beyond just the medication effect, a broader understanding of the role of specific neurotransmitters in the development of delirium would be beneficial.

19.2.3 Impaired Cerebral Energy Metabolism

The theory that cerebral metabolic insufficiency contributes to delirium dates back to the 1950s; at the time, the authors of a seminal paper proposed that a "derangement of functional metabolism underlies all instances of delirium" [28]. Their work described the progressive worsening of the electroencephalogram (EEG) in patients with delirium and the need for adequate glucose and oxygen levels to maintain mental acuity. While now understood to be just one of several mechanisms, dysfunction of cerebral metabolism remains a key component of the pathophysiology of delirium.

Dysregulated glucose metabolism is a cause of both acute and sustained brain injuries. Sustained hypoglycaemia can cause significant neurological injury, and both actual and relative hypoglycaemia have been associated with increased rates of delirium in both medical ICU and post-operative surgical populations [29–31]. Beyond the blood sugar measurement itself, deficits in the utilisation of glucose during acute illness and specifically brain insulin resistance may contribute significantly to the pathophysiology of delirium [32]. Evidence supporting this mechanism includes studies demonstrating elevated cerebrospinal fluid lactate levels and ketone bodies in patients with delirium, consistent with altered glucose metabolism and utilisation [32, 33]. More recently, FDG-PET scans which have previously demonstrated altered glucose metabolism in Alzheimer's disease have been performed in hospitalised patients with and without delirium and demonstrated cortical and subcortical hypometabolism during episodes of delirium. Thalamic hypometabolism, particularly, was a distinguishing feature of delirium, as this pattern is atypical in Alzheimer's dementia. The degree of hypometabolism correlated with the severity of delirium [34].

Hypoxia is frequently identified as a precipitating factor for delirium in humans [35], and a lower P/F (P_aO_2/F_iO_2) ratio has been associated with an increased rate of delirium in critically ill patients [36]. Direct causative research is lacking, but recent publications have focussed on non-invasive monitoring of regional cerebral oximetry using near-infrared spectroscopy (NIRS). A systematic review and separate meta-analysis of available trials suggested an association between lower levels of cerebral oxygenation and delirium; however, the studies were of insufficient size and significant variability to draw firm conclusions [37, 38]. NIRS is reflective not only of the oxygen content of blood but also of the blood flow and perfusion [39].

19.2.4 Hypoperfusion

Delivery of energy substrates as described above is dependent on the maintenance of adequate cerebral blood flow. Alterations in regional cerebral blood flow during delirium have been demonstrated by multiple imaging techniques in both medical and post-operative patients. Studies using technetium-enhanced single proton emission CT demonstrated that regional hypoperfusion occurred more frequently in patients with delirium than in those without. Demonstrated perfusion abnormalities resolved after the resolution of delirium in most cases. These studies described multiple affected cortical structures including the anterior temporal parietal regions and frontal and occipital lobes. Alternative techniques using xenon-enhanced computer tomography and transcranial Doppler have yielded similar findings [34, 40]. While a direct causative link is still not clear, and studies suffer from small patient numbers, variable imaging techniques and study designs, the demonstration of altered regional cerebral perfusion in patients provides a plausible mechanism in the pathophysiology of delirium.

19.2.5 Inflammation

Many of the precipitating factors associated with delirium are characterised by an inflammatory response, including infections, malignancy, surgery and trauma [41]. Despite the protection of the blood-brain barrier (which itself may be compromised in delirium), peripheral inflammation and circulating cytokines can alter brain function due to direct effects or alteration of neurotransmission or through activation of microglia to produce pro-inflammatory cytokines in the central nervous system (CNS) [42]. Due to the relative difficulty of accessing the CNS for the purposes of research, much of the evidence for peripheral and central inflammatory hypotheses of delirium comes from animal and post-mortem studies [43, 44]. An extensive systematic review of human trials looking for biomarkers supportive of an inflammatory mechanism of delirium did not identify any single marker which was consistently present in or predictive of delirium. Research in this area is hampered by small trials with heterogeneous methodologies and conflicting results. Although it is clearly evident that systemic inflammation can trigger delirium and that there are often high levels of circulating and CNS inflammatory markers in delirious patients, the challenge of identifying specific inflammatory pathways persists [14].

19.2.6 Failure of Neural Pathways

All of the previously described hypotheses and mechanisms may contribute to a final common pathway of delirium, that being a failure of functional connectivity in neural networks [45]. Adequate brain function relies on the interconnectivity of different regions of the brain, be they structurally or functionally linked [46]. This may account for the heterogeneity of results in previous trials and may account for the multitude of triggers and potential pathways to a persistent clinical phenotype. This final pathway would also help explain the significant correlation between pre-existing brain vulnerabilities and high rates of delirium, as alterations in brain network connectivity have been demonstrated in multiple forms of dementia [47, 48]. Techniques to study brain connectivity include functional magnetic resonance imaging (fMRI) and EEG. Small fMRI studies have demonstrated reversible changes in the functional connectivity between the pre-frontal cortex and posterior cingulated gyrus [49]. EEG studies of neural connectivity have consistently demonstrated decreased functional connections in patients with delirium. Different trials have demonstrated different patterns of reduced connectivity across multiple neural networks, but this may be reflective of different aetiological origins of delirium or differing underlying brain vulnerabilities across patients [50, 51].

Diminishing functional connectivity of various regions of the brain appears to be a key element and possibly a common final pathway in the pathophysiology of delirium. Larger studies will be crucial to further our understanding of how the theories of pre-existing brain vulnerability, systemic and intracerebral inflammation, neurotransmitter dysfunction and cerebral metabolism can be integrated into a unified understanding of the precipitation and pathophysiology of delirium.

19.3 The Epidemiology of Delirium

It cannot be denied that delirium is a major issue in hospitalised patients, with delirium occurring in up to 23% of adult medical patients in secondary care [52]. Estimates in the critically ill have suggested prevalence rates of up to 89% [6], making delirium an important and pervasive issue in the critically ill, given its association with adverse short- and long-term patient-centred outcomes.

19.3.1 Delirium in the ICU

In the literature, the incidence of delirium in the undifferentiated ICU population ranges from 19% [53] to 83% [54], with delirium occurrence ranging from 7% [16] to 89% in survivors of stupor or coma [55]. These estimates are now between 10 and 20 years old and fail to account for modern methods of delirium detection, study design or the changing populations of ICUs over this time frame. Many studies have focussed on patients over 65, but a recent systematic review suggests that more than a third of critically ill children will suffer from delirium during their ICU admission [56], so studies need to be representative of the entire ICU population.

Delirium occurrence has been demonstrated to vary significantly between diagnostic groups within the ICU. In the critically ill surgical population, estimates of delirium occurrence are relatively scarce and of low quality. Estimates of prevalence range from 24.4% to 73% [6, 57, 58]. Following cardiac surgery, the reported prevalence of delirium ranges from 11% to 73% [6]. In a recent large European retrospective cohort analysis, delirium occurred in 21.4% of post-operative cardiac surgical patients over the age of 65 and 33.5% of those over the age of 80 [59]. In neurocritically ill patients, the pooled prevalence rate of delirium ranges from 12% to 43% in a systematic review of relevant prospective cohort studies [60]. In neurosurgical populations, the pooled estimates of delirium incidence are 19% (95% CI: 12–26%) [61], with a prevalence of up to 42% in those patients requiring ICU admission [62]. The lone study of critically ill patients in a trauma ICU suggests an incidence of 67% [58].

Fewer studies have explored the occurrence of delirium by subtype. In a systematic review of the 18 clinically and statistically heterogeneous ICU studies reporting on the incidence of delirium by motoric subtype, the pooled incidence of hyperactive delirium was lowest at 4% (95% CI, 2–6%), then mixed delirium at 7% (95% CI, 4–11%), with hypoactive delirium having the highest pooled incidence at 11% (95% CI, 8–17%). The data in the 31 studies examining the prevalence of delirium in critically ill populations was similarly heterogeneous. The pooled prevalence of hyperactive delirium was 4% (95% CI, 3–6%), mixed delirium at 9% (95% CI, 6–13%) and highest for the hypoactive subtype at 17% (95% CI, 13–22%). However, a recent scoping review suggests that this may be a gross underestimate, reporting a prevalence of 22.7% (95% CI, 19.0–26.5) for hyperactive delirium and 50.3% (95% CI, 46.0–54.7) for hypoactive delirium [63]. All forms were particularly prevalent in those studies with a high proportion of ventilated patients with high illness severity scores [10].

19.3.2 Complexities of Delirium Estimation

Several issues limit the accurate epidemiological assessment of delirium in the critical care setting. These include the use of sedation interfering with assessment and the fact that the tools used to screen and diagnose delirium rely on symptomatology, not biomarkers or other objective markers of a pathophysiological condition, which can make case ascertainment challenging. The fluctuant nature of delirium means point prevalence estimates can be inaccurate, and the different features of the different motoric subtypes can further compromise positive identification of cases. Moreover, the heterogeneous population of ICUs, the differing populations of different types of ICUs and those in different jurisdictions can make defining a study population and choosing a sample size challenging to ensure external validity [64]. The true incidence and prevalence of delirium can be hard to identify, and the occurrence rate may be a more accurate measure of the burden of the condition [65]. Given the complexities of reliably identifying delirium, true estimates of delirium in the form of large, prospective, methodologically sound cohort studies are lacking.

19.4 Associations and Risk Factors

The clinical syndrome of delirium has been associated with multiple risk factors for more than two millennia, with fever, poisoning and trauma among the earliest described [3]. Risk factors have classically been divided into those characteristics of the patients which predispose them to the development of delirium and those features of their current illness, admission or intervention which risk precipitating delirium and are generally well described in the literature (Table 19.2).

19.4.1 The Undifferentiated Cohorts

Literally, hundreds of factors are associated with the development of delirium, with the most recent systematic review of hospitalised patients recognising 33 predisposing and 112 precipitating factors across more than 100,000 patients from over 300 studies of delirium in this population [35]. The clearest predisposing factors appear to be advanced age, cognitive impairment and functional impairment in the form of frailty or sensory impairment. The best summary of the evidence to date in the undifferentiated critically ill population is now almost a decade old. While this systematic review of 33 methodologically diverse studies is robust, it fails to capture the population of several modern studies now considered central to the management of delirium in the critically ill and the evolving population and demography of ICUs internationally. Increasing age, cognitive impairment and pre-existing hypertension are the predisposing features with the strongest association with delirium, while illness severity, metabolic acidosis, trauma, renal failure, coma, emergent surgery and mechanical ventilation had the strongest evidence as precipitating factors. Notably, while frequently described as being a strong deliriogenic, benzodiazepine use was inconclusively associated with delirium development [66].

19.4.2 Delirium Subtypes

While the existence of the motoric subtypes of delirium and the difference in their incidence and prevalence have been established, it is less clear if phenotype-specific risk factors exist. The identification of such potentially modifiable associations also offers

Table 19.2 Precipitating, predisposing, modifiable, and fixed risk factors for delirium

Risk factors for delirium			
Predisposing[a]		Precipitating[b]	
Fixed	Age Cognitive impairment/dementia Frailty/functional impairment Cumulative comorbidities Cardiovascular disease including AF and hypertension CNS disorder including stroke, PD, delirium Male sex Lower educational attainment Diabetes Psychiatric disorder including anxiety	Metabolic	Hypoalbuminaemia Dysnatraemias Dysglycaemias Electrolyte disturbance Metabolic acidosis Metabolic disorder
		Surgical	Type (emergent, open, invasive) Intraoperative bleeding/transfusion Intraoperative hypotension Operative duration Post-operative complication Surgical delay
Modifiable	Alcohol use Smoking Malnutrition Anaemia Multiple medications Psychoactive medications	Organ dysfunction	Neurological injury Anaemia High Illness Severity Score Infection Mechanical ventilation Acute kidney injury Pain Hypoxia Hypo/hyperthermia Stroke Elevated WCC Abnormal liver function
		Medications	Opioids Benzodiazepines Sedatives Analgesics Anticholinergics Multiple medications
		Trauma	
		Environment	Urinary catheter Physical restraints Increased length of stay ICU admission Sleep disturbance

Adapted from Ormseth CH, et al. Predisposing and Precipitating Factors Associated With Delirium: A Systematic Review. JAMA Netw Open. 2023;6(1):e2249950 [35]

AF atrial fibrillation; *CNS* central nervous system; *PD* Parkinson's disease; *WCC* white cell count

[a] Predisposing risk factors identified in aggregates of >1000 patient or >5 studies

[b] Precipitating risk factors identified in aggregates of >1000 patient or >5 studies

subtype-specific predictive and therapeutic options [9, 63]. Sex, age and illness severity (measured by Acute Physiology and Chronic Health Evaluation Score II) were the most commonly featured risk factors in the 20 studies, though these were of varying quality and demonstrated varying results. No association between sex and delirium subtype was demonstrated. The data regarding age was heterogeneous, but there is a suggestion that the hypoactive form of delirium may be more common in those over 65 years of age. Illness severity is associated with increasing delirium occurrence, but the evidence was inconsistent in relating it to a particular subtype. No strong or persistent signals for other risk factors were identified [67]. Future studies must consider motoric subtypes to allow the identification of subtype-specific risk factors, should they exist, to enhance our understanding of the epidemiology of delirium.

19.4.3   Specific Populations

Different patient groups will experience different constellations of risk factors, and these will be of differing significance as they negotiate their journey through the critical care service. For example, in the cardiac surgical population undergoing bypass graft surgery, predisposing factors appear to be pre-existing cognitive impairment, depression, previous stroke or higher European System for Cardiac Operative Risk Evaluation score, with probable precipitants including duration of intubation, length of ICU stay and presence of post-operative arrhythmia [68].

In a recent individual participant data meta-analysis of over 8000 patients undergoing non-cardiac surgery, post-operative delirium was associated with being male, being older (>65 years and >85 years of age), being underweight (BMI <18.5), being a smoker, having a history of prior delirium, institutionalisation, an increasing burden of comorbidities, increasing ASA status, increasing duration of anaesthesia or undergoing emergency surgery, as were polypharmacy (being on five or more medications) and elevation of C-reactive protein. Educational attainment appeared to be protective. However, only a limited number of studies identified by the search criteria provided data for the analysis, and the data set did not include any Middle Eastern or African cohorts, limiting external validity. In addition, a high rate of between-study missingness was demonstrated, which prevented the authors from commenting on the relationship between delirium and the use of analgosedative medications, choice of anaesthesia and reported pain [69]. Similar findings were reported in a systematic review of studies exploring delirium following major abdominal surgery. Increasing age, ASA status, duration of anaesthesia, hypoalbuminaemia, lower insulin-like growth factor-1 levels, and pre-existing cognitive impairment, or functional impairment as described by a preoperative Katz-ADL score <6 were associated with the development of delirium in the ten trials meeting inclusion criteria [70].

19.5   Delirium and Outcomes

The adverse patient-centred outcomes associated with the development of delirium in the critically ill are well established. While now approaching 10 years old, and lacking information from some landmark trials in the management of sedation and delirium in the ICU, robust systematic review data from 44 studies and more than 16,500 patients clearly identified the independent association between delirium and ICU or hospital mortality, after adjustment for sex, age and illness severity (adjusted risk 2.72, 95% CI: 1.75–3.69). Both ICU length of stay (standardised mean difference 1.38, 95% CI: 0.99–1.77 days) and hospital length of stay (standardised mean difference 0.97, 95% CI: 0.61–1.33 days) were significantly longer in patients with delirium. This may be explained, in part, by the significantly increased duration of mechanical ventilation experienced by such patients (standardised mean difference 1.79, 95% CI: 0.31–3.27 days) [71]. Similar findings were demonstrated more recently in the post-operative cardiac surgical population [72]. Delirious patients are more likely to be restrained or undergo tracheostomy [73]. Other neuropsychiatric conditions such as depression and post-traumatic stress disorder are also prevalent in post-ICU survivors, but the association with delirium is unclear [74, 75].

The adverse effects of delirium in the ICU are not limited to the proximate admission. A strong relationship between delirium and subsequent cognitive decline has been demonstrated in several studies of older adults [76–78], which can be persistent and lead to a diagnosis of dementia in this population [79]. The hugely influential BRAIN-ICU study demonstrated that, in a truly unwell population, independent of analgosedation strategy, age, baseline cognition or other potential confounding features, a longer duration of ICU delirium was associated with worse executive function and global cognition scores at 3 and 12 months [80]. In the surgical ICU population, delirium is an independent risk factor for physical dependence and a reduction in quality of life across multiple domains at 6 months post-discharge [81], with similar findings in survivors of mechanical ventilation [82]. The lasting impact on mortality has been more difficult to quantify, with some studies failing to show a persisting relationship [83] and others suggesting that the hospitalisation delirium burden of mechanically ventilated patients is an independent predictor of mortality and poor Glasgow Outcome Scores up to 2.5 years post-discharge [84].

In the studies exploring outcomes by delirium subtype, all of the motoric forms are associated with an increased risk of death, though several included in a recent systematic review suggest that the hypoactive subtype has the strongest association with mortality. Hyperactive and mixed forms are more likely to be associated with increased duration of mechanical ventilation and hospital and ICU length of stay [10]. There is a suggestion, from a post hoc analysis of a cohort comprised of patients from the BRAIN-ICU and MIND-ICU studies, that hypoactive delirium is associated with impaired global cognitive function and executive functioning at 3- and 12-month post-discharge from ICU, a phenomenon not observed with the hyperactive subtype in this study [85]. Future studies should address the core outcome set identified by international clinician and consumer group stakeholders in a Delhi process, later endorsed by several international societies and comprising delirium occurrence, severity and duration; health-related quality of life; emotional distress; cognition; and mortality [86]. It would seem that collecting by delirium subtype would be a useful addition to this process.

19.6   Predicting Delirium

Given the range of potential risk factors for developing delirium in different populations, the associated adverse outcomes and the ensuing costs to both the patient and the health service [87], the ability to reliably predict and potentially prevent delirium would lead to both benefits for patients and health services [88]. Developed in a single Dutch centre, the PRE-DELIRIC (Prediction of Delirium in ICU patients) delirium prediction model uses demographic (age), admission (admission group, emergent admission), clinical (presence of coma, infection), biochemical (urea concentration, metabolic acidosis) and treatment (use of sedatives or morphine) variables to predict the incidence of delirium 24 h after ICU admission. With an area under the receiver operator curve = 0.85 (0.84–0.87) on initial validation, PRE-DELIRIC appeared to be a reasonable method by which to predict the development of delirium and performed better than either doctors or nurses [89]. Issues with timing are a consistent feature of the delirium literature, and the PRE-DELIRIC model fails to capture those patients developing early delirium. Moreover, it demonstrated variable discrimination across a range of study populations at variable risk of bias [90–94], though it has been shown to be superior to other models in several studies [90, 91, 95]. The early prediction model for delirium (E-PRE-DELIRIC) was developed as a point-of-admission predictive tool using nine variables, including biochemical, demographics, admission and physiological indices [96]. With limited discriminative ability being shown on subsequent attempts to validate the model in other cohorts, it would seem to have a limited role in clinical decision-making in the critically ill [90, 91, 97, 98].

19.6.1   Recent Developments

Numerous other predictive models exist, with more than 23 models having been identified over the period 2015–2019, though none are in widespread use [99]. Attempting to predict the development of delirium is complex, given the sudden onset and fluctuant nature of the condition, the challenges in diagnosis and the myriad of associations encompassing patient, treatment and time course [88]. It perhaps remains most useful to be cognisant of the risk factors pertaining to your patient population and being aware of those predictors most commonly included in recent predictive modelling studies. Across all candidate studies over the same time period, the predictors most often included, in order of frequency, were age, need for mechanical ventilation, renal dysfunction, emergency admission/surgery, use of sedatives/antipsychotics/benzodiazepines and illness severity [99]. Clinically useful prediction models need to be dynamic and identify patients where intervention can lead to the prevention or amelioration of the subsequent pathological state [100]. Machine learning techniques offer techniques for dealing with these issues but have particular problems of their own in dealing with bias and adapting to new patient cohorts which have begun to be dealt with [101]. There is evidence that machine learning models for the prediction of delirium are evolving and have entered clinical workflow [102].

19.7 Diagnosis and Screening

The gold standard for the diagnosis of delirium is patient assessment by an expert clinician (often a geriatrician or neuropsychiatrist) assessing for the presence of diagnostic features as defined by the Diagnosis and Statistical Manual of Mental Illness [103]. The current fifth version defines delirium across five domains. The essential feature of delirium is an acute impairment of consciousness characterised by a disturbance in attention, accompanied by a reduced awareness of one's environment. The disturbance in consciousness must develop over a short period of time and represent a change from baseline. It tends to be fluctuant across the day. Beyond attention, there must be disturbance in other cognitive functions (e.g. memory or orientation), and these disturbances must not be better explained by a pre-existing or evolving neurocognitive disorder. Finally, these criteria must be met in the context of a medical illness, substance intoxication or withdrawal, exposure to a toxin or, frequently, a combination of these aetiologies.

19.7.1 Screening Assessments in the ICU

Given that the frequency of delirium in ICU routine and complex assessment of all patients by a geriatrician or neuropsychiatrist is unrealistic, most diagnosis occurs by means of screening assessments designed to be performed by nursing staff. Screening for the presence of delirium in critically ill patients is vital and recommended by multiple professional bodies, including the Australian Commission of Safety and Quality in Health Care, the National Institute for Health Care Excellence, the Scottish Intercollegiate Guideline Network and the Society of Critical Care Medicine [75, 104–106]. Despite guidelines from these professional bodies, adherence to screening is highly variable. Publications from multiple countries over the past two decades have described rates of screening with a validated tool as between 7% and 33% [107–109]. A more recent multinational survey of intensive care units reported higher rates of screening, with 70% of respondents describing regular screening of patients for delirium; however, only 42% reported the use of a validated delirium screening tool [110]. While these figures may suggest progressive improvements in delirium screening compliance, a number of potential barriers to implementation have been described. These include lack of knowledge, difficulty using screening tools, organisational cultures or individual clinician attitudes which are not conducive to delirium prevention, and competing clinical priorities [111–113].

There are many different delirium screening tools validated for use in ICU patients. These include the Confusion Assessment Method for the intensive care unit (CAM-ICU) [54], the Intensive Care Delirium Screening Checklist (ICDSC) [53], the Cognitive Test for Delirium (CTD) [114], the Nursing Delirium Scale (NuDESC) [115], the Delirium Detection Score [116] and the Neelon and Champagne Confusion Scale (NEECHAM) [117]. Despite all these screening tests being validated in ICU patients, by far the most used are the CAM-ICU and ICDSC, which warrant further description.

19.7.1.1 Confusion Assessment Method for the Intensive Care Unit (CAM-ICU)

CAM-ICU is the most frequently used screening tool in ICUs globally [118]. It has been validated in at least ten different languages and was specifically designed to allow use in lightly sedated and intubated patients [118, 119]. CAM-ICU was first validated in 2001 in an American medical ICU with intubated and non-intubated patients [54]. Many studies subsequently have validated the tool's ability to detect delirium in a variety of different critical care populations, and a recent meta-analysis demonstrated a pooled sensitivity of 0.85 and a pooled specificity of 0.95 [120]. It demonstrates reasonable inter-rater reliability between physicians and nurses at 86% and can be completed in less than 2 min [118].

The original Confusion Assessment Method (CAM) was first described in 1990, and the CAM-ICU is a modification which enhances its use in an ICU setting [121]. It assesses patients across four domains, as defined in the fourth edition of the DSM [122]. The domains are acute changes in mental status, inattention, disorganised thinking and altered level of consciousness. The test results in a binary outcome, with delirium being either present or absent. The assessment of a change in mental status is aided by the use of the Richmond Agitation and Sedation Scale [123]. Attention is assessed using the Attention Screening Examination, which uses both visual and auditory assessments of concentration [114]. These tests were validated prior to their inclusion in CAM-ICU.

19.7.1.2 Intensive Care Delirium Screen Checklist (ICDSC)

The ICDSC was originally designed and validated in 2001 in a French ICU with the aim of creating a delirium screening tool that did not require the patient to engage with the assessment [53]. It was designed to address what the authors identified as difficulty using language-based questions with intubated patients or any tasks which required good vision or intact motor skills. It was initially reported to have a sensitivity of 99% and a specificity of 64%. A recent meta-analysis described a somewhat lower, pooled sensitivity of 83% and specificity of 87% [120]. While much less frequently used than CAM-ICU, ICDSC was found in one study to be favoured among nurses, which was postulated to be due to its reliance on nuance and qualitative assessment over time [124].

It relies on serial observations of eight defined criteria derived from the DSM over the duration of a shift. The criteria include the level of consciousness—comatose or deeply sedated patients are eliminated from further screening, inattention, disorientation, presence of hallucinations, delusions or psychosis, psychomotor agitation or retardation, inappropriate speech or mood, sleep–wake cycle disturbance and fluctuance of symptoms. It results in a score out of eight, but still presents a binary diagnosis with a score greater than four representing the presence of delirium; higher scores are not indicative of greater delirium severity.

19.7.2   Clinical Investigations

Assessment of patients with delirium includes thorough examination and investigation for underlying precipitants. Diagnostic tests are primarily focussed on this, rather than contributing to the diagnosis of delirium. An evidence-based guide as to what tests should be included in an assessment of delirium is lacking, as most studies assume a fundamental baseline level of care and investigation will be performed for patients in acute settings [106]. Some delirium presentations are caused by disorders of the central nervous system, and these may warrant extensive investigation, including neuroimaging; however, in the absence of clinical suspicion, the yield from such investigations may be low [125].

While currently only relevant in the research setting, there is significant interest in diagnostic tests for delirium, including neuroimaging and specific biomarkers, warranting a brief mention here.

19.7.3   Neuroimaging

Various neuroimaging techniques have been vital in progressing our understanding of the pathophysiological mechanisms of delirium. These include functional magnetic resonance imaging, positron emission tomography and single photon emission computed tomography [126]. Cerebral perfusion scans using various techniques have demonstrated decreased cortical blood flow and perfusion in patients with delirium [40, 127], while functional MRI shows decreased functional connectivity between various subcortical brain regions in delirious patients [49]. Despite their role in research and contribution to our understanding of delirium, these techniques can be challenging to perform on delirious patients and are not currently used in clinical practice.

19.7.4 Biomarkers

To date, no biomarker has been determined as specific to delirium. A recent systematic review of biomarkers in delirium identified the most frequently studied including interleukin-6, C-reactive protein, cortisol, S-100B, insulin-like growth factor-1 and tumour necrosis factor alpha. Despite a wealth of studies, there is insufficient evidence to support the use of any single biomarker in the assessment of delirium [128]; they remain vital in the investigation of the pathophysiology of delirium and an area for further research into future clinical applications.

19.8 Delirium Management

19.8.1 Delirium Prevention

The prevention of delirium is an attractive proposition. By reducing delirium incidence, outcomes such as mortality, ICU and hospital length of stay, and duration of mechanical ventilation may improve. In addition, the long-term functional impact of delirium on ICU survivors can be attenuated, with a net benefit to patients and an economic benefit to health services. Given the nature of delirium as a neuropsychiatric clinical expression of a final common pathway of a variety of pathophysiological insults, it is no surprise that no single pharmacological or non-pharmacological agent has demonstrated a universal ability to reduce the incidence of delirium. Most clinical research has focussed on the limitation of exposure to known risk factors and proposed deliriogenic agents in an attempt to reduce the incidence of delirium. It has also historically been very difficult to compare the disparate interventions that have been used in an attempt to prevent the development of acute confusion.

19.8.1.1 Non-pharmacological Interventions

The mainstay of current international guidelines for the prevention of delirium in hospitalised patients is multicomponent, non-pharmacological bundles of interventions targeting multiple risk factors simultaneously [129, 130]. In non-critically ill patients, current evidence suggests that such approaches should incorporate attempts to keep patients orientated, stimulate memory and maintain sleep where possible [131]. In ICU populations, different approaches are required.

ICU Liberation Bundles

The ICU Liberation, or ABCDEF, Bundle of interventions (see Table 19.3) [132, 133] has been widely, though variably, implemented in an attempt to reduce the incidence of delirium in critically ill patients [110]. These evolved from the original

Table 19.3 The ABCDEF/ICU Liberation Bundle

Deliriogenic factors being addressed	Example interventions and approaches
A: Assess, prevent, and manage pain	
Untreated pain Over-sedation Medication side effects	Regular pain assessment with validated tool such as the BPS or CPOT Non-opioid analgesia Regional techniques Analgesia not sedation
B: Both spontaneous awakening and breathing trials	
Over-sedation Sedation accumulation Duration of mechanical ventilation Duration of restraint	Adapted from the ABC study Embed into routine practice MDT empowerment Protocolised sedation weans/holds
C: Choice of analgesia and sedation	
Over-sedation Medication side effects Medication interactions	Regular assessments with a validated tool such as RASS or SAS Avoid deliriogenic agents Target light sedation where possible Dexmedetomidine where delirium risk is high
D: Delirium: assess, prevent, manage	
Sleep-wake cycle Orientation and reorientation Sensory impairment	Regular assessments with a validated tool such as ICDSC or CAM-ICU Regular orientation Appropriate light and sound exposure Sensory aid provision Communication aid provision Sleep hygiene Dexmedetomidine if pharmacotherapy is required
E: Early mobility and exercise	
Immobility Day-night reinforcement	MDT assessment and intervention Progressive safe mobilisation Integrate with other aspects of the bundle such as awakening trials for optimal effect Target at functional goals
F: Family engagement and empowerment	
Reorientation	Cognitive stimulation for patient Ongoing reorientation Provision of emotional support and safety Increased understanding for family Free visiting for delirious patients

Adapted from www.icudelirium.org, accessed 30th January 2024; Girard et al. Lancet. 2008 Jan 12;371(9607):126–34; the Clinical Practice Guidelines for the Prevention and Management of Pain, Agitation/Sedation, Delirium, Immobility, and Sleep Disruption in Adult Patients in the ICU (PADIS) 2018 guidelines [75]; and the Rapid Practice Guideline from ICU [202]

BPS Behavioural Pain Scale; *CPOT* Cirtical Care Pain Observation Tool; *RASS* Richmond Agitation-Sedation Scale; *SAS* Riker Sedation Agitation Scale; *ICDSC* Intensive Care Delirium Screening Checklist; *CAM* Confusion Assessment Method for the ICU

Society of Critical Care Medicine's Clinical Practice Guidelines for the Management of Pain, Agitation and Delirium in Adult Patients in the Intensive Care Unit [134], the precursor to the current recommendations [75]. The Bundle and implementation resources can be found online at the Critical Illness, Brain Dysfunction and Survivorship Center (www.icudelirium.org).

In the critically ill, early evidence suggested that multicomponent programmes reduced ICU length of stay and mortality if employing six or more implementation strategies when they were based on these guidelines or similar bundles of care [135]. Patient-centred outcomes improve with improving compliance to these programmes [136]. However, recent attempts at evidence synthesis and review have demonstrated that the randomised controlled trials exploring preventative measures in ICU patients are heterogeneous in the study population, outcomes and intervention delivered [137]. No individual or multicomponent non-pharmacological approaches have been demonstrated to reduce the incidence of delirium with any confidence in the critically ill.

Light Therapy

Given the disturbance in circadian rhythm that accompanies delirium, the use of bright light therapy has been trialled as an intervention in delirium. Four heterogeneous trials, when their results were pooled, failed to show any difference in delirium duration or other patient-centred outcomes [137]. Guidelines recommend against using bright light therapies to prevent or reduce delirium [75]. However, the typical ICU patient has a reduced exposure to light in a non-circadian pattern [138]. It may be that maintenance of a more natural light exposure pattern over the period of ICU admission may influence the development of delirium. While several studies have explored this with disparate results, they have been underpowered or could only be considered hypothesis generating [139–143]. Further understanding of the delivery of light exposure as an intervention is required, as is an understanding of those patients likely to benefit, given the suggestion of heterogeneity of effect.

Sleep Interventions

Overlapping with light therapy and some forms of pharmacological intervention, sleep interventions are often considered as a subset of multicomponent treatment programmes. While an attractive target is a potentially modifiable risk factor for delirium development, the relationship between sleep and delirium is complicated. However, fractured sleep may be worth targeting for intervention independently due to its independent association with poor outcomes [75].

Consideration of sleep interventions often slices the literature in a different fashion than, say, determining the effectiveness of melatonin/melatonin receptor agonists (MRAs) in preventing delirium [144]. When only RCTs aimed at promoting sleep were considered, three pooled trials of pre-emptive dexmedetomidine use found it to be effective at reducing ICU delirium and length of stay. This drove the overall signal for benefit in the meta-analysis; when other sleep interventions, including light therapy, noise suppression, melatonin/MRAs and multicomponent interventions, were considered alone, no such benefit was observed [145]. It is challenging synthesising such a heterogeneous body of work in a meaningful fashion. Moreover, the ICU environment is complex and seems inherently designed to confound attempts to promote sleep, with disruptive interactions, noise, fluctuant light levels opposing normal circadian variation and medication administration associated with disrupted sleep architecture [146]. A recent scoping review reinformed these themes and identified the challenges of reporting and assessing the impact of differing bundles of care with variable compliance of different elements in this group of studies [147].

The Challenges of Complex Interventions

The reasons for this may be manifold. As the implementation literature demonstrates, such approaches are inconsistently applied, are often confounded by illness severity and are institution and resource dependent. By delivering multiple complex interventions simultaneously, it becomes challenging to identify which components are individually effective, which are synergistic and which may be harmful. High-level evidence is scarce, with most recommendations being made on observational data. This parallels the widespread adoption of the bundled interventions for sepsis and septic shock, and for ventilator-associated pneumonia, with many of the same concerns [148, 149]. There is emerging evidence that innovative use of technology may have a role to play in delirium prevention, with communication supports, music, recorded messages, dynamic light interventions and video game technologies being introduced to these bundles, though high-quality, high-level evidence remains lacking [150]. Given the heterogeneous nature of the critically ill population, the different risk factors these different groups experience and the constraints that exist at an institutional level, a uniformly effective, evidence-based, affordable and easy-to-implement approach may remain out of reach for some time.

19.8.1.2 Pharmacological Prevention

A network meta-analysis of pharmacotherapy for delirium treatment and prevention in any setting demonstrated the range of attempted interventions, including alpha-adrenergic agonists, melatonin and melatonin receptor antagonists (MRAs), antipsychotics (typical and atypical), benzodiazepines, acetylcholinesterase inhibitors, 5-HT3 antagonists, propofol and gabapentin. The atypical antipsychotics olanzapine and risperidone, dexmedetomidine and MRAs were all associated with a reduction in the occurrence of delirium, with the MRA ranked as the most effective. When only intravenous interventions were considered, dexmedetomidine reduced the incidence of delirium. It also had the least impact on all-cause mortality in this population, though both the atypical antipsychotics and the MRAs had a similar impact on mortality as placebo [151]. These groups of agents, and the specific populations they may benefit, are worth further consideration. The important features of each that must be considered when used in the critically ill are summarised in Table 19.4.

Table 19.4 Drugs for delirium management

	Route	Typical dosing[a]	Onset[b]	Half-life[c]	Practice points
α2-Agonists					
Dexmedetomedine	IV infusion	0.2–1.2 µg/kg/h	15–20 min	2 h	10–15% drop in heart rate and blood pressure at low doses May cause hypertension at higher doses Accumulates with hepatic impairment
Clonidine	IV bolus IV infusion	50–150 µg q6h 10–30 µg/h	10–15 min	6–7 h	Less neurospecific No evidence base Bradycardia, hypotension, rebound hypertension Accumulates with renal impairment
Antipsychotics					
Haloperidol	IV bolus PO	0.5–5 mg max 15 mg/24 h 1–5 mg q12h to q8h	3–20 min 2–6 h	20 h	Use lower doses in elderly patients Contraindicated in Parkinson's disease Risk of neuroleptic malignant syndrome Risk of QTc prolongation
Olanzapine	IM, SL	2.5–10 mg q12h to q8h	6 h	30 h	Contraindicated in Parkinson's disease Risk of neuroleptic malignant syndrome Risk of QTc prolongation
Quetiapine	PO	12.5–50 mg q12h	90 min	6 h	Use lower doses in elderly patients Higher doses with drug dependence Risk of neuroleptic malignant syndrome Risk of QTc prolongation

(continued)

Table 19.4 (continued)

	Route	Typical dosing[a]	Onset[b]	Half-life[c]	Practice points
Melatonin and melatonin receptor agonists					
Melatonin	PO	2–6 mg nocte	40–60 min	35–50 min	Wide variability in absorption and bioavailability Hepatic metabolism, uncertain elimination
Ramelteon	PO	4–16 mg nocte	5–20 min	1–2.5 h	No available toxicity data Hepatic metabolism, renal elimination Reduce dose in hepatic disease No evidence of respiratory depression

Dosing is given in around-the-clock format of qXh, where qXh refers to "quaque X hora," or "give every X hours"

IV intravenous; *PO* oral; *IM* intramuscular; *SL* sublingual

[a] Information from Australian Medicines Handbook, https://amhonline.amh.net.au.acs.hcn.com.au/, accessed 31st Jan 2024 and DRUGBANK Online, https://go.drugbank.com/, accessed 31st Jan 2024

[b] Time to onset of IV infusions will depend on a variety of patient, illness, and administration factors

[c] Half-life of bolus administration may represent distribution time; elimination half-life in critically ill patients will be subject to a variety of factors

Haloperidol and Atypical Antipsychotics

The Dutch REDUCE [152] and the EuRIDICE RCTs [153] demonstrated no difference in delirium occurrence between patients randomised to haloperidol or to placebo and actually had an arm [152], or the entire study [153], prematurely stopped for futility. Recent meta-analyses, including the recent AID-ICU data [26] from a methodologically sound Scandinavian multi-centre RCT of 1000 critically ill patients, suggest that, in the aggregate, haloperidol may be no more effective than placebo at reducing the occurrence of delirium [154, 155]. However, in no analyses is an excess of harm suggested, making it a potential choice for treatment of agitation, if not prophylactic for delirium.

While some evidence exists for the use of olanzapine as a prophylactic measure in elderly patients undergoing joint replacement surgery [156], in general, studies of atypical antipsychotic medications as delirium prophylaxis in the critically ill are underpowered and heterogeneous. Agents such as aripiprazole, risperidone and quetiapine have been used [157–159]; however, limited evidence exists to guide their use in this space.

Dexmedetomidine

The alpha-2 adrenergic agonist dexmedetomidine is the D-enantiomer of medetomidine [160] and has anti-nociceptive [161], sedative [162] and anxiolytic actions [163]. It is thought to decrease the need for opioid analgesia and gabaminergic agents, allowing arousal and sleep quality to be maintained while avoiding respiratory depression [164, 165].

In the 38 randomised/quasi-randomised trials of pharmacological interventions in critically ill populations in 2021, dexmedetomidine use probably reduced the occurrence of delirium compared to placebo with at least moderate certainty, with an odds ratio of 0.43 (95% credible interval 0.21–0.85). In smaller groups of studies and cohorts of patients, dexmedetomidine was shown to probably reduce both the ICU and hospital lengths of stay, presumably through delirium reduction [157]. Importantly, in network meta-analysis, no harm was demonstrated in these patients with the use of dexmedetomidine [166].

A network meta-analysis of over 25,000 post-operative patients comparing the efficacy of 18 different agents across 21 studies confirmed that dexmedetomidine, haloperidol and the atypical antipsychotics were also effective in reducing the incidence of delirium in this population, compared to placebo, clonidine and benzodiazepines. Dexmedetomidine had the highest probability to reduce delirium across this entire population, and more specifically in the non-cardiac surgery cohort. In the cardiac surgical subgroup, atypical antipsychotics may be more effective. The significant demonstrated heterogeneity between studies in delirium screening method, timing and patient demographics was explored but not explained using meta-regression [167]. The data in the cardiac surgical population is challenging to parse, with recent pooled estimates of trials at low risk of bias only suggesting a trend towards benefit for dexmedetomidine use—though optimal information size had not been reached on trial sequential analysis [168]. In critically ill adult patients admitted to the ICU following trauma and requiring sedation, the six RCTs comparing different pharmacological interventions are grossly underpowered, demonstrating no particular advantage for any specific agent in this subgroup.

Melatonin/Melatonin-Receptor Antagonists

Melatonin and melatonin receptor antagonists (MRAs) have been mooted as antideliriogenics by potentially preventing the sleep cycle disturbance that is a hallmark of delirium [16]. Given the currently understood pathogenic pathways resulting in delirium, the anti-inflammatory and antioxidant properties of MRAs are also of interest [169, 170]. Moreover, they lack the side-effect profile of the other agents used to prevent delirium. Early evidence in the generalised hospital population was mixed and of low quality [171]. There is a suggestion in the literature that ramelteon, an MRA, may be more effective than melatonin at reducing the incidence of delirium occurrence in this group of patients, but studies remain underpowered, in specific populations, and markedly heterogeneous, and a definitive trial has yet to be performed [172, 173].

The single largest RCT in a critically ill population encompassed more than 800 patients across 12 mixed Australian medical-surgical ICUs and demonstrated no difference in the incidence of delirium, or a variety of delirium-related and patient-centred outcomes, whether patients were randomised to 4 mg of melatonin or placebo within 48 h of admission at 2100 h for 14 consecutive nights or until ICU discharge [174]. The intervention and primary outcome assessment were limited to the ICU, making the data from the trial very specific to ICU practice, and the study was well conducted. Unfortunately, due to the nature of ICU practice, more than 15% of delirium assessments were missing, and this may have limited the ability to detect a treatment effect, despite an increase in the sample size over the original calculations [175]. Drug absorption was confirmed, but no evidence exists to guide optimal dosing or timing of melatonin in this population, and other dosing strategies may be more effective [176, 177]. Systematic review suggests that these drugs are unlikely to be helpful in the critically ill [144, 178], particularly if only trials at low risk of bias are considered. However, it is unlikely that sufficiently large studies have been performed to provide a definitive answer [178].

Given the heterogeneous nature of the ICU patient population, it seems exploration in specific populations would be worthwhile to identify the potential for heterogeneity of effect. Early trials in the post-operative population were small, methodologically and clinically heterogeneous, with conflicting results, though with a net suggestion of benefit in aggregate [179]. The most recent attempt to synthesise the post-operative adult data from RCTs at a low risk of bias suggests that, compared to a placebo, the use of melatonin or an MRA significantly reduces the risk of post-operative delirium with at least moderate certainty [180]. However, the variety of interventions used, the variable schedule and nature of delirium assessment, and the variety of outcome measures used in the included cohort of studies make the recommendation of a specific regimen challenging.

In patients undergoing cardiac surgery or percutaneous intervention, pooled estimates of the effect from RCTs and observational data suggest a reduction in the incidence of post-operative delirium with melatonin use but not MRAs [181, 182] and that this reduction may be more likely if short courses of the drug are given preoperatively. However, the trials were methodologically and clinically heterogeneous, and no reduction in the duration of mechanical ventilation or length of ICU or hospital stay was observed with either melatonin or MRAs [182]. Given the absence of improvement in patient-centred outcomes, it is difficult to conclusively adopt their use in this population, but no serious adverse events were evident from the trials [182]. Due to design limitations in the method of delirium screening and assessment, concurrent use of sedation and statistical heterogeneity, a large RCT of early dexmedetomidine for delirium prevention in the cardiothoracic surgical population is required [183].

19.8.2 Treatment of Active Delirium

Where prevention is aimed at reducing delirium occurrence, treatment is aimed at minimising the severity and duration of delirium, hence reducing mortality, increasing the number of delirium/coma-free days, shortening the duration of mechanical ventilation and length of intensive care or hospital stay, or decreasing the intermediate- to long-term harms associated with the development of the condition. Once delirium has been diagnosed, the strategies employed in its active management depend mainly on the motor subtype identified, as the treatment for hyperactive and hypoactive delirium is fundamentally different. Moreover, hypoactive delirium is less likely to be diagnosed [184], and these patients lack the features of psychomotor and behavioural agitation prompting medical review and intervention [185–187]. There are no published studies to guide the management of mixed states. No high-quality evidence exists to guide the pharmacological management of subsyndromal delirium [75]. In the absence of a discussion of the motoric subtype, there is likely to be a bias in most trials of delirium management towards the inclusion of patients with the potentially dangerous behavioural features of hyperactive delirium.

19.8.2.1 Demedicalisation and Non-pharmacological Treatments

The ICU Liberation Bundle's role in delirium prevention has already been discussed, but as a multicomponent, multistage complex intervention, there was hope that such process bundles would lead to a reduction in the duration and severity of delirium where it did occur. The results of the ICU Liberation ABCDEF Collaborative study are often used to justify the bundled approach to care in the critically ill population, given that patients completing every eligible component of the bundle on each eligible day demonstrated a significant reduction in the likelihood of delirium, mechanical ventilation, coma, physical restraint use within 24 h, hospital death within 7 days, ICU readmission or discharge to a care facility [136]. While it was carried out in a cohort of >15,000 patients from 68 centres, these were all within the United States, and so limit external validity. Moreover, while they are very suggestive of an association with improved outcomes, and these may pertain to delirium, the data are observational. While the association between Bundle completion and outcome persisted after adjustment for a variety of potential confounders and baseline characteristics, unusually cogent illness severity data was available for less than 7% of patients. When this group was examined in a sensitivity analysis, only the reduction in the likelihood of delirium, mechanical ventilation and physical restraint within 24 h remained significant, and this was acknowledged by the study authors as a limitation of their findings.

In a systematic review of randomised non-pharmacological interventions in critically ill patients, except for a lone study of family voice reorientation, neither multicomponent nor individual interventional trials were shown to reduce delirium duration [137]. A synthesis of the data from adult ICU studies describing the entirety of an ABCDEF Bundle and reporting delirium, functional outcomes or quality of life suggests that the use of the Bundle may reduce the duration of delirium, though with significant heterogeneity [188]. Notably in the wider hospital setting, the ability of multicomponent non-pharmacological interventions to prevent delirium in non-ICU patients does not translate into an improvement in mortality, or duration or severity of delirium with any degree of certainty [131].

Restraint is a complex topic, both ethically and clinically [189]. International guidelines fail to make recommendations regarding the use of physical restraint [75]. It contributes to moral distress for clinicians [190] and is deeply unpleasant for patients [191]. Rates of physical restraint use can vary between jurisdictions from 0 to >75% of mechanically ventilated admissions. While physical restraint may be necessary for patient safety during de-sedation or procedural work, its use is strongly associated with the development of delirium in the ICU [73]. It is unclear if the use of physical restraint compounds delirium, increasing its severity or duration. It may be associated with post-traumatic stress disorder in the critically ill [192]. Our understanding of the epidemiology and positive and negative impacts physical restraint may have on patient outcomes remains unclear and should be explored in well-conducted RCTs [193].

A key recent addition to the non-pharmacological ICU Liberation Bundle has been family engagement and empowerment. A recent systematic review suggests that unrestricted visiting policies, presumably with increased familiar contacts and ongoing reorientation, reduce the incidence of delirium and the duration of ICU, though it has no impact on ICU mortality or the rates of ICU-acquired infection [194]. Family participation in essential care activities has been demonstrated to be associated with a reduction in mental health symptoms, but further evidence is required to define both the intervention and its impact on patient-centred outcomes [195]. The wider impact of patient- and family-centred care interventions in the ICU remains uncertain, with the current collection of small trials producing heterogeneous results [196, 197]. It is likely that carefully conducted trials considering the cultural and socio-economic characteristics of the units and patients and utilising broader research approaches incorporating qualitative and quantitative methods will be required to truly unpick the potential benefits and harms to patients and their families from such interventions.

19.8.2.2 Dexmedetomidine Pharmacotherapy

Dexmedetomidine use has been conditionally recommended for the management of agitated delirium precluding ventilatory weaning or extubation in mechanically ventilated critically ill patients since the publications of the 2018 PADIS guidelines [75]. In 2019, the Sedation Practice in Intensive Care Evaluation (SPICE) III study, the largest RCT of sedation practice by an order of magnitude, randomising 4000 critically ill patients to receive open-label dexmedetomidine or clinician-determined analgosedation practice within 12 h of initiation of invasive ventilation, was published [198]. In this multi-centre, international cohort of patients, dexmedetomidine use was associated with meaningful reductions in the duration of mechanical ventilation (adjusted risk difference 1.0 day) and the number of days free from coma or delirium (adjusted risk difference 1.0 day). While no mortality difference was observed between groups overall, significant heterogeneity of effect was noted on pre-specified subgroup analysis for age, which persisted after adjustment. Older patients demonstrated a significant mortality advantage. Post hoc Bayesian analyses explored the observed heterogeneity of effect further, indicating that allocation to early dexmedetomidine treatment in post-operative general and cardiothoracic surgical patients lowered mortality and demonstrated a >99% probability of increasing coma-, ventilator- and delirium-free days in older patients [199].

Several further important pieces of guidance regarding the use of dexmedetomidine in the management of delirium have been published to incorporate the SPICE III data. A subsequent systematic review demonstrated that dexmedetomidine clearly reduces the occurrence of delirium and likely reduces the duration of mechanical ventilation and hence ICU stay compared to other agents, including benzodiazepines, propofol and opioids. While the risk of both bradycardia and hypotension was increased in patients treated with dexmedetomidine, the need for significant intervention as a consequence was not [200]. Consistent with the post hoc analyses of the SPICE III trial, where the mechanism of sedation management was found to mediate the heterogeneity of treatment effect observed between older and younger patients in the original trial [201], no relationship between age and treatment effect was demonstrated on meta-regression analysis [200].

The Rapid Practice Guideline issued alongside this systematic review highlighted the benefit of 108 fewer patients developing delirium for every 1000 treated with dexmedetomidine compared to other sedative agents. Recognising the consistent signal for benefit from and the limited potential for harm in appropriately selected patients, the authors recommended the use of dexmedetomidine over other agents in situations where a reduction in delirium was valued over the potential for the increased incidence of adverse events [202]. These adverse events did not lead to an excess of mortality [200, 202].

Dexmedetomidine may also have a unique role to play as a safe and effective agent in the unintubated, agitated patient in the ICU. In a non-randomised comparison, for patients non-responsive to haloperidol, dexmedetomidine seemed to achieve useful sedation results, with a better safety profile [203]. This study was carried out when dexmedetomidine remained on patent; generic forms of the drug are now available. It is possible that the mean cost savings of over $US4,000 per patient observed, primarily due to a reduction in ICU length of stay, would be even greater now. Two studies with similar methodology in this understudied population—the French 4D trial [204] and the Japanese DEX-HD trial [205]—have been registered and appear to be recruiting, and the results are awaited.

19.8.2.3　Haloperidol and Other Antipsychotic Agents

Returning to the AID-ICU study, there was no difference in the primary outcome, days alive and out of the hospital at 90 days, between groups [26]. The RECOVER cohort study demonstrated that this composite outcome may better reflect functional status at 12 months than standard clinical end points in the critically ill population, reflecting the complex nature of recovery from ICU admission and delirium [206]. While no significant difference in the number of days alive and delirium and coma free between groups was demonstrated on the initial frequentist analysis, the confidence interval around the point estimate suggested a clinically important benefit [207] with an adjusted absolute difference of 5.1 (99% CI: −1.2 to 11.3) days [26]. A secondary Bayesian analysis, using weakly informative priors, estimated a mean absolute difference of 5 more (95% credible interval: 0.3–9.7) days alive and delirium and coma free with a >95% probability of clinically important benefit and a <1% probability of clinically important harm in the haloperidol group [208].

The population recruited is unlikely to be the group at the most benefit from the intervention, given more than 20% of those screened were excluded for prior ICU exposure to antipsychotics, and the majority of treated patients (54.7%) had hypoactive delirium. Major protocol violations occurred in more than 20% of cases, 47.7% of patients in the haloperidol group and 52.1% of the placebo received α2-agonist rescue therapy for a median duration of 3 days. The placebo group also received more benzodiazepines (32.5% vs. 27.3%, median of 2 days of use). The distribution of these therapies and violations by subtype is not presented, but it may be that at least some of this benefit is due to these other agents in this study. In aggregate, no benefit over other agents or placebo was demonstrated [154]. These findings are consistent with those of the EuRIDICE study, which demonstrated a greater than 95% rescue medication use in each group, though this small 132-patient cohort was primarily mixed or hyperactive in nature [153].

While there is ongoing concern regarding the impact of haloperidol administration on ECG QTc interval prolongation, a systematic review suggests that this may not be clinically significant, as serious adverse events appear rare [154]. Further studies are required, with less than 5% of the required information size having been accrued on trial sequential analysis. A recent post hoc analysis of the MIND-USA study demonstrated a similar safety profile [209]. The evidence for other antipsychotics as a primary therapy is sparse, and the 2018 PADIS guidelines recommend against the routine use of antipsychotics in the management of delirium, though they may remain useful for the incident management of distressing neuropsychiatric symptoms or dangerous agitation [75].

19.8.3　*Hypoactive Delirium*

While hypoactive delirium may be the most prevalent form of delirium encountered in clinical practice and may be most strongly associated with mortality, data on effective interventions are limited. Patients with hypoactive delirium are significantly less likely to receive pharmacological intervention than agitated patients outside the context of an RCT, but many will still receive therapy [210, 211]. The MIND-USA trial, comparing haloperidol, ziprasidone or placebo, demonstrated no benefit for either agent in a large American cohort of predominantly mechanically ventilated critically ill patients with hypoactive delirium [25]. While not representative of standard international practice, it is the largest cohort of patients with recognised hypoactive delirium in the ICU setting treated with pharmacotherapy. Prophylactic intraoperative dexmedetomidine infusion has been demonstrated to reduce the incidence of delirium in patients recovering from elective brain tumour resection. Pain scores and sleep quality were also improved. Of note, this finding was driven by the significant reduction in the development of the hypoactive subtype [212]. Hypoactive delirium remains a state of neuropsychiatric distress. It is possible that the multimodal action of dexmedetomidine, through analgesia, anxiolysis and sparing deliriogenic exposure by reducing benzodiazepine and opioid exposure, may be an effective treatment. Larger, properly powered and controlled trials will be required to know definitively.

19.8.4 Steroids in Delirium

Corticosteroids have been associated with the development of delirium in mechanically ventilated patients [213], though the evidence is mixed [214]. Most RCTs of steroid use in the critically ill have not reported on the development of delirium as an outcome [215, 216]. The HYPRESS trial, including 380 patients from 34 German hospitals treated for severe sepsis with adjunctive hydrocortisone or placebo, demonstrated a 13.3% reduction in the occurrence of delirium in the treatment arm [217]. Only 56.6% of the study cohort required mechanical ventilation, and 6.5% received etomidate, meaning these results may be difficult to extrapolate to the broader critical care cohort in other jurisdictions.

19.9 The Economic Value of Clinical Interventions for Delirium

Estimates of the economic impact of delirium in the inpatient setting suggest a potential cost of between US$6.6 and US$82.4 billion, corrected to 2019 values, in the United States alone. In the ICU, each episode costs somewhere between approximately $1500 and $14,500 [87]. With the increasing number of elderly patients being hospitalised, and the changing demographic of patients admitted to the ICU [218–220], the cost of delirium and related care is an emerging international healthcare concern [221]. However, the literature is wildly heterogeneous, with significant differences between and within jurisdictions in how costs are measured, identified and analysed [87]. Moreover, the economic efficacy of interventions designed to prevent or reduce the duration of delirium is poorly described across a limited number of low-quality studies, preventing the most cost-effective interventions from being identified [222]. Future large randomised interventional trials in delirium management must include economic and cost-effectiveness analyses as an integral part of their data collection and follow-up design, in keeping with best practice recommendations and to provide data on patient-relevant outcomes [223].

19.10 A Future Without Delirium

Our understanding of delirium pathophysiology and triggers of delirium events has evolved over the past two decades. While it varies by setting, the incidence of delirium continues to be unacceptably high. Considering the short- and long-term consequences of delirium, it is therefore a clinical and a societal imperative to achieve a future with no delirium and, if it occurs, for it to be identified and resolved in the shortest duration possible.

To achieve this, we need a mindset shift in the design of future ICU rooms to be more family centric, with less pervasive machinery, smart remote monitoring and a reflection of normal daylight circadian rhythm. The combination of special lighting and separation of machine and technology from patient and family has achieved promising improvements in delirium occurrence in pilot studies [224]. This is an exciting future avenue for an ICU system redesign with cognitive wellness as a prime target.

Our future bundles of care should mandate minimal use of sedation, keeping patients awake, comfortable and communicating at most times. The universal use of assessment tools to monitor sedation levels and identify patients at high risk of delirium and those with delirium is pivotal to successful and early management of delirium [225].

In summary, we provide a suite of interventions that target delirium subtypes. We promote an individual personalised approach to the prevention and management of delirium using combinations of non-pharmacologic-based interventions and delirium-specific treatment options, in particular in hyperactive, agitated delirium, as outlined earlier in this chapter. In concert with the above, these can provide a cornerstone to an ICU with no delirium.

References

1. Andrews EA, Short C, Lewis CT, Freund W. Harpers' Latin dictionary. Copious and critical lexicon, vol. xiii, [1]. New York: American Book Company., 2019 p; 1907.
2. Schuurmans MJ, Duursma SA, Shortridge-Baggett LM. Early recognition of delirium: review of the literature. J Clin Nurs. 2001;10(6):721–9. https://doi.org/10.1046/j.1365-270 2.2001.00548.x.

3. Adamis D, Treloar A, Martin FC, Macdonald AJ. A brief review of the history of delirium as a mental disorder. Hist Psychiatry. 2007;18(72 Pt 4):459–69. https://doi.org/10.1177/0957154X07076467.

4. Boehm LM, Jones AC, Selim AA, Virdun C, Garrard CF, Walden RL, et al. Delirium-related distress in the ICU: a qualitative meta-synthesis of patient and family perspectives and experiences. Int J Nurs Stud. 2021;122:104030. https://doi.org/10.1016/j.ijnurstu.2021.104030.

5. Ni Chroinin D, Alexandrou E, Frost SA. Delirium in the intensive care unit and its importance in the post-operative context: a review. Front Med (Lausanne). 2023;10:1071854. https://doi.org/10.3389/fmed.2023.1071854.

6. Boettger S, Zipser CM, Bode L, Spiller T, Deuel J, Osterhoff G, et al. The prevalence rates and adversities of delirium: too common and disadvantageous. Palliat Support Care. 2021;19(2):161–9. https://doi.org/10.1017/S1478951520000632.

7. Wilson JE, Mart MF, Cunningham C, Shehabi Y, Girard TD, MacLullich AMJ, et al. Delirium. Nat Rev Dis Primers. 2020;6(1):1–26. https://doi.org/10.1038/s41572-020-00223-4.

8. Lipowski ZJ. Update on delirium. Psychiatr Clin North Am. 1992;15(2):335–46.

9. Liptzin B, Levkoff SE. An empirical study of delirium subtypes. Br J Psychiatry. 1992;161:843–5. https://doi.org/10.1192/bjp.161.6.843.

10. Krewulak KD, Stelfox HT, Leigh JP, Ely EW, Fiest KM. Incidence and prevalence of delirium subtypes in an adult ICU: a systematic review and meta-analysis. Crit Care Med. 2018;46(12):2029–35. https://doi.org/10.1097/CCM.0000000000003402.

11. Serafim RB, Soares M, Bozza FA, Lapa ESJR, Dal-Pizzol F, Paulino MC, et al. Outcomes of subsyndromal delirium in ICU: a systematic review and meta-analysis. Crit Care. 2017;21(1):179. https://doi.org/10.1186/s13054-017-1765-3.

12. Oldham MA, Holloway RG. Delirium disorder: integrating delirium and acute encephalopathy. Neurology. 2020;95(4):173–8. https://doi.org/10.1212/WNL.0000000000009949.

13. Oldham MA, Flaherty JH, Maldonado JR. Refining delirium: a transtheoretical model of delirium disorder with preliminary neurophysiologic subtypes. Am J Geriatr Psychiatry. 2018;26(9):913–24. https://doi.org/10.1016/j.jagp.2018.04.002.

14. European Delirium Association, American Delirium Society. The DSM-5 criteria, level of arousal and delirium diagnosis: inclusiveness is safer. BMC Med. 2014;12(1):141. https://doi.org/10.1186/s12916-014-0141-2.

15. Pendlebury S, Lovett N, Smith S, Dutta N, Bendon C, Lloyd-Lavery A, et al. Observational, longitudinal study of delirium in consecutive unselected acute medical admissions: age-specific rates and associated factors, mortality and re-admission. BMJ Open. 2015;5(11):e007808. https://doi.org/10.1136/bmjopen-2015-007808.

16. Inouye SK, Westendorp RG, Saczynski JS. Delirium in elderly people. Lancet. 2014;383(9920):911–22. https://doi.org/10.1016/S0140-6736(13)60688-1.

17. Persico I, Cesari M, Morandi A, Haas J, Mazzola P, Zambon A, et al. Frailty and delirium in older adults: a systematic review and meta-analysis of the literature. J Am Geriatr Soc. 2018;66(10):2022–30. https://doi.org/10.1111/jgs.15503.

18. Zhang X-M, Jiao J, Xie X-H, Wu X-J. The association between frailty and delirium among hospitalized patients: an updated meta-analysis. J Am Med Dir Assoc. 2021;22(3):527–34. https://doi.org/10.1016/j.jamda.2021.01.065.

19. Tsui A, Searle SD, Bowden H, Hoffmann K, Hornby J, Goslett A, et al. The effect of baseline cognition and delirium on long-term cognitive impairment and mortality: a prospective population-based study. Lancet Healthy Longev. 2022;3(4):e232–e41. https://doi.org/10.1016/S2666-7568(22)00013-7.

20. Fong TG, Inouye SK. The inter-relationship between delirium and dementia: the importance of delirium prevention. Nat Rev Neurol. 2022;18(10):579–96. https://doi.org/10.1038/s41582-022-00698-7.

21. Alagiakrishnan K, Wiens CA. An approach to drug induced delirium in the elderly. Postgrad Med J. 2004;80(945):388–93. https://doi.org/10.1136/pgmj.2003.017236.

22. Reisinger M, Reininghaus EZ, Biasi JD, Fellendorf FT, Schoberer D. Delirium-associated medication in people at risk: a systematic update review, meta-analyses, and GRADE-profiles. Acta Psychiatr Scand. 2023;147(1):16–42. https://doi.org/10.1111/acps.13505.

23. Hall RJ, Watne LO, Cunningham E, Zetterberg H, Shenkin SD, Wyller TB, et al. CSF biomarkers in delirium: a systematic review. Int J Geriatr Psychiatry. 2018;33(11):1479–500. https://doi.org/10.1002/gps.4720.

24. Sampson EL, West E, Fischer T. Pain and delirium: mechanisms, assessment, and management. Eur Geriatr Med. 2020;11(1):45–52. https://doi.org/10.1007/s41999-019-00281-2.

25. Girard TD, Exline MC, Carson SS, Hough CL, Rock P, Gong MN, et al. Haloperidol and ziprasidone for treatment of delirium in critical illness. N Engl J Med. 2018;379(26):2506–16. https://doi.org/10.1056/NEJMoa1808217.

26. Andersen-Ranberg NC, Poulsen LM, Perner A, Wetterslev J, Estrup S, Hästbacka J, et al. Haloperidol for the treatment of delirium in ICU patients. N Engl J Med. 2022;387(26):2425–35. https://doi.org/10.1056/NEJMoa2211868.

27. Chyou TY, Nishtala PS. Identifying frequent drug combinations associated with delirium in older adults: application of association rules method to a case-time-control design. Pharmacoepidemiol Drug. 2021;30(10):1402–10. https://doi.org/10.1002/pds.5292.

28. Engel GL, Romano J. Delirium, a syndrome of cerebral insufficiency. J Neuropsychiatry Clin Neurosci. 2004;16:526.

29. Sonneville R, De Montmollin E, Poujade J, Garrouste-Orgeas M, Souweine B, Darmon M, et al. Potentially modifiable factors contributing to sepsis-associated encephalopathy. Intensive Care Med. 2017;43(8):1075–84. https://doi.org/10.1007/s00134-017-4807-z.

30. Van Keulen K, Knol W, Belitser SV, Zaal IJ, Van Der Linden PD, Heerdink ER, et al. Glucose variability during delirium in diabetic and non-diabetic intensive care unit patients: a prospective cohort study. PLoS One. 2018;13(11):e0205637. https://doi.org/10.1371/journal.pone.0205637.

31. Zhao H, Ying H-L, Zhang C, Zhang S. Relative hypoglycemia is associated with delirium in critically ill patients with diabetes: a cohort study. DMSO. 2022;15:3339–46. https://doi.org/10.2147/DMSO.S369457.

32. Titlestad I, Watne LO, Caplan GA, McCann A, Ueland PM, Neerland BE, et al. Impaired glucose utilization in the brain of patients with delirium following hip fracture. Brain. 2024;147(1):215–23. https://doi.org/10.1093/brain/awad296.

33. Caplan GA, Kvelde T, Lai C, Yap SL, Lin C, Hill MA. Cerebrospinal fluid in long-lasting delirium compared with Alzheimer's dementia. J Gerontol Ser A Biol Med Sci. 2010;65A(10):1130–6. https://doi.org/10.1093/gerona/glq090.

34. Nitchingham A, Pereira JVB, Wegner EA, Oxenham V, Close J, Caplan GA. Regional cerebral hypometabolism on 18F-FDG PET/CT scan in delirium is independent of acute illness and dementia. Alzheimers Dementia. 2023;19(1):97–106. https://doi.org/10.1002/alz.12604.

35. Ormseth CH, LaHue SC, Oldham MA, Josephson SA, Whitaker E, Douglas VC. Predisposing and precipitating factors associated with delirium: a systematic review. JAMA Netw Open. 2023;6(1):e2249950. https://doi.org/10.1001/jamanetworkopen.2022.49950.

36. Gong F, Ai Y, Zhang L, Peng Q, Zhou Q, Gui C. Relationship between PaO_2/FiO_2 and delirium in intensive care: a cross-sectional study. J Intensive Med. 2023;3(1):73–8. https://doi.org/10.1016/j.jointm.2022.08.002.

37. Bendahan N, Neal O, Ross-White A, Muscedere J, Boyd JG. Relationship between near-infrared spectroscopy-derived cerebral oxygenation and delirium in critically ill patients: a systematic review. J Intensive Care Med. 2019;34(6):514–20. https://doi.org/10.1177/0885066618807399.

38. Wood MD, Boyd JG, Wood N, Frank J, Girard TD, Ross-White A, et al. The use of near-infrared spectroscopy and/or transcranial Doppler as non-invasive markers of cerebral perfusion in adult sepsis patients with delirium: a systematic review. J Intensive Care Med. 2022;37(3):408–22. https://doi.org/10.1177/0885066621997090.

39. Tosh W, Patteril M. Cerebral oximetry. BJA Educ. 2016;16(12):417–21. https://doi.org/10.1093/bjaed/mkw024.

40. Yokota H, Ogawa S, Kurokawa A, Yamamoto Y. Regional cerebral blood flow in delirium patients. Psychiatry Clin Neurosci. 2003;57(3):337–9. https://doi.org/10.1046/j.1440-1819.2003.01126.x.

41. Simone MJ, Tan ZS. The role of inflammation in the pathogenesis of delirium and dementia in older adults: a review. CNS Neurosci Ther. 2011;17(5):506–13. https://doi.org/10.1111/j.1755-5949.2010.00173.x.

42. Cerejeira J, Firmino H, Vaz-Serra A, Mukaetova-Ladinska EB. The neuroinflammatory hypothesis of delirium. Acta Neuropathol. 2010;119(6):737–54. https://doi.org/10.1007/s00401-010-0674-1.

43. Van Munster BC, Aronica E, Zwinderman AH, Eikelenboom P, Cunningham C, De Rooij SEJA. Neuroinflammation in delirium: a postmortem case-control study. Rejuvenation Res. 2011;14(6):615–22. https://doi.org/10.1089/rej.2011.1185.

44. Hoogland ICM, Houbolt C, Van Westerloo DJ, Van Gool WA, Van De Beek D. Systemic inflammation and microglial activation: systematic review of animal experiments. J Neuroinflammation. 2015;12(1):114. https://doi.org/10.1186/s12974-015-0332-6.

45. Van Montfort SJT, Van Dellen E, Stam CJ, Ahmad AH, Mentink LJ, Kraan CW, et al. Brain network disintegration as a final common pathway for delirium: a systematic review and qualitative meta-analysis. NeuroImage Clin. 2019;23:101809. https://doi.org/10.1016/j.nicl.2019.101809.

46. Babaeeghazvini P, Rueda-Delgado LM, Gooijers J, Swinnen SP, Daffertshofer A. Brain structural and functional connectivity: a review of combined works of diffusion magnetic resonance imaging and electro-encephalography. Front Hum Neurosci. 2021;15:721206. https://doi.org/10.3389/fnhum.2021.721206.

47. Hasani Seyede A, Mayeli M, Salehi Mohammad A, Barzegar Parizi R. A systematic review of the association between amyloid-β and τ pathology with functional connectivity alterations in the Alzheimer dementia spectrum utilizing PET scan and rsfMRI. Dement Geriatr Cogn Disord Extra. 2021;11(2):78–90. https://doi.org/10.1159/000516164.

48. Kucikova L, Kalabizadeh H, Motsi KG, Rashid S, O'Brien JT, Taylor J-P, et al. A systematic literature review of fMRI and EEG resting-state functional connectivity in dementia with Lewy Bodies: underlying mechanisms, clinical manifestation, and methodological considerations. Ageing Res Rev. 2024;93:102159. https://doi.org/10.1016/j.arr.2023.102159.

49. Choi S-H, Lee H, Chung T-S, Park K-M, Jung Y-C, Kim SI, et al. Neural network functional connectivity during and after an episode of delirium. Am J Psychiatry. 2012;169(5):498–507. https://doi.org/10.1176/appi.ajp.2012.11060976.

50. Boord MS, Moezzi B, Davis D, Ross TJ, Coussens S, Psaltis PJ, et al. Investigating how electroencephalogram measures associate with delirium: a systematic review. Clin Neurophysiol. 2021;132(1):246–57. https://doi.org/10.1016/j.clinph.2020.09.009.

51. Hanna A, Jirsch J, Alain C, Corvinelli S, Lee JS. Electroencephalogram measured functional connectivity for delirium detection: a systematic review. Front Neurosci. 2023;17:1274837. https://doi.org/10.3389/fnins.2023.1274837.

52. Gibb K, Seeley A, Quinn T, Siddiqi N, Shenkin S, Rockwood K, et al. The consistent burden in published estimates of delirium occurrence in medical inpatients over four decades: a systematic review and meta-analysis study. Age Ageing. 2020;49(3):352–60. https://doi.org/10.1093/ageing/afaa040.

53. Bergeron N, Dubois MJ, Dumont M, Dial S, Skrobik Y. Intensive Care Delirium Screening Checklist: evaluation of a new screening tool. Intensive Care Med. 2001;27(5):859–64. https://doi.org/10.1007/s001340100909.

54. Ely EW, Inouye SK, Bernard GR, Gordon S, Francis J, May L, et al. Delirium in mechanically ventilated patients: validity and reliability of the confusion assessment method for the intensive care unit (CAM-ICU). JAMA. 2001;286(21):2703–10. https://doi.org/10.1001/jama.286.21.2703.

55. McNicoll L, Pisani MA, Zhang Y, Ely EW, Siegel MD, Inouye SK. Delirium in the intensive care unit: occurrence and clinical course in older patients. J Am Geriatr Soc. 2003;51(5):591–8. https://doi.org/10.1034/j.1600-0579.2003.00201.x.

56. Semple D, Howlett MM, Strawbridge JD, Breatnach CV, Hayden JC. A systematic review and pooled prevalence of delirium in critically ill children. Crit Care Med. 2022;50(2):317–28. https://doi.org/10.1097/CCM.0000000000005260.

57. Chaiwat O, Chanidnuan M, Pancharoen W, Vijitmala K, Danpornprasert P, Toadithep P, et al. Postoperative delirium in critically ill surgical patients: incidence, risk factors, and predictive scores. BMC Anesthesiol. 2019;19(1):39. https://doi.org/10.1186/s12871-019-0694-x.

58. Pandharipande P, Cotton BA, Shintani A, Thompson J, Pun BT, Morris JA Jr, et al. Prevalence and risk factors for development of delirium in surgical and trauma intensive care unit patients. J Trauma. 2008;65(1):34–41. https://doi.org/10.1097/TA.0b013e31814b2c4d.

59. Kotfis K, Szylinska A, Listewnik M, Strzelbicka M, Brykczynski M, Rotter I, et al. Early delirium after cardiac surgery: an analysis of incidence and risk factors in elderly (>/=65 years) and very elderly (>/=80 years) patients. Clin Interv Aging. 2018;13:1061–70. https://doi.org/10.2147/CIA.S166909.

60. Patel MB, Bednarik J, Lee P, Shehabi Y, Salluh JI, Slooter AJ, et al. Delirium monitoring in neurocritically ill patients: a systematic review. Crit Care Med. 2018;46(11):1832–41. https://doi.org/10.1097/CCM.0000000000003349.

61. Kappen PR, Kakar E, Dirven CMF, van der Jagt M, Klimek M, Osse RJ, et al. Delirium in neurosurgery: a systematic review and meta-analysis. Neurosurg Rev. 2022;45(1):329–41. https://doi.org/10.1007/s10143-021-01619-w.

62. Wang J, Ji Y, Wang N, Chen W, Bao Y, Qin Q, et al. Risk factors for the incidence of delirium in cerebrovascular patients in a Neurosurgery Intensive Care Unit: a prospective study. J Clin Nurs. 2018;27(1–2):407–15. https://doi.org/10.1111/jocn.13943.

63. la Cour KN, Andersen-Ranberg NC, Weihe S, Poulsen LM, Mortensen CB, Kjer CKW, et al. Distribution of delirium motor subtypes in the intensive care unit: a systematic scoping review. Crit Care. 2022;26(1):53. https://doi.org/10.1186/s13054-022-03931-3.

64. Davis DH, Kreisel SH, Muniz Terrera G, Hall AJ, Morandi A, Boustani M, et al. The epidemiology of delirium: challenges and opportunities for population studies. Am J Geriatr Psychiatry. 2013;21(12):1173–89. https://doi.org/10.1016/j.jagp.2013.04.007.

65. Scott BN, Roberts DJ, Robertson HL, Kramer AH, Laupland KB, Ousman SS, et al. Incidence, prevalence, and occurrence rate of infection among adults hospitalized after traumatic brain injury: study protocol for a systematic review and meta-analysis. Syst Rev. 2013;2:68. https://doi.org/10.1186/2046-4053-2-68.

66. Zaal IJ, Devlin JW, Peelen LM, Slooter AJ. A systematic review of risk factors for delirium in the ICU. Crit Care Med. 2015;43(1):40–7. https://doi.org/10.1097/CCM.0000000000000625.

67. Krewulak KD, Stelfox HT, Ely EW, Fiest KM. Risk factors and outcomes among delirium subtypes in adult ICUs: a systematic review. J Crit Care. 2020;56:257–64. https://doi.org/10.1016/j.jcrc.2020.01.017.

68. Greaves D, Psaltis PJ, Davis DHJ, Ross TJ, Ghezzi ES, Lampit A, et al. Risk factors for delirium and cognitive decline following coronary artery bypass grafting surgery: a systematic review and meta-analysis. J Am Heart Assoc. 2020;9(22):e017275. https://doi.org/10.1161/JAHA.120.017275.

69. Sadeghirad B, Dodsworth BT, Schmutz Gelsomino N, Goettel N, Spence J, Buchan TA, et al. Perioperative factors associated with postoperative delirium in patients undergoing noncardiac surgery: an individual patient data meta-analysis. JAMA Netw Open. 2023;6(10):e2337239. https://doi.org/10.1001/jamanetworkopen.2023.37239.

70. Liu J, Li J, Wang J, Zhang M, Han S, Du Y. Associated factors for postoperative delirium following major abdominal surgery: a systematic review and meta-analysis. Int J Geriatr Psychiatry. 2023;38(6):e5942. https://doi.org/10.1002/gps.5942.

71. Salluh JI, Wang H, Schneider EB, Nagaraja N, Yenokyan G, Damluji A, et al. Outcome of delirium in critically ill patients: systematic review and meta-analysis. BMJ. 2015;350:h2538. https://doi.org/10.1136/bmj.h2538.

72. Lin L, Zhang X, Xu S, Peng Y, Li S, Huang X, et al. Outcomes of postoperative delirium in patients undergoing cardiac surgery: a systematic review and meta-analysis. Front Cardiovasc Med. 2022;9:884144. https://doi.org/10.3389/fcvm.2022.884144.

73. Mehta S, Cook D, Devlin JW, Skrobik Y, Meade M, Fergusson D, et al. Prevalence, risk factors, and outcomes of delirium in mechanically ventilated adults. Crit Care Med. 2015;43(3):557–66. https://doi.org/10.1097/CCM.0000000000000727.

74. Jackson JC, Pandharipande PP, Girard TD, Brummel NE, Thompson JL, Hughes CG, et al. Depression, post-traumatic stress disorder, and functional disability in survivors of critical illness in the BRAIN-ICU study: a longitudinal cohort study. Lancet Respir Med. 2014;2(5):369–79. https://doi.org/10.1016/S2213-2600(14)70051-7.

75. Devlin JW, Skrobik Y, Gélinas C, Needham DM, Slooter AJC, Pandharipande PP, et al. Executive summary: Clinical practice guidelines for the prevention and management of pain, agitation/sedation, delirium, immobility, and sleep disruption in adult patients in the ICU. Crit Care Med. 2018;46(9):1532–48. https://doi.org/10.1097/CCM.0000000000003259.

76. Richardson SJ, Davis DHJ, Stephan BCM, Robinson L, Brayne C, Barnes LE, et al. Recurrent delirium over 12 months predicts dementia: results of the Delirium and Cognitive Impact in Dementia (DECIDE) study. Age Ageing. 2021;50(3):914–20. https://doi.org/10.1093/ageing/afaa244.

77. Garcez FB, Apolinario D, Campora F, Curiati JAE, Jacob-Filho W, Avelino-Silva TJ. Delirium and post-discharge dementia: results from a cohort of older adults without baseline cognitive impairment. Age Ageing. 2019;48(6):845–51. https://doi.org/10.1093/ageing/afz107.

78. Goldberg TE, Chen C, Wang Y, Jung E, Swanson A, Ing C, et al. Association of delirium with long-term cognitive decline: a meta-analysis. JAMA Neurol. 2020;77(11):1373–81. https://doi.org/10.1001/jamaneurol.2020.2273.

79. Pereira JV, Aung Thein MZ, Nitchingham A, Caplan GA. Delirium in older adults is associated with development of new dementia: a systematic review and meta-analysis. Int J Geriatr Psychiatry. 2021;36(7):993–1003. https://doi.org/10.1002/gps.5508.

80. Pandharipande PP, Girard TD, Jackson JC, Morandi A, Thompson JL, Pun BT, et al. Long-term cognitive impairment after critical illness. N Engl J Med. 2013;369(14):1306–16. https://doi.org/10.1056/NEJMoa1301372.

81. Abelha FJ, Luis C, Veiga D, Parente D, Fernandes V, Santos P, et al. Outcome and quality of life in patients with postoperative delirium during an ICU stay following major surgery. Crit Care. 2013;17(5):R257. https://doi.org/10.1186/cc13084.

82. Brummel NE, Jackson JC, Pandharipande PP, Thompson JL, Shintani AK, Dittus RS, et al. Delirium in the ICU and subsequent long-term disability among survivors of mechanical ventilation. Crit Care Med. 2014;42(2):369–77. https://doi.org/10.1097/CCM.0b013e3182a645bd.

83. Wolters AE, van Dijk D, Pasma W, Cremer OL, Looije MF, de Lange DW, et al. Long-term outcome of delirium during intensive care unit stay in survivors of critical illness: a prospective cohort study. Crit Care. 2014;18(3):R125. https://doi.org/10.1186/cc13929.

84. Paixao L, Sun H, Hogan J, Hartnack K, Westmeijer M, Neelagiri A, et al. ICU delirium burden predicts functional neurologic outcomes. PLoS One. 2021;16(12):e0259840. https://doi.org/10.1371/journal.pone.0259840.

85. Girard TD, Thompson JL, Pandharipande PP, Brummel NE, Jackson JC, Patel MB, et al. Clinical phenotypes of delirium during critical illness and severity of subsequent long-term cognitive impairment: a prospective cohort study. Lancet Respir Med. 2018;6(3):213–22. https://doi.org/10.1016/S2213-2600(18)30062-6.

86. Rose L, Burry L, Agar M, Campbell NL, Clarke M, Lee J, et al. A core outcome set for research evaluating interventions to prevent and/or treat delirium in critically ill adults: an international consensus study (Del-COrS). Crit Care Med. 2021;49(9):1535–46. https://doi.org/10.1097/CCM.0000000000005028.

87. Kinchin I, Mitchell E, Agar M, Trepel D. The economic cost of delirium: a systematic review and quality assessment. Alzheimers Dement. 2021;17(6):1026–41. https://doi.org/10.1002/alz.12262.

88. Evered LA. Predicting delirium: are we there yet? Br J Anaesth. 2017;119(2):281–3. https://doi.org/10.1093/bja/aex082.

89. van den Boogaard M, Pickkers P, Slooter AJ, Kuiper MA, Spronk PE, van der Voort PH, et al. Development and validation of PRE-DELIRIC (PREdiction of DELIRium in ICu patients)

delirium prediction model for intensive care patients: observational multicentre study. BMJ. 2012;344:e420. https://doi.org/10.1136/bmj.e420.

90. Anton Joseph N, Poulsen LM, Maagaard M, Tholander S, Pedersen HBS, Georgi-Jensen C, et al. Validation of PRE-DELIRIC and E-PRE-DELIRIC in a Danish population of intensive care unit patients—a prospective observational multicenter study. Acta Anaesthesiol Scand. 2024;68(3):385–93. https://doi.org/10.1111/aas.14363.

91. Wassenaar A, Schoonhoven L, Devlin JW, van Haren FMP, Slooter AJC, Jorens PG, et al. Delirium prediction in the intensive care unit: comparison of two delirium prediction models. Crit Care. 2018;22(1):114. https://doi.org/10.1186/s13054-018-2037-6.

92. Linkaite G, Riauka M, Buneviciute I, Vosylius S. Evaluation of PRE-DELIRIC (PREdiction of DELIRium in ICu patients) delirium prediction model for the patients in the intensive care unit. Acta Med Litu. 2018;25(1):14–22. https://doi.org/10.6001/actamedica.v25i1.3699.

93. Liang S, Chau JPC, Lo SHS, Bai L, Yao L, Choi KC. Validation of PREdiction of DELIRium in ICu patients (PRE-DELIRIC) among patients in intensive care units: a retrospective cohort study. Nurs Crit Care. 2021;26(3):176–82. https://doi.org/10.1111/nicc.12550.

94. Miyamoto K, Nakashima T, Shima N, Kato S, Kawazoe Y, Morimoto T, et al. Utility of a prediction model for delirium in intensive care unit patients (PRE-DELIRIC) in mechanically ventilated patients with sepsis. Acute Med Surg. 2020;7(1):e589. https://doi.org/10.1002/ams2.589.

95. Amerongen HVN, Stapel S, Spijkstra JJ, Ouweneel D, Schenk J. Comparison of prognostic accuracy of 3 delirium prediction models. Am J Crit Care. 2023;32(1):43–50. https://doi.org/10.4037/ajcc2023213.

96. Wassenaar A, van den Boogaard M, van Achterberg T, Slooter AJ, Kuiper MA, Hoogendoorn ME, et al. Multinational development and validation of an early prediction model for delirium in ICU patients. Intensive Care Med. 2015;41(6):1048–56. https://doi.org/10.1007/s00134-015-3777-2.

97. Cowan SL, Preller J, Goudie RJB. Evaluation of the E-PRE-DELIRIC prediction model for ICU delirium: a retrospective validation in a UK general ICU. Crit Care. 2020;24(1):123. https://doi.org/10.1186/s13054-020-2838-2.

98. Gao W, Zhang Y, Jin J. Validation of E-PRE-DELIRIC in cardiac surgical ICU delirium: a retrospective cohort study. Nurs Crit Care. 2022;27(2):233–9. https://doi.org/10.1111/nicc.12674.

99. Ruppert MM, Lipori J, Patel S, Ingersent E, Cupka J, Ozrazgat-Baslanti T, et al. ICU delirium-prediction models: a systematic review. Crit Care Explor. 2020;2(12):e0296. https://doi.org/10.1097/CCE.0000000000000296.

100. Xie Q, Wang X, Pei J, Wu Y, Guo Q, Su Y, et al. Machine learning-based prediction models for delirium: a systematic review and meta-analysis. J Am Med Dir Assoc. 2022;23(10):1655–68.e6. https://doi.org/10.1016/j.jamda.2022.06.020.

101. Bhattacharyya A, Sheikhalishahi S, Torbic H, Yeung W, Wang T, Birst J, et al. Delirium prediction in the ICU: designing a screening tool for preventive interventions. JAMIA Open. 2022;5(2):ooac048. https://doi.org/10.1093/jamiaopen/ooac048.

102. Strating T, Shafiee Hanjani L, Tornvall I, Hubbard R, Scott IA. Navigating the machine learning pipeline: a scoping review of inpatient delirium prediction models. BMJ Health Care Inform. 2023;30(1) https://doi.org/10.1136/bmjhci-2023-100767.

103. American Psychiatric Association. Neurocognitive disorders. Diagnostic and statistical manual of mental disorders revised. 5th ed. DSM Library: American Psychiatric Association; 2022.

104. Australian Commission on Safety and Quality in Health Care. Delirium clinical care standard. Sydney: ACSQHC; 2021.

105. National Institute for Health and Care Excellence (NICE). Delirium: prevention, diagnosis and management in hospital and long-term care. NICE clinical guidelines. London: National Institute for Health and Care Excellence (NICE); 2023.

106. Scottish Intercollegiate Guidelines Network. Risk reduction and management of delirium. A national clinical guideline. Edinburgh: NHS Scotland; 2019.

107. Van Eijk MMJ, Kesecioglu J, Slooter AJC. Intensive care delirium monitoring and standardised treatment: a complete survey of Dutch intensive care units. Intensive Crit Care Nurs. 2008;24(4):218–21. https://doi.org/10.1016/j.iccn.2008.04.005.
108. MacSweeney R, Barber V, Page V, Ely EW, Perkins GD, Young JD, et al. A national survey of the management of delirium in UK intensive care units. QJM. 2010;103(4):243–51. https://doi.org/10.1093/qjmed/hcp194.
109. Shehabi Y, Botha JA, Boyle MS, Ernest D, Freebairn RC, Jenkins IR, et al. Sedation and delirium in the intensive care unit: an Australian and New Zealand perspective. Anaesth Intensive Care. 2008;36(4):570–8. https://doi.org/10.1177/0310057X0803600423.
110. Morandi A, Piva S, Ely EW, Myatra SN, Salluh JIF, Amare D, et al. Worldwide survey of the "assessing pain, both spontaneous awakening and breathing trials, choice of drugs, delirium monitoring/management, early exercise/mobility, and family empowerment" (ABCDEF) bundle. Crit Care Med. 2017;45(11):e1111–e22. https://doi.org/10.1097/CCM.0000000000002640.
111. Rowley-Conwy G. Barriers to delirium assessment in the intensive care unit: a literature review. Intensive Crit Care Nurs. 2018;44:99–104. https://doi.org/10.1016/j.iccn.2017.09.001.
112. Arachchi TMJ, Pinto V. Understanding the barriers in delirium care in an intensive care unit: a survey of knowledge, attitudes, and current practices among medical professionals working in intensive care units in teaching hospitals of Central Province, Sri Lanka. Indian J Crit Care Med. 2021;25(12):1413–20. https://doi.org/10.5005/jp-journals-10071-24040.
113. Ragheb J, Norcott A, Benn L, Shah N, McKinney A, Min L, et al. Barriers to delirium screening and management during hospital admission: a qualitative analysis of inpatient nursing perspectives. BMC Health Serv Res. 2023;23(1):712. https://doi.org/10.1186/s12913-023-09681-4.
114. Hart RP, Levenson JL, Sessler CN, Best AM, Schwartz SM, Rutherford LE. Validation of a cognitive test for delirium in medical ICU patients. Psychosomatics. 1996;37(6):533–46. https://doi.org/10.1016/S0033-3182(96)71517-7.
115. Abelha F, Veiga D, Norton M, Santos C, Gaudreau J-D. Delirium assessment in postoperative patients: validation of the Portuguese version of the Nursing Delirium Screening Scale in critical care. Braz J Anesthesiol. 2013;63(6):450–5. https://doi.org/10.1016/j.bjane.2012.09.003.
116. Otter H, Martin J, Bäsell K, von Heymann C, Hein OV, Böllert P, et al. Validity and reliability of the DDS for severity of delirium in the ICU. Neurocrit Care. 2005;2(2):150–8. https://doi.org/10.1385/NCC:2:2:150.
117. Van Rompaey B, Schuurmans MJ, Shortridge-Baggett LM, Truijen S, Elseviers M, Bossaert L. A comparison of the CAM-ICU and the NEECHAM Confusion Scale in intensive care delirium assessment: an observational study in non-intubated patients. Crit Care. 2008;12(1):R16. https://doi.org/10.1186/cc6790.
118. Gélinas C, Bérubé M, Chevrier A, Pun BT, Ely EW, Skrobik Y, et al. Delirium assessment tools for use in critically ill adults: a psychometric analysis and systematic review. Crit Care Nurse. 2018;38(1):38–49. https://doi.org/10.4037/ccn2018633.
119. Ely EW, Margolin R, Francis J, May L, Truman B, Dittus R, et al. Evaluation of delirium in critically ill patients: validation of the Confusion Assessment Method for the Intensive Care Unit (CAM-ICU). Crit Care Med. 2001;29(7):1370.
120. Chen T-J, Chung Y-W, Chang H-C, Chen P-Y, Wu C-R, Hsieh S-H, et al. Diagnostic accuracy of the CAM-ICU and ICDSC in detecting intensive care unit delirium: a bivariate meta-analysis. Int J Nurs Stud. 2021;113:103782. https://doi.org/10.1016/j.ijnurstu.2020.103782.
121. Inouye SK, van Dyck CH, Alessi CA, Balkin S, Siegal AP, Horwitz RI. Clarifying confusion: the confusion assessment method. Ann Intern Med. 1990;113(12):941–8. https://doi.org/10.7326/0003-4819-113-12-941.
122. American Psychiatric Association. Diagnostic and statistical manual of mental disorders. 4th ed. American Psychiatric Association; 1994.
123. Sessler CN, Gosnell M, Grap MJ, Brophy GT, O'Neal PV, Tesoro E, et al. A new agitation-sedation scale for critically ill patients: development and testing of validity and inter-rater reliability. Am J Respir Crit Care Med. 2000;161:A506.

124. Nielsen AH, Larsen LK, Collet MO, Lehmkuhl L, Bekker C, Jensen JF, et al. Intensive care unit nurses' perception of three different methods for delirium screening: a survey (DELIS-3). Aust Crit Care. 2023;36(6):1035–42. https://doi.org/10.1016/j.aucc.2022.12.008.

125. Hijazi Z, Lange P, Watson R, Maier AB. The use of cerebral imaging for investigating delirium aetiology. Eur J Intern Med. 2018;52:35–9. https://doi.org/10.1016/j.ejim.2018.01.024.

126. Haggstrom L, Welschinger R, Caplan GA. Functional neuroimaging offers insights into delirium pathophysiology: a systematic review. Australas J Ageing. 2017;36(3):186–92. https://doi.org/10.1111/ajag.12417.

127. Fong TG, Bogardus ST, Daftary A, Auerbach E, Blumenfeld H, Modur S, et al. Cerebral perfusion changes in older delirious patients using 99mTc HMPAO SPECT. J Gerontol Ser A Biol Med Sci. 2006;61(12):1294–9. https://doi.org/10.1093/gerona/61.12.1294.

128. Dunne SS, Coffey JC, Konje S, Gasior S, Clancy CC, Gulati G, et al. Biomarkers in delirium: a systematic review. J Psychosom Res. 2021;147:110530. https://doi.org/10.1016/j.jpsychores.2021.110530.

129. Seo Y, Lee HJ, Ha EJ, Ha TS. 2021 KSCCM clinical practice guidelines for pain, agitation, delirium, immobility, and sleep disturbance in the intensive care unit. Acute Crit Care. 2022;37(1):1–25. https://doi.org/10.4266/acc.2022.00094.

130. Care ACoSaQiH. Delirium clinical care standard. Sydney: ACSQHC; 2021.

131. Burton JK, Craig LE, Yong SQ, Siddiqi N, Teale EA, Woodhouse R, et al. Non-pharmacological interventions for preventing delirium in hospitalised non-ICU patients. Cochrane Database Syst Rev. 2021;7(7):CD013307. https://doi.org/10.1002/14651858.CD013307.pub2.

132. Barnes-Daly MA, Phillips G, Ely EW. Improving hospital survival and reducing brain dysfunction at seven California community hospitals: implementing PAD guidelines via the ABCDEF bundle in 6,064 patients. Crit Care Med. 2017;45(2):171–8. https://doi.org/10.1097/CCM.0000000000002149.

133. Vasilevskis EE, Pandharipande PP, Girard TD, Ely EW. A screening, prevention, and restoration model for saving the injured brain in intensive care unit survivors. Crit Care Med. 2010;38(10 Suppl):S683–91. https://doi.org/10.1097/CCM.0b013e3181f245d3.

134. Barr J, Fraser GL, Puntillo K, Ely EW, Gélinas C, Dasta JF, et al. Clinical practice guidelines for the management of pain, agitation, and delirium in adult patients in the intensive care unit. Crit Care Med. 2013;41(1):263–306. https://doi.org/10.1097/CCM.0b013e3182783b72.

135. Trogrlic Z, van der Jagt M, Bakker J, Balas MC, Ely EW, van der Voort PH, et al. A systematic review of implementation strategies for assessment, prevention, and management of ICU delirium and their effect on clinical outcomes. Crit Care. 2015;19(1):157. https://doi.org/10.1186/s13054-015-0886-9.

136. Pun BT, Balas MC, Barnes-Daly MA, Thompson JL, Aldrich JM, Barr J, et al. Caring for critically ill patients with the ABCDEF bundle: results of the ICU liberation collaborative in over 15,000 adults. Crit Care Med. 2019;47(1):3–14. https://doi.org/10.1097/CCM.0000000000003482.

137. Bannon L, McGaughey J, Verghis R, Clarke M, McAuley DF, Blackwood B. The effectiveness of non-pharmacological interventions in reducing the incidence and duration of delirium in critically ill patients: a systematic review and meta-analysis. Intensive Care Med. 2019;45(1):1–12. https://doi.org/10.1007/s00134-018-5452-x.

138. Fan EP, Abbott SM, Reid KJ, Zee PC, Maas MB. Abnormal environmental light exposure in the intensive care environment. J Crit Care. 2017;40:11–4. https://doi.org/10.1016/j.jcrc.2017.03.002.

139. Lee HJ, Bae E, Lee HY, Lee SM, Lee J. Association of natural light exposure and delirium according to the presence or absence of windows in the intensive care unit. Acute Crit Care. 2021;36(4):332–41. https://doi.org/10.4266/acc.2021.00556.

140. Smonig R, Magalhaes E, Bouadma L, Andremont O, de Montmollin E, Essardy F, et al. Impact of natural light exposure on delirium burden in adult patients receiving invasive mechanical ventilation in the ICU: a prospective study. Ann Intensive Care. 2019;9(1):120. https://doi.org/10.1186/s13613-019-0592-x.

141. Sonneville R, Smonig R, Dupuis C, Bouadma L, de Montmollin E, Timsit JF. Natural light exposure and delirium in ICU: does the dark side cloud everything? Ann Intensive Care. 2020;10(1):25. https://doi.org/10.1186/s13613-020-0643-3.
142. Vahedian-Azimi A, Bashar FR, Khan AM, Miller AC. Natural versus artificial light exposure on delirium incidence in ARDS patients. Ann Intensive Care. 2020;10(1):15. https://doi.org/10.1186/s13613-020-0630-8.
143. Zaal IJ, Spruyt CF, Peelen LM, van Eijk MM, Wientjes R, Schneider MM, et al. Intensive care unit environment may affect the course of delirium. Intensive Care Med. 2013;39(3):481–8. https://doi.org/10.1007/s00134-012-2726-6.
144. Aiello G, Cuocina M, La Via L, Messina S, Attaguile GA, Cantarella G, et al. Melatonin or ramelteon for delirium prevention in the intensive care unit: a systematic review and meta-analysis of randomized controlled trials. J Clin Med. 2023;12(2):435. https://doi.org/10.3390/jcm12020435.
145. Teng J, Qin H, Guo W, Liu J, Sun J, Zhang Z. Effectiveness of sleep interventions to reduce delirium in critically ill patients: a systematic review and meta-analysis. J Crit Care. 2023;78:154342. https://doi.org/10.1016/j.jcrc.2023.154342.
146. Hardin KA, Seyal M, Stewart T, Bonekat HW. Sleep in critically ill chemically paralyzed patients requiring mechanical ventilation. Chest. 2006;129(6):1468–77. https://doi.org/10.1378/chest.129.6.1468.
147. Wilcox ME, Burry L, Englesakis M, Coman B, Daou M, van Haren FM, et al. Intensive care unit interventions to promote sleep and circadian biology in reducing incident delirium: a scoping review. Thorax. 2024;79:988. https://doi.org/10.1136/thorax-2023-220036.
148. Lavallee JF, Gray TA, Dumville J, Russell W, Cullum N. The effects of care bundles on patient outcomes: a systematic review and meta-analysis. Implement Sci. 2017;12(1):142. https://doi.org/10.1186/s13012-017-0670-0.
149. Paul N, Buse ER, Knauthe A-C, Nothacker M, Weiss B, Spies CD. Effect of ICU care bundles on long-term patient-relevant outcomes: a scoping review. BMJ Open. 2023;13(2):e070962. https://doi.org/10.1136/bmjopen-2022-070962.
150. Kim CM, van der Heide EM, van Rompay TJL, Verkerke GJ, Ludden GDS. Overview and strategy analysis of technology-based nonpharmacological interventions for in-hospital delirium prevention and reduction: systematic scoping review. J Med Internet Res. 2021;23(8):e26079. https://doi.org/10.2196/26079.
151. Wu YC, Tseng PT, Tu YK, Hsu CY, Liang CS, Yeh TC, et al. Association of delirium response and safety of pharmacological interventions for the management and prevention of delirium: a network meta-analysis. JAMA Psychiatry. 2019;76(5):526–35. https://doi.org/10.1001/jamapsychiatry.2018.4365.
152. van den Boogaard M, Slooter AJC, Bruggemann RJM, Schoonhoven L, Beishuizen A, Vermeijden JW, et al. Effect of haloperidol on survival among critically ill adults with a high risk of delirium: the REDUCE randomized clinical trial. JAMA. 2018;319(7):680–90. https://doi.org/10.1001/jama.2018.0160.
153. Smit L, Slooter AJC, Devlin JW, Trogrlic Z, Hunfeld NGM, Osse RJ, et al. Efficacy of haloperidol to decrease the burden of delirium in adult critically ill patients: the EuRIDICE randomized clinical trial. Crit Care. 2023;27(1):413. https://doi.org/10.1186/s13054-023-04692-3.
154. Andersen-Ranberg NC, Barbateskovic M, Perner A, Oxenboll Collet M, Musaeus Poulsen L, van der Jagt M, et al. Haloperidol for the treatment of delirium in critically ill patients: an updated systematic review with meta-analysis and trial sequential analysis. Crit Care. 2023;27(1):329. https://doi.org/10.1186/s13054-023-04621-4.
155. Huang J, Zheng H, Zhu X, Zhang K, Ping X. The efficacy and safety of haloperidol for the treatment of delirium in critically ill patients: a systematic review and meta-analysis of randomized controlled trials. Front Med (Lausanne). 2023;10:1200314. https://doi.org/10.3389/fmed.2023.1200314.
156. Larsen KA, Kelly SE, Stern TA, Bode RH Jr, Price LL, Hunter DJ, et al. Administration of olanzapine to prevent postoperative delirium in elderly joint-replacement patients: a ran-

domized, controlled trial. Psychosomatics. 2010;51(5):409–18. https://doi.org/10.1176/appi. psy.51.5.409.

157. Burry LD, Cheng W, Williamson DR, Adhikari NK, Egerod I, Kanji S, et al. Pharmacological and non-pharmacological interventions to prevent delirium in critically ill patients: a systematic review and network meta-analysis. Intensive Care Med. 2021;47(9):943–60. https://doi. org/10.1007/s00134-021-06490-3.

158. Abraham MP, Hinds M, Tayidi I, Jeffcoach DR, Corder JM, Hamilton LA, et al. Quetiapine for delirium prophylaxis in high-risk critically ill patients. Surgeon. 2021;19(2):65–71. https://doi.org/10.1016/j.surge.2020.02.002.

159. Kim Y, Kim HS, Park JS, Cho YJ, Yoon HI, Lee SM, et al. Efficacy of low-dose prophylactic quetiapine on delirium prevention in critically ill patients: a prospective, randomized, double-blind, placebo-controlled study. J Clin Med. 2019;9(1):69. https://doi.org/10.3390/ jcm9010069.

160. Paris A, Tonner PH. Dexmedetomidine in anaesthesia. Curr Opin Anaesthesiol. 2005;18(4):412–8. https://doi.org/10.1097/01.aco.0000174958.05383.d5.

161. Fairbanks CA, Stone LS, Wilcox GL. Pharmacological profiles of alpha 2 adrenergic receptor agonists identified using genetically altered mice and isobolographic analysis. Pharmacol Ther. 2009;123(2):224–38. https://doi.org/10.1016/j.pharmthera.2009.04.001.

162. Nelson LE, Lu J, Guo T, Saper CB, Franks NP, Maze M. The alpha2-adrenoceptor agonist dexmedetomidine converges on an endogenous sleep-promoting pathway to exert its sedative effects. Anesthesiology. 2003;98(2):428–36. https://doi. org/10.1097/00000542-200302000-00024.

163. Aantaa R, Marjamäki A, Scheinin M. Molecular pharmacology of α2-adrenoceptor subtypes. Ann Med. 1995;27(4):439–49. https://doi.org/10.3109/07853899709002452.

164. Shehabi Y, Bellomo R, Kadiman S, Ti LK, Howe B, Reade MC, et al. Sedation intensity in the first 48 hours of mechanical ventilation and 180-day mortality: a multinational prospective longitudinal cohort study*. Crit Care Med. 2018;46(6):850–9. https://doi.org/10.1097/ CCM.0000000000003071.

165. Skrobik Y, Duprey MS, Hill NS, Devlin JW. Low-dose nocturnal dexmedetomidine prevents ICU delirium. A randomized, placebo-controlled trial. Am J Respir Crit Care Med. 2018;197(9):1147–56. https://doi.org/10.1164/rccm.201710-1995OC.

166. Zitikyte G, Roy DC, Tran A, Fernando SM, Rosenberg E, Kanji S, et al. Pharmacologic interventions to prevent delirium in trauma patients: a systematic review and network meta-analysis of randomized controlled trials. Crit Care Explor. 2023;5(3):e0875. https://doi. org/10.1097/CCE.0000000000000875.

167. Park SK, Lim T, Cho H, Yoon HK, Lee HJ, Lee JH, et al. Comparative effectiveness of pharmacological interventions to prevent postoperative delirium: a network meta-analysis. Sci Rep. 2021;11(1):11922. https://doi.org/10.1038/s41598-021-91314-z.

168. Patel M, Onwochei DN, Desai N. Influence of perioperative dexmedetomidine on the incidence of postoperative delirium in adult patients undergoing cardiac surgery. Br J Anaesth. 2022;129(1):67–83. https://doi.org/10.1016/j.bja.2021.11.041.

169. Galano A, Tan DX, Reiter RJ. Melatonin as a natural ally against oxidative stress: a physicochemical examination. J Pineal Res. 2011;51(1):1–16. https://doi.org/10.1111/j.1600-079 X.2011.00916.x.

170. Tan DX, Reiter RJ, Manchester LC, Yan MT, El-Sawi M, Sainz RM, et al. Chemical and physical properties and potential mechanisms: melatonin as a broad spectrum antioxidant and free radical scavenger. Curr Top Med Chem. 2002;2(2):181–97. https://doi. org/10.2174/1568026023394443.

171. Siddiqi N, Harrison JK, Clegg A, Teale EA, Young J, Taylor J, et al. Interventions for preventing delirium in hospitalised non-ICU patients. Cochrane Database Syst Rev. 2016;3(3):CD005563. https://doi.org/10.1002/14651858.CD005563.pub3.

172. Khaing K, Nair BR. Melatonin for delirium prevention in hospitalized patients: a systematic review and meta-analysis. J Psychiatr Res. 2021;133:181–90. https://doi.org/10.1016/j. jpsychires.2020.12.020.

173. Yu CL, Carvalho AF, Thompson T, Tsai TC, Tseng PT, Tu YK, et al. Ramelteon for delirium prevention in hospitalized patients: an updated meta-analysis and trial sequential analysis of randomized controlled trials. J Pineal Res. 2023;74(3):e12857. https://doi.org/10.1111/jpi.12857.
174. Wibrow B, Martinez FE, Myers E, Chapman A, Litton E, Ho KM, et al. Prophylactic melatonin for delirium in intensive care (Pro-MEDIC): a randomized controlled trial. Intensive Care Med. 2022;48(4):414–25. https://doi.org/10.1007/s00134-022-06638-9.
175. Martinez FE, Anstey M, Ford A, Roberts B, Hardie M, Palmer R, et al. Prophylactic melatonin for delirium in intensive care (Pro-MEDIC): study protocol for a randomised controlled trial. Trials. 2017;18(1):4. https://doi.org/10.1186/s13063-016-1751-0.
176. Bellapart J, Roberts JA, Appadurai V, Wallis SC, Nunez-Nunez M, Boots RJ. Pharmacokinetics of a novel dosing regimen of oral melatonin in critically ill patients. Clin Chem Lab Med. 2016;54(3):467–72. https://doi.org/10.1515/cclm-2015-0323.
177. Andersen LP, Gogenur I, Rosenberg J, Reiter RJ. Pharmacokinetics of melatonin: the missing link in clinical efficacy? Clin Pharmacokinet. 2016;55(9):1027–30. https://doi.org/10.1007/s40262-016-0386-3.
178. Yan W, Li C, Song X, Zhou W, Chen Z. Prophylactic melatonin for delirium in critically ill patients: a systematic review and meta-analysis with trial sequential analysis. Medicine (Baltimore). 2022;101(43):e31411. https://doi.org/10.1097/MD.0000000000031411.
179. Campbell AM, Axon DR, Martin JR, Slack MK, Mollon L, Lee JK. Melatonin for the prevention of postoperative delirium in older adults: a systematic review and meta-analysis. BMC Geriatr. 2019;19(1):272. https://doi.org/10.1186/s12877-019-1297-6.
180. Barnes J, Sewart E, Armstrong RA, Pufulete M, Hinchliffe R, Gibbison B, et al. Does melatonin administration reduce the incidence of postoperative delirium in adults? Systematic review and meta-analysis. BMJ Open. 2023;13(3):e069950. https://doi.org/10.1136/bmjopen-2022-069950.
181. Duan Y, Yang Y, Zhu W, Wan L, Wang G, Yue J, et al. Melatonin intervention to prevent delirium in the intensive care units: a systematic review and meta-analysis of randomized controlled trials. Front Endocrinol (Lausanne). 2023;14:1191830. https://doi.org/10.3389/fendo.2023.1191830.
182. Han Y, Tian Y, Wu J, Zhu X, Wang W, Zeng Z, et al. Melatonin and its analogs for prevention of post-cardiac surgery delirium: a systematic review and meta-analysis. Front Cardiovasc Med. 2022;9:888211. https://doi.org/10.3389/fcvm.2022.888211.
183. Sanders RD, Wehrman J, Irons J, Dieleman J, Scott D, Shehabi Y. Meta-analysis of randomised controlled trials of perioperative dexmedetomidine to reduce delirium and mortality after cardiac surgery. Br J Anaesth. 2021;127(5):e168–e70. https://doi.org/10.1016/j.bja.2021.08.009.
184. Albrecht JS, Marcantonio ER, Roffey DM, Orwig D, Magaziner J, Terrin M, et al. Stability of postoperative delirium psychomotor subtypes in individuals with hip fracture. J Am Geriatr Soc. 2015;63(5):970–6. https://doi.org/10.1111/jgs.13334.
185. Freeman S, Hallett C, McHugh G. Physical restraint: experiences, attitudes and opinions of adult intensive care unit nurses. Nurs Crit Care. 2016;21(2):78–87. https://doi.org/10.1111/nicc.12197.
186. Inouye SK, Foreman MD, Mion LC, Katz KH, Cooney LM Jr. Nurses' recognition of delirium and its symptoms: comparison of nurse and researcher ratings. Arch Intern Med. 2001;161(20):2467–73. https://doi.org/10.1001/archinte.161.20.2467.
187. Rice KL, Bennett M, Gomez M, Theall KP, Knight M, Foreman MD. Nurses' recognition of delirium in the hospitalized older adult. Clin Nurse Spec. 2011;25(6):299–311. https://doi.org/10.1097/NUR.0b013e318234897b.
188. Sosnowski K, Lin F, Chaboyer W, Ranse K, Heffernan A, Mitchell M. The effect of the ABCDE/ABCDEF bundle on delirium, functional outcomes, and quality of life in critically ill patients: a systematic review and meta-analysis. Int J Nurs Stud. 2023;138:104410. https://doi.org/10.1016/j.ijnurstu.2022.104410.

189. Smithard D, Randhawa R. Physical restraint in the critical care unit: a narrative review. New Bioeth. 2022;28(1):68–82. https://doi.org/10.1080/20502877.2021.2019979.

190. Lao Y, Chen X, Zhang Y, Shen L, Wu F, Gong X. Critical care nurses' experiences of physical restraint in intensive care units: a qualitative systematic review and meta-synthesis. J Clin Nurs. 2023;32(9–10):2239–51. https://doi.org/10.1111/jocn.16528.

191. Perez D, Murphy G, Wilkes L, Peters K. Being tied down—the experience of being physically restrained while mechanically ventilated in ICU. J Adv Nurs. 2022;78(11):3760–71. https://doi.org/10.1111/jan.15354.

192. Franks ZM, Alcock JA, Lam T, Haines KJ, Arora N, Ramanan M. Physical restraints and post-traumatic stress disorder in survivors of critical illness. A systematic review and meta-analysis. Ann Am Thorac Soc. 2021;18(4):689–97. https://doi.org/10.1513/AnnalsATS.202006-738OC.

193. Kooken RWJ, Tilburgs B, Ter Heine R, Ramakers B, van den Boogaard M, Group Ps. A multicomponent intervention program to Prevent and Reduce AgItation and phySical rEstraint use in the ICU (PRAISE): study protocol for a multicenter, stepped-wedge, cluster randomized controlled trial. Trials. 2023;24(1):800. https://doi.org/10.1186/s13063-023-07807-x.

194. Wu Y, Wang G, Zhang Z, Fan L, Ma F, Yue W, et al. Efficacy and safety of unrestricted visiting policy for critically ill patients: a meta-analysis. Crit Care. 2022;26(1):267. https://doi.org/10.1186/s13054-022-04129-3.

195. Dijkstra BM, Felten-Barentsz KM, van der Valk MJM, Pelgrim T, van der Hoeven JG, Schoonhoven L, et al. Family participation in essential care activities in adult intensive care units: an integrative review of interventions and outcomes. J Clin Nurs. 2023;32(17–18):5904–22. https://doi.org/10.1111/jocn.16714.

196. Liang S, Chau JPC, Lo SHS, Zhao J, Choi KC. Effects of nonpharmacological delirium-prevention interventions on critically ill patients' clinical, psychological, and family outcomes: a systematic review and meta-analysis. Aust Crit Care. 2021;34(4):378–87. https://doi.org/10.1016/j.aucc.2020.10.004.

197. Deng LX, Cao L, Zhang LN, Peng XB, Zhang L. Non-pharmacological interventions to reduce the incidence and duration of delirium in critically ill patients: a systematic review and network meta-analysis. J Crit Care. 2020;60:241–8. https://doi.org/10.1016/j.jcrc.2020.08.019.

198. Shehabi Y, Howe BD, Bellomo R, Arabi YM, Bailey M, Bass FE, et al. Early sedation with dexmedetomidine in critically ill patients. N Engl J Med. 2019;380(26):2506–17. https://doi.org/10.1056/NEJMoa1904710.

199. Shehabi Y, Serpa Neto A, Howe BD, Bellomo R, Arabi YM, Bailey M, et al. Early sedation with dexmedetomidine in ventilated critically ill patients and heterogeneity of treatment effect in the SPICE III randomised controlled trial. Intensive Care Med. 2021;47(4):455–66. https://doi.org/10.1007/s00134-021-06356-8.

200. Lewis K, Alshamsi F, Carayannopoulos KL, Granholm A, Piticaru J, Al Duhailib Z, et al. Dexmedetomidine vs other sedatives in critically ill mechanically ventilated adults: a systematic review and meta-analysis of randomized trials. Intensive Care Med. 2022;48(7):811–40. https://doi.org/10.1007/s00134-022-06712-2.

201. Shehabi Y, Serpa Neto A, Bellomo R, Howe BD, Arabi YM, Bailey M, et al. Dexmedetomidine and propofol sedation in critically ill patients and dose-associated 90-day mortality: a secondary cohort analysis of a randomized controlled trial (SPICE III). Am J Respir Crit Care Med. 2023;207(7):876–86. https://doi.org/10.1164/rccm.202206-1208OC.

202. Møller MH, Alhazzani W, Lewis K, Belley-Cote E, Granholm A, Centofanti J, et al. Use of dexmedetomidine for sedation in mechanically ventilated adult ICU patients: a rapid practice guideline. Intensive Care Med. 2022;48(7):801–10. https://doi.org/10.1007/s00134-022-06660-x.

203. Carrasco G, Baeza N, Cabre L, Portillo E, Gimeno G, Manzanedo D, et al. Dexmedetomidine for the treatment of hyperactive delirium refractory to haloperidol in nonintubated ICU patients: a nonrandomized controlled trial. Crit Care Med. 2016;44(7):1295–306. https://doi.org/10.1097/CCM.0000000000001622.

204. Louis C, Godet T, Chanques G, Bourguignon N, Morand D, Pereira B, et al. Effects of dexmedetomidine on delirium duration of non-intubated ICU patients (4D trial): study protocol for a randomized trial. Trials. 2018;19(1):307. https://doi.org/10.1186/s13063-018-2656-x.
205. Minami T, Watanabe H, Kato T, Ikeda K, Ueno K, Matsuyama A, et al. Dexmedetomidine versus haloperidol for sedation of non-intubated patients with hyperactive delirium during the night in a high dependency unit: study protocol for an open-label, parallel-group, randomized controlled trial (DEX-HD trial). BMC Anesthesiol. 2023;23(1):193. https://doi.org/10.1186/s12871-023-02158-1.
206. Taran S, Coiffard B, Huszti E, Li Q, Chu L, Thomas C, et al. Association of days alive and at home at day 90 after intensive care unit admission with long-term survival and functional status among mechanically ventilated patients. JAMA Netw Open. 2023;6(3):e233265. https://doi.org/10.1001/jamanetworkopen.2023.3265.
207. Hemming K, Taljaard M. Why proper understanding of confidence intervals and statistical significance is important. Med J Aust. 2021;214(3):116–8.e1. https://doi.org/10.5694/mja2.50926.
208. Andersen-Ranberg NC, Poulsen LM, Perner A, Hastbacka J, Morgan M, Citerio G, et al. Haloperidol vs. placebo for the treatment of delirium in ICU patients: a pre-planned, secondary Bayesian analysis of the AID-ICU trial. Intensive Care Med. 2023;49(4):411–20. https://doi.org/10.1007/s00134-023-07024-9.
209. Stollings JL, Boncyk CS, Birdrow CI, Chen W, Raman R, Gupta DK, et al. Antipsychotics and the QTc interval during delirium in the intensive care unit: a secondary analysis of a randomized clinical trial. JAMA Netw Open. 2024;7(1):e2352034. https://doi.org/10.1001/jamanetworkopen.2023.52034.
210. van Velthuijsen EL, Zwakhalen SMG, Mulder WJ, Verhey FRJ, Kempen G. Detection and management of hyperactive and hypoactive delirium in older patients during hospitalization: a retrospective cohort study evaluating daily practice. Int J Geriatr Psychiatry. 2018;33(11):1521–9. https://doi.org/10.1002/gps.4690.
211. Zipser CM, Knoepfel S, Hayoz P, Schubert M, Ernst J, von Kanel R, et al. Clinical management of delirium: the response depends on the subtypes. An observational cohort study in 602 patients. Palliat Support Care. 2020;18(1):4–11. https://doi.org/10.1017/S1478951519000609.
212. Li S, Li R, Li M, Cui Q, Zhang X, Ma T, et al. Dexmedetomidine administration during brain tumour resection for prevention of postoperative delirium: a randomised trial. Br J Anaesth. 2023;130(2):e307–e16. https://doi.org/10.1016/j.bja.2022.10.041.
213. Schreiber MP, Colantuoni E, Bienvenu OJ, Neufeld KJ, Chen KF, Shanholtz C, et al. Corticosteroids and transition to delirium in patients with acute lung injury. Crit Care Med. 2014;42(6):1480–6. https://doi.org/10.1097/CCM.0000000000000247.
214. Wolters AE, Veldhuijzen DS, Zaal IJ, Peelen LM, van Dijk D, Devlin JW, et al. Systemic corticosteroids and transition to delirium in critically ill patients. Crit Care Med. 2015;43(12):e585–8. https://doi.org/10.1097/CCM.0000000000001302.
215. Sprung CL, Annane D, Keh D, Moreno R, Singer M, Freivogel K, et al. Hydrocortisone therapy for patients with septic shock. N Engl J Med. 2008;358(2):111–24. https://doi.org/10.1056/NEJMoa071366.
216. Venkatesh B, Finfer S, Cohen J, Rajbhandari D, Arabi Y, Bellomo R, et al. Adjunctive glucocorticoid therapy in patients with septic shock. N Engl J Med. 2018;378(9):797–808. https://doi.org/10.1056/NEJMoa1705835.
217. Keh D, Trips E, Marx G, Wirtz SP, Abduljawwad E, Bercker S, et al. Effect of hydrocortisone on development of shock among patients with severe sepsis: the HYPRESS randomized clinical trial. JAMA. 2016;316(17):1775–85. https://doi.org/10.1001/jama.2016.14799.
218. Darvall JN, Bellomo R, Paul E, Subramaniam A, Santamaria JD, Bagshaw SM, et al. Frailty in very old critically ill patients in Australia and New Zealand: a population-based cohort study. Med J Aust. 2019;211(7):318–23. https://doi.org/10.5694/mja2.50329.

219. Rai S, Brace C, Ross P, Darvall J, Haines K, Mitchell I, et al. Characteristics and outcomes of very elderly patients admitted to intensive care: a retrospective multicenter cohort analysis. Crit Care Med. 2023;51(10):1328–38. https://doi.org/10.1097/CCM.0000000000005943.
220. Sahle BW, Pilcher D, Litton E, Ofori-Asenso R, Peter K, McFadyen J, et al. Association between frailty, delirium, and mortality in older critically ill patients: a binational registry study. Ann Intensive Care. 2022;12(1):108. https://doi.org/10.1186/s13613-022-01080-y.
221. Khachaturian AS, Hayden KM, Devlin JW, Fleisher LA, Lock SL, Cunningham C, et al. International drive to illuminate delirium: a developing public health blueprint for action. Alzheimers Dement. 2020;16(5):711–25. https://doi.org/10.1002/alz.12075.
222. Kinchin I, Edwards L, Hosie A, Agar M, Mitchell E, Trepel D. Cost-effectiveness of clinical interventions for delirium: a systematic literature review of economic evaluations. Acta Psychiatr Scand. 2023;147(5):430–59. https://doi.org/10.1111/acps.13457.
223. Taylor CB, Thompson KJ, Hodgson C, Liew C, Litton E, McGain F, et al. Economic evaluations for intensive care unit randomised clinical trials in Australia and New Zealand: practical recommendations for researchers. Aust Crit Care. 2023;36(3):431–7. https://doi.org/10.1016/j.aucc.2022.02.002.
224. Kotfis K, Van Diem-Zaal I, Williams Roberson S, Sietnicki M, Van Den Boogaard M, Shehabi Y, et al. The future of intensive care: delirium should no longer be an issue. Crit Care. 2022;26(1):200. https://doi.org/10.1186/s13054-022-04077-y.
225. Shehabi Y, Al-Bassam W, Pakavakis A, Murfin B, Howe B. Optimal sedation and pain management: a patient- and symptom-oriented paradigm. Semin Respir Crit Care Med. 2021;42(01):098–111. https://doi.org/10.1055/s-0040-1716736.

Part V
Gastrointestinal and Hepatic Critical Care

Chapter 20
Acute Pancreatitis

Kaitlin M. Alexander and Bethany R. Shoulders

20.1 Introduction

The pancreas is a vital organ with endocrine and exocrine functions in the body. It performs essential functions to maintain blood glucose homeostasis and support digestion through the secretion of digestive enzymes, including amylase, lipase, and proteases. Acute pancreatitis is caused by inflammation of the pancreas, leading to impaired pancreatic function. Acute pancreatitis is a significant medical challenge often encountered in the critical care setting, and pharmacists may be involved in the care of patients with this disease state. The chapter's primary objective is to equip pharmacists with foundational knowledge of acute pancreatitis management and offer insights into recent recommendations to be able to develop evidence-based recommendations for patients with acute pancreatitis.

20.2 Epidemiology

Acute pancreatitis is a gastrointestinal disorder caused by inflammation of the pancreas and, in severe cases, can lead to multi-organ failure. Although most cases of acute pancreatitis are mild and resolve on their own, individuals with severe pancreatitis, especially those with organ failure, experience substantial mortality risk ranging from 20% to 40% and require intensive care [1–3]. Recent findings from a systematic review and meta-analysis indicate an increasing trend in hospital admissions due to acute pancreatitis, particularly in Western countries [4]. The escalating

K. M. Alexander (✉) · B. R. Shoulders
University of Florida College of Pharmacy, Gainesville, FL, USA
e-mail: Kaitlin.alexander@cop.ufl.edu; brshoulders@cop.ufl.edu

Y. Alzaidi, M. A. Gebily (eds.), *The Pharmacist's Expanded Role in Critical Care Medicine*, https://doi.org/10.1007/978-3-031-77335-8_20

rate of hospitalization suggests a potential ongoing impact on healthcare resources in the United States and underscores the need for effective management strategies.

20.3 Etiology

The underlying cause of acute pancreatitis should be identified upon presentation [5]. Gallstones leading to pancreatic duct obstruction and alcohol abuse comprise the most common causes of acute pancreatitis in the United States. Other potential, albeit less common, causes include adverse reactions to medications, infection, hypertriglyceridemia, hypercalcemia, endoscopic retrograde cholangiopancreatography (ERCP), and malignancy [2, 6]. Other factors, modifiable and non-modifiable, contributing to the risk of acute pancreatitis include obesity, older age, trauma, and smoking [2].

20.4 Drug-Induced Pancreatitis

Drug-induced pancreatitis occurs rarely and, typically, accounts for less than 2% of cases [7]. Other causes of acute pancreatitis should be ruled out before medications can be identified as the causative factor. Pharmacists can play a crucial role in the identification and management of drug-induced pancreatitis. Numerous medications have been linked to acute pancreatitis, with varying degrees of certainty regarding the association. Data is limited to case reports, some showing positive rechallenge. Table 20.1 provides a list of medications utilized in the intensive care unit with associations with acute pancreatitis [2, 7]. Antidiabetic agents, such as metformin, sulfonylureas, and incretin mimetics, have also been linked to pancreatitis, but this association is controversial and not well established in the literature [8, 9]. Drug-induced pancreatitis can manifest at any point during treatment, posing a challenge for diagnosis. However, if rechallenged, the onset can occur more quickly (within hours) [7].

Table 20.1 Medications in the intensive care unit associated with drug-induced acute pancreatitis

Medication or drug class
ACE inhibitors (enalapril, captopril, lisinopril, ramipril)
Acetaminophen
Amiodarone
Azathioprine[a]
Carbamazepine
Cimetidine
Corticosteroids
Hydrochlorothiazide
Itraconazole
Interferon-alpha
Furosemide
Losartan
Mesalamine[a]
Metronidazole
Methylprednisolone, prednisone
Nitrofurantoin
Octreotide
Opiates
Pentamidine[a]
Procainamide
Propofol
Statin drugs (rosuvastatin, pravastatin, simvastatin)
Sulfasalazine
Sulfamethoxazole and trimethoprim
Tigecycline
Valproic acid[a]

[a] >20 case reports
Information from [7]

20.5 Pathophysiology

Pancreatitis is a condition that arises from exposure to elevated levels of pancreatic enzymes, namely amylase, lipase, and protease, that causes acinar cell damage. These enzyme levels can increase due to trypsin hyperstimulation or blockages in the ducts, leading to increased ductal pressure, edema, and inflammation.

In either case, these insults trigger the release of active enzymes, vasoactive substances, and inflammatory markers, resulting in acute inflammation and edema. If damage progresses, cell death can result in necrotizing pancreatitis and acute necrotic collections. In addition, the systematic inflammatory response as a result of acute pancreatitis can progress to cause multi-organ dysfunction, including acute respiratory distress syndrome (ARDS), acute kidney injury, or cardiovascular failure [2, 10]. Hypovolemia and hypoperfusion can lead to further injury, causing pancreatic necrosis.

20.6 Goals of Therapy

Initially, the causative factor of acute pancreatitis should be identified. Adequate hydration and nutrition should be maintained to avoid hypovolemia and malnutrition. The goals of treatment involve halting the progression of the disease, including preventing pancreatic necrosis. Additionally, the aim is to avoid organ failure and systemic complications through early identification and initial management strategies. Adequate pain control for patients is also a priority. Lastly, care should emphasize risk reduction strategies to prevent long-term consequences and the onset of chronic pancreatitis. Patient education, particularly for those requiring support in alcohol cessation, should be provided [2, 5, 6].

20.7 Clinical Presentation

A pharmacist's specific approach to this disease state includes a collection of data points. Clinical presentation is typically comprised of abdominal pain and gastrointestinal symptoms with subsequent diagnostics pinpointing pancreatitis as the etiology. Abdominal pain is typically epigastric with some radiation to the back or upper quadrants. Pain is often described as sudden and severe soon after initiation (~30 min) and can persist for days [10]. The patient's ability to indicate this pain may be masked by alcohol misuse, multi-organ failure, or sedation and/or analgesic medications provided in the ICU. Nausea and vomiting are also hallmark symptoms of acute pancreatitis. Vomiting and repositioning do not relieve the abdominal pain. Signs can include a distended abdomen with decreased or absent bowel sounds in severe disease. Pancreatic inflammation and necrosis can lead to hypotension, tachycardia, and fever, as well as respiratory complications such as dyspnea and tachypnea.

Since patients can present with acute pancreatitis either at admission or as a complication of their inpatient or ICU stay, a thorough medication review of home medications and inpatient medications should be conducted. This review helps to identify medications that can also cause gastrointestinal disturbances or are known to contribute to a drug-induced etiology of this disease. The severity of the clinical presentation ranges from acute mild symptoms to shock and respiratory distress from the severe inflammatory response.

20.8 Diagnosis

20.8.1 Laboratory Tests

Abdominal pain and elevated enzyme serum concentrations, amylase or lipase at least 3× the upper limit of normal (ULN), are the standard for pancreatitis diagnosis. Serum lipase provides more sensitivity and specificity than amylase. Both enzymes are elevated around 4–8 h after injury or aggravation of disease, will peak at 24 h, and will return to normal over 1–2 weeks. However, lipase will remain elevated until inflammation resolves and has a longer half-life than amylase. These properties contribute to its superiority as a diagnostic marker [10]. Hyperamylasemia is also indicative of other non-pancreatic diseases, including parotitis, Gullo's syndrome, and celiac disease, and elevated triglycerides can interfere with the assay. Despite these limitations, amylase greater than 3× ULN is highly suggestive of pancreatitis. While the degree of enzyme elevation is related to diagnosis, they do not predict prognosis for pancreatitis. Laboratory tests with prognostic value include hematocrit, blood urea nitrogen (BUN), calcium, and C-reactive protein. The outcomes associated with these lab abnormalities are in Table 20.2.

Other laboratory tests are associated with the diagnosis of acute pancreatitis, but the specificity of the diagnosis varies. For instance, leukocytosis, hyperglycemia, and hypoalbuminemia are associated with pancreatitis but are nonspecific in comparison to other common ICU disease states. On the other hand, lab abnormalities with more specificity can reveal etiology and targets for treatment. Elevated liver transaminases, alkaline phosphatase, and bilirubin indicate gallstone pancreatitis, and elevated serum triglycerides reveal hypertriglyceridemia as an etiology. Patients presenting with hypercalcemia should also be evaluated for primary hyperparathyroidism, malignancy, or thyrotoxicosis [2].

Table 20.2 Laboratory tests with prognostic value in acute pancreatitis

Labs	Rationale
Hemoconcentration	• HCT >44% predicts severe acute pancreatitis • Failure to reverse hemoconcentration has been associated with pancreatic necrosis
Blood urea nitrogen (BUN)	• >20 or rising in first 24 h associated with increased mortality • Every 5 mg/dL increase in 24 h associated with increase in odds ratio for mortality
Hypocalcemia	• Disproportionate to hypoalbuminemia • Indication of severe necrosis
C-reactive protein	• >190 mg/dL at 48 h predicts severe acute pancreatitis

Information from [10–14]

20.8.2 *Imaging*

While not required for a clinical diagnosis of acute pancreatitis, diagnostic imaging can assist with discerning the etiology and grading severity of disease. Ultrasound imaging and magnetic resonance cholangiopancreatography (MRCP) can detect dilated biliary ducts and gallstones. Contrast-enhanced computed tomography (CECT) imaging is generally delayed around 72–96 h to avoid missing necrosis and may be helpful in diagnosing patients with lower amylase and lipase (<3× ULN) or sedated patients unable to express abdominal pain. Magnetic resonance imaging (MRI) may be required for grading severity in patients with a contraindication to CECT or to further identify biliary duct problems unable to visualize on computed tomography (CT). Finally, a CT or endoscopic ultrasonography is recommended to evaluate for pancreatic malignancy in younger patients (age <40 years) with unknown etiology of the disease [10].

20.9 Classification

After collecting the essential diagnostics, patient assessment includes classification of the severity of the disease. The Revised Atlanta classification system stratifies acute pancreatitis according to organ failure and the presence of local or systemic complications. Local complications include acute peripancreatic and pancreatic fluid collections (APFCs) or mature collections, pseudocysts, and walled-off necrosis. Mature collections occur approximately 4 weeks after persistent acute collections. Extrapancreatic local complications also include gastric outlet obstruction, splenic or portal vein thrombosis, and colonic necrosis [15]. Systemic complications include respiratory, cardiovascular, or renal failure and exacerbations of a comorbid condition, such as chronic obstructive pulmonary disease, heart failure, or chronic liver disease [16]. Mild disease does not include organ failure or complications, while moderately severe disease is characterized by transient organ failure. Severe disease is classified by persistent organ failure. Transient organ failure resolves within 48 h, with persistent enduring beyond that time frame. This classification recommends the modified Marshall scoring system to assess organ failure. This scoring tool measures respiratory status via the $PaO_2{:}FiO_2$ ratio, renal function via serum creatinine (SCr), and cardiovascular function with systolic blood pressure (SBP). Scores representing the presence of organ failure in each category include the $PaO_2{:}FiO_2$ ratio 201–300, SCr 1.9–3.6 mg/dL, and SBP <90 mmHg that is not fluid responsive [15].

A more recently developed classification system utilizes a determinant-based classification including causal events associated with severity, organ dysfunction, and necrosis. Mild disease exhibits neither of these complications, while moderate is associated with sterile necrosis and/or transient organ dysfunction. Severe disease is comprised of infected necrosis or persistent organ dysfunction, and critical disease consists of both complications [17]. As expected, prognosis and mortality

Table 20.3 Components and scoring of the BISAP tool for predicted mortality in acute pancreatitis

Scoring parameter	Points assigned
BUN >25 mg/dL	1
Impaired mental status, Glasgow Coma Scale <15	1
Evidence of systemic inflammatory response syndrome (SIRS)	1
Age >60 years old	1
Pleural effusion on imaging	1
Total score: 0–2 points—<1% mortality 3–5 points—>20% mortality	

worsen with severity, and the first and second occurrences of pancreatitis are at a higher risk for mortality than later episodes [10].

A large amount of scoring tools for predicting outcomes in acute illness exist, but many have not been evaluated for acute pancreatitis or have poor predictability. Therefore, bedside use is limited, and guidelines from the American Gastroenterological Association (AGA) recommend a combination of clinical judgment and scoring tools for assessment of disease. Guidelines endorse combining demographic (advanced age, high BMI, comorbid conditions) and clinical factors (HCT, BUN, SCr) and the presence of systemic inflammatory response syndrome (SIRS) at admission to identify patients at the greatest need for high-intensity medical care [5, 6]. One bedside scoring tool, the Bedside Index for Severity in Acute Pancreatitis (BISAP), is more practical to calculate and can be done within 24 h of presentation. The components of the BISAP scoring tool are listed in Table 20.3 [18]. In one study, this score in combination with SIRS, transient organ failure, and an algorithm for treatment shortened hospital length of stay [19].

20.10 Treatment

20.10.1 Supportive Care

Fluid resuscitation is described as the "cornerstone" of acute pancreatitis management, and intravascular depletion is exacerbated by vomiting, reduced oral intake, and peripancreatic inflammation [2]. Hypovolemia can lead to organ dysfunction including microcirculatory defects in the pancreas that can progress to necrosis; however, overall evidence for fluid therapy remains low quality [20]. Studies have targeted types of crystalloid solutions, adjunctive use of colloids, and goal-directed therapy. Differences in outcomes have been seen with lactated Ringer's solution (LR), and, theoretically, it has the benefits of reducing pancreatic acidosis and trypsin activity. In a study comparing surrogate outcomes following resuscitation with LR versus normal saline, patients on LR demonstrated reduced incidence of SIRS at 24 h and lower CRP levels [12, 14]. Data are lacking on other balanced salt solutions, but, in theory, these fluids may also be preferred compared to normal saline.

There is insufficient evidence that goal-directed therapy to a specific clinical or biochemical target such as heart rate, mean arterial pressure, or urine output prevents multisystem organ failure or mortality, but AGA guidelines recommend this strategy without specific IV fluid dosing [6]. Other guidelines recommended the following dosing strategies for crystalloids: 5–10 mL/kg/h IV until one or more resuscitation goals are met, 250–500 mL/h for 12–24 h, or 150–600 mL/h [5, 21, 22]. Following a specified strategy can lead to a large variety in the fluid rate of administration and even overresuscitation; therefore, a personalized resuscitation approach is likely optimal with bedside monitoring, etc. Colloids are not specifically addressed by guidelines as a class. However, 6% hydroxyethyl starch may increase the risk of persistent multisystem organ failure, and its use is not recommended [20].

A recent randomized controlled trial conducted by de-Madaria et al. advocates for a moderate resuscitation approach as opposed to early aggressive fluid resuscitation. In this study, patients were randomly assigned to receive either 20 mL/kg of LR solution followed by a maintenance infusion of 3 mL/kg/h or a 10 mL/kg LR intravenous bolus followed by a 1.5 mL/kg/h maintenance infusion. Fluid volumes were adjusted as necessary. The study found no difference in outcomes between the two groups, regardless of the fluid resuscitation strategy used. This study suggests that a more conservative resuscitation approach may not worsen outcomes and could potentially limit complications related to volume overload [23].

Nutrition is the second major point of emphasis early in acute pancreatitis management. Historically, the rationale behind withholding nutrition and feeding was to "rest the pancreas" and reduce stimulation; however, the focus has shifted to protecting the gut mucosal barrier, which has brought enteral nutrition back as first line of nutrition support. Enteral nutrition in comparison to total parenteral nutrition (PN) has shown a decrease in the incidence of organ failure in both mild and severe disease [20]. In patients with mild disease, oral feeding can start prior to the resolution of pain or serum enzyme elevation. If oral feeding is not tolerated at 72 h, tube feeding may be initiated. PN should be reserved for patients with paralytic ileus, obstruction, or other causes of feeding intolerance.

Questions do exist regarding the ideal route of enteral feeding, oral, nasogastric, nasojejunal, or duodenal. Currently, there is insufficient evidence to identify a preference. Nasojejunal tube feeding theoretically helps to minimize pancreatic secretion, but nasogastric and nasoduodenal feeding have shown clinical equivalence in trials and in a meta-analysis [24]. In some cases, patients may struggle with malabsorption and develop steatorrhea. Diagnostic tests can confirm exocrine pancreatic insufficiency, and pancreatic enzymes can be considered for these patients with evidence of malabsorption; however, pancreatic enzyme supplementation is not required for patients able to tolerate tube feeding without malabsorption.

Relief of pain and nausea is another target of supportive care for acute pancreatitis. Parenteral opioid analgesics are often used for pain relief with minimal evidence to support their use over other agents [25]. Adjunctive agents such as nonsteroidal anti-inflammatory drugs (NSAIDs) can play a role in mild disease in patients without a contraindication [10]. There is promising evidence for mortality reduction for epidural analgesia use compared to standard management; however, this evidence is limited [26]. Nausea relief may require parenteral antiemetics, and guidelines do not reflect a preference for agent or dosing.

20.10.2 Antimicrobial Therapy

Pancreatic and extrapancreatic infections are diagnosed often in acute pancreatitis and are significant contributing factors to morbidity and mortality. Therefore, prophylactic antibiotics have been studied in severe disease or in those with established necrotizing pancreatitis prior to a documented infection. While positive outcomes were found in one study with imipenem-cilastatin, studies conducted with higher-quality methodology failed to confirm the benefit [27, 28] and, therefore, routine antimicrobial prophylaxis should not be prescribed for patients with necrotizing pancreatitis without evidence of active infection. Despite clear guidelines recommending against this practice, antibiotics are frequently prescribed. Pharmacists can play an important role in improving antimicrobial stewardship for patients who are prescribed inappropriate antibiotics [29, 30].

The bacterial contamination in acute pancreatitis likely originates from the colon, leading to the exploration of probiotics for prevention. However, randomized controlled trials assessing the benefits of probiotics have significant heterogeneity due to the use of various probiotic strains, dosing strategies, and treatment durations, resulting in conflicting outcomes. A systematic review and meta-analysis of the use of probiotics in severe acute pancreatitis did not show any benefit in terms of infection rate or mortality with probiotic treatment [31]. Consequently, current guidelines state that probiotics cannot be routinely recommended. However, future high-quality trials may provide additional data regarding the optimal dose and duration of therapy and validate previous results [5].

Broad-spectrum antimicrobials are indicated for infected pancreatic necrosis, including coverage of enteric gram-negative and anaerobic organisms. Common pathogens may include *E. coli*, *Klebsiella* spp., *Enterobacter* spp., *Proteus* spp., and *Streptococci*. Carbapenems have been used in prophylactic antimicrobial trials and are generally regarded as an agent of choice; however, guidelines do not endorse specific agents for empiric or definitive treatment. Fluoroquinolones or third- or fourth-generation cephalosporins plus metronidazole have also been included in trials and are reasonable choices for empiric regimens [20]. These regimens are likely preferred over carbapenems, such as meropenem or imipenem, due to the risk of developing antimicrobial resistance. Empiric regimens should take into account local and institutional antibiograms and resistance patterns as well.

Antibiotics may be sufficient alone or delay the need for an invasive procedure long enough for the necrotic areas to be walled off. A mature, walled necrosis is easier to drain and debride. In unstable patients, a percutaneous drain in the collection might be necessary to continue to wait 4 weeks for collection maturation. Drainage and debridement can be done via several minimally invasive techniques and are superior to the prior surgical technique of open necrosectomy. Fungal infections are also a concern at this stage in the disease, with *Candida albicans* most frequently isolated [32]. No large trials have addressed the use of empiric antifungal agents, and guidelines have not made specific recommendations regarding agents and duration [33]. Fluconazole is a reasonable antifungal agent if yeast is identified on culture unless resistance is suspected.

Once culture and sensitivity results are available, antibiotic therapy should be tailored to the isolated organism. Antimicrobial therapy should generally continue for 7–14 days from source control.

20.10.3 Etiology-Specific Therapy

Urgent endoscopic retrograde cholangiopancreatography (ERCP) may be needed for mild or severe disease when complicated by cholangitis or persistent biliary obstruction; however, ERCP use outside of this setting is discouraged. The timing of the intervention is recommended to be 24–48 h after diagnosis to allow time for spontaneous passages of stones, yet also avoid prolonged biliary obstruction [20].

Pharmacologic treatment with fibrates, HMG-CoA reductase inhibitors, niacin, or omega-3 fatty acids may be required to treat hypertriglyceridemia-associated acute pancreatitis [2, 34]. Insulin, heparin, and apheresis/plasmapheresis have been studied as additional therapy, in particular if triglycerides are elevated above 1000 mg/dL, but the literature is limited to case reports. Lipoprotein lipase (LPL) is involved in hydrolyzing triglycerides, and insulin and heparin lead to an increase in LPL activity. Heparin use is less favored as there has been shown to be an opposing effect with depletion of LPL. Therapeutic plasma exchange (TPE) rapidly removes triglycerides from the serum [35]. These therapies may be considered in specific patients, but general recommendations for their use are limited by available evidence.

20.11 Therapeutic Outcomes and Follow-Up

While the initial management of acute pancreatitis focuses on alleviating symptoms and addressing the underlying causes, the long-term therapeutic outcomes and the importance of follow-up care play a crucial role in preventing recurrent episodes.

The primary therapeutic goals are the resolution of the acute pancreatitis episode and the prevention of complications. Timely intervention, including pain management, fluid resuscitation, and nutritional support, as described previously, contributes to the reduction of inflammation and facilitates the healing process. Effective management aims to prevent complications such as pancreatic necrosis, pseudocysts, and systemic complications like sepsis and end-organ dysfunction. Interventional procedures, including drainage of fluid collections and surgical interventions when necessary, are integral components of the therapeutic strategy.

Identifying and addressing the underlying causes of acute pancreatitis are essential for preventing recurrence. This may involve lifestyle modifications, such as alcohol cessation or dietary changes, as well as addressing gallstone-related issues through cholecystectomy. Ideally, cholecystectomy should be done early (within 24–48 h of hospitalization). If the patient presents with peripancreatic fluid collections or poor visualization, cholecystectomy may be delayed. Yet, patients should be followed closely and plan for the procedure once complications resolve [2].

Patients with alcohol-related pancreatitis are at particular risk for recurrence and developing chronic pancreatitis. These patients should be administered a brief alcohol counseling intervention before discharge and provided resources for counseling and alcohol reduction strategies [6].

Other potentially impactful interventions include counseling patients on diet and nutrition, along with weight loss. Nutritional counseling is often part of the post-acute pancreatitis care plan. Ensuring adequate enteral nutrition early in the course of the disease can mitigate malnutrition and improve overall outcomes. Emphasizing lifestyle modifications, including dietary changes, avoiding alcohol, and maintaining a healthy weight, is vital for preventing recurrent episodes. Behavioral interventions, such as smoking cessation, may also be recommended. In addition, these interventions can be particularly impactful for patients with obesity or those presenting with hypertriglyceridemia [2].

Without proper intervention and follow-up, acute pancreatitis may progress to chronic pancreatitis. Recurrence, continued tobacco use, pancreatic necrosis, and alcohol-related acute pancreatitis are risk factors for chronic pancreatitis [2]. In cases of pancreatic dysfunction, patients may require pancreatic enzyme supplementation to manage symptoms of diarrhea or steatorrhea long-term. Pancreatic insufficiency can be confirmed through pancreatic function tests.

Therapeutic success in acute pancreatitis extends beyond the immediate management of the acute episode. Long-term outcomes depend on a comprehensive approach that includes addressing the underlying causes, preventing complications, and providing sustained follow-up care. Collaborative efforts between healthcare providers, pharmacists, and patients are crucial for achieving optimal therapeutic outcomes and improving the overall quality of life for individuals recovering from acute pancreatitis.

20.12 Conclusion

In summary, the management of acute pancreatitis is a multifaceted challenge that demands a collaborative effort from healthcare professionals, with pharmacists playing a pivotal role. Acute pancreatitis most commonly results from gallstones or is alcohol induced; however, many medications have also been implicated as the cause of acute pancreatitis. Therapy revolves around appropriate fluid management, nutritional support, and pain management. Pharmacists can play a key role in addressing long-term therapeutic outcomes and providing patient education on lifestyle modifications, nutritional counseling, and follow-up care. The pharmacist's role in acute pancreatitis management remains vital, with valuable contributions from initial management through long-term care and prevention.

References

1. Boxhoorn L, Voermans RP, Bouwense SA, Bruno MJ, Verdonk RC, Boermeester MA, van Santvoort HC, Besselink MG. Acute pancreatitis. Lancet. 2020;396(10252):726–34.
2. Mederos MA, Reber HA, Girgis MD. Acute pancreatitis: a review. JAMA. 2021;325(4):382–90.
3. Schepers NJ, Bakker OJ, Besselink MG, Ahmed Ali U, Bollen TL, Gooszen HG, van Santvoort HC, Bruno MJ, Dutch Pancreatitis Study Group. Impact of characteristics of organ failure and infected necrosis on mortality in necrotising pancreatitis. Gut. 2019;68(6):1044–51.
4. Iannuzzi JP, King JA, Leong JH, Quan J, Windsor JW, Tanyingoh D, Coward S, Forbes N, Heitman SJ, Shaheen AA, Swain M, Buie M, Underwood FE, Kaplan GG. Global incidence of acute pancreatitis is increasing over time: a systematic review and meta-analysis. Gastroenterology. 2022;162(1):122–34.
5. Working Group IAP/APA Acute Pancreatitis Guidelines. IAP/APA evidence-based guidelines for the management of acute pancreatitis. Pancreatology. 2013;13(4 Suppl 2):e1–15.
6. Crockett SD, Wani S, Gardner TB, Falck-Ytter Y, Barkun AN, American Gastroenterological Association Institute Clinical Guidelines Committee. American Gastroenterological Association Institute guideline on initial management of acute pancreatitis. Gastroenterology. 2018;154(4):1096–101.
7. Wolfe D, Kanji S, Yazdi F, Barbeau P, Rice D, Beck A, Butler C, Esmaeilisaraji L, Skidmore B, Moher D, Hutton B. Drug induced pancreatitis: a systematic review of case reports to determine potential drug associations. PLoS One. 2020;15(4):e0231883.
8. Li L, Shen J, Bala MM, Busse JW, Ebrahim S, Vandvik PO, Rios LP, Malaga G, Wong E, Sohani Z, Guyatt GH, Sun X. Incretin treatment and risk of pancreatitis in patients with type 2 diabetes mellitus: systematic review and meta-analysis of randomised and non-randomised studies. BMJ. 2014;348:g2366.
9. Azoulay L, Filion KB, Platt RW, Dahl M, Dormuth CR, Clemens KK, Durand M, Hu N, Juurlink DN, Paterson JM, Targownik LE, Turin TC, Ernst P, the Canadian Network for Observational Drug Effect Studies (CNODES) Investigators, Suissa S, Dormuth CR, Hemmelgarn BR, Teare GF, Caetano P, Chateau D, Henry DA, Paterson JM, LeLorier J, Levy AR, Ernst P, Platt RW, Sketris IS. Association between incretin-based drugs and the risk of acute pancreatitis. JAMA Intern Med. 2016;176(10):1464–73.
10. Bolesta S. Pancreatitis. In: DiPiro JT, Yee GC, Haines ST, Nolin TD, Ellingrod VL, Posey L, editors. DiPiro's pharmacotherapy: a pathophysiologic approach. 12th ed. McGraw Hill; 2023. Accessed 4 Jan 2024.
11. Wu BU, Johannes RS, Sun X, Conwell DL, Banks PA. Early changes in blood urea nitrogen predict mortality in acute pancreatitis. Gastroenterology. 2009;137(1):129–35.
12. Wu BU, Bakker OJ, Papachristou GI, Besselink MG, Repas K, van Santvoort HC, Muddana V, Singh VK, Whitcomb DC, Gooszen HG, Banks PA. Blood urea nitrogen in the early assessment of acute pancreatitis: an international validation study. Arch Intern Med. 2011;171(7):669–76.
13. Stirling AD, Moran NR, Kelly ME, Ridgway PF, Conlon KC. The predictive value of C-reactive protein (CRP) in acute pancreatitis—is interval change in CRP an additional indicator of severity? HPB (Oxford). 2017;19(10):874–80.
14. Wu BU, Hwang JQ, Gardner TH, Repas K, Delee R, Yu S, Smith B, Banks PA, Conwell DL. Lactated Ringer's solution reduces systemic inflammation compared with saline in patients with acute pancreatitis. Clin Gastroenterol Hepatol. 2011;9(8):710–717.e1.

15. Banks PA, Bollen TL, Dervenis C, Gooszen HG, Johnson CD, Sarr MG, Tsiotos GG, Vege SS, Acute Pancreatitis Classification Working Group. Classification of acute pancreatitis—2012: revision of the Atlanta classification and definitions by international consensus. Gut. 2013;62(1):102–11. https://doi.org/10.1136/gutjnl-2012-302779.
16. Forsmark CE, Vege SS, Wilcox CM. Acute pancreatitis. N Engl J Med. 2016;375(20):1972–81.
17. Dellinger EP, Forsmark CE, Layer P, Lévy P, Maraví-Poma E, Petrov MS, Shimosegawa T, Siriwardena AK, Uomo G, Whitcomb DC, Windsor JA, Pancreatitis Across Nations Clinical Research and Education Alliance (PANCREA). Determinant-based classification of acute pancreatitis severity: an international multidisciplinary consultation. Ann Surg. 2012;256(6):875–80.
18. Wu BU, Johannes RS, Sun X, Tabak Y, Conwell DL, Banks PA. The early prediction of mortality in acute pancreatitis: a large population-based study. Gut. 2008;57(12):1698–703.
19. Dimagno MJ, Wamsteker EJ, Rizk RS, Spaete JP, Gupta S, Sahay T, Costanzo J, Inadomi JM, Napolitano LM, Hyzy RC, Desmond JS. A combined paging alert and web-based instrument alters clinician behavior and shortens hospital length of stay in acute pancreatitis. Am J Gastroenterol. 2014;109(3):306–15.
20. Vege SS, DiMagno MJ, Forsmark CE, Martel M, Barkun AN. Initial medical treatment of acute pancreatitis: American Gastroenterological Association Institute technical review. Gastroenterology. 2018;154(4):1103–39.
21. Tenner S, Baillie J, DeWitt J, Vege SS, American College of Gastroenterology. American College of Gastroenterology guideline: management of acute pancreatitis. Am J Gastroenterol. 2013;108(9):1400–15; 1416.
22. Yokoe M, Takada T, Mayumi T, Yoshida M, Isaji S, Wada K, Itoi T, Sata N, Gabata T, Igarashi H, Kataoka K, Hirota M, Kadoya M, Kitamura N, Kimura Y, Kiriyama S, Shirai K, Hattori T, Takeda K, Takeyama Y, Hirota M, Sekimoto M, Shikata S, Arata S, Hirata K. Japanese guidelines for the management of acute pancreatitis: Japanese guidelines 2015. J Hepatobiliary Pancreat Sci. 2015;22(6):405–32.
23. de Madaria E, Buxbaum JL, Maisonneuve P, García García de Paredes A, Zapater P, Guilabert L, Vaillo-Rocamora A, Rodríguez-Gandía MÁ, Donate-Ortega J, Lozada-Hernández EE, Collazo Moreno AJR, Lira-Aguilar A, Llovet LP, Mehta R, Tandel R, Navarro P, Sánchez-Pardo AM, Sánchez-Marin C, Cobreros M, Fernández-Cabrera I, Casals-Seoane F, Casas Deza D, Lauret-Braña E, Martí-Marqués E, Camacho-Montaño LM, Ubieto V, Ganuza M, Bolado F, ERICA Consortium. Aggressive or moderate fluid resuscitation in acute pancreatitis. N Engl J Med. 2022;387(11):989–1000.
24. Chang YS, Fu HQ, Xiao YM, Liu JC. Nasogastric or nasojejunal feeding in predicted severe acute pancreatitis: a meta-analysis. Crit Care. 2013;17(3):R118.
25. Mahapatra SJ, Jain S, Bopanna S, Gupta S, Singh P, Trikha A, Sreenivas V, Shalimar, Garg PK. Pentazocine, a kappa-opioid agonist, is better than diclofenac for analgesia in acute pancreatitis: a randomized controlled trial. Am J Gastroenterol. 2019;114(5):813–21.
26. Jabaudon M, Belhadj-Tahar N, Rimmelé T, Joannes-Boyau O, Bulyez S, Lefrant JY, Malledant Y, Leone M, Abback PS, Tamion F, Dupont H, Lortat-Jacob B, Guerci P, Kerforne T, Cinotti R, Jacob L, Verdier P, Dugernier T, Pereira B, Constantin JM, Azurea Network. Thoracic epidural analgesia and mortality in acute pancreatitis: a multicenter propensity analysis. Crit Care Med. 2018;46(3):e198–205.
27. Lim CL, Lee W, Liew YX, Tang SS, Chlebicki MP, Kwa AL. Role of antibiotic prophylaxis in necrotizing pancreatitis: a meta-analysis. J Gastrointest Surg. 2015;19(3):480–91.
28. Jiang K, Huang W, Yang XN, Xia Q. Present and future of prophylactic antibiotics for severe acute pancreatitis. World J Gastroenterol. 2012;18(3):279–84.
29. Vlada AC, Schmit B, Perry A, Trevino JG, Behrns KE, Hughes SJ. Failure to follow evidence-based best practice guidelines in the treatment of severe acute pancreatitis. HPB (Oxford). 2013;15(10):822–7.
30. Sun E, Tharakan M, Kapoor S, Chakravarty R, Salhab A, Buscaglia JM, Nagula S. Poor compliance with ACG guidelines for nutrition and antibiotics in the management of acute pancre-

atitis: a North American survey of gastrointestinal specialists and primary care physicians. JOP. 2013;14(3):221–7.
31. Gou S, Yang Z, Liu T, Wu H, Wang C. Use of probiotics in the treatment of severe acute pancreatitis: a systematic review and meta-analysis of randomized controlled trials. Crit Care. 2014;18(2):R57.
32. Sahar N, Kozarek RA, Kanji ZS, Chihara S, Gan SI, Irani S, Larsen M, Ross AS, Gluck M. The microbiology of infected pancreatic necrosis in the era of minimally invasive therapy. Eur J Clin Microbiol Infect Dis. 2018;37(7):1353–9.
33. Firsova VG, Parshikov VV, Kukosh MV, Mukhin AS. Antibacterial and antifungal therapy for patients with acute pancreatitis at high risk of pancreatogenic sepsis (review). Sovrem Tekhnologii Med. 2020;12(1):126–36.
34. Rawla P, Sunkara T, Thandra KC, Gaduputi V. Hypertriglyceridemia-induced pancreatitis: updated review of current treatment and preventive strategies. Clin J Gastroenterol. 2018;11(6):441–8.
35. Gavva C, Sarode R, Agrawal D, Burner J. Therapeutic plasma exchange for hypertriglyceridemia induced pancreatitis: a rapid and practical approach. Transfus Apher Sci. 2016;54(1):99–102.

Chapter 21
Acute Liver Failure

Sajjadh M. J. Ali and Sanjiv Chopra

21.1 Introduction

Acute liver failure (ALF) is a clinical syndrome of rapid hepatocyte injury leading to increased susceptibility to multiorgan dysfunction. The syndrome has many etiologies. However, the clinical findings are similar leading to hospitalization with infection, bleeding, and other organ complications in a matter of days [1]. Prior to the transplantation era, mortality rates used to be as high as 90% [2]. Recent improvements in critical care management and liver transplantation have helped improve survival outcomes. ALF has an onset of less than 26 weeks, and it is used to differentiate between acute and chronic liver failure.

21.2 Definition

ALF is a clinical syndrome consisting of severe hepatic injury with altered sensorium and coagulation parameters in the absence of preexisting liver disease. The accepted definition now is the development of severe acute liver injury with any degree of hepatic encephalopathy and INR >1.5 in the absence of cirrhosis or preexisting liver disease with presumed onset of less than 26 weeks [3].

S. M. J. Ali (✉)
Beth Israel Deaconess Medical Center, Boston, MA, USA
e-mail: sjawahar@bidmc.harvard.edu

S. Chopra
Beth Israel Deaconess Medical Center, Boston, MA, USA

Harvard Medical School, Boston, MA, USA

© The Author(s), under exclusive license to Springer Nature Switzerland AG 2025 571
Y. Alzaidi, M. A. Gebily (eds.), *The Pharmacist's Expanded Role in Critical Care Medicine*, https://doi.org/10.1007/978-3-031-77335-8_21

The definition may have certain exceptions. Patients with severe alcoholic hepatitis often have a long history of alcohol use prior to presentation and are considered to be acute on chronic liver failure even with the onset of less than 26 weeks. On the other hand, certain fulminant manifestations of chronic liver disease are considered to be part of ALF provided that the onset has been recognized for less than 26 weeks: reactivation of chronic hepatitis B, acute presentation of Wilson disease, and de novo presentation of autoimmune hepatitis [4].

ALF may be subclassified into hyperacute (<7 days), acute (7–21 days), and subacute (>21 days and <26 weeks). The subclassifications tend to reflect presentation, complications, and prognosis. At presentation, hyperacute subtype generally has very high transaminase levels, elevated INR, and low bilirubin, while acute/subacute subtypes are associated with lower transaminases and higher bilirubin. Hepatic encephalopathy and cerebral edema are common in hyperacute/acute subtypes, while renal failure and portal hypertension are more frequent in subacute types. Etiologies of hyperacute subtype include acetaminophen or ischemic hepatopathy, and these have better prognosis compared to etiologies of subacute subtype such as Wilson disease [1, 3].

21.3 Epidemiology

Incidence in the Western world is estimated to be 1.4–5.5 cases per million habitants per year [5]. The annual incidence in the USA is estimated at around 2000–4000 cases per year [1]. Estimated incidence of etiologies in the USA includes acetaminophen overdose of 45%, drug-induced liver injury 10%, and hepatitis B 8%. Globally, incidence of viral hepatitis causing ALF is as high as 27% for hepatitis A and 22% for hepatitis B in countries without routine immunization [1]. About 5–10% of the patients may not have an identifiable cause and may be indeterminate ALF [1].

21.4 Pathophysiology

ALF is known to be associated with two different clinicopathologic mechanisms. The first mechanism is described as a consequence to insufficient hepatic parenchyma from necrosis, resulting in inadequate detoxification, and the second mechanism is described as insufficient hepatocyte metabolic function as a result of mitochondrial toxicity [6]. Resultant histological injury patterns include zone 3 necrosis with preserved zone 1 in acetaminophen toxicity, near-complete necrosis of hepatocytes in acute hepatitis B, microvesicular steatosis with certain drugs, and central vein occlusion by loose connective tissue in veno-occlusive disease [1].

21.5 Etiology

The etiologies of ALF are described in Table 21.1. Drug-induced liver injury predominates in Western countries, while infectious causes are common in other countries.

21.5.1 Drug Induced/Toxins

Acetaminophen is the most common cause of ALF in developed countries [4]. Cases occur by accidental or intentional ingestion. The toxicity is dose dependent and is rare with therapeutic doses (up to 4 g per day in a patient without preexisting liver disease and up to 2 g a day in patients with compensated liver disease). Patients taking medications known to induce the cytochrome P450 system such as anticonvulsants and alcohol

Table 21.1 Etiology of acute liver failure

A	Acetaminophen Autoimmune Hepatitis A Adenovirus *Amanita phalloides*
B	Hepatitis B Budd-Chiari
C	Hepatitis C Carcinoma Cytomegalovirus Chickenpox (varicella zoster)
D	Drugs/toxins Hepatitis D
E	Hepatitis E Epstein-Barr virus Esoteric liver disease • Wilson • Fanconi anemia
F	Fatty infiltration Acute fatty liver of pregnancy Jamaican vomiting sickness Reye syndrome
G	"God only knows"—indeterminate or cryptogenic
H	Herpes simplex Heat stroke HELLP syndrome (hemolysis, elevated liver enzyme levels, and low platelet levels) Hepatectomy Hemophagocytic lymphohistiocytosis Hydrocarbons
I	Ischemic Idiosyncratic

can have increased liver injury due to the formation of *N*-acetyl-*p*-benzoquinoneimine (NAPQI), which is toxic to the liver [7]. Other etiologies include mushroom poisoning (often *Amanita phalloides*) commonly in patients who participate in wild mushroom picking. Reports of entire families having ALF after a meal are not uncommon in mushroom poisoning. Idiosyncratic drug reactions can also occur, which is dose independent and often occurs within 6 months of drug initiation. Common culprits include antibiotics, anticonvulsants, and NSAIDs. Herbal and dietary supplements can also cause ALF.

21.5.2 Viral

Several viruses have been associated including hepatitis A, B, C, D, and E and other viruses including herpes simplex (HSV), cytomegalovirus (CMV), adenovirus, varicella zoster (VZV), and Epstein-Barr virus (EBV) [8]. Most common causes of ALF are hepatitis A and B and herpes viruses [9]. Patients with hepatitis B can have reactivation on immunosuppression. With recent advent of biologics and chemotherapy, care must be taken to screen patients for hepatitis B before starting such medications. Hepatitis B patients may also acquire hepatitis D at the same time (co-infection) or at a later date (superinfection) and may result in ALF [10]. Hepatitis E is a significant cause of mortality up to 30% in pregnant patients [11]. Other viral causes like varicella zoster, CMV, EBV, and adenovirus can cause significant liver injury in immunocompromised patients.

21.5.3 Hypoperfusion

Ischemic hepatitis can often result in ALF occurring from systemic hypoperfusion often from shock related to sepsis or cardiogenic dysfunction. Patients can have rapidly rising transaminases and rapid improvement often within days with improving mean arterial pressures. Drugs such as cocaine and methamphetamine can cause similar presentation due to hypoperfusion. Obstruction of blood outflow can cause hypoperfusion such as in hepatic vein thrombosis (Budd-Chiari) or veno-occlusive disease. Sudden thrombosis of the three hepatic veins or IVC thrombosis can occur in Budd-Chiari syndrome associated with Behcet's syndrome. Such patients can manifest with acute liver failure when there is not enough time for the collaterals to develop [12].

21.6 Clinical Manifestations

Patients will have encephalopathy and coagulopathy by definition. Patients will often present with jaundice, fatigue, malaise, right upper quadrant tenderness associated with nausea, and vomiting. They may have ascites, anorexia, lethargy, and confusion. Patients may have asterixis signifying hepatic encephalopathy, dry mucous membranes suggestive of intravascular depletion, fevers, and rashes in infective etiologies. Kayser-Fleischer rings may be seen in Wilson disease.

Recognizing hepatic encephalopathy is key to diagnosis. Encephalopathy is classified from grade I to IV, beginning with mild changes in behaviors and alteration in sleep cycle in grade I; lethargy, confusion, and obvious behavioral changes in grade II; somnolence/stupor and incoherent speech in grade III; and coma and unresponsiveness to pain in grade IV [13]. Progressive encephalopathy can lead to fixed and dilated pupils, which is a sign of brainstem herniation.

21.7 Laboratory and Imaging

INR is greater than 1.5 by definition. Other laboratory findings include elevated aminotransferases, elevated bilirubin, elevated creatinine, hypoglycemia, acidosis, elevated ammonia levels, and LDH. Patients with sepsis may have features of disseminated intravascular coagulation including low fibrinogen and low platelets. Pregnant patients may have hypertension and features of preeclampsia and HELLP syndrome (hemolysis, elevated liver enzyme levels, and low platelet levels) such as headaches, blurred vision, thrombocytopenia, proteinuria, and microangiopathic hemolytic anemia. Testing for etiologies including acetaminophen levels, phosphatidylethanol testing for alcohol, autoimmune markers, and viral hepatitis serologies may be helpful.

Imaging findings include ascites, hepatomegaly, and splenomegaly. Initial imaging evaluation is done with Doppler ultrasound as patients may have renal injury, and CT with contrast may be avoided. Doppler can be used to evaluate vessels for evidence of hepatic vein occlusion and signs of portal hypertension besides the liver parenchyma. CT and MRI imaging are more sensitive modalities for evaluation of malignancies and thrombus, and the benefits need to be balanced against the risk of contrast-induced renal injury. An echocardiogram may help evaluate cardiac dysfunction causing hepatic ischemia or congestion. Transplant candidates may also need echocardiogram prior to being considered for transplantation.

Imaging of the head may reveal signs of cerebral edema, which include flattening of the cerebral gyri and decrease in the size of ventricles. Patients may develop signs of acute hypoxia with volume overload/decreased urine output and may have pulmonary edema on chest imaging.

Liver biopsy along with portal pressure measurements may be an option if the etiology is undetermined after initial evaluation, and benefits should be balanced with the risks of bleeding. Transjugular biopsy has lesser bleeding risk and may be preferred. Biopsy may be an important tool to diagnose malignancy and nonhepatotropic viral infections such as CMV, HSV, and EBV and for patients with suspected autoimmune hepatitis [1].

21.8 Diagnosis

By definition, patients will have signs of hepatic encephalopathy and elevated INR greater than 1.5. The etiology can be determined in most cases by a through history and clinical evaluation. Timely evaluation is of essence as it will help improve prognosis. Initial workup with laboratory and imaging should be initiated as soon as possible and should not be delayed even if the patient is being transferred to a liver transplant center.

21.9   Diagnostic Challenges

Patients with severe hepatic injury and coagulopathy but no signs of hepatic encephalopathy have severe acute hepatitis and have good prognosis. In contrast, patients with signs of hepatic encephalopathy have ALF and may need liver transplant [14]. Patients with alcohol hepatitis have a long history of alcohol use and are classified as acute on chronic liver failure [15]. Unless the patient has a concomitant injury from another etiology like acetaminophen poisoning, alcoholic hepatitis patients may not have priority listing for transplant. In patients with Wilson disease, neurologic features like choreoathetosis, ataxia, tremors, and dystonia can help differentiate from hepatic encephalopathy, and often neurologic features may predate hepatic derangements [16].

21.10   Management

Patients with ALF are better managed in liver transplant centers because of the high risk of mortality. Patients with ALF in non-transplant centers should be transferred to a transplant center at the earliest including patients who appear to be stable and are minimally encephalopathic. Some medical conditions such as heart failure and malignancy with portal vein invasion may preclude transplant, and usually the physician may discuss with a transplant hepatologist prior to transfer.

Patients with ALF are managed in the ICU. Patients unable to protect airway may be intubated. Patients are at risk of rapid brainstem herniation, and frequent clinical evaluation may be necessary. It may be reasonable to monitor patients with grade 1 encephalopathy on the medical wards if they are able to receive close monitoring with frequent neuro checks as often as every 2 h.

Frequent serial laboratory is done to monitor the patient's clinical course, usually every 4–6 h. Liver function tests, coagulation panel, complete blood counts, metabolic panel, arterial blood gases, ammonia levels, and electrolytes are usually monitored. Finger sticks are done to monitor for hyperglycemia. Ammonia levels greater than 150 µg/dL have been associated with increased risk of cerebral herniation [17].

Bilirubin and INR will downtrend with improving liver failure. While bilirubin may take weeks to normalize, INR usually improves within days. Transaminases may downtrend with recovery but should be interpreted with caution as it may also signify hepatocyte burnout leading to decreased transaminases. Bleeding complications do not correlate with INR but rather low platelet counts [18]. INR is used for prognostication, and hence, blood products such as fresh frozen plasma should be given only when there is an implicit indication [3]. Patients with ALF may also develop renal injury with low fractional excretion of sodium in urine, which is similar to hepatorenal syndrome.

Patients with ALF often have intravascular volume depletion, and adequate fluid hydration is a must. It is important to monitor closely for volume overload as it may worsen cerebral edema and respiratory failure. Fluid of choice for resuscitation is normal saline [3]. Norepinephrine is the pressor of choice in patients needing vasopressors as it has better splanchnic blood flow, and vasopressin or terlipressin can be added on as the second line [4]. In patients with septic shock, steroids can be added to supplement possible adrenal insufficiency.

N-acetylcysteine is given to patients with acetaminophen toxicity and is continued till INR persistently normalizes. It may be of benefit to patients with non-acetaminophen toxicity-related ALF, and studies have shown benefit [18–20].

Correction of INR with blood products such as fresh frozen plasma is not recommended as it may interfere with monitoring of liver function and cause fluid overload. Patients with ALF should undergo infectious workup with chest X ray and pan cultures of urine, blood, respiratory tract, and ascitic fluid, as they are at increased risk of sepsis if present. Studies have shown no benefit of prophylactic antibiotics [19]. On the other hand, patients should be started on antibiotics for evidence of active infection, clinical deterioration, and positive cultures [3, 20]. Patients at risk for fungal infections such as those receiving hemodialysis, steroids, or parenteral nutrition should have a low threshold for antifungal therapy.

Nutrition is of essence in patients with ALF as with any other critically ill patient. Adequate protein intake is necessary to prevent protein catabolism. Enteral feeding is usually adequate; if not, parenteral nutrition may be needed.

Hypoglycemia, hypokalemia, and hyponatremia are common and require appropriate management. Hypokalemia can increase renal ammonia production and should be corrected. Hypophosphatemia is also seen but does not often require repletion. Fall in phosphate is a good prognostic sign due to the increased consumption of phosphate by a regenerating liver [21].

In general, ALF patients have decreased hepatic ability to clear sedative medications, and it may mask progression of encephalopathy. Hence, long-acting sedative medications should be minimized. Nephrotoxic medications should be avoided as ALF patients usually have renal injury.

21.10.1   Etiology-Specific Management

As discussed, *N*-acetylcysteine (NAC) is the treatment of choice in patients with acetaminophen toxicity, and severe hepatotoxicity is uncommon if administered within 10 h [22]. Sometimes, acetaminophen toxicity may not be apparent especially with concomitant alcohol use and CYP inducers like anticonvulsants, and there should be a low threshold for NAC drip. Hepatitis B patients will benefit from antiviral therapy. Similarly, HSV patients will benefit from acyclovir [3].

Patients with Budd-Chiari should be planned for TIPS placement, thrombolysis, or surgical decompression for hepatic outflow. Primary treatment of acute fatty liver of pregnancy includes early delivery of the fetus [3]. In patients with Wilson disease, plasma exchange to remove copper may help as a standby measure prior to liver transplant. Patients with autoimmune hepatitis with ALF usually proceed towards liver transplant. Steroids may be trialed in autoimmune hepatitis patients without hepatic encephalopathy [3]. In patients with *Amanita phalloides* poisoning, early administration of charcoal helps bind to toxins and improves survival. Silibinin is beneficial, but it may not be widely available. Penicillin G is another treatment for *Amanita phalloides* [23].

21.11 Complications

21.11.1 Neurological

Ammonia plays a central role in hepatic encephalopathy by causing glutamine-related osmotic cerebral edema, oxidative stress, and mitochondrial dysfunction [4]. Patients may have mild confusion to cerebral edema and raised intracranial pressure leading to brainstem herniation. Continuous renal replacement therapy (CRRT) is beneficial to remove ammonia and manage fluid balance and metabolic abnormalities. Patients should have a low threshold for being started on CRRT especially with increasing ammonia levels even in the absence of acute kidney injury [24]. Seizures may be common, and EEG may be used to monitor seizures. Phenytoin is the first-line medication for seizures, and short-acting benzodiazepines may be used as second line [3].

Cerebral edema is common in grade III and IV hepatic encephalopathy. Raised intracranial pressure elevation and brainstem herniation are one of the common causes of mortality in ALF, and liver transplant is the only definitive treatment. Cushing's triad of hypertension, bradycardia, and irregular respiration are the signs of raised ICP. ICP monitoring may be done in patients at high risk of cerebral edema. The benefits of ICP monitoring have to be balanced against the risk of infection and bleeding. ICP is usually monitored with spinal or cranial catheters. Noninvasive methods being studied include transcranial Doppler and optic nerve sheath diameter [1]. ICP elevation prevention includes optimizing fluid balance to avoid overhydration, hypertonic saline, elevation of head of bed to 30°, and minimizing sensory stimulation/agitation [1]. Hypertonic saline (3%) helps in the induction of hypernatremia with a goal of 145–150 mEq/L. This may decrease water influx to the brain, thereby reducing cerebral edema [25].

Treatment of ICP elevation includes mannitol and hyperventilation to reduce ICP below 20–25 mmHg. Hyperosmotic agents like mannitol are first-line therapy. Rebound ICP elevation and renal injury may occur with mannitol. It may lead to fluid retention and oliguria, and fluid should be removed by CRRT. Hyperventilation is used for patients with impending herniation. Decreasing $PaCO_2$ to 25–30 mmHg via hyperventilation helps in vasoconstriction and fall in ICP. Other therapies include induction of hypothermia with targeted temperature management, barbiturate coma with pentobarbital or thiopental, and use of indomethacin [1, 3].

21.11.2 Renal

Acute renal failure is common in up to 70% of patients, and about 30% may require CRRT [26]. Once renal failure develops, prognosis is poor without liver transplantation. Early initiation of CRRT such as continuous venovenous hemofiltration may be better tolerated than HD due to hemodynamics. Early initiation of CRRT improves outcomes [1].

21.11.3 Pulmonary

Endotracheal intubation should not be delayed especially in patients who are unable to maintain airway. Lung-protective ventilation with low PEEP and low tidal volumes may help minimize barotrauma [1].

21.12 Liver Transplant

Liver transplant is beneficial to patients with low chances of recovery. Patients should be monitored closely, and it is often clinical judgment that helps transplant hepatologists to decide. Patients with ALF are listed as Status 1A which is priority listing for transplant in the USA. Patients who recover spontaneously may avoid lifelong immunosuppression with transplant. Important prognostic factors for ALF include the severity of encephalopathy, age, and etiology. Patients less than 10 years of age or more than 40 years have lower likelihood of spontaneous recovery. In a study of 308 patients, etiologies like acetaminophen toxicity, hepatitis A, ischemia, and pregnancy-related ALF had >50% transplant-free survival rate as compared to less than <25% for patients with hepatitis B, autoimmune hepatitis, cancer, or indeterminate causes [27]. In patients who undergo transplant, survival rates are around 70–90% at 1 year [28, 29].

21.13 Prognostic Models

King's College Criteria and Model for End-Stage Liver Disease (MELD) score have been used to predict outcomes [30]. MELD 3.0 score uses serum bilirubin, creatinine, INR, sodium, albumin, and sex. King's College Criteria use different predictors based on the etiology being acetaminophen versus non-acetaminophen toxicity. In acetaminophen-based toxicity, criteria for referral for liver transplant include arterial pH <7.30 irrespective of the grade of encephalopathy or grade III/ IV encephalopathy with prothrombin time >100 s and creatinine >3.4 mg/dL. In non-acetaminophen toxicity, criteria for referral include PT >100 s irrespective of the grade of encephalopathy and any three of the criteria: age <10 or >40 years, PT >50 s, serum bilirubin >18 mg/dL, duration of jaundice before encephalopathy more than 7 days, and unfavorable etiology such as non-A and non-B viral hepatitis, idiosyncratic drug reactions, and Wilson disease.

21.14　Extracorporeal Liver Support

A number of approaches are being studied as a bridge from ALF to liver transplant or spontaneous liver recovery. Artificial devices use selective membranes of various pore sizes and affinities to remove toxins from blood, whereas bioartificial devices incorporate hepatocytes into a bioactive platform for endogenous hepatic function [1].

CRRT could be considered as the basic form of artificial devices. Therapeutic plasma exchange (PLEX) has been shown to improve transplant-free survival in studies [31]. Limitations of PLEX include increased risk of infection from treatment-induced immunosuppression and removing coagulopathy as a prognostic marker [4]. Molecular adsorbent systems (MARS) may be helpful in ALF patients, and it works by removing water-soluble and protein-bound toxins. A novel artificial multiorgan replacement system (AMOR) has shown good results in a limited study, and larger studies may be needed [32]. Bioartificial devices have failed to show survival benefits in studies. However, future bioartificial devices under development with production of high quality of human hepatocytes may show promise [1].

References

1. Stravitz RT, Fontana RJ, Karvellas C, Durkalski V, McGuire B, Rule JA, et al. Future directions in acute liver failure. Hepatology. 2023;78(4):1266–89.
2. Rakela J, Mosley JW, Edwards VM, Govindarajan S, Alpert E. A double-blinded, randomized trial of hydrocortisone in acute hepatic failure. The Acute Hepatic Failure Study Group. Dig Dis Sci. 1991;36(9):1223–8.
3. Lee WM, Stravitz TR, Larson AM. Introduction to the revised American Association for the Study of Liver Diseases position paper on acute liver failure 2011. Hepatology. 2012;55(3):965–7.
4. Vasques F, Cavazza A, Bernal W. Acute liver failure. Curr Opin Crit Care. 2022;28(2):198–207.
5. Chayanupatkul M, Schiano TD. Acute liver failure secondary to drug-induced liver injury. Clin Liver Dis. 2020;24(1):75–87.
6. Lefkowitch JH. The pathology of acute liver failure. Adv Anat Pathol. 2016;23(3):144–58.
7. Devarbhavi H. An update on drug-induced liver injury. J Clin Exp Hepatol. 2012;2(3):247–59.

8. Lee WM. Etiologies of acute liver failure. Semin Liver Dis. 2008;28(2):142–52.

9. Little L, Rule J, Peng L, Gottfried M, Lee WM, the Acute Liver Failure Study Group. Herpes simplex virus–associated acute liver failure often goes unrecognized. Hepatology. 2019;69(2):917–9.

10. Odenwald MA, Paul S. Viral hepatitis: past, present, and future. World J Gastroenterol. 2022;28(14):1405–29.

11. Pérez-Gracia MT, Suay-García B, Mateos-Lindemann ML. Hepatitis E and pregnancy: current state. Rev Med Virol. 2017;27(3):e1929.

12. Seyahi E, Caglar E, Ugurlu S, Kantarci F, Hamuryudan V, Sonsuz A, et al. An outcome survey of 43 patients with Budd–Chiari syndrome due to Behçet's syndrome followed up at a single, dedicated center. Semin Arthritis Rheum. 2015;44(5):602–9.

13. Weissenborn K. Hepatic encephalopathy: definition, clinical grading and diagnostic principles. Drugs. 2019;79(Suppl 1):5–9.

14. Gill RQ, Sterling RK. Acute liver failure. J Clin Gastroenterol. 2001;33(3):191–8.

15. Ballester MP, Sittner R, Jalan R. Alcohol and acute-on-chronic liver failure. J Clin Exp Hepatol. 2022;12(5):1360–70.

16. Bandmann O, Weiss KH, Kaler SG. Wilson's disease and other neurological copper disorders. Lancet Neurol. 2015;14(1):103–13.

17. Tofteng F, Hauerberg J, Hansen BA, Pedersen CB, Jørgensen L, Larsen FS. Persistent arterial hyperammonemia increases the concentration of glutamine and alanine in the brain and correlates with intracranial pressure in patients with fulminant hepatic failure. J Cereb Blood Flow Metab. 2006;26(1):21–7.

18. Stravitz RT, Ellerbe C, Durkalski V, Schilsky M, Fontana RJ, Peterseim C, et al. Bleeding complications in acute liver failure. Hepatology. 2018;67(5):1931–42.

19. Karvellas CJ, Cavazos J, Battenhouse H, Durkalski V, Balko J, Sanders C, et al. Effects of antimicrobial prophylaxis and blood stream infections in patients with acute liver failure: a retrospective cohort study. Clin Gastroenterol Hepatol. 2014;12(11):1942–1949.e1.

20. European Association for the Study of the Liver, Clinical practice guidelines panel, Wendon, Panel members, Cordoba J, Dhawan A, et al. EASL Clinical Practical Guidelines on the management of acute (fulminant) liver failure. J Hepatol. 2017;66(5):1047–81.

21. Baquerizo A, Anselmo D, Shackleton C, Chen TW, Cao C, Weaver M, et al. Phosphorus as an early predictive factor in patients with acute liver failure. Transplantation. 2003;75(12):2007–14.

22. Green J, Heard K, Reynolds K, Albert D. Oral and intravenous acetylcysteine for treatment of acetaminophen toxicity: a systematic review and meta-analysis. West J Emerg Med. 2013;14(3):218–26.

23. Ye Y, Liu Z. Management of Amanita phalloides poisoning: a literature review and update. J Crit Care. 2018;46:17–22.

24. Nanchal R, Subramanian R, Karvellas CJ, Hollenberg SM, Peppard WJ, Singbartl K, et al. Guidelines for the management of adult acute and acute-on-chronic liver failure in the ICU: cardiovascular, endocrine, hematologic, pulmonary, and renal considerations. Crit Care Med. 2020;48(3):e173–91.

25. Murphy N, Auzinger G, Bernel W, Wendon J. The effect of hypertonic sodium chloride on intracranial pressure in patients with acute liver failure. Hepatology. 2004;39(2):464–70.

26. Rovegno M, Vera M, Ruiz A, Benítez C. Current concepts in acute liver failure. Ann Hepatol. 2019;18(4):543–52.

27. Ostapowicz G. Results of a prospective study of acute liver failure at 17 tertiary care centers in the United States. Ann Intern Med. 2002;137(12):947.

28. Reddy KR, Ellerbe C, Schilsky M, Stravitz RT, Fontana RJ, Durkalski V, et al. Determinants of outcome among patients with acute liver failure listed for liver transplantation in the United States. Liver Transpl. 2016;22(4):505–15.

29. Germani G, Theocharidou E, Adam R, Karam V, Wendon J, O'Grady J, et al. Liver transplantation for acute liver failure in Europe: outcomes over 20 years from the ELTR database. J Hepatol. 2012;57(2):288–96.

30. Mishra A, Rustgi V. Prognostic models in acute liver failure. Clin Liver Dis. 2018;22(2):375–88.
31. Larsen FS, Schmidt LE, Bernsmeier C, Rasmussen A, Isoniemi H, Patel VC, et al. High-volume plasma exchange in patients with acute liver failure: an open randomised controlled trial. J Hepatol. 2016;64(1):69–78.
32. Ahmad S, Novokhodko A, Liou IW, Smith NC, Carithers RL, Reyes J, et al. Development and first clinical use of an extracorporeal artificial multiorgan system in acute-on-chronic liver failure patients. ASAIO J. 2024;70:690. https://doi.org/10.1097/MAT.0000000000002174.

Chapter 22
Decompensated Cirrhosis

Mauro Bernardi and Giacomo Zaccherini

22.1   Liver Cirrhosis: Essential Epidemiology

Liver cirrhosis is a potentially fatal disease diffused worldwide. It is the 11th most common cause of death, accounting for more than one million deaths per year [1]. The principal causes of cirrhosis are excessive alcohol intake; chronic infection from hepatitis C, B, and D viruses; and metabolic-associated liver disease due to obesity and type 2 diabetes mellitus, whose relative prevalence varies throughout the world regions. There are also several other etiologies due to genetic predisposition or autoimmunity, whose enumeration is beyond the scope of this chapter.

22.2   Natural History of Cirrhosis

The course of liver cirrhosis develops through subsequent stages that, in turn, are associated with progressive pathological events, clinical manifestations, and likelihood of mortality [2, 3]. Cirrhosis is the result of the evolution of progressing chronic liver diseases, irrespective of their etiology, and consists of the disruption of hepatic architecture due to diffuse fibrosis, disorganized regenerative nodules, microvascular alterations such as sinusoid capillarization and vessel occlusion, and parenchymal extinction [4, 5]. These abnormalities lead to portal hypertension due to increased intrahepatic vascular resistance and enhanced splanchnic inflow favored by arterial vasodilation in this vascular district [6, 7]. At this initial stage, despite the occurrence of these events, cirrhosis usually

M. Bernardi (✉) · G. Zaccherini
Department of Medical and Surgical Sciences, Alma Mater Studiorum—University of Bologna, Bologna, Italy
e-mail: mauro.bernardi@unibo.it

Y. Alzaidi, M. A. Gebily (eds.), *The Pharmacist's Expanded Role in Critical Care Medicine*, https://doi.org/10.1007/978-3-031-77335-8_22

remains asymptomatic and is defined as *compensated*, with an estimated mortality of 1% per year. Above a hepatic venous pressure gradient of 10 mmHg, portal hypertension leads to the formation of venous portosystemic shunts, among which esophageal, gastric, and rectal varices are the most frequent and clinically relevant (stage 2). Compensated cirrhosis remains asymptomatic, but the estimated annual mortality rises to 3.4%. The occurrence of clinically relevant complications, represented by ascites formation, bleeding from gastro-esophageal varices, development of hepatic encephalopathy, and progressive jaundice, heralds *decompensation*, beyond which cirrhosis becomes a systemic disease and 1-year mortality increases strikingly: in stage 3, characterized by either ascites formation or variceal bleeding, the estimated mortality is 20% and reaches 57% in stage 4, characterized by the simultaneous presence of ascites and bleeding. Patients with decompensated cirrhosis often suffer from bacterial infections and are prone to develop renal dysfunction. These conditions identify stage 5, whose 1-year mortality reaches 67%.

The course of decompensated cirrhosis often accelerates because of the acute development of one or more main complications within less than 2 weeks, such as clinically relevant ascites, overt hepatic encephalopathy, acute gastrointestinal bleeding, and acute bacterial infection. This condition is called *acute decompensation*, requires hospitalization, and often presents extrahepatic organ or system dysfunction and failure [8, 9]. Acute decompensation is defined as stable if it does not require rehospitalization within 3 months, unstable if at least one rehospitalization is needed, and pre-acute-on-chronic liver failure (ACLF) if ACLF occurs in the follow-up. Three- and 12-month mortality varies from 0% to 9.5%, respectively, in stable acute decompensation; 21% to 35.6% in the unstable type; 53.7% to 67.4% in patients developing ACLF.

According to the definition of the Chronic Liver Failure Consortium of the European Association of the Study of the Liver (EASL), ACLF results from the development of organ or system failure, including liver, kidney, brain, circulation, coagulation, and lung, and occurs in about 1/3 of patients with acute decompensation [10]. The presence of organ failure is identified by a SOFA score [11] specifically modified to fit the context of decompensated cirrhosis (Tables 22.1 and 22.2). ACLF is graded from 1 to 3 according to the number of organs or systems failing, from 1 to ≥3. To be noted, kidney failure is the sole organ failure that identifies ACLF grade 1. The other organ/system failures need the simultaneous presence of kidney dysfunction or mild hepatic encephalopathy. The 28- and 90-day mortality ranges from 23.3% to 40.8% in grade 1, 31.2% to 55.2% in grade 2, and 74.5% to 78.4% in grade 3.

From this succinct description, it emerges that patients affected by decompensated cirrhosis often develop clinical conditions that make them critically ill and at risk of short-term mortality. The following paragraphs will deal with the management of the most ominous complications that can jeopardize their survival. However, a brief presentation of the main aspects of the pathophysiological substrate of decompensated cirrhosis is necessary before addressing these topics.

Table 22.1 The CLIF-SOFA score

ORGAN / SYSTEM	0	1	2	3	4
Liver (*bilirubin, mg/dl*)	<1.2	≥1.2 to <2.0	≥2.0 to <6.0	≥6.0 to <12.0	≥12.0
Kidney (*creatinine, mg/dl*)	<1.2	≥1.2 to <2.0	≥2.0 to <3.5	≥3.5 to <5.0	≥5.0
Cerebral (*HE grade*)	absence of HE	I	II	III	IV
Coagulation (*INR*)	<1.1	≥1.1 to <1.25	≥1.25 to <1.5	≥1.5 to <2.5	≥2.5 or platelet count ≤20 x 10^9/L
Circulation (*MAP, mmHg*)	≥70	<70	Dopamine ≤5 or Dobutamine or Terlipressin	Dopamine >5 or Epinephrine ≤0.1 or Norepinephrine ≤0.1	Dopamine >15 or Epinephrine >0.1 or Norepinephrine >0.1
Lungs (*PaO2/FiO2 or SpO2/FiO2*)	>400 >512	>300 to ≤400 >357 to ≤512	>200 to ≤300 > 214 to ≤357	>100 to ≤200 >89 to ≤214	≤100 ≤89

Gray areas indicate organ/system failure
Dosages of vasoactive drugs are expressed as µg/kg/min
Abbreviations: *HE* hepatic encephalopathy, *MAP* mean arterial pressure, *PaO2* partial pressure of oxygen, *SpO2* oxygen saturation, *FiO2* fraction of inspired oxygen, *RRT* renal replacement therapy

Table 22.2 The simplified CLIF-SOFA score

ORGAN / SYSTEM	1	2	3
Liver (*bilirubin, mg/dl*)	<6.0	≥6.0 to <12.0	≥12
Kidney (*creatinine, mg/dl*)	<1.5 >1.5 to <2.0	≥2.0 to <3.5	≥3.5 or use of RRT
Cerebral (*HE grade*)	Absence of HE	I-II	III-IV or intubation
Coagulation (*INR*)	<2.0	≥2.0 to <2.5	≥2.5
Circulation (*MAP, mmHg*)	≥70	<70	Use of vasopressors
Lungs (*PaO2/FiO2 or SpO2/FiO2*)	>300 >357	>200 to ≤300 >214 to ≤357	≤200 ≤214 or mechanical ventilation

Light gray areas indicate organ/system dysfunction. Heavy gray areas indicate organ/system dysfunction
Dosages of vasoactive drugs are expressed as µg/kg/min
Abbreviations: *HE* hepatic encephalopathy, *MAP* mean arterial pressure, *PaO2* partial pressure of oxygen, *SpO2* oxygen saturation, *FiO2* fraction of inspired oxygen, *RRT* renal replacement therapy

22.3 Pathophysiology of Decompensated Cirrhosis: The Essentials

For decades, we have been used to consider the pathophysiological background of decompensated cirrhosis as the expression of peripheral arterial vasodilation mainly occurring in the splanchnic circulatory area due to the development of portal hypertension. The clinical expression of these events is a hyperdynamic circulatory syndrome characterized by reduced arterial pressure, tachycardia, and increased cardiac output. Arterial vasodilation can reach an extent that endangers effective volemia despite the activation of vasoconstrictor and sodium- and water-retaining systems, such as the renin-aldosterone axis, sympathetic nervous system, and secretion of arginine-vasopressin [12, 13]. Altogether, these events account for some cardinal features of decompensated cirrhosis, such as renal sodium and water retention leading to ascites formation and hyponatremia, reduced renal perfusion, impaired cardiovascular responsiveness to physiological and pharmacological stimuli, and increased susceptibility to shock.

Over the last decade, research activity enlightened the primary causes of the just-described abnormalities, even though other pathophysiological events still need clarification. Now, it is clear that the pathophysiological background of decompensated cirrhosis is characterized by a systemic inflammatory and prooxidant *milieu* [6, 14]. The systemic spread of pathogen-associated molecular patterns (PAMPs) due to abnormal translocation from the gut- and damage-associated molecular patterns (DAMPs) released by the liver because of local inflammation and cell necrosis, after recognition by specific receptors, the innate recognition receptors, activates immune cells that produce proinflammatory cytokines and chemokines, along with reactive oxygen and nitrogen species. This cascade of events contributes to the development of splanchnic arterial vasodilation and circulatory dysfunction, and both favor multiorgan dysfunction and failure (Fig. 22.1). Another aspect that waits for clarification is the role of immune metabolism [9, 15]. Indeed, the sustained activation of the immune cells enhances their energetic demand, so that the immune tissue can be prioritized for body nutrient allocation at the expense of nonimmune cells. The latter may adapt to nutrient scarcity by reducing mitochondrial oxidative phosphorylation and, therefore, ATP production contributing to organ dysfunction or failure.

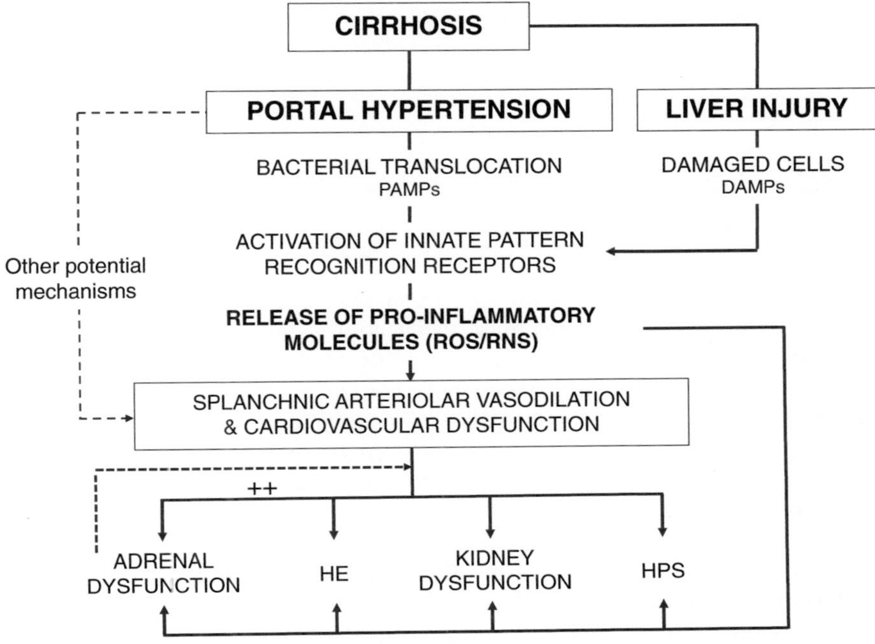

Fig. 22.1 Schematic representation of the pathophysiological background of advanced cirrhosis. *Abbreviations*: *PAMPs* pathogen-associated molecular patterns, *DAMPs* damage-associated molecular patterns. *ROS* reactive oxygen species, *RNS* reactive nitrogen species, *HE* hepatic encephalopathy, *HPS* hepato-pulmonary syndrome. (*Drawn from* [14])

22.4 Bleeding from Esophagogastric Varices

22.4.1 Introduction

Acute bleeding from esophageal and gastric varices is the most frequent type of upper gastrointestinal hemorrhage in patients with cirrhosis and portal hypertension [16]. Even though acute variceal bleeding mortality has substantially declined in the last decades, still overall in-hospital mortality can reach 20–30% [17]. The most relevant risk factors for variceal bleeding-induced mortality are the severity of cirrhosis, as assessed by Child-Pugh grade C[1] or MELD score[2] >20, and the development of extrahepatic organ failure [18]. Therefore, patients with ACLF are more at risk in case of acute variceal bleeding.

22.4.2 Mainstays for the Management of Acute Variceal Bleeding

Tissue perfusion requires immediate volume expansion with colloids and crystalloids, with the target to maintain mean arterial pressure above 65 mmHg. Advanced cirrhosis, especially during acute decompensation episodes, presents a complex hemostasis abnormality whose consequence is the disruption of the balance between impaired and enhanced coagulation activity [19] (see also Sect. 22.5). For this reason, routine fresh frozen plasma infusion should be avoided. The hemoglobin level achieved by blood transfusion should not exceed 7–8 g/dL [20].

Portal hypertension is the main factor favoring variceal rupture. Therefore, the pharmacological approach consists of drugs able to reduce it by promoting splanchnic arterial vasoconstriction [21]. The vasopressin analogue terlipressin is an effective drug, which can improve survival. However, the presence of cardiovascular diseases contraindicates its use. Then, somatostatin, which exerts a local mesenteric vasoconstrictive effect by inhibiting glucagon release, or its analogues octreotide and vapreotide can be employed. These treatments should start immediately and continue for 5 days after endoscopy. From 22% to 66% of patients with cirrhosis and acute variceal bleeding develop bacterial infections. Therefore, short-term antibiotic prophylaxis is recommended despite the risk of antibiotic resistance because there is evidence that it reduces the risk of infection and improves short-term survival [22]. Most studies employed quinolones or cephalosporin; the latter is preferred in patients with decompensated cirrhosis. However, the knowledge of the local microbial ecosystem and microbial stewardship assumes great relevance (see also Sect. 22.7).

---

[1] The Child-Pugh score is a system designed to predict mortality in patients with cirrhosis. It is articulated into three classes (A–C) indicating a progressive mortality risk. The parameters employed to assess classes are serum total bilirubin, serum albumin, prothrombin time (or INR), presence of ascites, and presence of hepatic encephalopathy. There are several online calculators for the Child-Pugh score. Among them: https://www.mdcalc.com/calc/340/child-pugh-score-cirrhosis-mortality

[2] The model for end-stage liver disease (MELD) is a numerical scale ranging from 6 to 40 originally designed to stratify cirrhosis severity in patients over 12 years enlisted for liver transplantation. It has become a universally used scoring system to predict the prognosis of patients with liver cirrhosis independently from being a candidate for liver transplantation. The parameters employed to assess classes are serum total bilirubin, INR for prothrombin time, and serum creatinine. There are several online calculators for the MELD score. Among them: https://www.mdcalc.com/calc/78/meld-score-model-end-stage-liver-disease-12-older

Endoscopy aims at stopping bleeding and should be performed as soon as possible, possibly in an intensive or emergency environment. Massive bleedings require orotracheal intubation and mechanical ventilation. Band ligation and sclerotherapy of the bleeding vessel are both effective, but band ligation ensures better bleeding control, improved survival, and fewer adverse events [21]. Cyanoacrylate is indicated to obliterate bleeding gastric varices [23].

22.4.3 The Role of Transjugular Portosystemic Shunt (TIPS[3]) in Patients with Acute Variceal Bleeding

Despite the improvement in pharmacological and endoscopic treatment of acute variceal bleeding, from 10% to 20% of patients experience treatment failure with continuous or early rebleeding, ominous events with an elevated short-term risk for severe complications, and death. Factors favoring treatment failure include the severity of cirrhosis, ongoing renal failure, bacterial infection, and active bleeding at endoscopy [24]. ACLF, as could be expected, further increases the probability of early rebleeding [8, 25].

To prevent treatment failure and its consequences, current guidelines recommend the placement of preemptive TIPS within 24–72 h from hospital admission in high-risk patients with cirrhosis [21, 26]. Child-Pugh score >7 and active bleeding at endoscopy or Child-Pugh class C (score <14) are the criteria to identify the candidates for this procedure, which improves patient survival [27]. More recent studies showed preemptive TIPS being also effective in patients with ACLF grade 1 or 2 [8, 25, 28]. In this context, both short- and long-term mortality could be reduced by 50%.

When endoscopic treatments or preemptive TIPS cannot immediately take place, salvage therapy aims at bridging patients with massive bleeding and hemodynamic instability to appropriate treatments. Balloon tamponade of esophageal (Sengstaken-Blakemore tube) or gastric (Linton tube) varices may help stop bleeding but should be put in place after patient intubation to avoid aspiration. A self-expanding esophageal metal stent is an alternative for bleeding esophageal varices, but its employment is still limited [29].

---

[3] The transjugular intrahepatic portosystemic shunt (TIPS) is a procedure creating a side-to-side shunt between the portal and hepatic (usually right) vein to reduce portal vein pressure. The shunt connects these veins by a self-expandable metal stent positioned via the jugular vein.

22.5 Abnormalities of Hemostasis

22.5.1 Introduction

The finding of prolonged prothrombin time and thrombocytopenia led to the traditional concept that patients with cirrhosis and portal hypertension are at increased risk of bleeding, which progresses in parallel with the severity of the disease. As a result, prophylactic and therapeutic use of fresh frozen plasma, concentrated platelet transfusion, and prothrombin complex concentrates became frequently employed in clinical practice. However, in the last decade, a different scenario emerged, and the concept of "rebalanced hemostasis" in cirrhosis replaced that of anticoagulative status, leading to relevant modifications in the approach to hemostasis abnormalities of advanced cirrhosis.

Indeed, we should consider that some hemorrhagic events, such as variceal or intraoperative bleeding, depend on portal hypertension or surgical techniques, respectively, rather than hemostatic deficiencies. Therefore, routine prophylactic or therapeutic administration of procoagulant treatments is unjustified. Hemostasis abnormalities are instead involved in hemorrhagic events such as oozing from venipuncture, bruising, and spontaneous mucosal bleeding [30].

22.5.2 Essential Pathophysiology

The concept of rebalanced hemostasis (Fig. 22.2) in cirrhosis leans on the findings that impaired hemostasis is limited or corrected by enhanced prohemostatic pathways. In advanced cirrhosis, impaired hepatic protein synthesis decreases the availability of most procoagulant factors. However, the same abnormality also involves anticoagulants such as antithrombin and protein C. As a result, thrombin generation can occur, as shown by in vitro tests. Similarly, due to the endothelial activation occurring in advanced cirrhosis, the increased availability of von Willebrand factor, which favors platelet adhesion and aggregation, and factor VIII counteracts the effects deriving from thrombocytopenia [31, 32].

The reach of rebalance does not mean that hemostasis is firmly restored. In contrast, the hemostatic system remains unstable due to the deficiencies involving both pro- and antihemostatic factors. Such instability increases in parallel with the severity of cirrhosis, peaking in ACLF, and is easily disrupted towards hemorrhage or thrombosis by intercurrent events, among which sepsis or acute kidney injury seems to exert the most relevant consequences [33, 34].

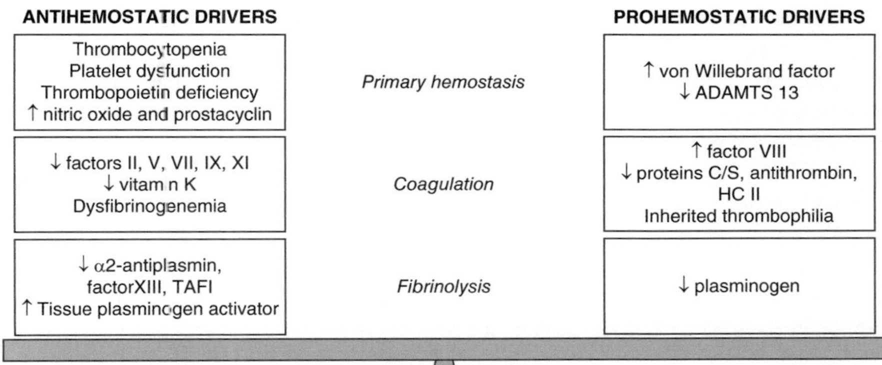

Fig. 22.2 Schematic representation of the rebalanced hemostasis in advanced cirrhosis. The changes in prohemostatic drivers balance the alterations occurring in antihemostatic drivers. *Abbreviations*: *TAFI* thrombin activatable fibrinolysis inhibitor, *ADAMST* a disintegrin and metalloproteinase with thrombospondin motifs, *HC* heparin cofactor II. (*Drawn from* [31])

22.5.3   *Prevention of Bleeding*

The fear of provoking bleeding secondary to invasive maneuvers in patients with advanced cirrhosis led to the widespread use of prophylactic treatments, mainly fresh frozen plasma and platelet concentrates. However, proof of the efficacy of these approaches is lacking, and the improved knowledge of the pathophysiology underlying hemostasis abnormalities does not justify them. Namely, the bleeding risk from procedures like paracentesis or thoracentesis, endoscopic variceal ligation, and venous and arterial catheterization present a low bleeding risk [30, 35].

A relevant aspect is the scarce reliability of routine tests assessing the coagulative status when employed in patients with advanced cirrhosis. The international normalized ratio (INR) relies on prothrombin time, which is influenced by procoagulant factors I, II, V, VII, and X, but does not perceive the deficiency of anticoagulation factors such as protein C. Therefore, an altered INR value in a patient with cirrhosis does not necessarily mean impaired coagulation. Thromboelastography (TEG) provides more comprehensive information about the status of pro- and anticoagulant pathways and detects hyperfibrinolysis or premature clot dissolution. Long employed during liver transplant surgery, TEG was used in patients with cirrhosis and significant coagulopathy based on INR assessment as a guide to bleeding prophylaxis with fresh frozen plasma or platelet concentrates. TEG-guided transfusion strategy significantly reduced blood product use compared to INR-guided transfusion without increasing the occurrence of bleeding complications [36].

Among patients admitted to intensive care, bleeding was more frequent in patients with cirrhosis than in those without and was associated with severe reductions in plasma fibrinogen concentration and platelet count [37]. The target values of fibrinogen plasma concentration and platelet count to be achieved before invasive procedures are not clearly defined. However, there is general agreement that platelet count of $50 \times 10^9/L$ and plasma fibrinogen concentration of 1.2 g/L ensure adequate protection from bleeding and should be achieved in patients showing severely impaired platelet count ($<20 \times 10^9/L$) and plasma fibrinogen (<1 g/L) [32, 38]. The use of prothrombin complex concentrates or thrombopoietin receptor agonists is generally discouraged because of their thrombotic risk in the context of the unstable hemostatic balance of advanced cirrhosis.

22.5.4 Treatment of Bleeding

Bleeding provoked by invasive procedures first requires local measures. In these contexts, interventional radiology is often resolutive. Fresh frozen plasma administration in variceal bleeding should be avoided, as there is evidence that volume expansion can fuel portal hypertension and prolong the bleeding. In both provoked and unprovoked bleeding associated with severe reductions in platelet count or coagulation factors, replacement treatments (see previous paragraph) can be considered and monitored using thromboelastography of other viscoelastic tests.

In patients developing hyperfibrinolysis, antifibrinolytic drugs such as e-aminocaproic acid and tranexamic acid can be employed [39] under close monitoring with viscoelastic tests.

22.5.5 Venous Thrombosis

Because of the unstable hemostasis balance, patients with cirrhosis are at risk of developing thrombosis besides the risk of bleeding. The awareness of this condition led to the progressive use of venous thromboembolism prophylaxis with fractionated heparins once their bleeding risk in patients with cirrhosis was convincingly excluded [40].

About 8% of patients with cirrhosis and portal hypertension per year develop portal vein thrombosis, which can extend to portal vein tributaries [41]. This event favors variceal bleeding and may negatively influence the progression of the disease. Treatment of portal vein thrombosis with fractionated heparins is now well established. A recent individual patient data meta-analysis of studies comparing anticoagulation with no treatment showed that anticoagulation reduces all-cause mortality independently of recanalization, even though the frequency of bleeding unrelated to portal hypertension increased [42]. Even the prophylaxis of portal vein thrombosis is now under scrutiny. Enoxaparin administration to patients with advanced cirrhosis prevented the occurrence of this complication, while 16% of untreated patients developed it. Interestingly, enoxaparin also reduced the incidence of acute decompensations and mortality [43].

22.6 Acute Kidney Injury

22.6.1 Introduction

As reported in the section dedicated to the pathophysiology of decompensated cirrhosis (Sect. 22.3), the combined effect of systemic inflammatory and prooxidant states and hemodynamic abnormalities leading to reduced effective volemia makes patients with advanced cirrhosis particularly prone to the development of acute kidney injury (AKI). Indeed, about 20% of hospitalized patients present AKI, either at admission or during the hospital stay [44]. Such a prevalence reaches 50% in patients with bacterial infection [45]. Among patients with AKI, most (68%) have prerenal AKI, about one-third have intrarenal AKI, and less than 1% present acute obstructive nephropathy. AKI in patients with decompensated cirrhosis increases their risk of mortality, which can reach about 25% within a month, and negatively influence the outcome of liver transplantation [46, 47].

22.6.2 Hepatorenal Syndrome

Hepatorenal syndrome (HRS) is a form of AKI peculiar to cirrhosis. It was initially considered a functional abnormality consequent to reduced renal perfusion caused by effective hypovolemia and intrarenal imbalance between activated vasoconstrictor and deficient vasodilator systems. Thus, HRS could be classified as a prerenal AKI with the peculiarity of being unresponsive to plasma volume expansion. More recently, the pathogenetic role of systemic inflammation and the pro-oxidative state that characterizes decompensated cirrhosis has emerged, so the concept of a purely functional nature of HRS is becoming outdated [48]. The prognosis of HRS-AKI is poor, as the median survival of untreated cases is shorter than 2 weeks [49].

22.6.3 Diagnosis of AKI in Cirrhosis

Before dealing with diagnosis, we must recall that serum creatinine concentration in patients with advanced cirrhosis can overestimate the glomerular filtration rate due to diminished creatinine production, protein malnutrition, and consequent muscle wasting. Such a shortcoming has not been overcome yet [50].

Table 22.3 Definition and diagnostic criteria of acute kidney injury in patients with cirrhosis (from [51])

	Acute kidney injury
Definition	Increase in Scr ≥0.3 mg/dL within 48 h or Percent increase in Scr ≥50% using the last available value of outpatient Scr within 3 months as the baseline or Urinary output ≤0.5 mL/kg b.w. for more than 6 h
Baseline Scr	Scr measured 48 h earlier than the assessment of AKI. If not available: Scr measured within the previous 3 months; use the value closest to the time of the assessment of AKI If no previous Scr is available, the Scr on admission to the hospital should be used
Staging	*Stage 1*: increase in Scr ≥0.3 mg/dL within 48 h, or an increase in Scr ≥1.5 to 2-folds from baseline *Stage 2*: increase in Scr >2 to 3-folds from baseline *Stage 3*: increase of Scr >3-fold from baseline or Scr ≥4.0 mg/dL with an acute increase ≥0.3 mg/dL or initiation of RRT
Evolution	*Progression*: reach of a higher stage and/or need for RRT *Regression*: reach of a lower stage
Response to Tx	*No response*: no regression *Partial response*: stage regression with a reduction of Scr to ≥0.3 mg/dL above the baseline value *Full response*: return of Scr to a value within 0.3 mg/dL from the baseline value

Scr serum creatinine, *RRT* renal replacement treatment

The diagnosis of AKI in patients with cirrhosis is based on criteria derived from the Kidney Disease Improving Global Outcomes (KDIGO) guidelines modified to adapt to the context of liver cirrhosis [51]. Its presence depends on absolute or relative increases in serum creatinine. Baseline serum creatinine values proximal to the time of patient evaluation are often unavailable. The agreement to employ the value measured within the previous 3 months, if available, or at the time of hospital admission allows us to overcome this shortcoming. Urine volume contraction also provides relevant information but is influenced by renal fluid retention typical of patients with advanced cirrhosis and concomitant use of diuretics. The extent of serum creatinine increase establishes the severity of AKI, defined in three stages. Table 22.3 reports the definition and diagnostic criteria of AKI in patients with cirrhosis.

The differential diagnosis (Fig. 22.3) of the various forms of AKI in patients with cirrhosis first requires the removal of potential risk factors and plasma volume expansion. The response to the infusion of 1 g/kg of body weight of human albumin for two consecutive days identifies prerenal AKI, while the lack of response requires distinguishing HRS-AKI from intrarenal AKI, mainly due to acute tubular necrosis (ATN). The diagnosis of HRS-AKI relies on the absence of proteinuria >500 mg/day, microhematuria, and/or abnormal renal ultrasonography. It is not always easy to distinguish HRS-AKI from ATN-AKI, especially in its early stage, considering

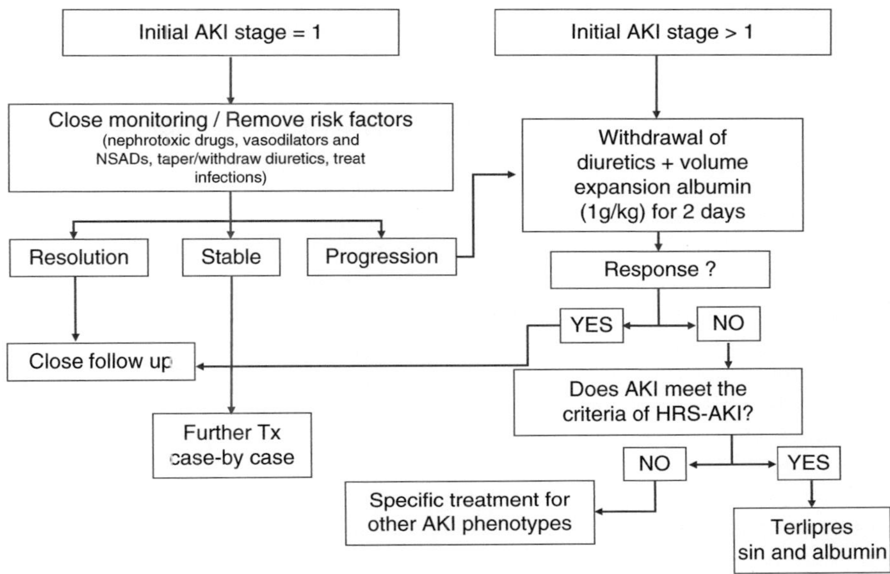

Fig. 22.3 Algorithm for the diagnosis of acute kidney injury in patients with cirrhosis. *Abbreviations*: *AKI* acute kidney injury, *NSAD* nonsteroidal ant-inflammatory drugs, *Tx* treatment, *HRS* hepatorenal syndrome. (*Drawn from* [51])

that HRS-AKI can seamlessly progress into ATN-AKI. Septic or hypovolemic shock or the assumption of nephrotoxic drugs may orient towards ATN from a clinical standpoint. Help can come from the measurement of urinary biomarkers of tubular damage. Among them, neutrophil gelatinase-associated lipocalin seems the most specific [52]. However, overlap areas remain, especially when AKI is induced by bacterial infections.

22.6.4 Management of Prerenal AKI

As reported above, the diagnosis of prerenal AKI descends from at least a partial response to blood volume expansion induced by human albumin administration. Potential precipitating factors, such as nephrotoxic drugs, nonsteroidal anti-inflammatory drugs, angiotensin-converting enzyme drugs, vasodilators, and diuretics, need to be removed, and fluid therapy should continue until normal serum creatinine is achieved and stabilized. Aside from human albumin, crystalloids can be employed, but sodium overload should be considered. However, they could be preferable in hypovolemia secondary to diarrhea, vomiting, or excessive diuretic-induced fluid loss. After resolution, patients who had developed prerenal AKI need close follow-up because of the risk of recidivism.

22.6.5 Medical Treatment of Hepatorenal Syndrome

The target of the medical treatment of HRS is to improve effective volemia, based on the concept that effective hypovolemia is the main pathogenetic event leading to this complication. As reported above, our knowledge of the pathophysiology of HRS has evolved, but still, current treatments rely on systemic vasoconstrictors to counteract arterial vasodilation and human albumin to expand plasma blood volume [53, 54] (Table 22.4). Ischemic heart disease, cerebrovascular disease, peripheral arterial disease, arterial hypertension, and asthma represent contraindications to the use of vasoconstrictors. Human albumin should be very cautiously if ever infused in patients with heart disease and pulmonary hypertension.

The most used vasoconstrictor is terlipressin. The initial dosage is 0.5–1 mg IV every 4–6 h and may increase any 48–72 h up to 2 mg/4–6 h. Terlipressin is associated with 20–40 g daily of human albumin. If human albumin was not already used for differential diagnosis (see above), a loading dose of 1 kg of body weight is infused on day 1. The treatment should continue until HRS resolution (stable reduction of serum creatinine below 1.5) or 14 days. Resolution occurs in 35–40% of cases, and partial response (reduction of serum creatinine >25%) in about 10% more cases. Recurrence of HRS occurs in about 20% of cases and requires re-treatment. Meta-analyses reported that this treatment can improve short-term survival. About 45% of patients treated with terlipressin develop side effects such as abdominal pain, diarrhea, and cardiac, intestinal, or peripheral ischemia, requiring dosage reduction or treatment interruption in about 20% of cases. Continuous terlipressin infusion (initial dose 2 g/day) is preferable to boluses as it is equally effective but ensures a lower incidence of ischemic side effects. Terlipressin plus albumin treatment implies close patient surveillance to avoid volume overload and pulmonary edema. Monitoring of central venous pressure may be helpful.

Table 22.4 Medical therapy of hepatorenal syndrome (HRS-AKI)

Treatment	Dose	Adjustments
Terlipressin	IV boluses starting from 0.5 to 1 mg/4–6 h Continuous infusion starting from 2 mg/day	Stepwise increases every 48–72 h up to 2 mg/4–6 h Stepwise increases every 48 h up to 12 mg/day
Noradrenaline	Continuous infusion starting from 0.5 mg/h	Stepwise 4-hourly increases up to 3 mg/h if a rise in MAP of ≥10 mmHg or diuresis >200 mL/h does not occur
Midodrine + octreotide	M: Starting oral dose 7.5 mg/8 h O: Starting s.c. dose 100 µg/8 h	Maximal dose 12.5 mg/8 h Maximal dose 200 µg/8 h
Human albumin	1 g/kg of body weight at diagnosis; then, 20–40 g/day	If possible, monitor CVP If not, close clinical surveillance to avoid overload

MAP mean arterial pressure, *CVP* central venous pressure, *M* midodrine, *O* octreotide

Continuous IV infusion of norepinephrine is an alternative to terlipressin. The baseline dosage is 0.5 mg/h with 4-hourly increases based on its impact on mean arterial pressure: changes smaller than 10 mmHg require increasing 0.5 mg/h up to a maximal dose of 3 mg/h. Human albumin infusion should maintain central venous pressure between 4 and 10 mmHg; the reach of higher values requires dose reductions or treatment withdrawal. The effects of this treatment seem to be similar to those obtained by terlipressin plus albumin. However, it is noteworthy that the studies reporting these effects had small sample sizes, so that equivalence was not warranted. Furthermore, norepinephrine administration would require to be monitored in intensive care rather than in general wards.

One of the first proposed treatments of HRS consists of the combination of midodrine, a prodrug of the α1-receptor agonist desglymidodrine, octreotide, and human albumin infusion. It can be easily managed in general wards, but its effects are inferior to the association between terlipressin and human albumin.

22.6.6 Renal Replacement Therapy

The decision to start with renal replacement therapy (RRT) in patients with decompensated cirrhosis and AKI is most challenging, as the potential candidates present HRS-AKI nonresponding to vasoconstrictors plus human albumin or severe ATN-AKI. Furthermore, the patients at this stage of cirrhosis often are hemodynamically unstable, so their tolerance to standard intermittent RRT is poor. Data from studies dealing with the outcomes of patients with cirrhosis undergoing RRT are often conflicting, as many reported a poor prognosis, especially in patients with multiorgan failure [55], while others testified acceptable results, especially in candidates for liver transplantation [56].

An in-depth discussion of this matter is outside the purpose of this chapter. However, some general aspects merit mention. RRT must be considered in front of volume overload, inability to maintain daily fluid balance, severe electrolyte abnormalities (hyponatremia, hyperkalemia), metabolic acidosis, and diuretic resistance. Given the results obtained in other clinical contexts [57], early initiation of RRT provides better outcomes. Therefore, patients with cirrhosis could also benefit from this policy. Lastly, continuous RRT is likely preferable to intermittent hemodialysis, as it ensures better hemodynamic stability and slower correction of electrolyte imbalances [58].

22.7 Bacterial Infections

22.7.1 Introduction

Quantitative and qualitative changes in gut microbiota, altered intestinal permeability, and reduced mucosal defenses, ultimately leading to abnormal bacterial translocation, along with a complex dysfunction endangering innate and adaptive immunity make patients with cirrhosis highly susceptible to bacterial infections [59]. As a result, about 1/3 of hospitalized patients are affected by bacterial infections, which have many adverse consequences: they induce complications of cirrhosis, including ACLF, prolong the hospital stay, increase costs, and lead patients awaiting liver transplantation to be delisted. Finally, bacterial infections are a leading cause of mortality in end-stage liver disease, as in-hospital mortality of patients with severe sepsis and septic shock is higher than in general patients (see Sect. 22.8). Once an infection has occurred, 1-year mortality increases fourfold [2, 60].

22.7.2 Recognizing Bacterial Infections in Patients with Cirrhosis

It is important to recognize patients at high risk of developing infections: they have advanced cirrhosis, comorbidities, and a low protein concentration in ascitic fluid, particularly if associated with renal dysfunction. Further conditions increasing the risk of infections are gastrointestinal bleeding, prior spontaneous bacterial peritonitis, instrumentation, and use of proton pump inhibitors [61, 62]. Infections by multidrug-resistant microorganisms are an ominous threat, as their resolution rate is inferior, about 70%, to infections with negative cultures or sustained by susceptible bacteria (92%). Furthermore, they more often lead to septic shock (26% vs. 10%) and in-hospital death, which reaches 25% vs. 12% of patients infected by susceptible strains [63]. The probability of contracting an infection by multidrug-resistant bacteria is enhanced by a recent hospitalization, staying in bed in a crowded room or intensive care unit, especially under ventilation, recent use of antibiotics, or ongoing antibiotic prophylaxis. Antibiotic-resistant bacteria frequently cause nosocomial, healthcare-associated, and second infections, especially in patients with high MELD scores and hepatic encephalopathy [64, 65].

Identifying sepsis in patients with cirrhosis may be difficult, as many features can be misleading and interfere with the recognition of systemic inflammatory response syndrome (SIRS) and, therefore, sepsis: arterial hypotension and tachycardia can be part of the hyperdynamic circulatory syndrome or tachycardia can be prevented by β-blockers, hyperventilation can be due to hepatic encephalopathy and hypersplenism, and relative hypothermia may prevent full-blown leukocytosis and fever. As a result, more than one-third of patients with infection do not present the features of SIRS, which, on the other side, are present in up to one-third of noninfected patients. In any case, the recognition of SIRS is relevant, as hospitalized patients with cirrhosis and SIRS more often present complications, such as gastrointestinal bleeding, hepatorenal syndrome, and hepatic encephalopathy, and have a higher death rate [66].

Even though C-reactive protein synthesis can be impaired in patients with cirrhosis, its diagnostic accuracy seems to be maintained and comparable to procalcitonin, but with conflicting reports. Whether C-reactive protein and procalcitonin are reliable to guide antibiotic therapy in patients with cirrhosis remains uncertain.

However, in the specific context of acute alcoholic hepatitis and SIRS, serum procalcitonin, but not high-sensitivity C-reactive protein, was able to distinguish patients with and without infection, with best cutoffs of 29 ng/mL to rule out infection and 45 ng/mL for diagnosing infection [67].

22.7.3 Assessing Prognosis in Patients with Bacterial Infection

Although the MELD score retains its prognostic power in the setting of sepsis, we should consider that short-term mortality is related to extrahepatic organ failure rather than to the severity of liver disease. Therefore, scoring systems related to organ dysfunction, such as SOFA, seem to perform better than "liver disease" scores [68]. Specific prognostic scores to be employed in the acute deterioration of cirrhosis with or without ACLF, often precipitated by bacterial infections, are available[4] [69, 70]. They perform better than the well-established liver disease prognostic scores, so help in identifying patients with an adverse prognosis and guiding their early admission to intensive care.

The reliability of the sepsis-3 criteria and quick-SOFA [71] has been tested in patients with cirrhosis, showing that they discriminate for in-hospital mortality significantly better than the SIRS criteria. Furthermore, sepsis-3 criteria were able to identify quite nicely those patients doomed to develop acute-on-chronic liver failure and septic shock or needing the transfer to an intensive care unit, mechanical ventilation, or renal replacement therapy [72] (Fig. 22.4). Once septic shock has developed, the mottling score, a marker of microcirculation abnormalities assessable at the bedside, seems to be superior to other well-established prognostic factors such as lactate, urine output, or venous oxygen saturation in patients with cirrhosis [73]. Indeed, none of the patients with a mottling score greater than 1 survived 2 weeks.

22.7.4 Management of Bacterial Infections

The management of bacterial infections is based on antibiotic treatment, and a de-escalation approach is recommended. Empirical antibiotic therapy should start immediately. As in other clinical settings, time delay to antibiotic treatment was a

---

[4] Specific prognostic scores to be employed in the acute deterioration of cirrhosis with or without ACLF are Chronic Liver Failure Consortium acute-on-chronic liver failure (CLIF-C ACLF) and Chronic Liver Failure Consortium acute decompensation (CLIF-C AD). The parameters employed to assess CLIF-C ACLF are simplified SOFA score (see Table 22.2), age, and white cell count. The parameters employed to assess CLIF-C AC are age, white cell count, serum creatinine, INR, and serum sodium. Both scores can be calculated at https://efclif.com/research-infrastructure/score-calculators/clif-c-of-aclf-ad/#calculator

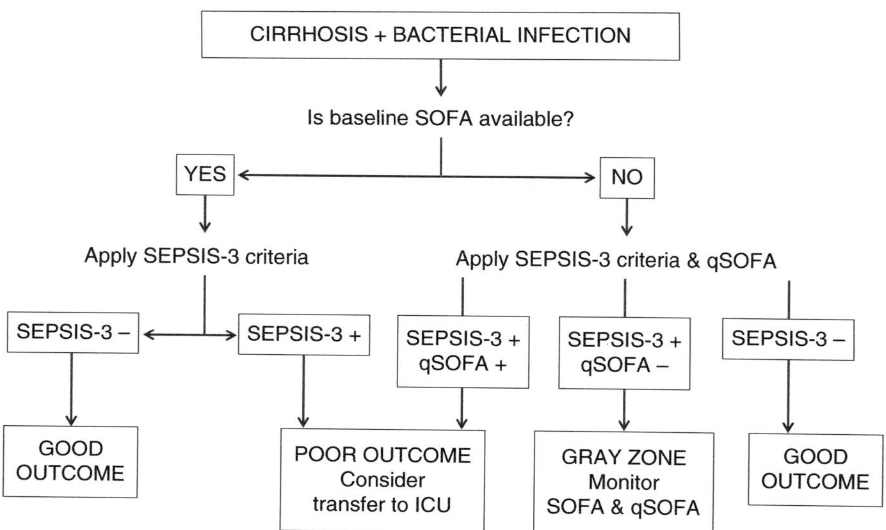

Fig. 22.4 Algorithm for predicting the outcome of patients with cirrhosis affected by bacterial infections employing sepsis-3 criteria and qSOFA. *Abbreviations*: *qSOFA* quick sequential organ failure assessment; *ICU* intensive care unit. (*Drawn from* [76])

strong independent predictor of in-hospital mortality in cirrhotic patients with septic shock [74].

The empirical choice of antibiotics is also crucial, as an initial inappropriate antibiotic therapy is associated with increased patient mortality [75]. Nephrotoxic agents, such as aminoglycosides, whenever possible, drugs prolonging QT interval, and recently used antibiotics should be avoided. We should recall that patients with decompensated cirrhosis are often under prophylaxis with fluoroquinolones, and resistance to these antibiotics is extremely frequent worldwide [76]. Other factors that should guide the choice of antibiotics are the type of infection and, equally important, the site of acquisition. Namely, the probability of facing an infection due to multidrug-resistant microorganisms should be carefully considered (see above).

Due to translocation from the gut, bacterial infections in patients with cirrhosis are often due to Gram-negative microorganisms. However, such a prevalence has decreased in favor of Gram-positive bacteria over the last decade. Namely, community-acquired pneumonia is largely due to Gram-positive bacteria, while Gram-negative bacteria and mixed infections prevail in the nosocomial setting. However, Gram-positive microorganisms are almost always involved in iatrogenic bacteremia following invasive procedures. It is also important to recall that strains producing extended-spectrum β-lactamase are more and more often reported in nosocomial infections. Therefore, the knowledge of the local microbial ecosystem and microbial stewardship assumes great relevance. For this reason, specific antibiotic regimes cannot be advised. Third-generation cephalosporins or amoxicillin/clavulanic acid were first-line antibiotics in the past. Now, piperacillin-tazobactam,

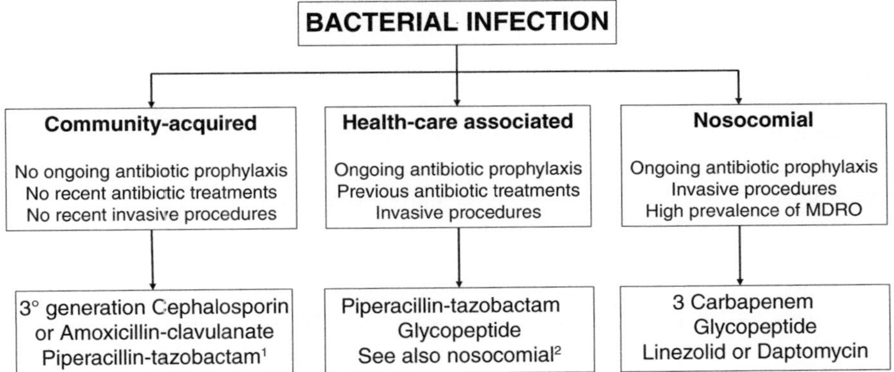

Fig. 22.5 Algorithm for the choice of empiric antibiotic therapy. Please note that the reported choices represent suggestions and not indications. The choice of empiric antibiotic therapy is substantially guided by the knowledge of the local microorganism ecosystem. (1) Piperacillin-tazobactam preferred in case of high prevalence of β-lactamase-producing microorganisms; (2) follow suggestions for nosocomial infections if high prevalence of MDRO; (3) linezolid or daptomycin suggested if high prevalence of MDR Gram+ microorganisms. *Abbreviations*: *MDRO* multidrug-resistant organism

administered through continuous infusion, when possible, is preferable. Glycopeptides should be added when Gram-positive microorganisms are likely into play. In contexts with a high prevalence of multidrug resistance, carbapenems may represent the first-line empirical approach, especially in nosocomial infections. Linezolid or daptomycin should be considered in patients with prior infection from or harboring vancomycin-resistant *Enterococcus* or in areas with a high prevalence of multidrug-resistant *Staphylococci* (Fig. 22.5).

Both HRS-AKI and ATN-AKI frequently occur in patients with cirrhosis and bacterial infections and are cause of mortality. Therefore, prophylactic treatments are warranted. In patients with spontaneous bacterial peritonitis, human albumin infusions (1.5 g/kg bw at diagnosis and 1 g/kg bw at day 3) reduce the incidence of AKI and improve survival [77]. Unfortunately, this is not true in other bacterial infections [78].

22.8 Sepsis and Septic Shock

22.8.1 Introduction

As described in the section dealing with the pathophysiology of decompensated cirrhosis (Sect. 22.3), hemodynamic abnormalities at this stage of the disease are responsible for effective hypovolemia and, therefore, imperfect organ perfusion and decreased oxygen extraction, and diffuse activation of immune cells provoking organ and system dysfunction or failure mediated by immunopathologic mechanisms. Given this background, the systemic response to infection is enhanced, and the effects on vasomotion are potentially catastrophic. Thus, it is not surprising that patients with decompensated cirrhosis are prone to developing sepsis, septic shock, and multiorgan failure, with a higher in-hospital mortality than the general population: about 40% in the case of severe sepsis and up to 70% once the septic shock has developed. Unfortunately, these values did not substantially change over time [79, 80].

Early goal-directed therapy targeting specific objectives in cardiovascular function, oxygenation, and renal function, widely used in patients admitted to intensive care units [81], also applies to decompensated cirrhosis. The principal targets to achieve are mean arterial pressure $\geq$65 mmHg, central venous pressure between 8 and 12 mmHg, central venous oxygen saturation $\geq$70%, and urine output $\geq$0.5 mL/kg/h. However, in advanced cirrhosis, these and other targets can be misleading due to the background of the disease, as reported in Table 22.5. Unfortunately, specific goals for patients with cirrhosis are still lacking.

Of course, antibiotic treatment plays a most relevant role in patients with sepsis and septic shock. This matter is discussed in the previous paragraph, as well as renal replacement therapy is dealt with in the section dedicated to acute kidney injury.

22.8.2 *Fluid Therapy*

The type of shock following severe sepsis is distributive in most cases. The first step is fluid administration, avoiding overload. Excessive fluid infusion enhances tissue edema, facilitating organ dysfunction [82]. In patients with cirrhosis, extracellular edema can ensue, increasing ascites, which aggravates intra-abdominal pressure and facilitates pulmonary edema. Tense ascites require paracentesis followed by human albumin infusion (8 g/L of ascites removed) [53] to reduce the risk of abdominal compartment syndrome. Mean arterial pressure above 65 mmHg is the

Table 22.5 Sepsis and septic shock in cirrhosis: shortcomings of currently employed target parameters in early goal directed therapy

Parameter	Potential limitation
Arterial pressure	Often reduced in advanced cirrhosis
Heart rate	Reduced in patients treated with β-blockers
Central venous pressure	Influenced by large ascites and pleural effusion
Vena cava diameter	Influenced by large ascites
Volume infusion challenge	Enhanced shear stress response
Effect of vasopressors	Impaired cardiovascular responsiveness
Changes in body weight	Influenced by ascites and edema
Urine output	Influenced by secondary hyperaldosteronism and diuretic therapy
Blood lactate	Impaired hepatic clearance
Central venous oxygen saturation	Reduced O_2 extraction ratio due to hyperdynamic circulatory syndrome

standard target in general patients admitted to intensive care. Patients with advanced cirrhosis usually present reduced arterial pressure, and the target of 60 mmHg has been proposed [83], but there is no general agreement on this parameter. Treatment effects can be monitored by assessing arterial lactate concentration, peripheral perfusion, echocardiography, or invasive methods.

The first-line fluid therapy in general patients is the infusion of crystalloids. In the absence of hyperkalemia, balanced solutions are preferred to 0.9% saline to avoid hyperchloremic acidosis and renal failure [84]. The reach of central venous pressure >12 mmHg should lead to stop fluid infusion. Human albumin is the sole colloid indicated in severe sepsis and septic shock because of the risk of severe allergic reactions and AKI shown by gelatins, dextran, and starches [85]. Human albumin use is recommended after initial crystalloid infusion when high volumes of fluids are needed [86]. The distribution volume of albumin is lower than crystalloids, representing an advantage in patients with advanced cirrhosis and ACLF, showing effective hypovolemia and hypoalbuminemia. A further advantage derives from albumin non-oncotic properties [87]. Indeed, antioxidation, immunomodulation, scavenging activity, and endothelium protection may help in counteracting the consequences of the proinflammatory and prooxidant milieu that characterizes patients with advanced cirrhosis and reaches its peak in ACLF (see Sect. 22.3). These properties likely contributed to cardiac workload improvement and peripheral vascular resistance increase in patients with spontaneous bacterial peritonitis enrolled in a pilot study comparing the efficacy of human albumin and hydroxyethyl starch. Interestingly, the starch solution did not achieve such effects [88].

Contrasting results emerged from two studies that compared the effects of human albumin and crystalloid infusions in patients with ACLF and septic shock. In one case, 5% human albumin was more effective than 9% saline solution in improving arterial pressure in the short-term and 1-week survival [89]. In the other case, 20% human albumin again was more effective in the early resuscitation (reach of mean arterial pressure >65 mmHg after 3 h) than Plasmalyte but led to a higher number of pulmonary complications and had no effect on survival [90]. Further investigation on this matter is needed.

22.8.3 Vasoactive Therapy

Upon failure of fluid therapy, the vasopressor infusion should start. According to current guidelines, the α1-β-1 receptor agonist norepinephrine is the first-line drug [86]. Poor response to 0.25–0.5 μg/kg/min of epinephrine requires the addition of vasopressin or terlipressin. This combination allows sparing catecholamines and reduces the risk of arrhythmias. Epinephrine administration is limited to patients who did not respond to the combination of norepinephrine and vasopressin because of the risk of ischemia. Dopamine is not used anymore due to the risk of arrhythmias.

Information about the efficacy of the different vasopressors in the specific context of advanced cirrhosis is scanty. The comparison between norepinephrine at a dose varying from 7.5 to 69 µg/min and terlipressin at a dose from 2 to 8 mg/24 h was reported by an open-label study that enrolled patients with cirrhosis and septic shock [91]. Terlipressin was more effective in ensuring hemodynamic stabilization, reducing variceal bleeding, and improving 48-h survival. However, its administration was associated with a higher rate of adverse events, mainly represented by ischemic events and lactic acidosis. Therefore, this matter requires further evaluation. However, there is a consensus that the continuous terlipressin infusion may represent the first-line vasoactive treatment in patients affected by HRS-AKI [53].

22.8.4 Corticosteroids

Relative adrenal insufficiency (RAI), a condition characterized by inadequate production of cortisol to face organ demand, is frequent in patients with advanced cirrhosis (26%). Such a prevalence increases strikingly in patients with sepsis or septic shock and in those with ACLF (up to 75%) [92, 93]. RAI carries a high risk of refractory shock and mortality. An increase of total serum cortisol of less than 9 µg/dL 1 h after the administration of 250 µg of cosyntropin or total serum cortisol <10 µg/dL at a random evaluation is the most accepted way to make a diagnosis [94].

The efficacy of steroid administration to patients with septic shock is debated. In a large prospective controlled trial, hydrocortisone administration at a dose of 50 mg six hourly to patients with septic shock accelerated the resolution of shock but increased the risk of infections without improving survival [95]. As in the general population, a study addressing patients with cirrhosis and septic shock reported favorable effects of hydrocortisone (200 mg/day) on hemodynamics, with higher rates of shock reversal. However, a higher rate of shock relapse and more gastrointestinal bleeding occurred, and survival did not improve [96].

Current guidelines only indicate stress dose steroid administration in patients with vasopressor-resistant shock needing norepinephrine ≥0.25 µg/kg/min [86]. This position is shared for patients with advanced cirrhosis [83]. To avoid side effects, steroid administration should not exceed 10 days, and the dosage tapering should immediately start at shock resolution.

22.9 Hepatic Encephalopathy

22.9.1 Introduction

Hepatic encephalopathy is defined as a spectrum of potentially reversible neuropsychiatric abnormalities in patients with liver dysfunction, characterized by personality changes, intellectual impairment, and a depressed level of consciousness. It derives from the systemic diffusion of neurotoxins from the gut through portosystemic shunts due to portal hypertension, among which ammonia plays the most relevant role, and systemic inflammation and oxidative state characterizing advanced cirrhosis [97]. Precipitating events such as upper gastrointestinal bleeding, renal failure, hyponatremia, and bacterial infections lead to the appearance or worsening of hepatic encephalopathy. In general, hepatic encephalopathy is not a direct cause of death but worsens the prognosis of the condition with which it is associated, especially ACLF [98]. Several diagnostic criteria, among which the West-Haven criteria (Table 22.6) are the most widely employed, can be used to grade its severity.

22.9.2 Approach to Patients with Hepatic Encephalopathy

The diagnosis of hepatic encephalopathy mainly relies on clinical examination and requires meticulous differentiation to exclude organic damage or assumption of drugs interfering with cerebral functions. Thus, in case of suspicion, a cerebral CT scan, lumbar puncture, and blood assessment of benzodiazepines are warranted. An electroencephalogram can also help to exclude other causes of altered mental status. Fasting blood ammonia levels are not closely related to the presence of hepatic encephalopathy and its degree. However, finding normal levels in a patient with cirrhosis and neuropsychiatric symptoms should raise the suspicion of causes other than hepatic encephalopathy.

Severe hepatic encephalopathy in grade 3 or 4 makes intubation necessary for airway protection, especially in patients with upper gastrointestinal bleeding. In this circumstance, propofol or dexmedetomidine administration is advisable because of their short action. Great attention to hemodynamic side effects is needed [99].

22.9.3 Treatment

After the ascertainment of the diagnosis of hepatic encephalopathy, an effort should be made to identify and correct potential precipitating events. Control of gastrointestinal bleeding, correction of electrolyte imbalance, fluid infusion to improve

Table 22.6 The West-Haven criteria for grading the severity of hepatic encephalopathy

Stage	Consciousness	Intellect and behavior	Neurological findings
0	Normal	Normal	Normal
I	Mild lack of awareness Personality changes	Impaired concentration Mild confusion	Apraxia, mild asterixis or tremor
II	Lethargy	Disorientation Inappropriate behavior	Obvious asterixis, dysarthria (slurred speech)
III	Somnolence	Gross disorientation, aggressivity	Muscular rigidity and clonus, hyperreflexia, Babinski sign
IV	Coma (awakening impossible)	Coma	Decerebrate posturing, rigidity

renal function, starting antibiotic therapy, and supplying nutritional support are examples of the first-line approaches. In the past, patients with episodic hepatic encephalopathy usually received a drastic reduction in protein assumption or administration to lower intestinal ammonia production. However, patients with cirrhosis have increased protein requirements to achieve balanced nitrogen metabolism, and low-protein diets can enhance malnutrition that, in turn, is associated with reduced survival. After demonstrating that a diet providing normal protein content (at least 1.5 g/kg bw) is well tolerated by patients with hepatic encephalopathy [100], low-protein diets are not recommended anymore.

Lactulose and its derivative lactitol are nonabsorbable synthetic disaccharides. Through metabolization in the colon by bacteria, they give rise to volatile fatty acids, hydrogen, and methane, thus increasing osmolality and reducing intraluminal pH. As a result, they facilitate evacuation and impair ammonia reabsorption. Their dosage in patients with episodic hepatic encephalopathy is 40–60 g/day for lactulose and 30–50 g/day for lactitol, with the target of inducing 2–3 evacuations of soft stools daily, taking care to avoid diarrhea. Comatose patients require lactulose administration by one to three enemas per day [101].

Rifaximin, a derivative of rifamycin, is a nonabsorbable antimicrobial with few side effects, a broad spectrum of activity against Gram-negative and Gram-positive anaerobic and aerobic bacteria, and a low risk of developing bacterial resistance. It can be used to treat acute hepatic encephalopathy with effects similar to or better than nonabsorbable disaccharides [102, 103], but it is mainly employed to prevent recidivism of encephalopathy at the dose of 550 mg twice daily [104].

Patients who developed hepatic encephalopathy following benzodiazepine assumption should receive IV flumazenil at the dose of 1 mg.

L-Ornithine-L-aspartate (LOLA) reduces serum ammonia by stimulating the urea cycle and glutamine synthesis. Its use is still experimental, but there is growing evidence of its potential efficacy in treating overt and minimal hepatic encephalopathy [105]. Recently, a double-blind randomized controlled trial that enrolled patients with cirrhosis and severe hepatic encephalopathy (grade 3 or 4) reported that the combination of LOLA with lactulose and rifaximin reduced the severity of and shortened the recovery time from encephalopathy more effectively than lactulose and rifaximin. Furthermore, this treatment was associated with 28-day survival.

There is some evidence that extracorporeal albumin dialysis ensures a more rapid reduction of the severity of acute overt hepatic encephalopathy but is not associated with an improvement in survival [106].

References

1. Ginés P, Krag A, Abraldes JG, et al. Liver cirrhosis. Lancet. 2021;398:1359–76.
2. Arvaniti V, D'Amico G, Fede G, et al. Infections in patients with cirrhosis increase mortality four-fold and should be used in determining prognosis. Gastroenterology. 2010;39:1246–56.
3. D'Amico G, Garcia-Tsao G, Pagliaro L. Natural history and prognostic indicators of survival in cirrhosis: a systematic review of 118 studies. J Hepatol. 2006;44:217–331.

4. Gracia-Sancho J, Marrone G, Fernandez-Iglesias A. Hepatic microcirculation and mechanisms of portal hypertension. Nat Rev Gastroenterol Hepatol. 2019;6:221–34.
5. Pinzani M, Rosselli M, Zuckermann M. Liver cirrhosis. Best Pract Res Clin Gastroenterol. 2011;25:281–90.
6. Engelmann C, Clària J, Szabo G, et al. Pathophysiology of decompensated cirrhosis: portal hypertension, circulatory dysfunction, inflammation, metabolism and mitochondrial dysfunction. J Hepatol. 2021;75(Suppl 1):S49–66.
7. García-Pagán JC, Gracia-Sancho J, Bosch J. Functional aspects on the pathophysiology of portal hypertension in cirrhosis. J Hepatol. 2012;57:458–61.
8. Trebicka J, Fernandez J, Papp M, et al. The PREDICT study uncovers three clinical courses of acutely decompensated cirrhosis that have distinct pathophysiology. J Hepatol. 2020;73:842–54.
9. Arroyo V, Angeli P, Moreau R, et al. The systemic inflammation hypothesis: towards a new paradigm of acute decompensation and multiorgan failure in cirrhosis. J Hepatol. 2021;74:670–85.
10. Moreau R, Jalan R, Gines P, et al. Acute-on-chronic liver failure is a distinct syndrome that develops in patients with acute decompensation of cirrhosis. Gastroenterology. 2013;144:1426–37.
11. Vincent JL, Moreno R, Takala J, et al. The SOFA (Sepsis-related Organ Failure Assessment) score to describe organ dysfunction/failure. Intensive Care Med. 1966;22:707–10.
12. Iwakiri Y, Groszmann RJ. The hyperdynamic circulation of chronic liver diseases: from the patient to the molecule. Hepatology. 2006;43(2 Suppl 1):S121–31.
13. Schrier RW, Arroyo V, Bernardi M, et al. Peripheral arterial vasodilation hypothesis: a proposal for the initiation of renal sodium and water retention in cirrhosis. Hepatology. 1988;8:1151–7.
14. Bernardi M, Moreau R, Angeli P, et al. Mechanisms of decompensation and organ failure in cirrhosis: from peripheral arterial vasodilation to systemic inflammation hypothesis. J Hepatol. 2015;63:1272–84.
15. Moreau R, Clària J, Aguilar F, et al. Blood metabolomics uncovers inflammation-associated mitochondrial dysfunction as a potential mechanism underlying ACLF. J Hepatol. 2020;72:688–701.
16. Bosch J, Abraldes JG, Albillos A, et al. Portal hypertension: recommendations for evaluation and treatment. Consensus document sponsored by the Spanish Association for the Study of the Liver (AEEH) and the Biomedical Research Network Center for Liver and Digestive Diseases (CIBERehd). Gastroenterol Hepatol. 2012;35:421–50.
17. Carbonell N, Pauwels A, Serfaty L, et al. Improved survival after variceal bleeding in patients with cirrhosis over the past two decades. Hepatology. 2004;40:652–9.
18. García-Tsao G, Bosch J, Groszmann RJ. Portal hypertension and variceal bleeding-unresolved issues. Summary of an American Association for the Study of Liver Diseases and European Association for the Study of the Liver single-topic conference. Hepatology. 2008;47:1764–72.
19. Tripodi A, Primignani M, Chantarangkul V, et al. An imbalance of pro- vs anti-coagulation factors in plasma from patients with cirrhosis. Gastroenterology. 2009;137:2105–11.
20. Villanueva C, Colomo A, Bosch A, et al. Transfusion strategies for acute upper gastrointestinal bleeding. N Engl J Med. 2013;368:11–21.
21. de Franchis R, Bosch J, Garcia-Tsao G. Baveno VII—renewing consensus in portal hypertension. J Hepatol. 2022;76:959–74.
22. Chavez-Tapia NC, Barrientos-Gutierrez T, Tellez-Avila FI, et al. Antibiotic prophylaxis for cirrhotic patients with upper gastrointestinal bleeding. Cochrane Database Syst Rev. 2010;2010:CD002907.
23. Lo GH, Lai KH, Cheng JS, et al. A prospective, randomized trial of butyl cyanoacrylate injection versus band ligation in the management of bleeding gastric varices. Hepatology. 2001;33:1060–4.
24. Cabrera L, Tandon P, Abraldes JG. An update on the management of acute esophageal variceal bleeding. Gastroenterol Hepatol. 2017;40:34–40.
25. Trebicka J, Gu W, Ibáñez-Samaniego L, et al. Rebleeding and mortality risk are increased by ACLF but reduced by pre-emptive TIPS. J Hepatol. 2020;73:1082–91.

26. García-Pagán JC, Caca K, Bureau C, et al. Early use of TIPS in patients with cirrhosis and variceal bleeding. N Engl J Med. 2010;362:2370–9.
27. Deltenre P, Trépo E, Rudler M, et al. Early transjugular intrahepatic portosystemic shunt in cirrhotic patients with acute variceal bleeding: a systematic review and meta-analysis of controlled trials. Eur J Gastroenterol Hepatol. 2015;27:e1–9.
28. Kumar R, Kerbert AJC, Sheikh MF, et al. Determinants of mortality in patients with cirrhosis and uncontrolled variceal bleeding. J Hepatol. 2021;74:66–79.
29. Marot A, Trépo E, Doerig C, et al. Systematic review with meta-analysis: self-expanding metal stents in patients with cirrhosis and severe or refractory oesophageal variceal bleeding. Aliment Pharmacol Ther. 2015;42:1250–60.
30. Northup PG, Garcia-Pagan JC, Garcia-Tsao G, et al. Vascular liver disorders, portal vein thrombosis, and procedural bleeding in patients with liver disease: 2020 Practice Guidance by the American Association for the Study of Liver Diseases. Hepatology. 2021;73:366–413.
31. Tripodi A, Mannucci PM. The coagulopathy of chronic liver disease. N Engl J Med. 2011;365:147–56.
32. Lisman T, Caldwell SH, Intagliata NM. Haemostatic alterations and management of haemostasis in patients with cirrhosis. J Hepatol. 2022;76:1291–305.
33. Lisman T, Arefaine B, Adelmeijer J, et al. Global haemostatic status in patients with acute-on-chronic liver failure and septics without underlying liver disease. J Thromb Haemost. 2021;19:85–95.
34. Zanetto A, Rinder HM, Campello E, et al. Acute kidney injury in decompensated cirrhosis is associated with both hypo-coagulable and hyper-coagulable features. Hepatology. 2020;72:1327–40.
35. Schepis F, Turco L, Bianchini M, et al. Prevention and management of bleeding risk related to invasive procedures in cirrhosis. Semin Liver Dis. 2018;38:215–29.
36. De Pietri L, Bianchini M, Montalti R, et al. Thrombelastography-guided blood product use before invasive procedures in cirrhosis with severe coagulopathy: a randomized, controlled trial. Hepatology. 2016;63:566–73.
37. Drolz A, Horvatits T, Roedl K, et al. Coagulation parameters and major bleeding in critically ill patients with cirrhosis. Hepatology. 2016;64:556–68.
38. Tripodi A, Primignani M, Chantarangkul V, et al. Global hemostasis tests in patients with cirrhosis before and after prophylactic platelet transfusion. Liver Int. 2013;33:362–67.
39. Gunawan B, Runyon B. The efficacy and safety of epsilon-aminocaproic acid treatment in patients with cirrhosis and hyperfibrinolysis. Aliment Pharmacol Ther. 2006;23:115–20.
40. Shatzel J, Dulai PS, Harbin D, et al. Safety and efficacy of pharmacological thromboprophylaxis for hospitalized patients with cirrhosis: a single-center retrospective cohort study. J Thromb Haemost. 2015;13:1245–53.
41. Francoz C, Belghiti J, Vilgrain V, et al. Splanchnic vein thrombosis in candidates for liver transplantation: usefulness of screening and anticoagulation. Gut. 2005;54:691–7.
42. Guerrero A, Campo LD, Piscaglia F, et al. Anticoagulation improves survival in patients with cirrhosis and portal vein thrombosis: the IMPORTAL competing-risk meta-analysis. J Hepatol. 2023;79:69–78.
43. Villa E, Cammà C, Marietta M, et al. Enoxaparin prevents portal vein thrombosis and liver decompensation in patients with advanced cirrhosis. Gastroenterology. 2012;143:1253–60.
44. Garcia-Tsao G, Parikh CR, Viola A. Acute kidney injury in cirrhosis. Hepatology. 2008;48:2064–77.
45. Wong F, O'Leary JG, Reddy KR, et al. New consensus definition of acute kidney injury accurately predicts 30-day mortality in patients with cirrhosis and infection. Gastroenterology. 2013;145:1280–08.
46. Bahirwani R, Campbell MS, Siropaides T, et al. Transplantation: impact of pretransplant renal insufficiency. Liver Transpl. 2008;14:665–71.
47. Tsien CD, Rabie R, Wong F. Acute kidney injury in decompensated cirrhosis. Gut. 2013;62:131–7.

48. Angeli P, Garcia-Tsao G, Nadim MK, et al. News in pathophysiology, definition and classification of hepatorenal syndrome: a step beyond the International Club of Ascites (ICA) consensus document. J Hepatol. 2019;71:811–22.
49. Ginés P, Schrier RW. Renal failure in cirrhosis. N Engl J Med. 2009;361:1279–90.
50. Davenport A, Cholongitas E, Xirouchakis E, et al. Pitfalls in assessing renal function in patients with cirrhosis—potential inequity for access to treatment of hepatorenal failure and liver transplantation. Nephrol Dial Transplant. 2011;26:2735–42.
51. Angeli P, Ginés P, Wong F, et al. Diagnosis and management of acute kidney injury in patients with cirrhosis: revised consensus recommendations of the ICA. J Hepatol. 2015;62:968–74.
52. Allegretti AS, Solà E, Ginès P. Clinical application of kidney biomarkers in cirrhosis. Am J Kidney Dis. 2020;76:710–9.
53. European Association for the Study of the Liver. EASL Clinical Practice Guidelines for the management of patients with decompensated cirrhosis. J Hepatol. 2018;69:406–60.
54. Biggins SW, Angeli P, Garcia-Tsao G, et al. Diagnosis, evaluation, and management of ascites, spontaneous bacterial peritonitis and hepatorenal syndrome: 2021 Practice Guidance by the American Association for the Study of Liver Diseases. Hepatology. 2021;74:1014–48.
55. Staufer K, Roedl K, Kivaranovic D, et al. Renal replacement therapy in critically ill cirrhotic patients. Outcome and clinical implications. Liver Int. 2017;37:843–50.
56. Wong LP, Blackley MP, Andreoni KA, et al. Survival of liver transplant candidates with acute renal failure receiving renal replacement therapy. Kidney Int. 2005;68:362–70.
57. Zarbock A, Kellum JA, Schmidt C, et al. Effect of early vs delayed initiation of renal replacement therapy on mortality in critically ill patients with acute kidney injury: the ELAIN randomized clinical trial. JAMA. 2016;315:2190–9.
58. Bellomo R, Cass A, Cole L, et al. Intensity of continuous renal-replacement therapy in critically ill patients. N Engl J Med. 2009;361:162–1638.
59. Jalan R, Fernandez J, Wiest R, et al. Bacterial infections in cirrhosis: a position statement based on the EASL Special Conference 2013. J Hepatol. 2014;60:1310–24.
60. Fasolato S, Angeli P, Dallagnese L, et al. Renal failure and bacterial infections in patients with cirrhosis: epidemiology and clinical features. Hepatology. 2007;45:223–9.
61. Fernández J, Navasa M, Planas R, et al. Primary prophylaxis of spontaneous bacterial peritonitis delays hepatorenal syndrome and improves survival in cirrhosis. Gastroenterology. 2007;133:818–24.
62. O'Leary JG, Reddy KR, Wong F, et al. Long-term use of antibiotics and proton pump inhibitors predict development of infections in patients with cirrhosis. Clin Gastroenterol Hepatol. 2015;13:753–9.
63. Fernández J, Acevedo J, Castro M, et al. Prevalence and risk factors of infections by multiresistant bacteria in cirrhosis: a prospective study. Hepatology. 2012;55:1551–61.
64. Merli M, Lucidi C, Giannelli V, et al. Cirrhotic patients are at risk for health-care associated bacterial infections. Clin Gastroenterol Hepatol. 2020;8:979–85.
65. Bajaj JS, O'Leary JG, Reddy KR, et al. Second infections independently increase mortality in hospitalized patients with cirrhosis: the North American consortium for the study of end-stage liver disease (NACSELD) experience. Hepatology. 2023;56:2328-2335.).
66. Fernández J, Gustot T. Management of bacterial infections in cirrhosis. J Hepatol. 2012;56(Suppl 1):S1–12.
67. Michelena J, Altamirano J, Abraldes JG, et al. Systemic inflammatory response and serum lipopolysaccharide levels predict multiple organ failure and death in alcoholic hepatitis. Hepatology. 2015;62:762–72.
68. Wehler M, Kokoska J, Reulbach U, et al. Short-term prognosis in critically ill patients with cirrhosis assessed by prognostic scoring systems. Hepatology. 2001;34:255–61.
69. Jalan R, Saliba F, Pavesi M, et al. Development and validation of a prognostic score to predict mortality in patients with acute-on-chronic liver failure. J Hepatol. 2014;61:1038–47.
70. Jalan R, Pavesi M, Saliba F, et al. The CLIF Consortium Acute Decompensation score (CLIF-C ADs) for prognosis of hospitalised cirrhotic patients without acute-on-chronic liver failure. J Hepatol. 2015;62:831–40.

71. Singer M, Deutschman CS, Seymour CW, et al. The Third International Consensus definitions for sepsis and septic shock (Sepsis-3). JAMA. 2016;315:801–10.
72. Piano S, Bartoletti M, Tonon M, et al. Assessment of Sepsis-3 criteria and quick SOFA in patients with cirrhosis and bacterial infections. Gut. 2018;67:1892–9.
73. Galbois A, Bigé N, Pichereau C, et al. Exploration of skin perfusion in cirrhotic patients with septic shock. J Hepatol. 2015;62:549–55.
74. Karvellas CJ, Abraldes JG, Arabi YM, et al. Appropriate and timely antimicrobial therapy in cirrhotic patients with spontaneous bacterial peritonitisassociated septic shock: a retrospective study. Aliment Pharmacol Ther. 2015;41:747–57.
75. Bartoletti M, Giannella M, Caraceni P, et al. Epidemiology and outcomes of bloodstream infection in patients with cirrhosis. J Hepatol. 2014;61:51–8.
76. Piano S, Singh V, Caraceni P, et al. Epidemiology and effects of bacterial infections in patients with cirrhosis worldwide. Gastroenterology. 2019;156:1368–80.
77. Sort P, Navasa M, Arroyo V, et al. Effect of intravenous albumin on renal impairment and mortality in patients with cirrhosis and spontaneous bacterial peritonitis. N Engl J Med. 1999;341:403–9.
78. Thévenot T, Bureau C, Oberti F, et al. Effect of albumin in cirrhotic patients with infection other than spontaneous bacterial peritonitis. A randomized trial. J Hepatol. 2015;62:822–30.
79. Moreau R, Hadengue A, Soupison T, et al. Septic shock in patients with cirrhosis: hemodynamic and metabolic characteristics and intensive care unit outcome. Crit Care Med. 1992;20:746–50.
80. Weil D, Levesque E, McPhail M, et al. Prognosis of cirrhotic patients admitted to intensive care unit: a meta-analysis. Ann Intensive Care. 2017;7:33.
81. Dellinger RP, Levy MM, Carlet JM, et al. Surviving Sepsis Campaign: international guidelines for management of severe sepsis and septic shock. Crit Care Med. 2008;36:296–327.
82. Vincent JL. Fluid management in the critically ill. Kidney Int. 2019;96:52–7.
83. Bernal W, Karvellas C, Saliba F, et al. Intensive care management of acute-on-chronic liver failure. J Hepatol. 2021;75(Suppl 1):S163–77.
84. Semler MW, Self WH, Wanderer JP, et al. Balanced crystalloids versus saline in critically ill adults. N Engl J Med. 2018;378:829–39.
85. Brown RM, Semler MW. Fluid management in sepsis. J Intensive Care Med. 2019;34:364–73.
86. Evans L, Rhodes A, Alhazzani W, et al. Surviving Sepsis Campaign: international guidelines for the management of sepsis and septic shock 2021. Crit Care Med. 2021;49:1974–82.
87. Bernardi M, Angeli P, Claria J, et al. Albumin in decompensated cirrhosis: new concepts and perspectives. Gut. 2020;69:1127–38.
88. Fernández J, Monteagudo J, Bargallo X, et al. A randomized unblinded pilot study comparing albumin versus hydroxyethyl starch in spontaneous bacterial peritonitis. Hepatology. 2005;42:627–34.
89. Philips CA, Maiwall R, Sharma MK, et al. Comparison of 5% human albumin and normal saline for fluid resuscitation in sepsis induced hypotension among patients with cirrhosis (FRISC study): a randomized controlled trial. Hepatol Int. 2021;15:983–94.
90. Maiwall R, Kumar A, Pasupuleti SSR, et al. A randomized-controlled trial comparing 20% albumin to plasmalyte in patients with cirrhosis and sepsis-induced hypotension [ALPS trial]. J Hepatol. 2022;77:670–82.
91. Choudhury A, Kedarisetty CK, Vashishtha C, et al. A randomized trial comparing terlipressin and noradrenaline in patients with cirrhosis and septic shock. Liver Int. 2017;37:552–61.
92. Acevedo J, Fernández J, Prado V, et al. Relative adrenal insufficiency in decompensated cirrhosis: relationship to short-term risk of severe sepsis, hepatorenal syndrome, and death. Hepatology. 2013;58:1757–65.
93. Piano S, Favaretto E, Tonon M, et al. Including relative adrenal insufficiency in definition and classification of acute-on-chronic liver failure. Clin Gastroenterol Hepatol. 2020;18:1188–96.
94. Annane D, Pastores SM, Rochwerg B, et al. Guidelines for the diagnosis and management of critical illness-related corticosteroid insufficiency (CIRCI) in critically ill patientys (Part I). Intensive Care Med. 2017;43:1751–63.

95. Sprung CL, Annane D, Keh D, et al. Hydrocortisone therapy for patients with septic shock. N Engl J Med. 2008;358:111–24.
96. Arabi YM, Aljumah A, Dabbagh O, et al. Low-dose hydrocortisone in patients with cirrhosis and septic shock: a randomized controlled trial. CMAJ. 2010;182:1971–7.
97. Rose CF, Amodio P, Bajaj JS, et al. Hepatic encephalopathy: novel insights into classification, pathophysiology and therapy. J Hepatol. 2020;73:1526–47.
98. Cordoba J, Ventura-Cots M, Simon-Talero M, et al. Characteristics, risk factors, and mortality of cirrhotic patients hospitalized for hepatic encephalopathy with and without acute-on-chronic liver failure (ACLF). J Hepatol. 2014;60:275–81.
99. Shehabi Y, Bellomo R, Reade MC, et al. Early goal directed sedation versus standard sedation in mechanically ventilated critically ill patients: a pilot study. Crit Care Med. 2013;41:1983–91.
100. Córdoba J, López-Hellín J, Planas M, et al. Normal protein diet for episodic hepatic encephalopathy: results of a randomized study. J Hepatol. 2004;41:38–43.
101. European Association for the Study of the Liver. EASL Clinical Practice Guidelines on the management of hepatic encephalopathy. J Hepatol. 2022;77:807–24.
102. Mas A, Rodés J, Sunyer L, et al. Comparison od rifaximin and lactitol in the treatment of acute hepatic encephalopathy: results of a randomized, double-blind, double-dummy, controlled clinical trial. J Hepatol. 2003;38:51–8.
103. Sharma BC, Sharma P, Lunia MK, et al. A randomized, double-blind, controlled trial comparing rifaximin plus lactulose with lactulose alone in treatment of overt hepatic encephalopathy. Am J Gastroenterol. 2013;108:1458–63.
104. Bass NM, Mullen KD, Sanyal A, et al. Rifaximin treatment in hepatic encephalopathy. N Engl J Med. 2010;362:1071–81.
105. Butterworth RF, McPhail MJW. L-Ornithine L-Aspartate (LOLA) for hepatic encephalopathy in cirrhosis: results of randomized controlled trials and meta-analyses. Drugs. 2019;79(Suppl 1):31–7.
106. Bañares R, Nevens F, Larsen FS, et al. Extracorporeal albumin dialysis with the molecular adsorbent recirculating system in acute-on-chronic liver failure: the RELIEF trial. Hepatology. 2013;57:1153–62.

Chapter 23
Acute Upper Gastrointestinal Bleeding in Adults

Alicia H. Muratore and Lisa M. Gangarosa

23.1 Introduction

Gastrointestinal bleeding (GIB) is one of the most common gastrointestinal diagnoses. It accounts for over 500,000 hospitalizations in the United States every year [1]. Gastrointestinal bleeding can result in an intensive care unit (ICU) stay or occur in patients with other critical illness and is a major source of morbidity and mortality. In this chapter, we will provide an overview of acute upper GI bleeds (UGIBs) and specifically focus on the role of the ICU pharmacist in helping to manage these patients. UGIBs are bleeds that originate from the esophagus, stomach, or duodenum. Resuscitation, empiric medical therapy, and early endoscopy constitute the basis of management for patients with UGIB. The ICU pharmacist plays an integral role in ensuring that proper empiric medical therapy is started and that appropriate targeted therapy is implemented once a bleeding source is delineated. This chapter provides you with the knowledge and framework to approach a patient with acute UGIB in the ICU.

23.2 Differential Diagnosis

There are many different causes of UGIB. There are erosive or inflammatory causes including peptic ulcer disease, esophagitis, and acute erosive gastropathy. There are vascular causes such as esophageal and gastric varices, Dieulafoy lesions (focal erosion exposing submucosal artery), and arteriovenous malformations (AVMs) also

A. H. Muratore · L. M. Gangarosa (✉)
Division of Gastroenterology and Hepatology, Department of Medicine, UNC Chapel Hill School of Medicine, Chapel Hill, NC, USA
e-mail: lisa_gangarosa@med.unc.edu

Y. Alzaidi, M. A. Gebily (eds.), *The Pharmacist's Expanded Role in Critical Care Medicine*, https://doi.org/10.1007/978-3-031-77335-8_23

called angiodysplasias. Bleeds can be secondary to neoplasms. They can be due to traumatic etiologies such as a Mallory-Weiss tear (a condition in which a sudden and severe rise in esophageal intraluminal pressure causes a mucous membrane laceration across the gastroesophageal junction).

Typically, UGIB is categorized as variceal or non-variceal as the management for these etiologies differs. Initially, it may not be known which type of UGIB a patient is presenting with; thus, initial empiric treatment will be based on clinical suspicion. Obtaining a detailed history and assessing for risk factors can help in assessing the most likely etiology of the UGIB. It is important to determine if the patient has had prior episodes of GIB, review other comorbidities (cirrhosis, UGI surgery, AAA repair, alcohol use), and obtain a detailed medication history with specific focus on the following: aspirin, nonsteroidal anti-inflammatory medications (NSAIDS), checkpoint inhibitors, steroids, anticoagulants, antiplatelets, and known causes of pill esophagitis.

Some of the more common causes are further discussed in the next sections.

1. **Peptic** (gastric and duodenal) **ulcers** are the most common source of UGIB comprising 65% of UGIB and noted to have ~6 million cases annually in the USA [2]. Ulcers involve damage to the mucosa that extends beyond the muscularis mucosa layer into the submucosa (Fig. 23.1). Peptic ulcer disease (PUD) can be caused by *Helicobacter pylori* (*H. pylori*) infection (most common), prolonged NSAID use, hypersecretory states, and stress. *H. pylori* and NSAIDs both damage the protective mucosal lining of the stomach and duodenum allowing acidic parietal cell secretion to erode the mucosa. In the stomach, *H. pylori* secretes urease which is an enzyme that converts urea to ammonia, raising the pH leading to alkalinization and improved survival of the bacteria in the gastric lumen. Bacterial colonization and attachment to epithelial cells result in the release of cytotoxins causing disruption of the mucosal

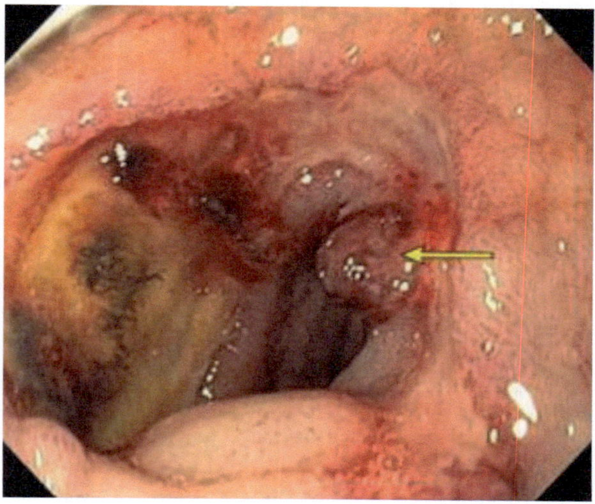

Fig. 23.1 Duodenal ulcer with a nonbleeding visible vessel (arrow)

barrier and damage underlying cells. NSAIDs inhibit cyclooxygenase-1 and -2, which leads to a decrease in prostaglandin synthesis. Prostaglandins decrease gastric acid secretion and increase bicarbonate and mucus secretion. Over time, the decrease in the protective effects of the prostaglandins can lead to the erosion of mucosa.

2. **Mallory-Weiss tears** are lacerations that occur vertically across the gastro-esophageal junction. Risk factors include forceful vomiting and other activities that cause increased abdominal pressure (lifting, etc.). This sudden rise in esophageal intraluminal pressure results in tearing of esophageal mucous membrane, as well as submucosal arteries and veins. Patients typically present with epigastric pain and hematemesis. The patient may report of a history of repeated vomiting episodes with the initial episodes non-bloody, followed by hematemesis.

3. **Acute variceal hemorrhage** is a life-threatening condition. Gastroesophageal varices are present in ~50% of patients with cirrhosis, 30–40% of patients with compensated cirrhosis, and up to 85% of patients with decompensated cirrhosis [3]. Variceal hemorrhage occurs at a rate of 10–15% per year [3].

   Varices occur when the normally small veins that line the esophagus and/or stomach become engorged from portal hypertension, a condition that is primarily associated with chronic liver disease (though can be seen in patients without cirrhosis due to vascular problems, for example splenic or portal vein thrombosis) (Fig. 23.2). Portal pressure increases through increased intrahepatic resistance to portal flow secondary to structural components (fibrous tissue, vascular distortion, etc.) and increased intrahepatic vascular tone from decreased nitric oxide bioavailability. Portal hypertension leads to formation of portosystemic collaterals. Varices are classified based on size on endoscopy (grades 1–3), degree of extension into stomach, and presence or absence of bleeding. Isolated gastric varices can be seen when there is splenic vein thrombosis.

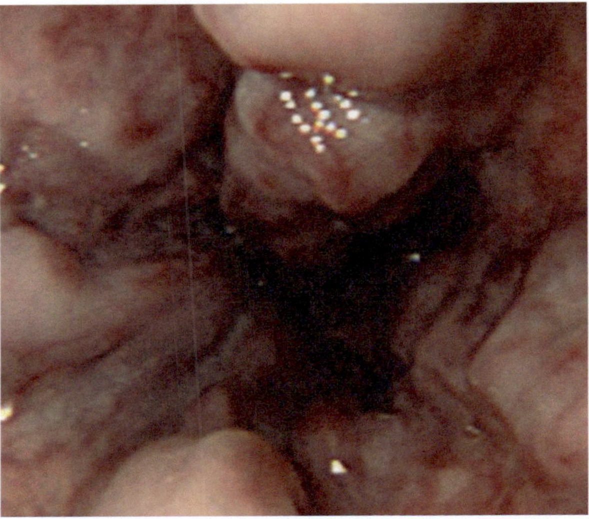

Fig. 23.2 Esophageal varices

23.3 Initial Assessment

Regardless of etiology, the initial management of a patient who presents with a gastrointestinal bleed begins with adequate resuscitation. Simultaneously, providers should obtain a history, perform a physical examination including vital signs, and send appropriate laboratory testing to guide next steps regarding triage, empiric therapy, and further diagnostic/therapeutic interventions. It is here that the pharmacist can play a pertinent role in careful review of medications, with particular attention to the use of anticoagulants and antiplatelets. Initial laboratory testing includes complete blood count, blood urea nitrogen (BUN), PT (INR)/PTT, and type and cross for blood products. Other labs that may be useful include albumin, liver panel, and lactate.

The BUN is often elevated in UGIB due to intestinal absorption and metabolism of hemoglobin as well as decreased urea excretion secondary to hypovolemia. Hemoglobin levels will be followed to assess for ongoing bleeding.

1. **Presentation**: Patients with acute UGIBs usually present with hematemesis, melena, or hematochezia [4]. Hematemesis can be described as bright red blood emesis or emesis that is "coffee ground" in appearance. Melena is defined as black and tarry stool, which is a result of the degradation of blood to hematin by gut bacteria [5]. Hematochezia is defined as red or maroon blood passed per rectum. While hematochezia is usually suggestive of lower gastrointestinal bleed, it can also be a sign of a brisk, rapid UGIB. Identifying current or recent medications that may increase the risk of bleeding is of the utmost importance. This includes nonsteroidal anti-inflammatory drugs, antiplatelets, and anticoagulants.

2. **Initial Management**: All patients with UGIB should be risk stratified to guide diagnostic and therapeutic measures, timing of endoscopy, and patient disposition. The most important first step is assessment of hemodynamic stability of the patient. For unstable patients, follow an ABCDE approach: airway, breathing, circulation, disability/drugs, and endoscopy. The medical team should first ensure that the patient has airway patency and secure this as needed to protect against aspiration and evaluate breathing and treat with respiratory support accordingly. The next priority is circulatory assessment and initiation of hemodynamic support. Resuscitation of the hemodynamically unstable patient takes precedence. Patients should be evaluated for appropriateness of administration of crystalloid fluid and packed red blood cells (PRBCs). Simultaneously, initiation of acid suppression medication and vasoactive medications (if concern for variceal bleed) should be considered. Tracheal intubation may be used to protect the airway in patients with severe ongoing hematemesis [4]. Sufficient IV access is required (for example two large-bore (16–18 Gauge) IVs). For patients in hemorrhagic shock, crystalloid fluid should only be used as a temporizing measure until blood products are available. Packed red blood cells should be given to unstable bleeding patients regardless of initial hemoglobin. In these patients, the initial hemoglobin may not reflect the degree of acute hemorrhage. We do not

recommend using nasogastric aspirate in those with suspected UGIB, and it has poor sensitivity; ~15% with UGIB can have a false-negative result [6].

3. **Risk Stratification**: There are several patient factors that are considered high risk: age >60, chronic comorbidities (such as cirrhosis, congestive heart failure, malignancy), and history of AAA graft. Several clinical features are also high risk: hemodynamic instability, ongoing bleeding, anemia, coagulopathy, elevated BUN, and need to transfuse >6 units PRBC. If more than one feature is present, this is associated with the risk of severe or recurrent bleeding. There are three well-established risk assessment scores: The Glasgow-Blatchford score (GBS), pre-endoscopic Rockall Score, and AIM65 score (albumin <3 mg/dL, INR >1.5, altered mental status (AMS), SBP <90 mmHg, age >65). The GBS stratifies upper GI bleeding patients who are "low risk" and candidates for outpatient management. However, these risk assessment scores cannot predict individual high-risk patients without endoscopic assessment. They do appear to have a clinical role in identifying patients who are very low risk [4]. Thus, these would not be applicable in an ICU-level patient. Patients in an ICU are already considered critically ill. In patients with variceal bleed, those who present with a hepatic venous pressure gradient >20 mmHg are at greater risk for early rebleeding and death. However, this measurement is not easily available at many locations; thus, patients can be risk stratified with Child-Pugh score or MELD score [7].

23.4 Empiric Pharmacological Interventions and Pre-endoscopy Management

There are certain measures that should be initiated as soon as possible prior to any procedures (such an endoscopy, angioembolization, and transjugular intrahepatic portosystemic shunt (TIPS)). These measures may vary based on the suspected cause of the UGIB. These include high-dose IV proton pump inhibitors if peptic ulcer disease is suspected and antibiotics and vasoactive agents if concern for variceal bleeding. Providers also need to discuss the management of antithrombotic and antiplatelet medications and the need for reversal agents if appropriate.

For all patients with UGIB:

1. **Packed Red Blood Cells (PRBCs)**: As discussed above, resuscitation is the most important first step. Guidelines from the American College of Gastroenterology (ACG) recommend restrictive transfusion for PRBC defined as Hgb threshold of 7 g/dL in most hospitalized patients including critical care patients and a threshold of 8 g/dL in those undergoing orthopedic or cardiac surgery and those with known cardiovascular disease [8]. An RCT in 2013 showed that a restrictive transfusion strategy significantly improves mortality in patients with acute UGIB [9]. The restrictive strategy showed significantly better 6-week survival, less rebleeding, no increase in portal-pressure gradient, and

reduced need for additional transfusion. This restrictive transfusion threshold is also supported by the European Society of Gastrointestinal Endoscopy (ESGE) Guidelines [10]. Furthermore, a review of RBC Transfusion Strategies in the ICU in the Journal of Critical Care Medicine also supported the use of restrictive transfusion strategies in the majority of critically ill populations [11]. Using PRBC more liberally increased the risk of transfusion-related reactions and volume overload. This does not apply to patients in hemorrhagic shock. Massive transfusion protocols (MTPs) are the standard of care for managing hemorrhagic shock.

2. **Proton Pump Inhibitors (PPIs)**: Proton pump inhibitors suppress acid secretion by irreversibly binding H^+/K^+ ATPase in the parietal cells of the gastric epithelium. Decreasing gastric acid is thought to promote clotting as gastric acid can inhibit platelet aggregation. In vitro data suggest that intragastric pH >6 may be required to promote clot formation and stability. Preprocedural PPI has not been shown to reduce mortality rates, but in the subcategory of PUD may improve clinically relevant outcomes such as rebleeding and need for surgical intervention. Thus, ACG guideline currently makes no recommendation for or against pre-endoscopic PPI [8]. Similarly, in the SUP-ICU study published in NEJM [12], adult patients admitted to the ICU for an acute condition who were at risk for gastrointestinal bleeding randomized to pantoprazole or placebo had no significant differences in either 90-day mortality or a composite outcome of four clinically important events. Although no mortality benefit was demonstrated, the incidence of clinically important GI bleeds (secondary outcome) was lower in the pantoprazole group. PPI use is recommended in Critical Care Guidelines for patients with acute-on-chronic liver failure (ACLF) and portal hypertensive bleeding [13].

   If PPI is ordered pre-endoscopy, it can be ordered as a continuous infusion or bolus dosing. A bolus IV dose followed by infusion was the recommended course of therapy, but a recent study suggests that twice-daily IV bolus dosing is noninferior in outcomes of rebleeding, mortality, and length of hospital stay [14]. Intermittent dosing may be preferred to decrease resource use and overall costs. No conclusions could be made regarding oral vs. IV dosing though oral administration does provide antisecretory effect comparable to equivalent doses of IV PPI [15]. Though the optimal PPI therapy pre-endoscopy is uncertain, if chosen to initiate, the following dosing options are reasonable: If planning for continuous infusion, give 80 mg IV PPI bolus followed by 8 mg/h. If planning for intermittent dosing, give a one-time 80 mg IV bolus, followed by 40 mg IV every 12 h.

   When compared to IV H2 antagonists, a 2015 meta-analysis showed the difference in mortality rate to be nonsignificant but did show that PPIs were superior regarding recurrent bleeding rate and surgical intervention [16].

3. **Prokinetic**: To prepare for endoscopy, GI promotility agents such as metoclopramide (given at a dose of 10 mg IV) and/or erythromycin (at a dose of 250 mg IV) can be given 30–90 min prior to procedure to enable increased visualization of gastric mucosa. Data is lacking regarding the benefit of reduction in further

bleeding and mortality, but prokinetics do show reductions in repeat endoscopies and length of hospitalization. Erythromycin has prokinetic properties secondary to motilin agonism that promotes GI peristalsis. ACG guidelines recommend IV erythromycin infusion of 250 mg given over 20–30 min [8] followed by endoscopy 90 min later. Azithromycin appears to be noninferior and may logistically be easier as it does not require reconstitution and is generally more available [17]. Metoclopramide increases sensitivity to acetylcholine in GI tract. Given that erythromycin is not usually readily available in the hospital, metoclopramide is often substituted in practice but not currently in guidelines. It is usually dosed at 10 mg IV 30–60 min before endoscopy.

4. **Anticoagulants**: Decisions to withhold or adjust and when to resume antithrombotic agents should be made in conjunction with specialist teams. These decisions should balance a patient's risk of bleeding with the risk of thromboembolic events. In general, for life-threatening bleeding, anticoagulant reversal should be considered. The ACG and Canadian Association of Gastroenterology 2022 [18] have provided guidance on management of anticoagulation. If on warfarin or DOAC with life-threatening bleed (defined as decrease in Hgb >5 g/dL, requiring >5 U PRBC, or hypotension requiring pressors) or supratherapeutic INR, give reversal agent. Otherwise, there is low evidence and thus no recommendation. The reversal agent is based on the specific antithrombotic agent.

   (a) Warfarin: There are several agents that can be used for reversal of warfarin including FFP, PCC, and vitamin K. The ACG guideline recommends against using FFP unless the patient has a life-threatening bleed. Guidelines could not reach consensus for or against PCC, though again it could be considered for life-threatening bleed in the setting of supratherapeutic INR. The guideline recommends PCC over FFP, as PCC has a more rapid and reliable correction of INR. The guideline recommends against vitamin K as there is no clinical evidence that this prevents further bleeding or improves mortality.

   (b) Dabigatran: Idarucizumab is the reversal agent for dabigatran. The ACG guideline recommends against routine idarucizumab given the limited evidence of benefit and high cost but it can be considered in life-threatening bleed and if dabigatran is taken within the past 24 h. If given, recommended dosing is 2.5 g IV ×2 doses, 15 min apart.

   (c) Apixaban/rivaroxaban: Andexanet alfa can be used as a reversal agent for apixaban and rivaroxaban. The ACG guideline recommends against routine use; however, it can be considered if there is life-threatening bleed and apixaban or rivaroxaban is taken within 24 h. If given, there are two dosing options: low dose 400 mg IV bolus and then 4 mg/min for 120 min or high dose 800 mg IV bolus and then 8 mg/min for 120 min.

5. **Antiplatelets and Thrombocytopenia**: Regarding antiplatelet management, first review the indication for therapy. If used for primary prevention, consider discontinuing aspirin. If used for secondary prevention, consider continuing or resuming within 24 h of endoscopic hemostasis [18].

It is recommended to only transfuse with platelets if the patient is thrombocytopenic (platelet level <50,000) or in those with other indications for platelet transfusions [1]. There is a possible mortality increase and lack of benefit of decreasing further bleeding unless thrombocytopenic. In those with cirrhosis and thrombocytopenia, RCTs with recombinant factor VIIa have not shown clear benefit. Thus, it is not recommended to correct INR with FFP or factor VIIa, especially since INR is not a reliable indicator of coagulation status in cirrhosis [3].

23.5 Endoscopy

Esophagogastroduodenoscopy (EGD) endoscopy allows for bleeding source identification, diagnostic biopsies, and hemostatic interventions. An endoscopy should ideally be performed within 24 h of admission. Studies have looked at the impact of performing endoscopic procedures earlier and showed that endoscopy performed within 6 h of gastroenterology consultation rather than 6–24 h did not reduce 30-day mortality [19]. Additionally, in patients with high-risk UGIB, those who were treated with pre-endoscopy PPI and were not in persistent shock, endoscopy performed at a median of 10 h vs. a median of 25 h post-presentation did not reduce 30-day mortality. However, if variceal bleeding is suspected, then EGD should be performed as soon as possible in unstable patients and within 12 h in all other patients [6]. Prior to EGD, a patient should ideally be fasting (NPO) for >2 h for clear liquids and >6–8 h for solids. As discussed above, consider a promotility agent to improve visualization.

Further management is based on findings on EGD. If endoscopy did not identify a source of the bleeding, it is said to be nondiagnostic. In these cases, if a patient is hemodynamically stable but has hematochezia or melena, a colonoscopy and/or small bowel evaluation may be considered. In patients that are hemodynamically unstable with ongoing bleeding, angioembolization may be considered. If a source of GI bleeding is identified on endoscopy, the endoscopist will attempt endoscopic hemostasis. Endoscopic hemostasis is indicated if any high-risk endoscopic findings are seen such as signs of active bleeding (e.g., bleeding peptic ulcer, angiodysplasia), nonbleeding visible vessel, and adherent clot [6, 18]. Endoscopists can use several types of therapies often in combination which include injection therapy with epinephrine, cauterization, and/or mechanical therapy with clips. For variceal bleeds, variceal ligation is the preferred intervention, but sclerotherapy (injection of sclerosant into or adjacent to the varix) can be used when ligation is technically difficult. Self-expanding metal stents may also be used in variceal bleeds as a bridge therapy to TIPS in refractory bleeding.

In patients with ongoing GI bleeding and hemodynamic instability refractory to resuscitation or in those with rebleeding or ongoing bleeding despite endoscopic hemostasis, angiography with interventional radiology is indicated. If other therapeutic options have failed and in hemodynamically unstable patients with ongoing bleed, surgery with exploratory laparotomy and surgical hemostasis is indicated.

23.6   Tranexamic Acid

Evidence does not support the routine use of tranexamic acid (TXA) in patients with acute UGIB. TXA inhibits fibrinolytic activity of plasmin. A meta-analysis reported reduced mortality with TXA in patients with UGIB, but many of these studies were of poor quality and done before widespread use of PPI and endoscopic therapy [20]. The HALT-IT trial showed that TXA does not reduce death from GIB [21].

For patients with suspected variceal bleed:

1. **Splanchnic Vasoconstriction**: Vasoactive medications reduce mortality and the need for blood transfusion by reducing splanchnic blood flow. These agents consist of octreotide, vasopressin, terlipressin, and somatostatin. Vasopressin is not used due to adverse side effects. A 2014 study showed no significant difference among somatostatin, octreotide, and terlipressin [22]. However, until recently, octreotide was the only available of the three in the USA (terlipressin was FDA approved in September 2022 for use in patients with cirrhosis and hepatorenal syndrome). Critical Care Guidelines [13] and 2016 AASLD Guidelines recommend octreotide. This is a long-acting analogue of somatostatin, a natural hormone that regulates the release of serotonin, gastrin, glucagon, insulin, and growth hormone. Because glucagon is a vasodilator, octreotide indirectly decreases splanchnic blood flow by inhibiting the release of glucagon. However, it does not provide a mortality benefit. The recommended dosage is to initiate with a 50 mcg IV bolus followed by 50 mcg/h continuous infusion. A 50 mcg IV bolus can be repeated for uncontrolled hemorrhage. The infusion should be continued for 5 days.
2. **Antibiotics**: Antibiotics should be used for any type of GI bleed in a patient with cirrhosis. Antibiotic prophylaxis is associated with decreased rates of infection, recurrent hemorrhage, and death [23]. Most commonly used is ceftriaxone 1 g every 24 h for 7 days, but antibiotic choice should be tailored based on local resistance patterns. IV ceftriaxone was shown to be more effective at preventing infection than oral norfloxacin, though that difference is largely explained based on individuals with high prevalence of quinolone-resistant bacterial infections.

23.7   Post-EGD Pharmacologic Management: Targeted Therapy

Once hemostasis has been achieved, therapy should be targeted to the underlying cause.

1. **Peptic Ulcer Disease**: If endoscopy confirms peptic ulcer disease, all patients should be counseled on avoiding NSAIDs and restricting alcohol and tobacco

products. Pharmacologic management includes acid-suppressive therapy with a PPI and, if *H. pylori* is detected, eradication therapy. Patients should be started on or continued on PPI IV BID therapy to complete a total of 72 h of treatment. Then patients can be transitioned to twice-daily oral acid suppression medication for 2 weeks. After this, patients should continue on oral daily medication for 4–8 weeks. If patients test positive for *H. pylori*, they should be treated for eradication based on current guidelines [24].

2. Mallory-Weiss tear: Endoscopic interventions to treat Mallory-Weiss tears include injection of epinephrine, electrocoagulation, and hemostatic clip placement. Post-endoscopy, the overall goal of pharmacological treatment is to promote mucosal healing [18]. This consists of acid suppression medication with PPI therapy, which can be continued daily for 2 weeks.

3. **Variceal Bleed**

   (a) Octreotide: If variceal bleed is identified, continue for 5 days based on the European Acute Bleeding Esophageal Variceal Episodes (ABOVE) Trial [25]. Octreotide can be stopped if EGD reveals non-variceal bleed.

   (b) Antibiotics: Continue up to 7 days in patients with cirrhosis and UGIB regardless of sources of bleed.

   (c) Beta-blocker: Nonselective beta-blockers are used for primary and secondary prophylaxis. These medications block beta-1 adrenergic receptors in the heart and beta-2 receptors in splanchnic venous system. Beta-1 blockade decreases splanchnic blood flow by decreasing cardiac output. Beta-2 blockade directly promotes splanchnic vasoconstriction. The AASLD recommends carvedilol, nadolol, or propranolol. It is essential that the medication is nonselective: beta-1 adrenergic blockade decreases portal flow through splanchnic vasoconstriction by unopposed alpha-adrenergic activity. However, NSBB effects are more related to beta-2-blocking effect. Carvedilol also has anti-alpha 1 adrenergic activity and thus also acts as a vasodilator. Beta-blockers should be started after octreotide is used for 2–5 days. The goal should be a target heart rate of 55–60 bpm. Monitor SBP (goal >90 mmHg). The beta-blocker should be continued indefinitely.

   (d) Anticoagulation: If and when patients are restarted on their anticoagulation and antiplatelet agents, they should also be continued on a PPI. Aspirin should be restarted if it is indicated for secondary prevention. The benefit of secondary prevention is greater than primary (NNT to prevent MI, stroke, vascular death 67 vs. 1745 for primary) [26]. Continue (or reintroduce within 3 days with higher-risk endoscopic lesions) once hemostasis has been achieved. Stop if for primary prophylaxis as the risk of bleed is probably greater than benefit.

   (e) TIPS: This can be considered if pharmacological and endoscopic treatment are unsuccessful. Additionally, early TIPS can be considered within 72 h of esophageal varix ligation in patients at high risk of bleeding who are Child-Pugh class C or Child-Pugh class B with active bleeding on endoscopy.

23.8 ICU-Specific Considerations

One thing to consider in an ICU setting is prevention of upper GI bleeds by means of prophylaxis. Stress-induced erosive gastropathy/ulcers are a consequence of gut ischemia in the context of multiorgan failure. This is further exacerbated by the use of opiate sedatives (decrease gut motility and venous return). Risk factors for developing GI bleed in ICU also include mechanical ventilation, coagulopathy, and hepatic or kidney failure. One study showed no significant difference in 90-day mortality, infectious adverse events, and serious adverse events between PPI and placebo [12]. However, fewer patients in PPI group had clinically important GIB in ICU.

References

1. Peery AF, Crockett S, et al. Burden and cost of gastrointestinal, liver, and pancreatic diseases in the United States: update 2021, vol. 162. Gastroenterology; 2022. p. 621–44.
2. Sandler RS, Everhart JE, et al. The burden of selected digestive diseases in the United States. Gastroenterology. 2002;122:1500.
3. Garcia-Tsao G, Abraldes JG, Berzigotti A, Bosch J. Portal hypertensive bleeding in cirrhosis risk stratification, diagnosis, and management 2016 practice guidance by the American Association for the study of liver diseases. Hepatology. 2017;65:310–35.
4. Stanley AJ, Laine L. Management of acute upper gastrointestinal bleeding. BMJ. 2019;364:l536.
5. Feldman M, Friedman L, Brandt L. Sleisenger and Fordtran's gastrointestinal and liver disease E-book. 10th ed. New York: Elsevier Health Sciences; 2015.
6. Hwang JH, Fisher DA, et al. The role of endoscopy in the management of acute non-variceal upper GI bleeding. Gastrointest Endosc. 2012;75:1132–8.
7. Zhao JR, Wang GC, Hu JH, Zhang CQ. Risk factors for early rebleeding and mortality in acute variceal hemorrhage. World J Gastroenterol. 2014;20(47):17941–8. https://doi.org/10.3748/wjg.v20.i47.17941. PMID: 25548492; PMCID: PMC4273144.
8. Laine LM, Barkun AN, Saltzman JR, Martel MM, Leontiadis GI. ACG clinical guideline: upper gastrointestinal and ulcer bleeding. Am J Gastroenterol. 2021;116(5):899–917.
9. Villanueva C, et al. Transfusion strategies for acute upper gastrointestinal bleeding. N Engl J Med. 2013;368:11–21.
10. Gralnek IM, Dumonceau JM, Kuipers EJ, et al. Diagnosis and management of nonvariceal upper gastrointestinal hemorrhage: European Society of Gastrointestinal Endoscopy (ESGE) Guideline. Endoscopy. 2015;47(10):a1–a46. https://doi.org/10.1055/s-0034-1393172.
11. Cable CA, Razavi SA, Roback JD, Murphy DJ. RBC transfusion strategies in the ICU: a concise review. Crit Care Med. 2019;47(11):1637–44. https://doi.org/10.1097/CCM.0000000000003985.
12. Krag M. Pantoprazole in patients at risk for gastrointestinal bleeding in the ICU. N Engl J Med. 2018;379:2199–208.
13. Nanchal RM-C, Subramanian RM-C, Alhazzani WM-C, Dionne JC, Peppard WJ, Singbartl KM. Guidelines for the management of adult acute and acute-on-chronic liver failure in the ICU: neurology, peri-transplant medicine, infectious disease, and gastroenterology considerations. Crit Care Med. 2023;51:657–76.
14. Sachar H, Vaidya K, Laine L. Intermittent vs continuous proton pump inhibitor therapy for high-risk bleeding ulcers. JAMA Intern Med. 2014;174:1755–62.

15. Freston J, Pilmer B, Chiu Y-L, Wang Q, Stolle J, Griffin J, Lee C. Evaluation of the pharmacokinetics and pharmacodynamics of intravenous lansoprazole. Aliment Pharmacol Ther. 2004;19:1111–22.
16. Zhang Y-S, Li Q, He B-S, Li Z-J. Proton pump inhibitors therapy vs H2 receptor antagonists therapy for upper gastrointestinal bleeding after endoscopy: a meta-analysis. World J Gastroenterol. 2015;21:6341–51.
17. Issa D, et al. Azithromycin versus erythromycin infusions prior to endoscopy in upper gastrointestinal bleeding. Transl Gastroenterol Hepatol. 2022;7:35.
18. Abraham NS, Barkun AN, et al. American College of Gastroenterology-Canadian Association of Gastroenterology Clinical Practice Guideline: management of anticoagulants and antiplatelets during acute gastrointestinal bleeding and the periendoscopic period. Am J Gastroenterol. 2022;117:542–58.
19. Lau JYW, Yu Y, et al. Timing of endoscopy for acute upper gastrointestinal bleeding. N Engl J Med. 2020;382:1299–308.
20. Gluud L, Klingenberg S, Langholz E. Tranexamic acid for upper gastrointestinal bleeding. Cochrane Database Syst Rev. 2012;1:CD006640.
21. HALT-IT Trial Collaborators. Effects of a high-dose 24-h infusion of tranexamic acid on death and thromboembolic events in patients with acute gastrointestinal bleeding (HALT-IT): an international randomized, double-blind, placebo-controlled trial. Lancet. 2020;395:1927–36.
22. Seo YS, Park SY, et al. Lack of difference among terlipressin, somatostatin, and octreotide in the control of acute gastroesophageal variceal hemorrhage. Hepatology. 2014;60:954–63.
23. Chavez-Tapia NC, et al. Meta-analysis: antibiotic prophylaxis for cirrhotic patients with upper gastrointestinal bleeding—an updated Cochrane review. Aliment Pharmacol Ther. 2011;34:509–18.
24. Chey WD, Howden CW, Moss SF, Morgan DR, Greer KB, Grover S, Shah SC. ACG Clinical Guideline: Treatment of Helicobacter pylori Infection. Am J Gastroenterol. 2024 Sep 1;119(9):1730–753. https://doi.org/10.14309/ajg.0000000000002968. Epub 2024 Sep 4. PMID: 39626064.
25. Avgerinos A. Early administration of somatostatin and efficacy of sclerotherapy in acute oesophageal variceal bleeds: the European Acute Bleeding Oesophageal Variceal Episodes (ABOVE) randomized trial. Lancet. 1997;350:1495–9.
26. Laine L. Upper gastrointestinal bleeding due to a peptic ulcer. N Engl J Med. 2016;374:2367–76.

Chapter 24
Abdominal Compartment Syndrome

Poornima Lakshmi Tamma, Yuhamy Curbelo-Pena, Emaad J. Iqbal, Mona K. Patel, and Beth Hochman ⓘ

Abbreviations

ACS	Abdominal compartment syndrome
AKI	Acute kidney injury
APP	Abdominal perfusion pressure
BPS	Behavioral Pain Scale
CPOT	Critical Care Pain Observation Tool
IAH	Intra-abdominal hypertension
IAP	Intra-abdominal pressure
ICU	Intensive care unit
LOS	Length of stay
MAP	Mean arterial pressure
NRS	Numerical Rating Scale
RASS	Richmond Agitation-Sedation Scale
SAS	Riker Sedation-Agitation Scale

P. L. Tamma · Y. Curbelo-Pena · E. J. Iqbal
New York-Presbyterian Hospital, Columbia University Irving Medical Center,
New York, NY, USA
e-mail: ktn9007@nyp.org; yc4356@cumc.columbia.edu

M. K. Patel
Pulmonary, Critical Care & Sleep Medicine, NYU Langone Health, NYU Grossman School
of Medicine, New York, NY, USA
e-mail: Mona.Patel2@nyulangone.org

B. Hochman (✉)
General Surgery & Critical Care Medicine, New York-Presbyterian Hospital, Columbia
University Irving Medical Center, New York, NY, USA

Acute Care Surgery & Surgical Critical Care, NYU Langone Health,
NYU Grossman School of Medicine, New York, NY, USA
e-mail: beth.hochman@nyulangone.org

Y. Alzaidi, M. A. Gebily (eds.), *The Pharmacist's Expanded Role in Critical
Care Medicine*, https://doi.org/10.1007/978-3-031-77335-8_24

24.1 Introduction

Abdominal compartment syndrome occurs when pressures within the abdominal cavity rise to the point of causing organ dysfunction [1]. The abdomen can be conceptualized as a semirigid closed space. When the volume of its contents increases acutely, the pressure within the entire cavity also rises. The resultant intra-abdominal hypertension (IAH) can decrease abdominal perfusion pressure (APP), which in turn can lead to organ injury with dysfunction and failure.

Abdominal compartment syndrome is most commonly seen as an iatrogenic problem in critically ill surgical patients who have received aggressive crystalloid resuscitation to address their initial pathology. Other patients at increased risk include those with ascites, hemoperitoneum, bowel distension, and large tumors [2, 3]. While the rate of ACS in critically ill patients has been noted in several single-center studies to be as low as 2–3% [4], its presence has been associated with mortality as high as 75–90% [4]. These stark numbers have prompted great interest in supporting timely recognition and intervention.

Pharmacists are essential members of the interdisciplinary care team, and their involvement in clinical care has been shown to improve safety and reduce cost by providing drug information, optimizing drug dosing, identifying and addressing drug interactions, and recommending pharmacologic therapies [5, 6]. The presence of specialty critical care pharmacists in adult ICUs has also been associated with decreased mortality, ICU length of stay, and adverse effects [7, 8]. Pharmacists can help with both the prevention and treatment of ACS through identification of patients at risk; management of fluid balance, pain, agitation, and delirium; antimicrobial therapy; prevention of venous thromboembolism; and optimization of drug dosing and delivery of medications.

24.2 Pathophysiology of Abdominal Compartment Syndrome

Compartment syndrome may manifest in any anatomical region where increased pressure within a confined body space leads to compromised blood flow, cellular damage, and subsequent organ dysfunction. Rising pressures override the relatively low pressure in the venous system, leading to congestion of involved organs. As pressures remain elevated or continue to rise, arterial inflow to the involved space also becomes impeded, precipitating organ ischemia. The duration of ischemia in concert with baseline underlying organ function determines whether any organ injury sustained can be reversed. This translates to the threat of limb loss with extremity compartment syndrome and the threat of multisystem organ failure with abdominal compartment syndrome [9]. For this reason, timeliness of identification and intervention for compartment syndrome directly determines clinical outcomes. Intervention may involve a combination of temporizing measures to acutely address the need to restore organ perfusion as well as treatment for the underlying cause of the rising pressures. In primary ACS, underlying etiologies include rapid accumulation of free fluid such as ascites or blood, expansion of solid organs or tumors, or dilation of hollow viscera. These pathologies often warrant invasive intervention. Secondary ACS arises from conditions outside the abdomen including conditions that decrease abdominal wall compliance like extensive burns, and recurrent ACS may develop following prior treatment [9–11].

The World Society of the Abdominal Compartment Syndrome has established the definition for ACS as sustained intra-abdominal pressure (IAP) $\geq$20 mmHg (with or without an APP <60 mmHg), coupled with the onset of new organ dysfunction or failure. Abdominal perfusion pressure is calculated by subtracting IAP from mean arterial pressure (MAP). An elevated IAP alone will not inherently meet the criteria for ACS as long as MAP is sufficiently high for the patient to maintain appropriate organ perfusion. Mitigating risk for ACS relies on having an appropriate level of suspicion to warrant measuring IAP and shared nomenclature that can prompt preventive measures when IAP becomes supranormal. Normal IAP typically ranges from 5 to 7 mmHg, consistent with the normal pressure in the vena cava. Intra-abdominal hypertension is stratified as shown in Box 24.1, where grades I and II reflect increased risk for progression to ACS, and grade III or higher should raise concern for the presence of ACS [10, 11].

> **Box 24.1 Intra-abdominal Hypertension Grading Scale**
> - Grade I: 12–15 mmHg
> - Grade II: 16–20 mmHg
> - Grade III: 21–25 mmHg
> - Grade IV: $\geq$25 mmHg

24.3 Risk Factors for Developing Abdominal Compartment Syndrome

Abdominal compartment syndrome is most commonly associated with large-volume crystalloid resuscitation. This association was first formally defined in 1989 in a small series of patients with significant abdominal distension after receiving more than 25 L of fluid for ruptured abdominal aortic aneurysm repairs [12], though large fluid resuscitation is not limited to surgical patients with abdominal catastrophe. A systematic review of studies from 1950 to 2013 found that among mixed surgical and medical intensive care unit patients, large-volume crystalloid resuscitation (defined as more than 3.5 L in 24 h), mechanical ventilation, and hypotension were the most common risk factors for developing IAH and ACS, and obesity, sepsis, abdominal surgery, and ileus were identified as additional risk factors for IAH [13].

IAH and ACS have also been reported in severely burned patients both as a consequence of the large fluid resuscitation required to replace insensible losses from injured tissue and decreased abdominal wall compliance in the setting of truncal burns with eschar formation. Up to 75% of patients with greater than 20% total body surface area burns have some grade of IAH [13, 14].

24.4 Diagnosis of ACS

The definitive diagnosis of ACS, which is sustained grade III or IV IAH with new organ dysfunction, requires precise measurement of IAP in conjunction with clinical assessment and evaluation of end-organ function. Complementary imaging studies, such as ultrasound or computed tomography, can play a supportive role in the diagnostic process by helping to identify the underlying cause of the elevated IAP and facilitate appropriate management strategies. IAP can be assessed using a pressure-sensitive catheter placed in the bladder (Fig. 24.1). Intermittent measurements in mmHg are recorded from the emptied bladder instilled with 25 mL of sterile saline when the patient is at end expiration in the supine position without interference of abdominal muscle contractions. This approach supports consistency and accuracy of individual measurements and their trends. Measurements taken in patients who are extubated and awake are more difficult to interpret given the challenge in controlling for abdominal wall contractions and timing of the measurement with end expiration [9, 11, 15].

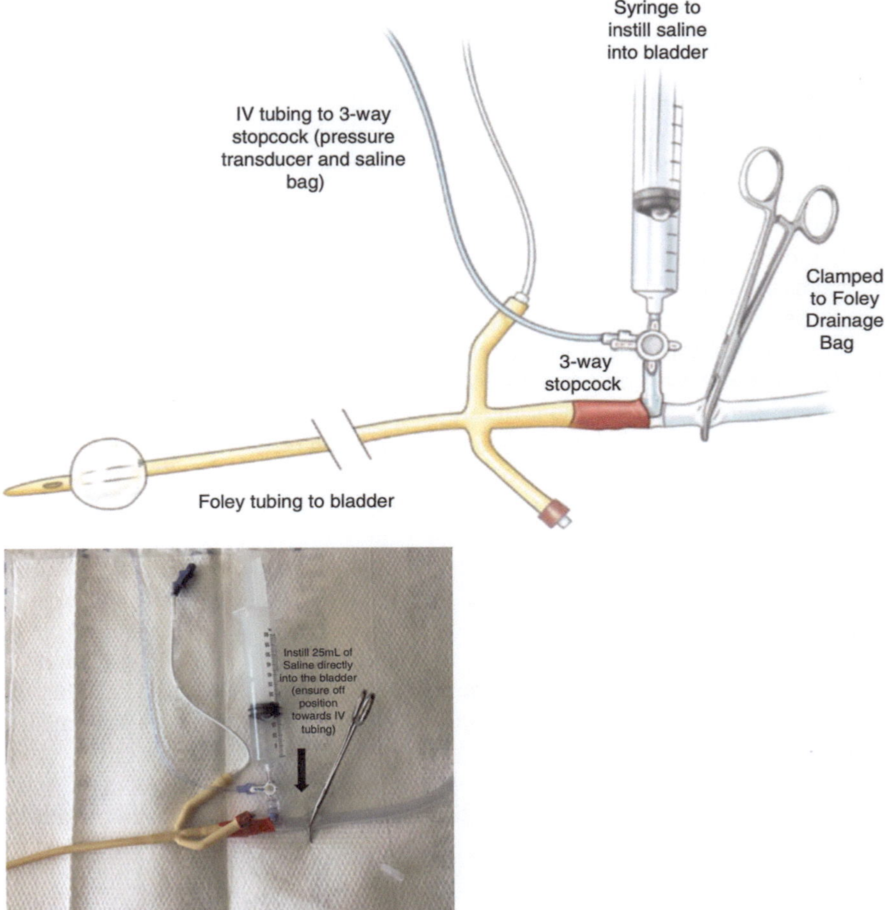

Fig. 24.1 Intra-abdominal pressure monitoring. (Source: https://link.springer.com/chapter/10.100 7/978-3-319-78367-3_26)

24.5 Manifestations of ACS by Organ System

Cardiovascular System: Inferior vena cava compression reduces venous return not only from the abdominal viscera and lower extremities, but also to the heart. This decrease in cardiac preload directly results in decreased cardiac output, which manifests as hypotension. Ongoing hypotension compromises blood flow and oxygen delivery to all organs and peripheral tissues [9]. Decreasing cardiac output is further exacerbated by direct pressure transmitted through the diaphragm onto the mediastinum, which limits ventricular compliance [16].

Pulmonary System: Elevated intrathoracic pressures transmitted from the abdomen across the diaphragm restrict pulmonary compliance, reducing tidal volume and functional residual capacity while increasing pulmonary vascular resistance. This manifests as increased airway pressures and difficulty ventilating. As ACS progresses, alveolar atelectasis increases dead space, impairing gas exchange, resulting in hypoxemia and hypercarbia [9, 16].

Renal System: Increased renal vein pressure, decreased arterial blood flow, and compensatory increases in renal vascular resistance all collectively impair renal glomerular and tubular function and increase the renal filtration gradient. This manifests as a reduction in urinary output. Oliguria can occur at an IAP of 15 mmHg and progress to anuria at an IAP of 30 mmHg. Recent research underscores the association between IAH and a heightened risk of acute kidney injury across diverse patient populations, with no discernible influence from age, body mass index, burns, or cardiac surgery [15, 16].

Gastrointestinal System: Decreased splanchnic blood flow results in both intestinal and hepatic malperfusion. Intestinal ischemia elevates the risk of bacterial translocation and infection, while hepatic ischemia results in metabolic acidosis and impaired toxin metabolism and clearance [16].

Nervous System: Elevated intrathoracic pressures transmitted from the abdomen across the diaphragm compromise venous drainage from the brain, leading to increased intracranial pressure and reduced cerebral blood flow. Compensatory increases in cerebral arterial flow further increase intracranial pressure [9, 16].

General: Polycompartment syndrome is characterized by elevated pressures in two or more anatomical compartments. In this condition, the increased abdominal pressure from ACS is transmitted to extra-abdominal compartments, resulting in thoracic compartment syndrome, intracranial compartment syndrome, and extremity compartment syndrome [17]. Overall, untreated ACS can lead to multi-organ dysfunction as described throughout this section and ultimately death [9].

24.6 Management of Abdominal Compartment Syndrome

Strategies to manage ACS revolve around preventing the evolution of IAH to ACS. For immediate measures, this translates to any interventions that can decrease the volume of abdominal contents or increase the compliance of the abdomen. Bladder decompression with Foley is a mainstay not only to directly address IAH but also to facilitate IAP measurements. Enteric decompression can be achieved with gastric and rectal tubes, laxative enemas, and cessation of enteral nutrition. Pharmacists should review medication profiles and facilitate discontinuation of enterally administered medications, not only to minimize enteric volume but also because absorption of enteric medications may be compromised in patients with IAH. Medication regimens should be converted to injectable formulations as appropriate. If large-volume ascites is present, teams might consider paracentesis to acutely decrease volume and relieve pressure and then review opportunities to limit ascites reaccumulation, including titrating diuretics and concentrating medications when able, in addition to treating the underlying cause for ascites. Diuretic protocols led by pharmacists have been associated with significantly lower median cumulative fluid balance 72 h post-shock compared to standard of care in a pilot study with 364 medical ICU patients [−2257 (−5676 to 920) mL vs. 265 (−2283 to 3025) mL, $p < 0.0001$] [18]. If a temporary abdominal dressing is present, surgical teams might consider decreasing the degree of negative pressure being applied or changing the dressing altogether to directly improve abdominal wall compliance.

Pharmacists are critical to helping optimize sedation and pain control, which increases abdominal wall compliance. Deep sedation using sedatives and analgesics is often required. A trial of paralysis to maximally relax abdominal wall musculature may be needed to reduce IAP if deep sedation alone is insufficient. Prior to initiating paralysis, pharmacists and interdisciplinary team members must ensure that patients are deeply sedated (i.e., Richmond Agitation Sedation Scale score of −5) with sedatives such as propofol and/or benzodiazepines to prevent patient awareness during paralysis. Since sedation depth is not assessable in the setting of paralysis, pharmacists must ensure that all team members know not to wean sedatives while patients are chemically paralyzed. This can be done through education, modifying orders that eliminate titration of sedatives, and establishing best practice alerts in the electronic medical record.

Beyond directly reducing compartment volume and increasing compliance of the abdomen, the care team, including pharmacists, must also consider their overall approach to resuscitation and whether fluid-sparing strategies with early use of vasopressors are feasible for the patient's pathology. Limiting crystalloid infusion prevents fluid overload and stems IAH by limiting visceral edema and ascites. In patients who have hypovolemia due to significant blood loss, balanced transfusion of products rather than crystalloid is preferred and will also prevent coagulopathy that would otherwise exacerbate or prolong blood loss. Common sources of volume include maintenance fluids, resuscitation fluids, nutrition, and medications via all routes. In a single-center cohort study with over 14,000 critically ill patients, maintenance and replacement fluids accounted for approximately 25% of the total daily fluid volume while resuscitation fluids accounted for only 6.5%. Fluid creep, defined as unintentional fluid administration, accounted for 33% of the total daily fluid volume [19]. An observational study including 426 medical ICU patients revealed that medication diluents accounted for up to 63% of the total fluid volume administered to patients [20]. Pharmacists can assist with fluid stewardship through assessment of fluid balance, laboratory data, hemodynamics, and fluid responsiveness (Box 24.2) [21, 22]. As mentioned earlier, pharmacists can help implement multimodal diuretic regimens that optimize fluid removal when indicated. There is no conclusive data supporting the use of routine diuretic, renal replacement therapy, or hypertonic fluids to prevent progression to ACS.

> **Box 24.2 Pharmacist Interventions for Fluid Stewardship**
> - Initiate/discontinue or adjust doses of maintenance fluids and enteral water
> - Initiate/discontinue or adjust dose of diuretics
> - Initiate/discontinue nutrition (TPN, enteral)
> - Adjust doses of enteral and IV-administered medications
> - Concentrate medications
> - Adjust administration routes of medications (intravenous, enteral)
> - Choose the type of IV fluids (crystalloids, colloids)
> - Recommend evaluation of volume responsiveness (hemodynamic monitoring, SVV, PPV, fluid challenge, PLR)
>
> *IV* intravenous, *PLR* passive leg raise, *PPV* positive-pressure ventilation, *SVV* stroke volume variation, *TPN* total parenteral nutrition

Once IAH is sustained and progresses to ACS, definitive management involves laparotomy to open the abdominal compartment and thereby relieve deleterious pressure. Patients need not be transported to the operating room for a decompressive laparotomy, and in fact generally they are not stable enough to tolerate such transport. Instead, the minimal equipment needed for decompressive laparotomy (scalpel, cautery, suction, and temporary closure device/dressings) can be brought to the intensive care unit and used bedside. After the abdominal cavity has been opened, a temporary abdominal closure dressing is applied that effectively enlarges the abdominal compartment and can be kept in place or changed at intervals until the underlying pathology for ACS and need for an enlarged abdominal compartment have resolved. At that point, the temporary abdominal closure dressing can be removed, and the abdominal wound formally closed.

For patients who undergo operations for trauma or other intra-abdominal catastrophes, surgical teams should consider temporary abdominal closure dressings as a preventative measure if there is excessive tension with attempted fascial closure or if the team anticipates that risk factors for IAH and ACS are likely to occur postoperatively, specifically large-volume crystalloid resuscitation or ongoing shock that may precipitate significant bowel edema and abdominal distension.

24.7   Management of Patients with an Open Abdomen for Abdominal Compartment Syndrome

Patients with ACS or at high risk for postoperative ACS are managed with an open abdominal wound with a temporary abdominal closure dressing. These patients are described as having an open abdomen. There are a number of considerations to keep in mind when caring for patients with an open abdomen. These are explored in detail below.

24.7.1 *Sedation and Analgesia*

As with all critically ill patients, pain should be routinely assessed in all critically ill patients using validated scales. The Numerical Rating Scale (NRS) is applicable to patients who are able to self-report their pain, whereas the Behavioral Pain Scale (BPS) or Critical Care Pain Observation Tool (CPOT) can be used for patients who are unable to communicate their pain. Uncontrolled pain must always be treated before sedatives are added or increased. Multimodal analgesic regimens that optimize non-pharmacologic and opioid and non-opioid pharmacologic therapies are recommended [23]. Routine assessment and management of pain are associated with decreased sedative use, shorter duration of mechanical ventilation, and decreased intensive care unit (ICU) length of stay (LOS) [24].

Similarly, sedation should be routinely assessed using validated scales such as the Richmond Agitation Sedation Scale (RASS) or Riker Sedation Agitation Scale (SAS) and titrated to achieve a calm state unless the patient's hemodynamics necessitate a different sedation goal. Care teams should avoid using benzodiazepines for routine sedation due to the associated increased risk for delirium, longer duration of mechanical ventilation, and increased ICU and hospital LOS compared to alternative options. When sedation is needed, agents such as propofol or dexmedetomidine should be preferentially used [23, 25]. Deep sedation is associated with increased duration of mechanical ventilation, increased ICU and hospital LOS, and mortality and therefore should generally be avoided without a clear indication. The presence of an open abdomen does not inherently warrant deep sedation as long as the temporary abdominal closure dressing is secure. If IAP increases or patients themselves are at high risk of inducing self-harm by removing their own dressings, then deepened sedation is indeed indicated.

Pharmacist-developed and -enforced sedation protocols and guidelines have been associated with decreased drug costs, shorter duration of mechanical ventilation, increased patient comfort, better compliance with care protocols, and decreased ICU and hospital LOS [26–30]. Pharmacists can create these helpful algorithms as well as help establish daily sedation goals and ensure that those goals are met.

24.7.2 *Nutrition and Gastrointestinal Function*

The catabolic state imposed by any critical illness makes nutrition administration particularly important to enhance recovery, and ACS requiring an open abdomen is no exception. The presence of an open abdomen is not in itself a contraindication to enteral nutrition. However, it is important to confirm with surgical teams whether the patient's gastrointestinal tract is intact or "in continuity" and able to tolerate inflow before starting any form of enteral medications or nutrition. The American Society for Parenteral and Enteral Nutrition and the Society of Critical Care Medicine recommend early enteral nutrition within 24–48 h of presentation in patients with open abdomen without bowel injury [31]. Benefits of early enteral nutrition include protection from nosocomial infections, maintenance of the enteral mucosal lining, higher success at fascial closure, and decreased mortality [32, 33]. Guidelines recommend that patients with an open abdomen should receive an additional 15–30 g of protein per liter of exudate lost [31].

Pharmacists can help assess the likelihood of absorption of enterally administered medications. Medications should be changed to parenteral formulations if concerns for malabsorption exist due to the patient's overall clinical picture and organ function. The prolonged presence of an open abdomen may be accompanied by the evolution of an entero-atmospheric fistula, whereby the gastrointestinal tract opens into the wound, and intraluminal contents are secreted in the same manner as an ostomy. In these circumstances, pharmacists can assist with determining enteral medication absorption based on the location and volume of output of fistulas and can devise pharmacologic options to slow fistula output as well as propose parenteral medication alternatives if enteral absorption will still be insufficient. Pharmacists can also assist with electrolyte replacement, which may be particularly complex in the setting of high-output fistulas or renal dysfunction requiring an extra layer of cautious dosing. Similarly, in patients with acute or chronic hepatic dysfunction, pharmacists are critical in helping adjust medication regimens or devise alternatives that reduce the risk for accumulation and adverse effects in the face of enteral malabsorption and/or ongoing impaired hepatic blood flow [34].

24.7.3 Fluid Balance and Renal Function

As described earlier in this chapter, fluid resuscitation is directly related to the risk for ACS. It should be no surprise, then, that the ability to successfully and safely close an open abdomen is also directly related to fluid balance. As with all critically ill patients, fluid resuscitation should be guided by the patient's hemodynamics. This generally requires close monitoring and careful titration, as hypovolemia threatens organ perfusion and function, while fluid overload is also associated with increased morbidity and mortality [35–38].

The open abdomen allows for significant loss of fluid that would normally be reabsorbed by an intact peritoneal lining. This amounts to 500–2000 mL of nitrogen-rich losses [39]. Replacement strategies for these losses remain controversial. There is no difference in clinical outcomes in critically ill patients who receive crystalloids versus colloids for replacement; however, this data is not specific to patients with open abdomens [40, 41]. Due to the higher costs associated with albumin and lack of data supporting superiority, crystalloids are preferred. Pharmacists can help create guidelines that outline fluid administration and reduce inappropriate albumin use [42]. As a patient recovers from ACS and its precipitating pathology with resolving hypotension and organ dysfunction, active diuresis may become indicated, and doing so can help facilitate abdominal closure as the edema within the abdominal compartment decreases.

Acute kidney injury (AKI) associated with IAH and ACS can result in alterations in metabolism and excretion of many drugs including sedatives, opioids, anticoagulants, and antimicrobials. Pharmacists can provide dosing recommendations to prevent drug accumulation and associated adverse effects. Pharmacists can also help prevent new or worsening AKI by identifying nephrotoxic agents or doses and providing alternative regimens, as approximately 20–25% of AKI in critically ill patients may be caused by medications [43].

24.7.4 Antimicrobial Use

Prophylactic antimicrobials are not indicated for open abdomen. If infection is present related to the underlying pathology of ACS, then empiric antimicrobials should be selected based on the presumed source and tailored based on the status of source control and culture data [44–46]. Antibiotic stewardship, involving the conscientious selection of antibiotic regimens to ensure appropriate treatment while minimizing complications including emergence of resistant microbes, has long been prioritized by the Infectious Disease Society of America and major health agencies such as the World Health Organization and Centers for Disease Control [47, 48]. This relies on expertise that the pharmacist is particularly well positioned to provide. Pharmacists can apply pharmacokinetic and pharmacodynamic principles to create dosing regimens that will maximize time and/or drug concentrations above the minimum inhibitory concentration for a given organism while preventing further harm through therapeutic drug monitoring of nephrotoxic agents like aminoglycosides and vancomycin, particularly in the setting of pre-existing renal dysfunction. Intensive care units with pharmacists helping to care for patients with severe infections have been shown to have shorter ICU LOS, less total cost, and lower mortality. Mortality in patients with nosocomial infections who received care in ICUs without pharmacists had 23.6% higher mortality compared to ICUs with pharmacists [49].

24.8 Summary

Patients with intra-abdominal hypertension and abdominal compartment syndrome require prompt diagnosis and management. Clinicians can prevent and mitigate the impact of these conditions by understanding their risk factors. A multidisciplinary approach involving surgeons, intensivists, and pharmacists can optimize patient outcomes and facilitate timely abdominal closure for those patients requiring an open abdomen.

References

1. Malbrain MLNG, Cheatham ML, Kirkpatrick A, et al. Results from the International Conference of Experts on Intra-abdominal Hypertension and Abdominal Compartment Syndrome. I. Definitions. Intensive Care Med. 2006;32:1722–32. https://doi.org/10.1007/s00134-006-0349-5.
2. Balogh ZJ, Lumsdaine W, Moore EE, Moore FA. Postinjury abdominal compartment syndrome: from recognition to prevention. Lancet. 2014;384(9952):1466–75. https://doi.org/10.1016/S0140-6736(14)61689-5.
3. Leon M, Chavez L, Surani S. Abdominal compartment syndrome amongst surgical patients. World J Gastrointest Surg. 2021;13:330–9.
4. Padar M, Reintam Blaser A, Talving P, et al. Abdominal compartment syndrome: improving outcomes with a multidisciplinary approach—a narrative review. J Multidiscip Healthc. 2019;12:1061–74. https://doi.org/10.2147/jmdh.s205608.
5. Lat I, Paciullo C, Mitchell D, et al. Position paper on critical care pharmacy services: 2020 update. Crit Care Med. 2020;48:e813–34.
6. Leape LL, Cullen DJ, Clapp MD, et al. Pharmacist participation on physician rounds and adverse drug events in the intensive care unit. JAMA. 1999;282:267–70.
7. Bond CA, Raehl CL. Clinical pharmacy services, pharmacy staffing, and hospital mortality rates. Pharmacotherapy. 2007;27:481–93.
8. Lee H, Ryu K, Sohn Y, et al. Impact on patient outcomes of pharmacist participation in multidisciplinary critical care teams: a systematic review and meta-analysis. Crit Care Med. 2019;47:1243–50.
9. De Laet IE, Malbrain MLNG, De Waele JJ. A clinician's guide to management of intra-abdominal hypertension and abdominal compartment syndrome in critically ill patients. Crit Care. 2020;24:97. https://doi.org/10.1186/s13054-020-2782-1.
10. Khot Z, Murphy PB, Ball IM, et al. Incidence of intra-abdominal hypertension and abdominal compartment syndrome: a systematic review. J Intensive Care Med. 2021;36(2):197–202. https://doi.org/10.1177/0885066619892225.
11. Kirkpatrick AW, Roberts DJ, De Waele J, et al. Intra-abdominal hypertension and the abdominal compartment syndrome: updated consensus definitions and clinical practice guidelines from the World Society of the Abdominal Compartment Syndrome. Intensive Care Med. 2013;39:1190–206. https://doi.org/10.1007/s00134-013-2906-z.
12. Fietsam R, Villalba M, Glover JL, Clark K. Intra-abdominal compartment syndrome as a complication of ruptured abdominal aortic aneurysm repair. Am Surg. 1989;55(6):396–402.
13. Holodinsky JK, Roberts DJ, Ball CG, et al. Risk factors for intra-abdominal hypertension and abdominal compartment syndrome among adult intensive care unit patients: a systematic review and meta-analysis. Crit Care. 2013;17(5):R249. https://doi.org/10.1186/cc13075.
14. Strang SG, Van Lieshout EMM, Breederveld RS, Van Waes OJF. A systematic review on intra-abdominal pressure in severely burned patients. Burns. 2014;40(1):9–16. https://doi.org/10.1016/j.burns.2013.07.001.
15. Sun J, Sun H, Sun Z, et al. Intra-abdominal hypertension and increased acute kidney injury risk: a systematic review and meta-analysis. J Int Med Res. 2021;49(5):3000605211016627. https://doi.org/10.1177/03000605211016627.
16. Rajasurya V, Surani S. Abdominal compartment syndrome: often overlooked conditions in medical intensive care units. World J Gastroenterol. 2020;26(3):266–78. https://doi.org/10.3748/wjg.v26.i3.266.
17. Malbrain ML, Roberts DJ, Sugrue M, et al. The polycompartment syndrome: a concise state-of-the-art review. Anaesthesiol Intensive Ther. 2014;46(5):433–50. https://doi.org/10.5603/AIT.2014.0064.
18. Bissell BD, Laine ME, Bastin ML, et al. Impact of protocolized diuresis for de-resuscitation in the intensive care unit. Crit Care. 2020;24:70.

19. Van Regenmortel N, Verbrugghe W, Roelant E, et al. Maintenance fluid therapy and fluid creep impose more significant fluid, sodium, and chloride burdens than resuscitation fluids in critically ill patients: a retrospective study in a tertiary mixed ICU population. Intensive Care Med. 2018;44:409–17.
20. Magee CA, Bastin MLT, Laine ME, et al. Insidious harm of medication diluents as a contributor to cumulative volume and hyperchloremia: a prospective, open-label, sequential period pilot study. Crit Care Med. 2018;46:1217–23.
21. Bissell BD, Mefford B. Pathophysiology of volume administration in septic shock and the role of the clinical pharmacist. Ann Pharmacother. 2020;54:388–96.
22. Hawkins AW, Butler SA, Poirier N, et al. From theory to bedside: implementation of fluid stewardship in a medical ICU pharmacy practice. Am J Health Syst Pharm. 2022;79:984–92.
23. Devlin JW, Skrobik Y, Gélinas C, et al. Management of pain, agitation/sedation, delirium, immobility, and sleep disruption in adult patients in the ICU. Crit Care Med. 2018;46:e825–73.
24. Payen JF, Bosson JL, Chanques G, et al. Pain assessment is associated with decreased duration of mechanical ventilation in the intensive care unit: a post hoc analysis of the DOLOREA study. Anesthesiology. 2009;111:1308–16.
25. Hughes CG, Mailloux PT, Devlin JW, et al. Dexmedetomidine vs propofol for sedation in mechanically ventilated adult patients with sepsis. N Engl J Med. 2021;384:1424–36.
26. Devlin JW, Holbrook AM, Fuller HD. The effect of ICU sedation guidelines and pharmacist interventions on clinical outcomes and drug cost. Ann Pharmacother. 1997;31:689–95.
27. Louzon P, Jennings H, Ali M, et al. Impact of pharmacist management of pain, agitation, and delirium in the intensive care unit through participation in multidisciplinary bundle rounds. Am J Health Syst Pharm. 2017;74:253–62.
28. MacLaren R, Plamondon JM, Ramsay KB, et al. A prospective evaluation of empiric versus protocol-based sedation and analgesia. Pharmacotherapy. 2000;20:662–72.
29. Marshall J, Finn CA, Theodore AC. Impact of a clinical pharmacist-enforced intensive care unit sedation protocol on duration of mechanical ventilation and hospital stay. Crit Care Med. 2008;36:427–33.
30. Stollings JL, Foss JJ, Ely EW, et al. Pharmacist leadership in ICU quality improvement: coordinating spontaneous awakening and breathing trials. Ann Pharmacother. 2015;49:883–91.
31. McClave SA, Taylor BE, Martindale RG, et al. Guidelines for the provision and assessment of nutrition support therapy in the adult critically ill patient: Society of Critical Care Medicine (SCCM) and American Society for Parenteral and Enteral Nutrition (ASPEN). JPEN J Parenter Enteral. 2016;40 159–211.
32. Burlew CC, Moore EE, Cuschieri J, et al. Who should we feed? Western Trauma Association multi-institutional study of enteral nutrition in the open abdomen after injury. J Trauma Acute Care Surg. 2012;73(6):1380–7; discussion 1387–8. https://doi.org/10.1097/TA.0b013e318259924c.
33. Dissanaike S, Pham T, Shalhub S, et al. Effect of immediate enteral feeding on trauma patients with an open abdomen: protection from nosocomial infections. J Am Coll Surg. 2008;207(5):690–7. https://doi.org/10.1016/j.jamcollsurg.2008.06.332.
34. Verbeeck RK. Pharmacokinetics and dosage adjustment in patients with hepatic dysfunction. Eur J Clin Pharmacol. 2008;64:1147–61.
35. Balakumar V, Murugan R, Sileanu FE, et al. Both positive and negative fluid balance may be associated with reduced long-term survival in the critically ill. Crit Care Med. 2017;45(8):e749–57.
36. Kelm DJ, Perrin JT, Cartin-Ceba R, et al. Fluid overload in patients with severe sepsis and septic shock treated with early goal-directed therapy is associated with increased acute need for fluid-related medical interventions and hospital death. Shock. 2015;43(1):68–73.
37. Mitchell KH, Carlbom D, Caldwell E, et al. Volume overload: prevalence, risk factors, and functional outcome in survivors of septic shock. Ann Am Thorac Soc. 2015;12(12):1837–44.
38. Ostermann M, Straaten HM, Forni LG. Fluid overload and acute kidney injury: cause or consequence? Crit Care. 2015;19:443.

39. Cheatham ML, Safcsak K, Brzezinski SJ, Lube MW. Nitrogen balance, protein loss, and the open abdomen. Crit Care Med. 2007;35(1):127–31. https://doi.org/10.1097/01. CCM.0000250390.49380.94.

40. Annane D, Siami S, Jaber S, et al. Effects of fluid resuscitation with colloids vs. crystalloids on mortality in critically ill patients with hypovolemic shock: the CRISTAL randomized trial. JAMA. 2013;310:1809–17.

41. Finfer S, Bellomo R, Boyce N, et al. A comparison of albumin and saline for fluid resuscitation in the intensive care unit. N Engl J Med. 2004;350:2247–56.

42. Buckley MS, Knutson KD, Agarwal SK, et al. Clinical pharmacist-led impact on inappropriate albumin use and costs in the critically ill. Ann Pharmacother. 2020;54:105–12.

43. Brivet FG, Kleinknecht DJ, Loirat P, et al. Acute renal failure in intensive care units—causes, outcome, and prognostic factors of hospital mortality; a prospective, multicenter study. French Study Group on Acute Renal Failure. Crit Care Med. 1996;24:192–8.

44. Mazuski JE, Tessier JM, May AK, et al. The Surgical Infection Society Revised Guidelines on the management of intra-abdominal infection. Surg Infect (Larchmt). 2017;18(1):1–76. https:// doi.org/10.1089/sur.2016.261.

45. Montravers P, Tubach F, Lescot T, et al. Short-course antibiotic therapy for critically ill patients treated for postoperative intra-abdominal infection: the DURAPOP randomised clinical trial. Intensive Care Med. 2018;44(3):300–10. https://doi.org/10.1007/s00134-018-5088-x.

46. Solomkin JS, Mazuski JE, Bradley JS, et al. Diagnosis and management of complicated intra-abdominal infection in adults and children: guidelines by the Surgical Infection Society and the Infectious Diseases Society of America. Clin Infect Dis. 2010;50(2):133–64. https://doi. org/10.1086/649554.

47. Dyar OJ, Huttner B, Schouten J, Pulcini C, ESGAP (ESCMID Study Group for Antimicrobial stewardshiP). What is antimicrobial stewardship? Clin Microbiol Infect. 2017;23(11):793–8. https://doi.org/10.1016/j.cmi.2017.08.026.

48. Pulcini C, Binda F, Lamkang AS, et al. Developing core elements and checklist items for global hospital antimicrobial stewardship programmes: a consensus approach. Clin Microbiol Infect. 2019;25(1):20–5. https://doi.org/10.1016/j.cmi.2018.03.033.

49. MacLaren R, Bond CA, Martin SJ, et al. Clinical and economic outcomes of involving pharmacists in the direct care of critically ill patients with infections. Crit Care Med. 2008;36:3184–9.

Chapter 25
Critical Care of the Abdominal Surgery Patient

Malerie Pratt, Grace Lee, Alex Panuccio, Aulina Chowdhury, and Kristin Madenci

25.1 Introduction

Managing abdominal surgery patients in the intensive care unit (ICU) involves a variety of unique challenges and benefits from a multidisciplinary approach. Critical care physicians, surgeons, advanced practitioners, nurses, nutritionists, and pharmacists are just some of the many team players who must work collaboratively to provide the best comprehensive care. A basic understanding of the complexities of abdominal surgery patients provides a foundation to best care for this group of patients. In this chapter, we will describe some of the surgical procedures that you may encounter while caring for these patients and how that can influence their treatment in the ICU. Specifically, we will discuss the open abdomen, ileostomies, colostomies, enterocutaneous fistulas, NSTIs, tracheostomies, and gastrostomy feeding tubes.

M. Pratt
Brigham and Women's Hospital, Boston, MA, USA

G. Lee · A. Panuccio
Los Angeles Medical Center, Kaiser Permanente, Los Angeles, CA, USA

A. Chowdhury
Boston Children's Hospital, Boston, MA, USA

K. Madenci (✉)
Brigham and Women's Hospital, Harvard Medical School, Boston, MA, USA
e-mail: kmadenci@bwh.harvard.edu

25.2 Open Abdomen

The term "open abdomen" refers to not closing the fascia after an operation, as a temporary measure. At the end of the procedure, the abdomen is temporarily closed to help minimize the loss of domain, protect the abdominal contents, decrease the infection risk, minimize fluid losses, and allow for quick reentry of the abdomen. One of the more common techniques used for temporary abdominal closure includes a barrier protecting the viscera, a sponge, and then another thin drape forming a closed system. The device is then hooked up to suction to isolate and protect the abdominal contents. A common medical device that uses this negative-pressure system is called an abthera (Fig. 25.1).

The most common indications for an open abdomen include trauma damage control procedures, abdominal compartment syndrome, or patients who are intraoperatively unstable and require a second-look procedure for re-evaluation. In trauma, damage control surgery involves creating a laparotomy in a severely injured patient with the goal of temporizing life-threatening injuries such as controlling hemorrhage and spillage of enteric contents. These patients are typically unstable, coagulopathic, and acidotic and likely will continue to bleed until warmed and coagulopathy is corrected. Therefore, the priority is getting them out of the OR for further resuscitation. The patient is then transferred to the intensive care unit for resuscitation until they are stable enough to undergo definitive repair if needed and abdominal closure.

Abdominal compartment syndrome is defined as an increase in intra-abdominal pressure (IAP) that can lead to multisystem organ failure. IAP can be measured indirectly most readily by measuring bladder pressure using a Foley catheter. Abdominal compartment syndrome occurs when intra-abdominal pressure is sustained >20 mmHg. The abdomen is a fixed space, and the accumulation of fluid, air, or blood in the abdomen can compress organs and blood vessels leading to decreased

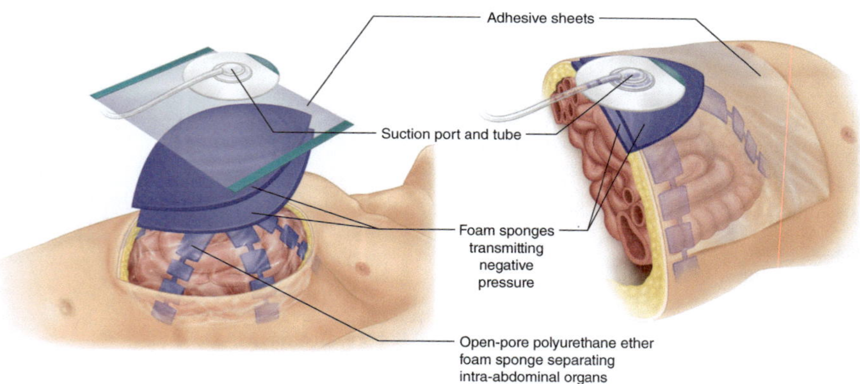

Fig. 25.1 Abthera

blood flow, oxygen delivery, and organ dysfunction. For these patients, what they need is decompression of their abdominal cavity by opening the abdominal fascia. The underlying etiology must also then be addressed prior to closure. Risk factors for abdominal compartment syndrome include but are not limited to abdominal trauma, abdominal surgery, intra-abdominal inflammation or infection (e.g., pancreatitis), and high-volume fluid resuscitation.

Damage control surgery is not limited to trauma patients. Other indications for temporarily leaving the abdomen open are patients who are unstable due to septic shock or intra-abdominal hemorrhage and require a second look. In acute care surgery, patients who benefit from this lifesaving method are patients with intestinal perforation, such as perforated diverticulitis, patients in septic shock on multiple pressors, and OB-GYN patients who have significant bleeding and develop coagulopathy or abdominal vascular surgery emergencies where this is a concern about hemostasis or organ perfusion. This approach limits operative time in unstable patients and allows for control of hemorrhage, contamination, and sepsis while allowing for subsequent surgeries.

25.3 ICU Considerations

Leaving the abdomen open while the patient stabilizes in the ICU can increase the patient's risk for infection. The abdomen is physiologically a sterile space; leaving the cavity open to air can expose it to pathogens. A temporary abdominal closure device helps to prevent this exposure. Furthermore, in critically ill patients, gut microbes that normally live inside the intestines can translocate through leaky intestinal walls into the bloodstream and cause sepsis. If there was an intestinal injury leading to contamination of the abdomen with stool during the initial operation, there is an increased risk of infection due to spillage of gut microbes. To prevent sepsis from infection from an open abdomen, patients may be placed on prophylactic antibiotics until the abdomen is closed. Prophylactic antibiotics should have broad gram-positive, gram-negative, and anaerobic coverage to cover gut microbes as well as organisms that can cause hospital-acquired infections.

25.3.1 Enterocutaneous Fistulas and Incisional Hernias

Although temporarily leaving a patient's abdomen open can be lifesaving, it can also create complex long-term complications that may have lasting implications. Two common complications from an open abdomen are enterocutaneous fistulas (ECF) and incisional hernias. An ECF is an abnormal epithelial-lined connection from the intestine to the skin that causes leakage of enteric or bowel contents through the abdominal wall. Frequent bowel manipulation and injury during repeat trips to the operating room increase the incidence of ECF to as high as 20% in patients with an open abdomen. ECF fistulas are characterized by low-output (enteric content drainage of less than 200 mL/day), moderate-output (200–500 mL/day), and high-output fistulas (more than 500 mL/day). Patients with high-output fistulas are at an increased risk of dehydration, electrolyte derangements, and malnutrition. Once the patient is stabilized by sepsis management, replacing fluid and electrolyte loss from the fistula, it is recommended to trial a short period of bowel rest with or without total parenteral nutrition (TPN) to evaluate if the fistula output will decrease or spontaneously close. If output continues, then enteral feeding is trialed and continued as long as output does not exceed more than 1.5 L a day. Different drug therapies such as anticathartics, histamine-2 receptor antagonists, antisecretories, somatostatin analogs, and cholestyramine may be tried to decrease output. If fistula output increases with oral intake to greater than 1.5 L a day, then TPN is initiated. Operative management is offered at a minimum of 6 months after fistula diagnosis when infection and malnutrition have been resolved.

Another notable complication in patients with an open abdomen is an incisional hernia from the abdominal wall muscles retracting the fascia laterally causing a loss of domain. After effective management of the initial insult for an open abdomen has been addressed, early abdominal closure between 24 and 48 h is preferred. The surgical intensive care team focuses on volume resuscitation, reversal of coagulopathy, and correction of acidosis to optimize the patient for fascial closure. If the fascia cannot be primarily closed even after an abdominal muscle release, the abdomen may be closed with a functional bridge such as a biological mesh that bridges the facial defect. If either of these options are not possible, then the patient may or the abdominal viscera may be covered with a skin-only or split-thickness skin graft closure as a planned ventral hernia.

25.3.2 Ileostomy and Colostomy

During the abdominal closure, the patient may receive a stoma. This involves exteriorizing a portion of the intestine to the surface of the abdominal wall to divert bowel contents and facilitate recovery. An ostomy is indicated in patients who are hemodynamically unstable and at a high risk of anastomotic failure. Enteric diversion may benefit patients with inflammatory bowel disease, malignancy, bowel obstruction, or congenital anomalies. Understanding the anatomy of these stomas is crucial and requires individualizing resuscitation and nutrition strategies that match the patients' new digestion and absorption patterns. A temporary or permanent ostomy can be made anywhere throughout the gastrointestinal tract. Careful selection of the stoma site is key as the patient must be able to access it without difficulty for daily care. It should be located preferably in the rectus where it is free from skin folds, umbilicus, or belt lines.

An ileostomy is an anastomosis between the ileum and the abdominal wall that completely bypasses the large intestine (Fig. 25.2). These are often created to protect a distal high-risk anastomosis. There are different ways to create an ileostomy.

Fig. 25.2 Ileostomy
anatomy

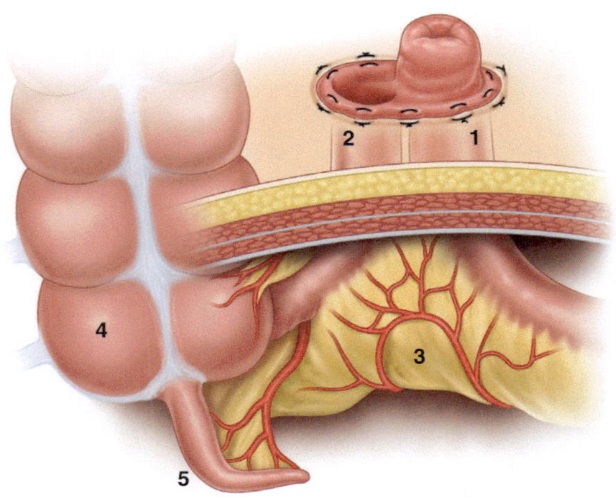

The most common are diverting loop ileostomy (Fig. 25.2) and an end ileostomy. A diverting loop ileostomy is when a loop of the terminal ileum is exteriorized through the abdominal wall, whereas an end ileostomy refers to when only the afferent or proximal limb of the ileum is exteriorized. Some complications of ileostomies include dehydration, electrolyte imbalances, malnutrition, and parastomal hernias.

A colostomy is an anastomosis between the large intestine and the abdominal wall that bypasses the distal colon, rectum, and anus (Fig. 25.3). Indications for a colostomy include protecting a distal high-risk anastomosis, distal obstructions or perforations, malignancy, or sacral ulcers. Due to being more distal in the gastrointestinal tract, they have a decreased risk of dehydration, metabolic derangements, and malnutrition compared to ileostomies. However, they may be harder to reverse due to adhesions. Colostomies, similar to ileostomies, are created as a diverting loop, which allows for a proximal fecal diversion and distal decompression, or an end colostomy.

Ostomies can be reversed when intestinal continuity can safely be restored. Ostomy closure can occur as early as 6–8 weeks; however, some advocate for closer to 3–6 months to allow for a decrease in residual adhesions.

25.3.3   Necrotizing Soft Tissue Infections

Necrotizing soft tissue infections (NSTIs) are surgical emergencies that frequently require intensive care unit management. NSTIs are severe infections with a rapid onset that can involve not only the skin and soft tissue but also the subcutaneous fat, fascia,

Fig. 25.3 Colostomy anatomy

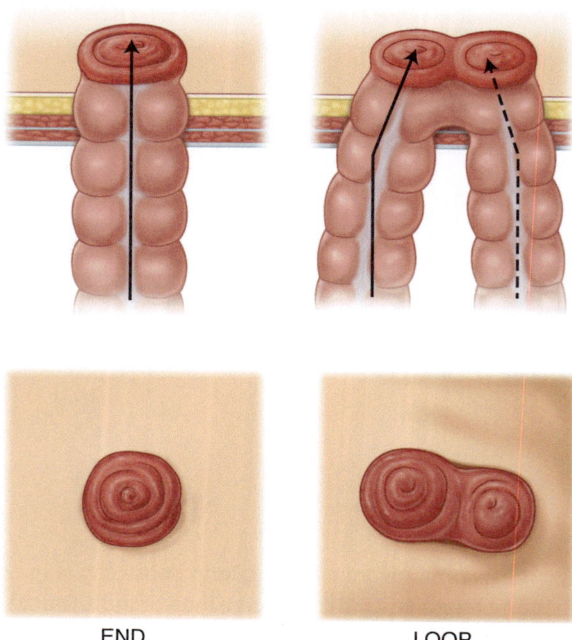

and muscle. The diagnosis of NSTIs is primarily a clinical diagnosis with mortality rates as high as 20% in the United States. Early recognition and prompt surgical debridement can decrease morbidity and improve overall survival. After the initial operation, these patients require a second-look surgery within 24 h and may require multiple trips to the operating room for infection source control and debridement of necrotic tissue. NSTIs are often associated with septic shock that requires aggressive fluid resuscitation, broad-spectrum antibiotics, and vasopressors. A multidisciplinary approach is recommended for proper pain and anxiolytic management due to the multiple debridements and dressing changes. Patients who undergo extensive debridement may necessitate complex surgical reconstruction requiring a collaboration of various surgical specialties.

25.3.4 Tracheostomy

Critically ill patients may require prolonged intubation which can lead to complications such as pneumonia, tracheal stenosis, and vocal cord injury. A tracheostomy is a connection between the anterior neck and the trachea between the second and third tracheal rings that allows for mechanical ventilation without an oral airway (Fig. 25.4). A tracheostomy may improve patient comfort and aid in recovery of speech, swallowing, and oral hygiene. A tracheostomy may be placed in patients with severe upper airway obstruction or who are unable to be liberated from mechanical ventilation. It is recommended that tracheostomies are performed between 10 days and 3 weeks of mechanical ventilation. As the patient starts to wean off the ventilator, a tracheostomy may be downsized and eventually capped as steps towards decannulation.

25.3.5 Percutaneous Endoscopic Gastrostomy Tube

A percutaneous endoscopic gastrostomy (PEG) tube is a feeding tube that is placed from the stomach to the abdominal wall to allow for enteral feeds or hydration that bypasses the oropharynx and esophagus or allows for gastric decompression

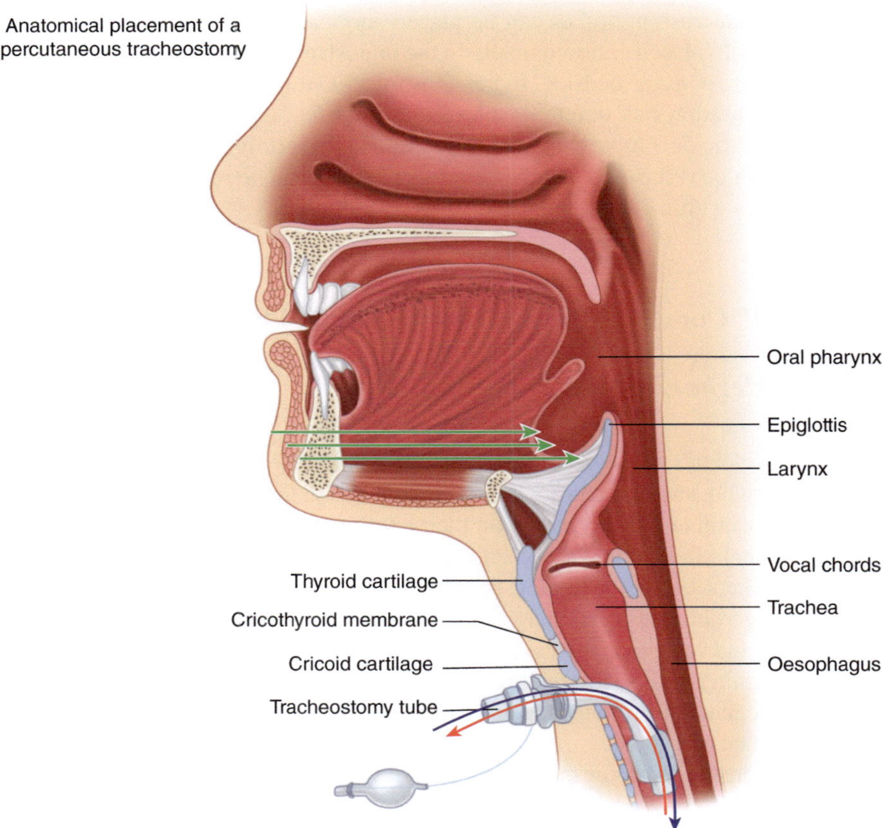

Fig. 25.4 Tracheostomy

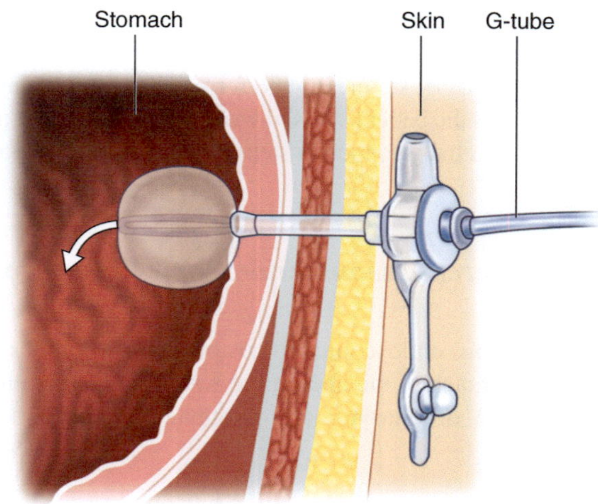

Fig. 25.5 Percutaneous endoscopic gastrostomy tube

(Fig. 25.5). Gastrostomy tubes can be placed surgically, or radiologically, but are most commonly placed endoscopically in the intensive care unit setting either in the operating room or at the bedside. Indications for PEG tubes include patients with an increased aspiration risk due to dysphagia, dysmotility, or malignancy or patients who need gastric decompression due to prolonged ileus or intestinal obstruction. If oral feeds can be restarted, then the gastrostomy tube can be removed and the tract usually closes within 72 h.

25.4 ICU Considerations of the Abdominal Surgery Patient

25.4.1 Mechanical Ventilation

The same principles of mechanical ventilation in critically ill patients apply to those in the ICU who have undergone abdominal surgery. Patients who are unable to adequately ventilate and oxygenate on their own require mechanical ventilation. In general, patients should be weaned off the ventilator as soon as possible. The longer patients are kept on the ventilator, they are at an increased risk of complications from prolonged intubation such as ventilator-acquired pneumonia, delirium, laryngeal edema, and ventilator-induced lung injury. Patients should undergo daily spontaneous breathing trials to test their readiness for extubation, and if they are expected to remain dependent on mechanical ventilation for a prolonged period, tracheostomy should be considered.

Special consideration for the trauma patient includes an increased risk for acute respiratory distress syndrome (ARDS), which is a life-threatening lung injury that is characterized by inflammation and fluid accumulation in the lung. This significantly impairs gas exchange, decreases compliance of the lungs, and ultimately leads to hypoxia and respiratory failure. Mortality is high in patients with ARDS—between 20% and 50%. Lung-protective ventilation settings are recommended for trauma patients to prevent and treat ARDS. The ARDSnet protocol developed by the ARDS network is commonly cited and guides mechanical ventilation in critically ill patients.

Lastly, it is important to note that an open abdomen alone does not mandate mechanical ventilation. Sometimes, a patient with an open abdomen may be kept intubated in anticipation of a second-look laparotomy or abdominal closure soon. The patient should otherwise be weaned as soon as possible to breathe spontaneously on the ventilator; neither deep sedation nor paralysis is required in an open abdomen. Patients with an open abdomen do not need to be kept intubated.

25.4.2 Fluid Management

Determining the right amount of fluid to give to a critically ill patient remains a challenging task. On the one hand, if too little fluids are administered, the patient can experience hypovolemia-related complications such as kidney injury and hypotension. If too much is given, cerebral, pulmonary, or intestinal edema can ensue and can cause ventilator dependence or abdominal compartment syndrome. Determining fluid status is the first step—serum markers of adequate perfusion, imaging, dynamic hemodynamic monitoring, daily ins and outs, and physical exams are used to evaluate for adequate resuscitation. Determination of fluid balance can be obscured by poor urine output due to kidney damage, extremity edema due to prolonged bed rest, or hemodynamic changes due to shock.

Larger fluid losses are expected in patients who have undergone abdominal surgery or who remain in the ICU with an open abdomen. These patients have "insensible" fluid losses, as the fluid that evaporates from the abdomen is not easily quantified like urine or blood loss. Open abdominal operations have greater insensible fluid losses compared to minimally invasive operations. Patients who undergo abdominal surgery undergo a phenomenon called "auto-diuresis"—they tend to retain fluid and then have increased urine output about 3 days after surgery. If they remain with an open abdomen, they can have insensible fluid loss up to 1 mL/kg/h. Fever increases insensible fluid loss.

Fluid resuscitation should aim to restore organ perfusion and correct electrolyte derangements. Replacement fluids of crystalloids, colloids, and blood projects are replaced postoperatively depending on the fluid lost. The REstrictive versus LIbEral Fluid therapy (RELIEF) is an international, multicenter study published in 2018 that evaluated the restrictive versus liberal fluid therapy during and up to 24 h after surgery. They found that restrictive fluid was not associated with a difference in the rate of pulmonary edema or duration of mechanical ventilation versus liberal fluid. Restrictive fluid was not associated with higher rates of disability-free survival but was associated with higher rates of acute kidney injury.

25.4.3 Complications

Understanding possible complications of abdominal surgery in critically ill patients is imperative to patient outcomes. Infection is a common complication, and the risk can increase with greater contamination (e.g., higher wound classification) at the initial surgery. Patients with gross contamination of the abdomen with enteric contents in damage control trauma surgery are more likely to develop infection after surgery. Infections can range from superficial surgical site infections to deep infections that include intra-abdominal abscesses. Infection can lead to wound dehiscence and, if severe, can lead to evisceration. Feared risks in those who have had intestinal surgery are intestinal anastomotic leak and enterocutaneous fistulas. These complications can be challenging to treat and often require prolonged antibiotics, source control, and possible parenteral nutrition before possible definitive repair. In the critically ill patient who is already in a catabolic state, the inability to be fed enterally can be an additional hit that increases morbidity.

Early diagnosis, appropriate diagnostic testing, adequate source control, and optimal antimicrobial therapy are key to reducing morbidity and mortality of surgical patients.

Close monitoring of surgical wounds, vitals, and labs should be performed to assess for complications on a daily basis. While prophylactic antibiotic agents reduce postsurgical wound infections, they can breed multidrug resistance.

Traditionally, once physicians have diagnosed a clinical infection, they have given antibiotics until resolution of symptoms of infection. This has led to longer courses of antibiotics that expose the patient to possible multidrug resistance. The STOP-IT trial was a randomized study that assessed a fixed duration of 4 days of antibiotic treatment after source control versus the traditional longer course of antibiotics until symptom resolution. They found that 4 days of antibiotics were non-inferior to a longer duration, and the study suggests that after adequate source control, the benefits of systemic antimicrobial therapy may be limited to the first few days.

When patients are diagnosed with an abdominal infection, source control should be obtained and the source should be sent for aerobic, anaerobic, and fungal cultures and gram stains, which can help guide antibiotic therapy. Empiric antibiotics should be started based on local epidemiology, infection source, severity of the infection, and patient's risk factors for multidrug resistance. If there is complete source control, antibiotics should only be given for a short course (3–5 days). If there is a persistent infection without adequate source control, clinical judgment and objective laboratory data should be used to make an individual assessment on when to stop antibiotics. Results of the cultures as well as the patient's clinical progress should guide antibiotic de-escalation, and antibiotics should be de-escalated as soon as clinically possible. Multidisciplinary assessment is critical in guiding the care of these particular patients.

25.5 Nutrition

The timing to begin enteric feed postoperatively has been debated over the years. Older protocols recommended delaying the initiation of feeds postoperatively. This was primarily out of concern for complications caused by postoperative ileus. Newer guidelines recommend initiation of feeds within the first 48 h following surgery with advancement of diet, as tolerated by patients [1–3]. Enteral feeds can reduce the risk of postoperative infectious complications [4] and can aid in wound healing [5]; they should be initiated as early as possible [6].

Enteral feeds are usually the preferred method for ensuring nutritional intake in patients as this route of administration has been shown to prevent gastric mucosal atrophy and and stress ulcers and has a reduced risk of other infectious complications when compared to parenteral nutrition [3, 7, 8]. In most patients, gastric feeding tubes are appropriate with post-pyloric tubes being used for patients with gastroparesis [3].

Protein administration is essential for critical care patients as proteins directly contribute to a patient's nitrogen balance with a negative nitrogen balance leading to a catabolic state [9]. Monitoring carbohydrate feeding is equally incredibly important for intubated patients. Too low a carbohydrate content can put a patient in starvation ketoacidosis leading to shifts in blood pH and electrolytes [3]. Conversely, an excess of carbohydrate administration will result in increased CO_2 production and hyperglycemia as well as make it difficult to wean the patient from a ventilator [3].

While enteral feeds are typically the preferred method of administration of nutrients, parenteral nutrition is preferred for a few specific clinical indications such as obstructions (i.e., malignancies), mesenteric ischemia, perforations, those on high levels of vasopressors, and those with high-output fistulas [10, 11].

Abdominal surgery patients may require repeat operations or procedures. The goal is to minimize interruptions in enteral feeds around these procedures. For intubated patients who will undergo a procedure that involves manipulation of their airway (such as changing their endotracheal tube or a laryngoscopy), tube feeds should be stopped no earlier than 6 h before the start of their procedure. For all other intubated patients with gastric feeding tubes (either orogastric or nasogastric), feeds can be stopped the morning of the procedure, with the tubes being set to wall suction to remove residual gastric contents before the procedure. If enteral feeds are paused for a procedure, it is crucial to communicate with the entire team to resume feeds as early as possible to minimize nutritional disruption.

A key element in the care of critically ill patients is nutrition optimization. Gastroparesis, slow gastric emptying, can be a limiting factor with enteral nutrition. Within the critical care population, several factors can contribute to decreased gastrointestinal motility including head injury, abdominal surgery, sepsis, hyperglycemia, recumbent position, narcotics, and catecholamines. The result of gastroparesis in these patients can be impaired drug and nutrition absorption as well as a predisposition for reflux and aspiration [12–16]. Prokinetic agents can be used to improve gastric emptying and aid in correcting gastroparesis.

The current agents in use include motilin receptor agonists (erythromycin, azithromycin), 5-HT4 receptor agonists (metoclopramide), D2 receptor antagonists (domperidone), Mu receptor antagonists (methylnaltrexone, alvimopan, naloxegol), and laxatives/secretagogues (lubiprostone, linaclotide) [17].

The mechanism of erythromycin is stimulation of the migrating motor complex. However, it has been found to lose its efficacy in as few as 72 h as motilin receptors become downregulated [10]. Side effects include gastrointestinal intolerance, prolonged QTc interval, and CYP3A-associated drug interactions [18]. Erythromycin has fewer side effects, though cardiac arrhythmias have been described with its use [19]. Metoclopramide stimulates gastroduodenal activity by stimulating the release of acetylcholine from myenteric cholinergic neurons [20]. Its side effects may also be short-lived. The drug also acts as a D2-receptor antagonist. Consequently, side effects include extrapyramidal symptoms, including tardive dyskinesia. These side effects are related to the duration of exposure to metoclopramide, and they are generally irreversible [21]. Domperidone improved upper gut motility by stimulating cholinergic activity [22]. However, it is not approved in the USA due to its cardiovascular side effects, including QT prolongation and cardiac arrhythmias [9]. Mu receptor antagonists act peripherally; they do not cross the blood-brain barrier. In effect, the centrally acting analgesic effects of narcotics are not reversed. Methylnaltrexone has shown benefits in treating opioid-induced constipation in advanced illness [23]. Alvimopan has been shown to improve the return of bowel function and reduce the length of stay in patients who underwent major abdominal surgery [24].

Prophylactic promotility medications can be considered in this high-risk population, potentially averting complications.

25.5.1   DVT

Venous thromboembolism (VTE) is a common event seen during hospitalization. Deep-vein thrombosis (DVT) and pulmonary embolism (PE) contribute significantly to morbidity and mortality seen with critical illness. Many patients admitted to the ICU arrive with risk factors predisposing them to these adverse events. Such risk factors include advanced age, serious medical illness, recent surgery, trauma, orthopedic fractures, sepsis, heart failure, malignancy, burns, immobilization/stroke/spinal cord injury, pregnancy, estrogens, and previous VTE. Additional ICU-related factors that increase these patients' risks include prolonged hospitalization, mechanical ventilation, central venous lines, and use of paralytic drugs [13, 14, 16, 17, 19, 25]. In a meta-analysis reviewing VTEs among the critically ill, reportedly the rate of confirmed DVTs ranged from 13% to 31% among those who did not receive chemoprophylaxis [25].

Several populations to account for that may have specific anticoagulation needs include trauma, surgical, neurosurgical, and COVID patients [12, 13, 15]. A meta-analysis from JAMA looking at data from 1990 to 2015 concluded that emergency surgery patients have a moderate VTE risk. Consequently, they should receive pharmacologic prophylaxis in the form of unfractionated (UFH) or low-molecular-weight heparin (LMWH) unless there is an absolute contraindication. The first dose should be given on admission and continued until discharge without missed doses. Additionally, all should be considered for mechanical prophylaxis [12]. The American Association for the Surgery of Trauma (AAST) Critical Care Committee Clinical Consensus Document released consensus guidelines in 2021 for the use of chemoprophylaxis in the critically ill trauma population. In patients with blunt solid-organ injury undergoing nonoperative management, the recommendation is to start LMWH within 48 h from the time of injury barring any active bleeding or other contraindications. Among patients with a traumatic brain injury (TBI), it is recommended that chemoprophylaxis is started 24–72 h following admission in the form of UFH or LMWH. However, this is pending the stability of intracranial/extracranial hemorrhage. This decision should be made with the assistance of a neurosurgeon [13]. COVID patients are another population with an elevated risk of VTE. Several society guidelines have recommended chemoprophylaxis in these patients when there is no contraindication. However, even with the usual doses of chemoprophylaxis agents, there are still notable high VTE rates, though there is conflicting data on the use of higher doses as prophylaxis in critically ill patients [15]. In patients who cannot tolerate chemoprophylaxis, pneumatic compression should be utilized [10].

When choosing a prophylactic agent, the decision must be individualized to the patient. Currently, the American Society of Hematology guidelines are that LMWH should be considered UFH in critically ill patients [18]. LMWH probably reduces the incidence of DVT compared to UFH [10, 18]. LMWH has a higher bioavailability after subcutaneous dosing and a longer plasma half-life. One does not seem to have a higher rate of bleeding than the other, though the incidence of HIT appears lower in LMWH compared to UFH [10, 19]. Renal failure may be a reason to use UFH over LMWH as there is possibly bioaccumulation associated with LMWH in this setting [10].

A meta-analysis that reviewed several randomized control trials specific to the critical care setting made several recommendations regarding this population and the use of chemoprophylaxis. In short, the use of chemoprophylaxis agents should be initiated early, individualized, and regularly reviewed. Interruptions should be minimal. Many institutions have standardized guidelines for the administration of VTE prophylaxis. Refer to institution guidelines when starting chemoprophylaxis in patients while individualizing their care to their specific needs.

25.6 Conclusion

Managing abdominal surgery patients in the ICU requires a personalized and collaborative multidisciplinary approach, considering the multidimensional nature of their needs. Specifically, we discussed management of the open abdomen, ileostomies, colostomies, enterocutaneous fistulas, NSTIs, tracheostomies, and gastrostomy feeding tubes. This chapter highlights the unique challenges of managing patients with an open abdomen and emphasizes the importance of early enteral nutrition initiation and vigilant infection control measures. Early enteral feeding can aid in wound healing and reduce the risk of postoperative infectious complications. Infections can range from superficial wound infections to deeper intra-abdominal infections. Source control with careful antibiotic stewardship is essential. Emergency general surgery and trauma patients are at an increased risk of acute respiratory distress syndrome, and ventilation settings must be adjusted to reduce ventilator-induced lung injury. Fluid resuscitation is nuanced; there are many confounding variables to consider when determining a patient's fluid status. Insensible fluid losses in abdominal surgery or in the open abdomen, acute kidney injury causing poor urine output, and states of shock that alter hemodynamics can obscure the determination of fluid status. Critically ill abdominal surgery patients are at a heightened risk of venous thromboembolism; therefore, DVT prophylaxis is recommended. Incorporating these principles in parallel with interdisciplinary collaboration, evidence-based medicine, and developing personalized treatment plans will optimize the quality of care for abdominal surgery patients in the critical care setting.

References

1. Reignier J, Boisramé-Helms J, Brisard L, et al. Enteral versus parenteral early nutrition in ventilated adults with shock: a randomised, controlled, multicentre, open-label, parallel-group study (NUTRIREA-2). Lancet. 2018;391(10116):133–43. https://doi.org/10.1016/S0140-6736(17)32146-3.
2. Morlion BJ, Stehle P, Wachtler P, Siedhoff HP, Koller M, Konig W, Furst P, Puchstein C. Total parenteral nutrition with glutamine dipeptide after major abdominal surgery. Ann Surg. 1998;227:302–8. https://doi.org/10.1097/00000658-199802000-00022.
3. Lambell KJ, Tatucu-Babet OA, Chapple LA, Gantner D, Ridley EJ. Nutrition therapy in critical illness: a review of the literature for clinicians. Crit Care. 2020;24(1):35. https://doi.org/10.1186/s13054-020-2739-4.
4. Jiang ZM, Cao JD, Zhu XG, Zhao WX, Yu JC, Ma EL, Wang XR, Zhu MW, Shu H, Liu YW. The impact of alanyl-glutamine on clinical safety, nitrogen balance, intestinal permeability, and clinical outcome in postoperative patients: a randomised, double-blind, controlled study of 120 patients. JPEN J Parenter Enteral Nutr. 1999;23:S62–6.
5. Singer P, Blaser AR, Berger MM, et al. ESPEN guideline on clinical nutrition in the intensive care unit. Clin Nutr. 2019;38(1):48–79. https://doi.org/10.1016/j.clnu.2018.08.037.
6. Ward N. Nutrition support to patients undergoing gastrointestinal surgery. Nutr J. 2003;2:18. https://doi.org/10.1186/1475-2891-2-18.
7. Reissman P, Teoh TA, Cohen SM, Weiss EG, Nogueras JJ, Wexner SD. Is early oral feeding safe after elective colorectal surgery? A prospective randomized trial. Ann Surg. 1995;222:73–7.
8. Braga M, Gianotti L, Gentilini S, Liotta S, Di Carlo V. Feeding the gut early after digestive surgery: results of a nine-year experience. Clin Nutr. 2002;21:59–65. https://doi.org/10.1054/clnu.2001.0504.
9. Li J, Ren J, Zhu W, Yin L, Han J. Management of enterocutaneous fistulas: 30-year clinical experience. Chin Med J. 2003;116(2):171–5.
10. Villet S, Chiolero RL, Bollmann MD, Revelly J-P, Marie Christine Cayeux RN, Delarue J, Berger MM. Negative impact of hypocaloric feeding and energy balance on clinical outcome in ICU patients. Clin Nutr. 2005;24(4):502–9.

11. Preiser JC, Arabi YM, Berger MM, et al. A guide to enteral nutrition in intensive care units: 10 expert tips for the daily practice. Crit Care. 2021;25(1):424. https://doi.org/10.1186/s13054-021-03847-4.

12. Nimmagadda K, et al. Virtual multidisciplinary rounds to reduce length of stay, decrease variation, and promote accountability. Jt Comm J Qual Patient Saf. 2023;49(9):450–7. https://doi.org/10.1016/j.jcjq.2023.04.006.

13. Roberts DJ, Ball CG, Feliciano DV, Moore EE, Ivatury RR, Lucas CE, Fabian TC, Zygun DA, Kirkpatrick AW, Stelfox HT. History of the innovation of damage control for management of trauma patients: 1902–2016. Ann Surg. 2017;265(5):1034–44. https://doi.org/10.1097/SLA.0000000000001803.

14. Kirkpatrick AW, Roberts DJ, De Waele J, Jaeschke R, Malbrain ML, De Keulenaer B, Duchesne J, Bjorck M, Leppaniemi A, Ejike JC, Sugrue M, Cheatham M, Ivatury R, Ball CG, Reintam Blaser A, Regli A, Balogh ZJ, D'Amours S, Debergh D, Kaplan M, Kimball E, Olvera C, Pediatric Guidelines Subcommittee for the World Society of the Abdominal Compartment Syndrome. Intra-abdominal hypertension and the abdominal compartment syndrome: updated consensus definitions and clinical practice guidelines from the World Society of the Abdominal Compartment Syndrome. Intensive Care Med. 2013;39(7):1190–206. https://doi.org/10.1007/s00134-013-2906-z. Epub 2013 May 15.

15. Karageorgos V, Proklou A, Vaporidi K. Lung and diaphragm protective ventilation: a synthesis of recent data. Expert Rev Respir Med. 2022;16(4):375–90. https://doi.org/10.1080/17476348.2022.2060824. Epub 2022 Apr 5.

16. Zielinski MD, Jenkins D, Cotton BA, Inaba K, Vercruysse G, Coimbra R, Brown CV, Alley DE, DuBose J, Scalea TM, AAST Open Abdomen Study Group. Adult respiratory distress syndrome risk factors for injured patients undergoing damage-control laparotomy: AAST multicenter post hoc analysis. J Trauma Acute Care Surg. 2014;77(6):886–91. https://doi.org/10.1097/TA.0000000000000421.

17. Dubose JJ, Scalea TM, Holcomb JB, Shrestha B, Okoye O, Inaba K, Bee TK, Fabian TC, Whelan J, Ivatury RR. Open abdominal management after damage-control laparotomy for trauma: a prospective observational American Association for the Surgery of Trauma multicenter study. J Trauma Acute Care Surg. 2013;74:113–20. https://doi.org/10.1097/TA.0b013e31827891ce.

18. Ho C, Culhane J. Reduced fasting protocol for endoscopic percutaneous gastrostomy in intubated patients. Int J Clin Med. 2013;4(8):48066.

19. Brady M, Kinn S, Stuart P. Preoperative fasting for adults to prevent perioperative complications. Cochrane Database Syst Rev. 2003;2003:CD004423.

20. Douglas MJ, Ciraulo D. Variability in perioperative fasting practices negatively impacts nutritional support of critically ill intubated patients. Am Surg. 2017;83(8):895–900.

21. Fekaj E, Salihu L, Morina A. Treatment of enterocutaneous fistula with total parenteral feeding in combination with octreotide: a case report. Cases J. 2009;2:177. https://doi.org/10.1186/1757-1626-2-177.

22. Polk TM, Schwab CW. Metabolic and nutritional support of the enterocutaneous fistula patient: a three-phase approach. World J Surg. 2012;36(3):524–33. https://doi.org/10.1007/s00268-011-1315-0.

23. Badrasawi M, Shahar S, Sagap I. Nutritional management in enterocutaneous fistula. What is the evidence? Malays J Med Sci. 2015;22(4):6–16.

24. Wischmeyer PE. Overcoming challenges to enteral nutrition delivery in critical care. Curr Opin Crit Care. 2021;27(2):169–76. https://doi.org/10.1097/MCC.0000000000000801.

25. Mishima Y, Nawa N, Asada M, Nagashima M, Aiso Y, Nukui Y, Fujiwara T, Shigemitsu H. Impact of antibiotic time-outs in multidisciplinary ICU rounds for antimicrobial stewardship program on patient survival: a controlled before-and-after study. Crit Care Explor. 2023;5(1):e0837. https://doi.org/10.1097/CCE.0000000000000837.

Part VI
Critical Care Nephrology

Chapter 26
Acute Kidney Injury

Andrea M. Nei, Nikitha Yagnala, Hailey A. Thompson, Brandy N. Hernandez, and Erin F. Barreto

26.1 Introduction

Acute kidney injury (AKI) is defined as an acute change to kidney structure or function that occurs over hours to days. AKI may lead to accumulation of urea, electrolyte derangements, acid-base abnormalities, and fluid accumulation. It is a diagnosis with multiple causes and profound implications on short- and long-term outcomes, especially in the critically ill. As medications are one of the few modifiable risk factors for AKI, and dynamically affected by changes in kidney function, pharmacists in the intensive care unit (ICU) are uniquely positioned to improve AKI prevention and management in the critically ill.

26.2 Epidemiology

The incidence of AKI varies depending on the definition used, the patient population assessed, and the underlying severity of illness. In low- to middle-income settings, community-acquired AKI is most common, accounting for upwards of 70% of cases [1]. Conversely, hospital-acquired AKI is more common in high-income settings, with a higher incidence in the ICU (upwards of 30–60%) compared to the

A. M. Nei · B. N. Hernandez · E. F. Barreto (✉)
Department of Pharmacy, Mayo Clinic Hospital—Rochester, Rochester, MN, USA
e-mail: nei.andrea@mayo.edu; hernandez.brandy@mayo.edu; barreto.erin@mayo.edu

H. A. Thompson
Department of Pharmacy, UW Health, Madison, WI, USA

N. Yagnala
Department of Pharmacy, Hospital of University of Pennsylvania, Philadelphia, PA, USA
e-mail: nikitha.yagnala@pennmedicine.upenn.edu

© The Author(s), under exclusive license to Springer Nature Switzerland AG 2025
Y. Alzaidi, M. A. Gebily (eds.), *The Pharmacist's Expanded Role in Critical Care Medicine*, https://doi.org/10.1007/978-3-031-77335-8_26

ward (3–18%) [2]. In large multicenter studies of critically ill patients with AKI, approximately 10–15% of patients required kidney replacement therapy (KRT). Unfortunately, the incidence of AKI and use of KRT in critically ill patients have increased over time [2].

In critically ill patients, AKI is typically attributed to complications of severe illness, with a small percentage of cases caused by primary kidney diseases such as vasculitis or glomerulonephritis [2]. Sepsis is a leading cause of AKI in the critically ill. Additional risk factors for AKI include hypotension, exposure to nephrotoxins, and major surgery. Chronic medical conditions such as history of chronic kidney disease (CKD), congestive heart failure, and diabetes are also risk factors. In low- to middle-income settings, community-acquired AKI tends to impact young, previously healthy patients. Sepsis remains a common cause, but other causes such as obstetric complications, animal venom, HIV infection, hantavirus, malaria, and dengue may be implicated depending on local prevalence [2].

Reported short-term mortality in critically ill patients with AKI ranges from 20% to 60%, with patients requiring KRT at the high end of this range [2, 3]. The long-term health consequences of AKI have been increasingly recognized. Estimates indicate that among the 80–90% of individuals that survive after an episode of AKI during a hospitalization, there is a 15–30% incidence of chronic kidney disease and a 1.9-fold higher risk of cardiovascular disease [4–6]. Fifty percent of moderate-to-severe AKI survivors are rehospitalized in the first year, most within the first 90 days [7]. The increased burden of care contributes to substantially worse quality of life for AKI survivors [8].

26.3   AKI Definition

The evolution of AKI definitions began in 2004 with the landmark RIFLE (risk, injury, failure, loss, end-stage renal disease) classification, defining AKI based on a ≥50% rise in creatinine, a ≥25% decline in glomerular filtration rate (GFR), and/or decreased urine output [9]. The RIFLE criteria also included two clinical outcomes based on the duration of loss of kidney function. Subsequent studies highlighted the independent association between small creatinine increases and long-term adverse events [10]. The AKI Network (AKIN) criteria, introduced in 2007, therefore refined and simplified the RIFLE criteria into three stages of AKI, omitted the outcome classifications of loss and end stage, and added a rise in serum creatinine of ≥0.3 mg/dL within 48 h to the stage 1 AKI criteria [11]. Despite these updates, both RIFLE and AKIN had limitations in their sensitivity for detecting AKI [12]. The contemporary Kidney Disease Improving Global Outcomes (KDIGO) criteria merged the RIFLE and AKIN definitions, allowing for both a rise in creatinine of ≥0.3 mg/dL over 48 h or increase of ≥1.5 times baseline within 7 days [13]. Stage 3 AKI was updated for greater parity to include an increase in ≥0.3 mg/dL or ≥1.5 baseline if creatinine is >4 mg/dL. For a comparison of the AKI definitions, refer Table 26.1.

Table 26.1 Definitions of acute kidney injury [9, 11, 13]

	RIFLE	AKIN	KDIGO
Stage	**Risk[a]**	**Stage 1**	**Stage 1**
SCr criteria	Increase to ≥1.5× baseline	Increase to 1.5 to 2× from baseline or by ≥0.3 mg/dL within 48 h	Increase to 1.5 to <2× from baseline over 7 days or by ≥0.3 mg/dL within 48 h
GFR criteria	GFR decrease >25% from baseline	None	None
UOP criteria	UOP <0.5 mL/kg/h for 6–12 h	UOP <0.5 mL/kg/h for 6–12 h	UOP <0.5 mL/kg/h for 6–12 h
Stage	**Injury**	**Stage 2**	**Stage 2**
SCr criteria	Increase to ≥2× baseline	Increase to ≥2 to 3× from baseline	Increase to ≥2 to <3× from baseline
GFR criteria	GFR decrease >50% from baseline	None	None
UOP criteria	UOP <0.5 mL/kg/h for ≥12 h	UOP <0.5 mL/kg/h for ≥12 h	UOP <0.5 mL/kg/h for ≥12 h
Stage	**Failure**	**Stage 3**	**Stage 3**
SCr criteria	Increase to ≥3× baseline, or SCr ≥4 mg/dL (acute increase of at least 0.5 mg/dL)	Increase >3× from baseline or ≥4 mg/dL with an acute rise of ≥0.5 mg/dL	Increase ≥3× from baseline or ≥4 mg/dL
GFR/KRT criteria UOP criteria	GFR decrease >75% from baseline UOP <0.3 mL/kg/h for ≥24 h or anuria for ≥12 h	Initiation of KRT UOP <0.3 mL/kg/h for ≥24 h or anuria for ≥12 h	Initiation of KRT UOP <0.3 mL/kg/h for ≥24 h or anuria for ≥12 h
Clinical outcome	**Loss**	**None**	**None**
	Complete loss of function for >4 weeks	NA	NA
Clinical outcome	**End-stage kidney disease**	**None**	**None**
	Complete loss of function for >3 months	NA	NA

AKIN AKI Network, *GFR* glomerular filtration rate, *KDIGO* Kidney Disease Improving Global Outcomes, *KRT* kidney replacement therapy, *NA* not applicable, *RIFLE* risk, injury, failure, loss, end stage, *SCr* serum creatinine, *UOP* urine output
[a] Criteria met within 7 days

In 2012, KDIGO also proposed a standard nomenclature to capture the full spectrum of kidney function. The spectrum includes no kidney disease, AKI defined by kidney injury or dysfunction over hours to days, acute kidney disease (AKD) defined as kidney injury or dysfunction for less than 3 months, or CKD defined as kidney damage or dysfunction for more than 3 months (Fig. 26.1) [14]. The harmonized nomenclature standardizes care and criteria across the kidney spectrum [15]. Nevertheless, controversies and uncertainty remain. Patients meeting AKI/AKD criteria may not meet CKD parameters at 3 months, and further study is needed into the long-term health implications in this subgroup. The

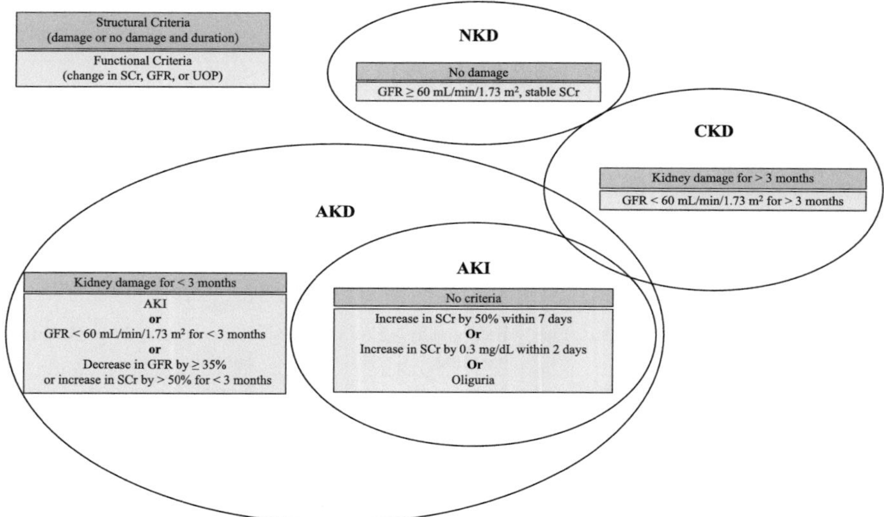

Fig. 26.1 Spectrum of kidney disease: definitions and criteria for NKD, AKI, AKD, and CKD [13]. *AKD* acute kidney disease, *AKI* acute kidney injury, *CKD* chronic kidney disease, *GFR* glomerular filtration rate, *NKD* no kidney disease, *SCr* serum creatinine, *UOP* urine output

optimal approach to establishing baseline serum creatinine concentrations for AKI and AKD definitions is uncertain. Use of novel biomarkers and multi-omics for defining, diagnosing, and staging AKI is an area of interest and need for future study [16].

26.4 Diagnostic Workup and Evaluation

26.4.1 Diagnosis

No one single test can be used to diagnose AKI. A thorough history that includes comorbidities, time course of symptoms, and changes to drug therapy, as well as a physical examination, laboratory workup, and rarely kidney biopsy, should be considered. Clinical symptoms of AKI can include fluid balance abnormalities (e.g., overload due to accumulation, or decreased intravascular volume due to dehydration), hypertension, or decreased urination or may be asymptomatic with small initial changes in creatinine.

The existing diagnostic criteria for AKI rely on functional biomarkers including serum creatinine and urine output, each of which has limitations in the critically ill. As the terminal byproduct of skeletal muscle catabolism, nonrenal factors influence serum creatinine concentrations including age, sex, diet, muscle mass, and weight [17–20]. Serum creatinine lags by as much as 48–72 h from the onset of kidney damage and is insensitive to small changes in kidney function [21]. Urine output can be confounded by diuretic use and fluid status and is dependent on accurate charting, which is often difficult if the patient does not have an indwelling urinary catheter.

Alternative functional biomarkers have also been evaluated in AKI in the critically ill. Serum cystatin C is a low-molecular-weight protein, produced from all nucleated cells, that is freely filtered at the glomerulus. Serum cystatin C may exhibit a more favorable kinetic profile in the setting of AKI than creatinine [22]. However nonrenal determinants of cystatin C concentrations (e.g., inflammation, certain medications) are prevalent in ICU patients, which may impact its utility for AKI evaluation and GFR assessment [23]. Proenkephalin is a molecule in the enkephalin family that is not plasma protein bound and is extensively filtered in the glomerulus. It has shown promise as a functional biomarker due to strong correlation of plasma levels with iohexol plasma clearance in critically ill patients with sepsis ($R^2 = 0.90$, $p < 0.0001$) and its ability to predict AKI in the critically ill [24, 25]. Alternative approaches to assessing kidney structure and function have been proposed. One strategy is the "furosemide stress test" (FST) [1 mg/kg (loop diuretic naïve) or 1.5 mg/kg (loop diuretic past 7 days)]. In the early stages of AKI, the FST has been shown to predict AKI progression [26]. A post-FST test 2-h urine output of 200 mL or less had the best sensitivity (87.1%) and specificity (84.1%) for predicting AKI progression. Another small pilot study of postoperative critically ill patients showed a negative FST (<200 mL/h urine output for 2 h) combined with the biomarker C-C motif chemokine ligand 14 (CCL14) that had a high negative predictive value for the development of an indication for KRT [area under the curve (AUC) 0.87, 95% CI 0.82–0.92] [27].

Novel blood or urine structural biomarkers of kidney stress, damage, or dysfunction may be useful for risk stratification, AKI diagnosis, and prognostication and have been applied in the context of sepsis, drug-induced nephrotoxicity, and major surgery [28–31]. Tissue inhibitor of metalloproteinase-2 (TIMP-2) and insulin-like growth factor-binding protein 7 (IGFBP7) are a US Food and Drug Administration (FDA)-approved combination of two urinary cell cycle arrest biomarkers, released during kidney stress and injury. TIMP-2•IGFBP7 is strongly associated with the development of stage 2 or 3 AKI within 12 h in the critically ill (AUC 0.80, $p < 0.002$). A TIMP-2•IGFBP7 cutoff of >0.3 has shown to be predictive of AKI with high sensitivity. A cutoff of 2 or higher has a high specificity for the risk of AKI [2, 32, 33]. Neutrophil gelatinase-associated lipocalin (NGAL) is produced with proximal or distal tubular kidney injury. Although NGAL can be measured in the serum, there is a lack of specificity to kidney damage, making urine the preferred option [34, 35]. In 2023, urinary NGAL received FDA approval for use in ICU patients, to identify those at higher risk for AKI within 48–72 h. CCL14 is a chemokine involved in immune cell recruitment and chemotaxis. The role of CCL14 in AKI is still being elucidated, but as an inflammatory marker, it may signal ongoing kidney inflammation, damage, and dysfunction. Elevated levels of urinary CCL14 predict the persistence of severe (KDIGO stage 3) AKI (AUC 0.83, 95% CI 0.78–0.87) [36,

37]. Many other structural markers have been explored in preclinical drug development and research. The FDA now allows for the use of six urinary biomarkers to be considered in conjunction with traditional assessments of kidney function in early-phase clinical trials to detect drug-induced kidney injury. These biomarkers include clusterin (CLU), cystatin C, kidney injury molecule-1 (KIM-1), *N*-acetyl-beta-D-glucosaminidase (NAG), neutrophil gelatinase-associated lipocalin (NGAL), and osteopontin (OPN).

Use of these novel biomarkers in critical care is limited, particularly in low- to middle-income countries. Among them, serum cystatin C is the most commonly used in the ICU, albeit still rarely, catalyzed by greater accessibility than the other tests and increased use in the community setting [38–40]. Implementation of novel structural and functional kidney biomarkers remains a challenge [41]. Best practice would be to consider these tools as adjuncts rather than alternatives to creatinine-based assessment in AKI. Forthcoming guidelines will likely provide additional consideration about the role for these biomarkers in AKI prediction, prognostication, and management [30].

26.4.2   Causes and Mechanisms of AKI

Historically, the etiologies of AKI have been classified based on three general pseudo-anatomical categories: prerenal, intrarenal, and post-renal (Table 26.2). In prerenal AKI, decreased kidney perfusion leads to a decrease in GFR. Note that hypovolemia is only a small subset of the cases with prerenal AKI as many factors can alter kidney perfusion including hypervolemia. Intrarenal AKI is secondary to parenchymal or vascular disease, with ATN being the most common example. Post-renal AKI occurs because of acute urinary tract obstruction [42].

Table 26.2 Prerenal, intrarenal, and post-renal causes of acute kidney injury [1]

Classification	Causes with examples
Prerenal	• Low effective arterial blood volume (hypovolemia, acute decompensated heart failure, abdominal compartment syndrome) • Peripheral vasodilation (sepsis) • Renal vasoconstriction (hepatorenal syndrome) • Renal occlusion (arterial thrombus)
Intrarenal	• Acute tubular necrosis • Vasculitis • Glomerulonephritis • Interstitial nephritis • Infections • Connective tissue disease • Crystalluria
Post-renal	• Prostatic hypertrophy • Nephrolithiasis • Tumor obstruction

Urine indices such as the fractional excretion of sodium (FeNa) and fractional excretion of urea (FeUrea) may be useful in distinguishing between prerenal and intrinsic AKI. A FeNa cutoff of <1% has been used to distinguish prerenal from intrarenal AKI, with the greatest sensitivity and specificity seen in oliguric patients without CKD and without recent diuretic use [43]. Diuretic exposure alters urinary sodium handling and compromises FeNa performance, so use of a FeUrea cutoff of <35% may have a greater positive predictive value [44]. While FeNa and FeUrea may provide conditional evidence to distinguish prerenal vs. intrarenal AKI, the variables required for their calculations may be altered by medications, disease states, and variations in normal physiology, as outlined in Table 26.3 [45]. Therefore, if used, FeNa and FeUrea should be accompanied by a thorough history, physical exam, comprehensive medication review, and urinalysis with sediment microscopy to determine AKI etiology [46].

While the traditional classification of AKI into these three large categories may be useful in forming an initial differential diagnosis, it is important to recognize that AKI is a heterogeneous syndrome, with various etiologies, exposures, and complex intertwined pathophysiological pathways. For example, critically ill patients with sepsis experience a complex interaction of inflammatory, ischemic, and nephrotoxic insults to their kidneys, ultimately resulting in a paradigm of AKI that is unique at a molecular level from a prerenal AKI due to ischemia or hypovolemia. As such, shifting the classification of AKI to better align with the underlying pathology may

Table 26.3 Variables affecting FeNa and FeUrea[a] calculations [45]

Scenarios causing FeNa <1% (not due to prerenal AKI)	Scenarios causing FeNa >2% (not true intrarenal AKI)
Normal kidney function with low salt intake	Normal kidney function with high salt intake
Acute glomerulonephritis	Normal kidney function after administration of sodium-containing IV fluids
Acute urinary obstruction	Resolving urinary obstruction
Early acute interstitial nephritis	Bicarbonaturia
Transplant rejection	Glucosuria (SGLT2 inhibitor use)
FeNa <1% despite intrarenal AKI	**FeNa >2% despite prerenal AKI**
AKI with liver failure or CHF	Administration of sodium-containing IV fluids
Early sepsis-associated AKI	Diuretics (loop, thiazides)
Radiocontrast nephropathy	Chronic kidney disease
Pigment nephropathy (myoglobinuria or hemoglobinuria)	Glucosuria
	Bicarbonaturia
	Salt-wasting nephropathies (Bartter, Gitelman syndrome)

FeNa and FeUrea calculations:
FeNa = [(urinary sodium × serum creatinine)/(urinary creatinine × serum sodium)] × 100
FeUrea = [(urinary urea × serum creatinine)/(urinary creatinine × serum urea)] × 100

AKI acute kidney injury, *CHF* congestive heart failure, *FeNa* fractional excretion of sodium, *FeUrea* fractional excretion of urea, *IV* intravenous, *SGLT2* sodium-glucose transport protein 2
[a]Table displays factors that primarily affect FeNa. Factors that can falsely elevate FeUrea despite prerenal AKI include administration of mannitol, acetazolamide, high-protein diet, or excessive catabolism

better inform the therapeutic approach. The dominant AKI paradigms in critically ill patients include sepsis-, ischemia-, and drug-associated AKI, each of which will be discussed in slightly more detail [47, 48].

Almost 50% of patients with severe AKI in the ICU have sepsis [48]. Sepsis triggers a systemic inflammatory response, leading to the release of pro-inflammatory cytokines and immune cell activation. The dysregulated immune response leads to alterations in renal blood flow, glomerular filtration, and tubular function. The activation of toll-like receptors and nuclear factor-kappa B leads to the release of damage-associated molecular patterns, contributing to renal microcirculatory dysfunction and endothelial injury. Direct tubular damage and apoptosis, coupled with impaired autoregulation and microvascular dysfunction, further exacerbate kidney injury in the setting of sepsis [47, 48].

The incidence of ischemic AKI requiring KRT is approximately 20% [48]. Any class of shock—cardiogenic, distributive, hypovolemic, and obstructive—could lead to kidney ischemia. Ischemic AKI arises from reduced renal blood flow, leading to impaired oxygen delivery, and hypoxic injury to the kidneys. The initial insult triggers a cascade of events including vasoconstriction, inflammation, oxidative stress, and cellular apoptosis, ultimately resulting in tubular injury and dysfunction. The activation of various pathways, such as the renin-angiotensin-aldosterone system and release of inflammatory mediators, further perpetuates renal injury and contributes to the pathophysiology of ischemic AKI [47].

Medications are associated with roughly one-third of hospital AKI cases. Recently, an innovative framework for drug-induced kidney disease (DIKD) classification was proposed [49, 50]. This 2 × 2 table incorporates functional and damage biomarkers alongside predominant mechanisms of nephrotoxicity to categorize medications into four categories: dysfunction without damage, damage without dysfunction, dysfunction and damage, and neither dysfunction nor damage (Fig. 26.2). Drugs that cause an increase in serum creatinine without causing renal damage or dysfunction, commonly termed pseudo-AKI, fit into the "neither dysfunction nor damage" category. Some medications that act on systemic or intraglomerular hemodynamics may lead to worsening kidney function without causing direct kidney damage. Conversely, many medications can cause kidney damage through various mechanisms, without immediately causing kidney dysfunction, as outlined in Table 26.4. Drugs that cause both kidney dysfunction and damage are typically associated with both hemodynamically and non-hemodynamically related AKI mechanisms. This novel classification system of DIKD allows for movement between categories, as patient-specific scenarios may accelerate the transformation between categories. Early AKI detection and management are imperative in preventing the progression of "damage without dysfunction" and "dysfunction without damage" to the "damage and dysfunction" category [49].

Of the various potentially nephrotoxic drugs detailed in Table 26.4, contrast exposure is somewhat controversial among clinicians. Contrast-associated AKI is thought

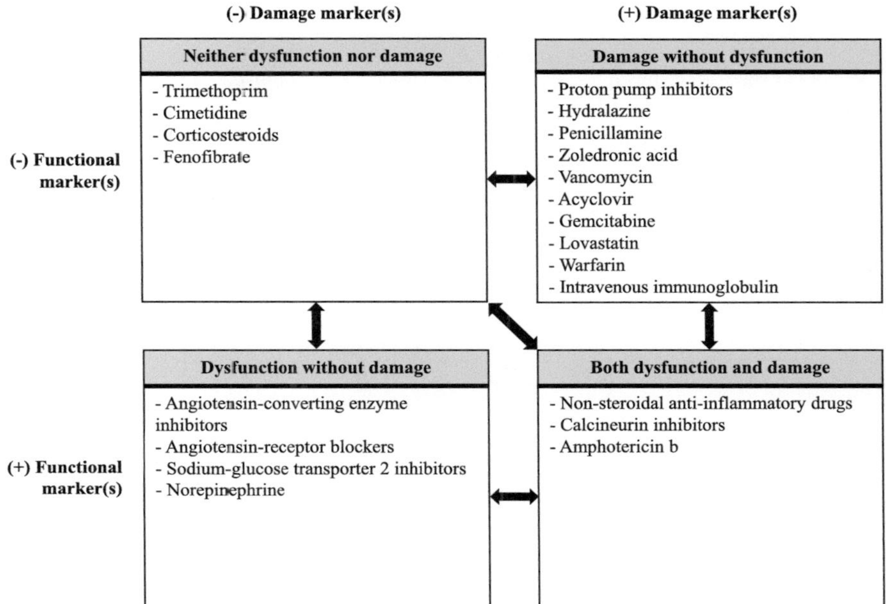

Fig. 26.2 Classification of drug-induced kidney injury [49, 50]. Classification of drug-induced kidney injury based on damage and functional markers, initially proposed by Ostermann et al. and modified by Karimzadeh et al. Examples of medications or medication classes are provided for each category and are not all-inclusive. The arrows depict opportunity for movement between categories based on patient susceptibility factors and time course, including both progression and recovery of injury or functional markers

to occur within 48–72 h of iodinated contrast exposure, through mechanisms of osmotic nephrosis, renal vasoconstriction, renal medullary ischemia, and generation of reactive oxygen species, ultimately resulting in direct tubular necrosis [52]. While patients with renal insufficiency (eGFR <30 mL/min) and reduced effective arterial volume remain at the highest risk of contrast-associated AKI, recent literature indicates that the overall incidence has declined with the use of low-osmol contrast agents, supportive care with volume expansion, and updated medical practices [50]. In patients with an indication for contrast exposure that would impact treatment decisions, it should not be withheld because of concerns about AKI.

It is well established that AKI is a heterogeneous syndrome, with various etiologies, clinical presentations, and outcomes. Sub-phenotyping AKI, beyond the classic pseudo-anatomical groups, using clinical and biological features may help differentiate patients with unique pathophysiology, mechanisms of disease, severity of illness, treatment response, and outcomes [53].

Table 26.4 Medications associated with kidney injury [49, 51]

Type of damage	Mechanism	Medication examples	Suggestive features
Acute tubular necrosis	Dose-dependent toxicity resulting in direct tubular damage and subsequent cell apoptosis	Aminoglycosides, vancomycin, amphotericin B, colistin, antiviral agents, platinum chemotherapy, IV contrast	Muddy brown casts or renal tubular epithelial cells on urinalysis
Acute interstitial nephritis	Cell-medicated immune response	Penicillins, cephalosporins, sulfonamides, ciprofloxacin, vancomycin, NSAIDs, COX-2 inhibitors, proton pump inhibitors, immune checkpoint inhibitors, phenytoin, valproic acid, ranitidine, diuretics, cocaine	Proteinuria on urinalysis "Clinical triad" of eosinophilia, fever, and rash
Glomerular diseases	Idiopathic, dose-independent, potentially irreversible toxicities divided into immune-mediated (ANCA-associated vasculitis, drug-induced lupus, drug-associated membranous nephropathy, and direct glomerular toxicities (focal segmental glomerulosclerosis)	*Immune-mediated*: Hydralazine, propylthiouracil *Direct glomerular cell toxicity*: Lithium, NSAIDs, anabolic steroids, anti-angiogenesis drugs, chemotherapeutics, calcineurin inhibitors, interferon, thienopyridines, quinine, sirolimus	Kidney biopsy
Crystalluria/ nephrolithiasis	Drug crystal deposition in collecting tubules results in intraparenchymal obstructive nephropathy	Acyclovir, methotrexate, antiretrovirals, triamterene	Crystalluria on urinalysis or obstruction on ultrasound
Altered electrolyte handling/ tubular dysfunction	Alteration of tubular electrolyte handling resulting in conditions similar to SIADH, Fanconi syndrome, or nephrogenic diabetes insipidus	Lithium, SSRIs, antiepileptics, vincristine, antiretrovirals	Assessment of serum and urine electrolytes and osmolality
Osmotic nephrosis	Process of pinocytosis causes cellular swelling and tubular lumen obstruction	Mannitol, hydroxyethyl starch, dextrans, sucrose-containing immunoglobulins	Tubular vacuolization in urine cytology

ANCA antineutrophilic cytoplasmic antibody, *COX* cyclooxygenase, *IV* intravenous, *NSAIDs* non-steroidal anti-inflammatory drugs, *SIADH* syndrome of inappropriate antidiuretic hormone, *SSRIs* selective serotonin reuptake inhibitors

26.5 Management: The Pharmacist's Role

Pharmacists can be involved with the care of patients with AKI before, during, and after the event. Therapeutic interventions focused on prevention in high-risk patients may reduce the incidence and severity of AKI. Despite preventative efforts, AKI will inevitably occur in some patients. Critical care pharmacists may facilitate AKI management through treatment of the underlying cause, appropriate monitoring, hemodynamic optimization, and medication safety assessment. Illustrative examples from the literature summarize areas where pharmacists could be involved including in the use of KDIGO AKI prevention bundles, nephrotoxin stewardship, and fluid and electrolyte management.

26.5.1 KDIGO Bundles

AKI guidelines recommend a stage-based bundled approach to early recognition and intervention (Fig. 26.3). In clinical trials which used novel kidney biomarkers to enrich the study population for moderate- or high-risk patients, the KDIGO AKI prevention bundle has shown benefit. The single-center Prev-AKI randomized controlled trial in postoperative cardiovascular surgery patients with a TIMP-2•IGFBP7 ≥0.3 found that use of the KDIGO prevention bundle resulted in less AKI of any stage and less stage 2 or 3 AKI compared to usual care [54]. The Prev-AKI multi-center study in cardiovascular surgery and the BigpAK study in major non-cardiovascular surgery corroborated these findings [55, 56]. A larger quality improvement initiative in on-pump cardiac surgery patients compared outcomes before and after implementation of TIMP-2•IGFBP7 and protocolized care. The post-implementation group experienced less stage 2 and 3 AKI events [57]. Based on these available studies, cardiovascular surgery guidelines suggest screening with urinary biomarkers to identify high-risk patients who benefit from preventive care bundles [58, 59]. Although bundle implementation is observed to be beneficial, the impact of individual bundle components is unclear. In addition, prevention bundle elements and adherence vary across studies and patient populations. A retrospective analysis of the two Prev-AKI studies suggested that among the bundle components, prevention of hypotension and low cardiac index and avoidance of nephrotoxic drugs were the most important in preventing AKI [60]. In a broader, general ICU

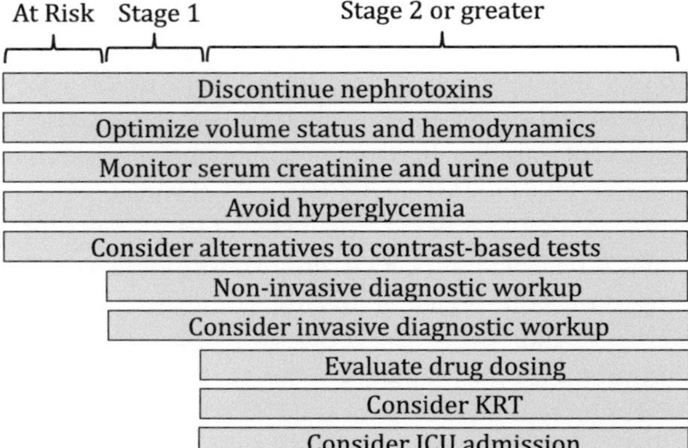

Fig. 26.3 KDIGO Bundle for stage-based management of acute kidney injury [13]. *ICU* intensive care unit, *KRT* kidney replacement therapy

population, a quality improvement project aimed to assess real-world implementation of KDIGO bundle interventions based on TIMP-2•IGFBP7 result. In patients with TIMP-2•IGFBP7 >0.3, 75% received at least one component of the KDIGO bundle, with 51% having at least one medication management intervention used [61]. This highlights an important opportunity for pharmacist involvement in the creation and implementation of urinary biomarker-based AKI prevention algorithms with embedded pharmacotherapy recommendations for renally active drugs.

26.5.2 Nephrotoxin Stewardship

Drugs are frequently implicated as a contributor to AKI in hospitalized patients. Additionally, prescribing of excess nephrotoxic drugs is associated with increased mortality in the critically ill [62]. Nephrotoxin stewardship is a concept analogous to antimicrobial stewardship. It involves coordinated interventions to promote safe use of nephrotoxic and kidney eliminated medications, optimize patient outcomes and kidney health, and avoid unnecessary costs [63]. Components of nephrotoxin stewardship are outlined in Table 26.5. These interventions should be automated when able with accurate clinical decision support.

An example of a successful approach to nephrotoxin stewardship is the Nephrotoxic Injury Negated by Just-in time Action (NINJA) quality improvement program. Pharmacist-led systematic screening identified hospitalized, non-critically ill pediatric patients at high risk for AKI, defined as three or more high-risk nephrotoxic medications or an aminoglycoside for more than 3 days. Pharmacists acted in these high-risk patients to promote daily kidney function monitoring. Nephrotoxic medication discontinuation or pharmacokinetic drug monitoring was undertaken per care team preference. The NINJA project demonstrated a sustained decrease in nephrotoxin exposure by 38% and decrease in AKI rate of 64% [64]. The benefits of this single-center intervention were confirmed through a multicenter initiative, which observed a sustained 24% decrease in nephrotoxic medication-associated AKI [65].

Stress or damage biomarkers could be integrated with clinical decision support systems (CDSSs) to promote nephrotoxin stewardship in the highest risk patients. A quality improvement project in the ICUs at the University of Pittsburgh Medical Center used CDSS to alert pharmacists of patients with prescriptions for three or more nephrotoxins. In patients without existing AKI, urinary TIMP-2•IGFBP7 was ordered [66]. If TIMP-2•IGFBP7 was elevated (>0.3), the pharmacist provided recommendations for nephrotoxin stewardship including discontinuation of candidate nephrotoxins and, if needed, drug substitution, avoidance of new nephrotoxins, and drug dose adjustment of renally eliminated medications. Other elements of the KDIGO bundle were also provided by the care team. Pharmacists documented 191 interventions on 81 patients in the quality project. The number of interventions per patient increased with associated TIMP-2•IGFBP7 risk category [1.64 for low risk (≤0.3), 3.43 for moderate risk (0.4–2), and 3.75 for high risk (>2)]. The practical

Table 26.5 Nephrotoxin stewardship [63]

Intervention focus	Example actions
Goal 1: Coordinated patient care strategies providing actions to enhance medication safety	
Safe use of nephrotoxins, renally eliminated medications, and kidney disease treatments	• Medication safety (prevention of medication errors, adverse drug events, and therapeutic failure)
Optimize use of renally cleared medications	• Standardized list of renally cleared medications for surveillance, update annually • Evaluate functional biomarkers, provide recommendations on initial and maintenance dosing • Recheck medication dosages with changes in kidney function • Optimize medication dosing in patients requiring kidney replacement therapy • Therapeutic drug monitoring for non-nephrotoxic medications
Goal 2: Coordinated patient care strategies providing actions to ensure kidney health	
Safe medication use of nephrotoxins and kidney disease treatments	• Prevention of AKI or worsening of kidney function
Minimize nephrotoxins	• Standardized list of nephrotoxins for surveillance, combine with reliable renal risk assessment tool • Evaluate damage biomarkers to determine risk before nephrotoxin administration • Use of evidence-based strategies for prevention of AKI (e.g., hydration for medications causing crystalluria, KDIGO AKI prevention bundle) • Monitor for drug-drug interactions that may impact nephrotoxicity risk • Use of functional biomarkers for appropriate initial and maintenance dosing of nephrotoxic medications • Therapeutic drug monitoring of nephrotoxic medications • Avoid unnecessary nephrotoxins post-AKI
Goal 3: Avoiding unnecessary costs	
Use of automated clinical decision support combined with quality assurance and minimizing alert fatigue	• Surveillance monitoring of renally cleared medications and nephrotoxins • Drug interaction monitoring • Automated detection of drug-associated acute kidney injury • Reassess medication dosing with changes in kidney function

(continued)

Table 26.5 (continued)

Intervention focus	Example actions
Choosing wisely to avoid unnecessary tests, treatment, and procedures	• Stewardship of frequency of monitoring biomarkers • Appropriate use of therapeutic drug monitoring • Minimizing non evidence-based practices
Cost of stewardship program relative to the impact on outcomes	• Assess impact on outcomes such as AKI incidence, AKI severity, progression to CKD, hospital length of stay, and readmission

Each goal within a nephrotoxin stewardship program has multiple elements. Actionable patient care strategies must be undertaken to successfully achieve each goal. The table provides a few example actions within each goal

AKI acute kidney injury, *CKD* chronic kidney disease, *KDIGO* Kidney Disease Improving Global Outcomes

approach lays the groundwork for further study of CDSS use to identify patients at high risk of AKI warranting nephrotoxin stewardship and to assess the link between pharmacist-guided medication management in high-risk patients and clinical outcomes.

Vancomycin is a common nephrotoxin used in the ICU, which can be minimized through therapeutic drug monitoring and appropriate antimicrobial de-escalation. Use of vancomycin de-escalation protocols with methicillin-resistant *Staphylococcus aureus* (MRSA) nasal swabs has been shown to decrease vancomycin use and exposure. MRSA nasal swabs have a high negative predictive value, particularly for pneumonia (>95%), which allows for early de-escalation of vancomycin [67]. Use of MRSA de-escalation protocols has decreased the risk for AKI, making it a viable intervention for nephrotoxin stewardship [68].

26.5.3 Other Issues in AKI

Appropriate fluid management is essential in the critically ill patient to prevent organ failure and adverse outcomes. While hypovolemia as a cause of AKI should be intervened on with appropriate intravascular resuscitation, patients with AKI are also at high risk for volume overload associated with oligoanuria. Fluid overload may propagate AKI due to decreased renal blood flow in the setting of increased venous pressure [69]. A pilot study evaluating a pharmacist-led de-resuscitation protocol, using diuretics where necessary, in mechanically ventilated patients with fluid overload or positive fluid balance significantly decreased cumulative fluid balance [72-h post-shock median fluid balance -2257 (-5676–920) mL vs. 265 (-2283–3025) mL; $p < 0.0001$] [70]. The intervention group also had a lower mortality (5.5 vs. 16.1%; $p = 0.008$), higher ICU-free days [19 (13–22) days vs. 17 (7–21) days; $p = 0.030$], and reduced need for KRT in ICU (0 vs. 6.2%; $p < 0.0001$) and at hospital discharge (0 vs. 5.1%; $p = 0.025$). There was higher incidence of hypokalemia and hypernatremia in the intervention group, but no difference in

AKI. Notably, patients with a creatinine >2 mg/dL or urinary output <30 mL/h were excluded from this study.

Electrolyte disturbances are also common in AKI, most concerning of which is hyperkalemia given the risk of cardiac conduction abnormalities or arrhythmias. Pharmacists can promote successful acute management of hyperkalemia to limit downstream complications. Treatment of acute hyperkalemia involves acute cardiac stabilization with calcium administration and administration of medications to decrease extracellular potassium concentration acutely, through promoting intracellular shifts, or sustainably by facilitating renal or gastrointestinal potassium elimination. A list of therapeutic interventions is included in Table 26.6. Patiromer and sodium zirconium cyclosilicate (SZC) are newer potassium binders, FDA approved for the management of chronic hyperkalemia. Data are limited for the management of acute hyperkalemia and should not be administered as monotherapy in severe, life-threatening hyperkalemia due to delayed onset of action. These therapies are appealing given the concern of variable absorption and efficacy and severe adverse GI events reported with the historical standard, sodium polystyrene sulfate (SPS). SZC has a favorable onset (Table 26.6) and has been shown to effectively lower potassium acutely, including additive benefit when administered with insulin and dextrose [71–73]. While patiromer's onset is somewhat slower than SZC, it has been shown to be effective at acutely lowering potassium, including one study which showed a reduction in potassium within 2 h of administration [74–76]. One retrospective analysis suggested similar efficacy of SZC to patiromer in potassium reduction with no major difference in adverse effects [77]. Another study suggested a larger decrease in potassium and improved hyperkalemia resolution associated with SPS compared to SZC, but these findings were likely due to differences in dose intensity [78]. Continued study of the efficacy of potassium lowering, cost-effectiveness of therapy, optimal dosing, and adverse effects of SZC and patiromer for acute hyperkalemia is needed [79, 80].

Another prominent challenge with AKI is dosing of renally eliminated medications. Typical clearance equations including the Cockcroft-Gault (CG), Modification of Diet in Renal Disease (MDRD), and Chronic Kidney Disease Epidemiology Collaboration (CKD-EPI) are designed for use at a steady state and constrained by the use of creatinine with previously noted limitations in the critically ill. Alternative methods for medication dosing in the ICU such as measured creatinine clearance and measured GFR are technically complex, costly, and time consuming. Measured clearance may also lag, depending on the timeframe of urinary collection. The kinetic eGFR (KeGFR) formula uses the change in creatinine over time to dynamically estimate GFR [81]. A study comparing KeGFR with CKD-EPI and CG showed that calculation of KeGFR in patients with AKI suggested a need for change in medication dosing category of 33.5% (95% CI 29.3–37.6%) when compared to CG [82]. Similarly, KeGFR outperformed traditional steady-state eGFR equations in a population pharmacokinetic model as a covariate for vancomycin clearance [83]. Use of an alternative functional biomarker such as cystatin C is of interest to estimate GFR for medication dosing. A standardized vancomycin dosing protocol based on $CKD\text{-}EPI_{cystatin\ C}$ and $CKD\text{-}EPI_{creatinine\text{-}cystatin\ C}$ in hospitalized patients

Table 26.6 Treatment of hyperkalemia

Medication	Mechanism	Dose	Pharmacokinetic considerations	Therapeutic considerations
Calcium gluconate	Cardiac stabilization through decreasing the threshold potential of cardiac myocytes, resulting in restoration of the transmembrane voltage gradient	1000 mg IV over 2–3 min	Onset: Immediate duration: 30–60 min *Does not impact potassium levels	Calcium chloride is an alternative (central line administration) and provides approximately three times the amount of elemental calcium
Insulin regular + dextrose	Enhances activity of Na-K-ATPase pump to shift potassium intracellularly Glucose administration to prevent hypoglycemia	Insulin IV 0.1 units/kg (up to 10 units); consider 0.05 units/kg (up to 5 units for non-DM history) Dextrose IV 25 g, (unless glucose >250 mg/dL); consider 10% dextrose IV infusion for 3–4 h after	Onset: 10–20 min Duration: 4–6 h	May also be given as fixed dose of 10 units; however weight-based dosing vs. fixed dosing may achieve similar potassium-lowering effects, with lower risk of hypoglycemia
Albuterol	Beta-2 adrenergic agonist, enhances Na-K-ATPase pump to shift potassium intracellularly	10–20 mg inhalation over 10 min	Onset: 30 min Duration: 2 h	May induce tachycardia or angina in susceptible individuals; inconsistent efficacy; IV administration may be considered, where available
Sodium bicarbonate	Hydrogen ion release from cells for buffering with exchange to move potassium intracellularly	IV bolus 50 mEq/50 mL over 15 min or continuous infusion 150 mEq in 1 L D5W over 2–4 h (infusion may be preferred)	Onset: 30 min Duration: 1–2 h or duration of infusion	Controversial data for efficacy and safety; risk of hypernatremia, metabolic alkalosis

(continued)

Table 26.6 (continued)

Medication	Mechanism	Dose	Pharmacokinetic considerations	Therapeutic considerations
Loop diuretic	Inhibition of Na-K-Cl cotransporter in thick ascending limb of loop of Henle, causing potassium excretion in urine	Furosemide IV 40–80 mg push, higher dose depending on kidney function	Onset: 15–60 min Duration: 4–6 h	Consider volume status of the patient, may require fluid administration due to diuretic effects
Sodium polystyrene sulfonate (SPS)	Binds potassium in GI tract and enhances fecal elimination in exchange for sodium counterions	15 g/dose enterally once, up to four times daily	Onset: >2 h Duration: 6–24 h	High sodium load; should not be used in patients at risk for constipation or obstruction; serious and fatal adverse effects including colonic necrosis and other GI effects, especially when administered with sorbitol
Sodium zirconium cyclosilicate	Binds potassium in GI tract and enhances fecal elimination in exchange for sodium and hydrogen counterions	10 g enteral once, up to three times daily	Onset: 1 h Duration: Not well defined	High sodium load (less than SPS), caution in patients at risk of edema; avoid with severe constipation, bowel obstruction or impaction
Patiromer	Binds potassium in GI tract and enhances fecal elimination through non-absorbed potassium-binding polymer with calcium-sorbitol counterion	8.4–25.2 g enteral once	Onset: 2–7 h Duration: 24 h after last dose (2-day administration)	Delayed onset; avoid with severe constipation, bowel obstruction, or impaction; may also bind magnesium

D5W dextrose 5% in water, *DM* diabetes mellitus, *IV* intravenous, *GI* gastrointestinal, *Na-K-ATPase* sodium-potassium adenosine triphosphatase, *Na-Cl-K* sodium-potassium-chloride, *SPS* sodium polystyrene sulfonate

without AKI was shown to increase achievement of goal trough levels [84, 85]. Although cystatin C is somewhat more dynamic in AKI than creatinine, GFR estimation equations like the CKD EPI eGFR$_{cysC}$ have similar steady-state limitations as creatinine-based equations [86]. Change in kidney elimination is not the only factor increasing the complexity of medication dosing in AKI. Patients with AKI have changes in drug volume of distribution, protein binding, and metabolism. The addition of KRT, discussed in a separate chapter, further augments the complexity of medication dosing and monitoring. Ultimately, pharmacists must consider the clinical scenario, drug therapeutic index, pharmacokinetic changes, residual kidney function, nonrenal elimination, and KRT elimination when determining medication dose adjustments.

26.6 AKI Survivorship

The long-term health consequences of AKI survivors have garnered increased recognition. In part, the morbidity with AKI survivorship could be mitigated with improvements in healthcare delivery quality, particularly at transitions from hospital to home. Recent estimates suggest that up to one-third of individuals who survive moderate-to-severe AKI fail to receive even the most basic elements of follow-up care (a serum creatinine assessment, and a clinical visit with a healthcare provider) in the 30 days after discharge [87]. Urine protein evaluation, a key prognostic indicator and surveillance marker for CKD, is checked in less than 50% of AKI survivors [88, 89]. Medications like renin-angiotensin system inhibitors, sodium glucose cotransporter 2 inhibitors, or oral anti-diabetes medications like metformin or glyburide are often held during an AKI episode, but frequently not restarted at discharge leading to undertreated health conditions and medication errors [90, 91]. Other medications like gabapentin or antimicrobials are often dose adjusted for the reduced eGFR in AKI but, with the dynamic course of recovery, require iterative re-evaluation [86, 92]. Pharmacists are uniquely well positioned to improve AKI survivor care through optimal medication management.

The favorable impact of pharmacists on the care of patients with kidney disease has been demonstrated, particularly for patients with CKD and end-stage kidney disease [93]. Less clear is the role for pharmacists to improve AKI survivor care, although there is broad support for their involvement [94]. In one randomized controlled trial of 98 stage 3 AKI survivors, patients were randomized to usual care or care delivered in a nephrologist-led AKI survivor clinic by a multidisciplinary team inclusive of a pharmacist. In the intervention arm, pharmacists completed a medication review and reconciliation within approximately 4 weeks of discharge, delivered education on nephrotoxins, and provided recommendations to the attending nephrologist. The frequency of medication reconciliation and medication alert for potential harmful medication was significantly higher in the intervention arm with a pharmacist compared to usual care (medication reconciliation 100 vs. 0%, $P < 0.001$; medication alert care 33.3 vs. 0%, $P < 0.001$) [95]. In another report, pharmacists provided structured follow-up care for 11 AKI survivors within 2 weeks of discharge as part of a primary care-based model. Pharmacists identified a median of three medication therapy problems per patient, about 20% of which were related to nephrotoxic and renoprotective medication optimization. At least one medication discrepancy or medication therapy problem was noted in 100% of patients, and in 86% of cases, pharmacist recommendations were accepted and enacted by providers within 7 days [96]. Additional high-quality evidence is expected in the next several years as ongoing trials that involve pharmacists in AKI survivor care are published [97].

While we have only begun to understand the role of pharmacists in AKI survivor care, one can envision numerous pathways for involvement in the future. Pharmacists could facilitate hospital dismissal medication reconciliation and ensure that comprehensive dismissal follow-up plans are in place for renally active medication use (renally eliminated, nephrotoxic, and nephroprotective) [98]. Medication-specific education could be provided to AKI survivors and their loved ones. Pharmacists could complete clinical encounters with AKI survivors independently, through comprehensive medication management services, or collaboratively through practice agreements. In these visits, pharmacists could focus on the core elements of AKI survivor care as highlighted in the KAMPS framework—kidney function monitoring (i.e., serum creatinine, urine protein), advocacy/education about kidney health, medication review, individualized blood pressure evaluation, and discussion about safe sick day behaviors [99, 100]. Pharmacists in ICU recovery centers have demonstrated an integral role in identifying and preventing medication-related problems in post-critical illness follow-up [101, 102]. This setting may be another opportunity for AKI survivors to interface with pharmacists post-critical illness for medication optimization.

26.7 Conclusion

Defining, diagnosing, and managing AKI are an evolving field. Incorporating functional and structural biomarkers to better predict the course of AKI and patient prognosis is an exciting area of research. A more precise understanding of AKI allows for personalized intervention targeting the underlying pathophysiology and identifying patients most likely to benefit from therapeutic interventions. Pharmacists and care teams must continue to work to identify opportunities and strategies for preventing AKI in the critically ill. In addition, vigilance in early identification and management is of clinical importance. Finally, given the long-term health implications of AKI, special attention to the entire spectrum of AKI management including transitions of care is an important research priority.

References

1. Kellum JA, Romagnani P, Ashuntantang G, et al. Acute kidney injury. Nat Rev Dis Primers. 2021;7:52. https://doi.org/10.1038/s41572-021-00284-z.
2. Hoste EAJ, Kellum JA, Selby NM, et al. Global epidemiology and outcomes of acute kidney injury. Nat Rev Nephrol. 2018;14:607–25. https://doi.org/10.1038/s41581-018-0052-0.
3. Uchino S, Kellum JA, Bellomo R, et al. Acute renal failure in critically ill patients: a multinational, multicenter study. JAMA. 2005;294:813–8. https://doi.org/10.1001/jama.294.7.813.

4. Heung M, Steffick DE, Zivin K, et al. Acute kidney injury recovery pattern and subsequent risk of CKD: an analysis of veterans health administration data. Am J Kidney Dis. 2016;67:742–52. https://doi.org/10.1053/j.ajkd.2015.10.019.

5. James MT, Pannu N, Hemmelgarn BR, et al. Derivation and external validation of prediction models for advanced chronic kidney disease following acute kidney injury. JAMA. 2017;318:1787–97. https://doi.org/10.1001/jama.2017.16326.

6. Odutayo A, Wong CX, Farkouh M, et al. AKI and long-term risk for cardiovascular events and mortality. J Am Soc Nephrol. 2017;28:377–87. https://doi.org/10.1681/ASN.2016010105.

7. Siew ED, Parr SK, Abdel-Kader K, et al. Predictors of recurrent AKI. J Am Soc Nephrol. 2016;27:1190–200. https://doi.org/10.1681/ASN.2014121218.

8. Rewa O, Bagshaw SM. Acute kidney injury-epidemiology, outcomes and economics. Nat Rev Nephrol. 2014;10:193–207. https://doi.org/10.1038/nrneph.2013.282.

9. Bellomo R, Ronco C, Kellum JA, et al. Acute renal failure—definition, outcome measures, animal models, fluid therapy and information technology needs: the second international consensus conference of the acute dialysis quality initiative (ADQI) group. Crit Care. 2004;8:R204–12. https://doi.org/10.1186/cc2872.

10. Priyanka P, Zarbock A, Izawa J, et al. The impact of acute kidney injury by serum creatinine or urine output criteria on major adverse kidney events in cardiac surgery patients. J Thorac Cardiovasc Surg. 2021;162:143–151.e7. https://doi.org/10.1016/j.jtcvs.2019.11.137.

11. Mehta RL, Kellum JA, Shah SV, et al. Acute kidney injury network: report of an initiative to improve outcomes in acute kidney injury. Crit Care. 2007;11:R31. https://doi.org/10.1186/cc5713.

12. Xiong J, Tang X, Hu Z, et al. The RIFLE versus AKIN classification for incidence and mortality of acute kidney injury in critical ill patients: a meta-analysis. Sci Rep. 2015;5:17917. https://doi.org/10.1038/srep17917.

13. KDIGO AKI Work Group. KDIGO clinical practice guideline for acute kidney injury. Kidney Inter Suppl. 2012;2:1–138.

14. Levey AS. Defining AKD: the spectrum of AKI, AKD, and CKD. Nephron. 2022;146:302–5. https://doi.org/10.1159/000516647.

15. Lameire NH, Levin A, Kellum JA, et al. Harmonizing acute and chronic kidney disease definition and classification: report of a kidney disease: improving global outcomes (KDIGO) consensus conference. Kidney Int. 2021;100:516–26. https://doi.org/10.1016/j.kint.2021.06.028.

16. Stanski NL, Rodrigues CE, Strader M, et al. Precision management of acute kidney injury in the intensive care unit: current state of the art. Intensive Care Med. 2023;49:1049–61. https://doi.org/10.1007/s00134-023-07171-z.

17. Doi K, Yuen PST, Eisner C, et al. Reduced production of creatinine limits its use as marker of kidney injury in sepsis. J Am Soc Nephrol. 2009;20:1217–21. https://doi.org/10.1681/ASN.2008060617.

18. Levey AS, Becker C, Inker LA. Glomerular filtration rate and albuminuria for detection and staging of acute and chronic kidney disease in adults: a systematic review. JAMA. 2015;313:837–46. https://doi.org/10.1001/jama.2015.0602.

19. Rule AD, Bailey KR, Schwartz GL, et al. For estimating creatinine clearance measuring muscle mass gives better results than those based on demographics. Kidney Int. 2009;75:1071–8. https://doi.org/10.1038/ki.2008.698.

20. Salazar DE, Corcoran GB. Predicting creatinine clearance and renal drug clearance in obese patients from estimated fat-free body mass. Am J Med. 1988;84:1053–60. https://doi.org/10.1016/0002-9343(88)90310-5.

21. Haase M, Kellum JA, Ronco C. Subclinical AKI—an emerging syndrome with important consequences. Nat Rev Nephrol. 2012;8:735–9. https://doi.org/10.1038/nrneph.2012.197.

22. Nejat M, Pickering JW, Walker RJ, Endre ZH. Rapid detection of acute kidney injury by plasma cystatin C in the intensive care unit. Nephrol Dial Transplant. 2010;25:3283–9. https://doi.org/10.1093/ndt/gfq176.

23. Knight EL, Verhave JC, Spiegelman D, et al. Factors influencing serum cystatin C levels other than renal function and the impact on renal function measurement. Kidney Int. 2004;65:1416–21. https://doi.org/10.1111/j.1523-1755.2004.00517.x.

24. Beunders R, van Groenendael R, Leijte GP, et al. Proenkephalin compared to conventional methods to assess kidney function in critically ill sepsis patients. Shock. 2020;54:308–14. https://doi.org/10.1097/SHK.0000000000001510.

25. Caironi P, Latini R, Struck J, et al. Circulating proenkephalin, acute kidney injury, and its improvement in patients with severe sepsis or shock. Clin Chem. 2018;64:1361–9. https://doi.org/10.1373/clinchem.2018.288068.

26. Chawla LS, Davison DL, Brasha-Mitchell E, et al. Development and standardization of a furosemide stress test to predict the severity of acute kidney injury. Crit Care. 2013;17:R207. https://doi.org/10.1186/cc13015.

27. Meersch M, Weiss R, Gerss J, et al. Predicting the development of renal replacement therapy indications by combining the furosemide stress test and chemokine (C-C motif) ligand 14 in a cohort of postsurgical patients. Crit Care Med. 2023;51:1033–42. https://doi.org/10.1097/CCM.0000000000005849.

28. Kane-Gill SL, Smithburger PL, Kashani K, et al. Clinical relevance and predictive value of damage biomarkers of drug-induced kidney injury. Drug Saf. 2017;40:1049–74. https://doi.org/10.1007/s40264-017-0565-7.

29. Murray PT, Mehta RL, Shaw A, et al. Potential use of biomarkers in acute kidney injury: report and summary of recommendations from the 10th acute dialysis quality initiative consensus conference. Kidney Int. 2014;85:513–21. https://doi.org/10.1038/ki.2013.374.

30. Ostermann M, Zarbock A, Goldstein S, et al. Recommendations on acute kidney injury biomarkers from the acute disease quality initiative consensus conference: a consensus statement. JAMA Netw Open. 2020b;3:e2019209. https://doi.org/10.1001/jamanetworkopen.2020.19209.

31. Poston JT, Koyner JL. Sepsis associated acute kidney injury. BMJ. 2019;364:k4891. https://doi.org/10.1136/bmj.k4891.

32. Bihorac A, Chawla LS, Shaw AD, et al. Validation of cell-cycle arrest biomarkers for acute kidney injury using clinical adjudication. Am J Respir Crit Care Med. 2014;189:932–9. https://doi.org/10.1164/rccm.201401-0077OC.

33. Kashani K, Al-Khafaji A, Ardiles T, et al. Discovery and validation of cell cycle arrest biomarkers in human acute kidney injury. Crit Care. 2013;17:R25. https://doi.org/10.1186/cc12503.

34. Albert C, Zapf A, Haase M, et al. Neutrophil gelatinase-associated lipocalin measured on clinical laboratory platforms for the prediction of acute kidney injury and the associated need for dialysis therapy: a systematic review and meta-analysis. Am J Kidney Dis. 2020;76:826–841.e1. https://doi.org/10.1053/j.ajkd.2020.05.015.

35. Haase M, Bellomo R, Devarajan P, et al. Accuracy of neutrophil gelatinase-associated lipocalin (NGAL) in diagnosis and prognosis in acute kidney injury: a systematic review and meta-analysis. Am J Kidney Dis. 2009;54:1012–24. https://doi.org/10.1053/j.ajkd.2009.07.020.

36. Bagshaw SM, Al-Khafaji A, Artigas A, et al. External validation of urinary C-C motif chemokine ligand 14 (CCL14) for prediction of persistent acute kidney injury. Crit Care. 2021;25:185. https://doi.org/10.1186/s13054-021-03618-1.

37. Hoste E, Bihorac A, Al-Khafaji A, et al. Identification and validation of biomarkers of persistent acute kidney injury: the RUBY study. Intensive Care Med. 2020;46:943–53. https://doi.org/10.1007/s00134-019-05919-0.

38. Delgado C, Baweja M, Crews DC, et al. A unifying approach for GFR estimation: recommendations of the NKF-ASN task force on reassessing the inclusion of race in diagnosing kidney disease. J Am Soc Nephrol. 2021;32:2994–3015. https://doi.org/10.1681/ASN.2021070988.

39. Kidney Disease: Improving Global Outcomes (KDIGO) CKD Work Group. KDIGO 2024 clinical practice guideline for the evaluation and management of chronic kidney disease. Kidney Int. 2024;105:S117–314. https://doi.org/10.1016/j.kint.2023.10.018.

40. Teaford HR, Rule AD, Mara KC, et al. Patterns of cystatin C uptake and use across and within hospitals. Mayo Clin Proc. 2020;95:1649–59. https://doi.org/10.1016/j.mayocp.2020.03.030.

41. Miano TA, Barreto EF, McNett M, et al. Toward equitable kidney function estimation in critical care practice. Guidance from the Society of Critical Care Medicine's diversity, equity,

and inclusion in renal clinical practice task force. Crit Care Med. 2024;52:951–62. https://doi.org/10.1097/CCM.0000000000006237.

42. Turgut F, Awad AS, Abdel-Rahman EM. Acute kidney injury: medical causes and pathogenesis. J Clin Med. 2023;12:375. https://doi.org/10.3390/jcm12010375.

43. Abdelhafez M, Nayfeh T, Atieh A, et al. Diagnostic performance of fractional excretion of sodium for the differential diagnosis of acute kidney injury: a systematic review and meta-analysis. Clin J Am Soc Nephrol. 2022;17:785–97. https://doi.org/10.2215/CJN.14561121.

44. Seethapathy H, Fenves AZ. Fractional excretion of sodium (FENa): an imperfect tool for a flawed question. Clin J Am Soc Nephrol. 2022;17:777–8. https://doi.org/10.2215/CJN.04750422.

45. Perazella MA, Coca SG. Traditional urinary biomarkers in the assessment of hospital-acquired AKI. Clin J Am Soc Nephrol. 2012;7:167–74. https://doi.org/10.2215/CJN.09490911.

46. Brown RS. Fractional excretion of sodium and urea are useful tools in the evaluation of AKI: COMMENTARY. Kidney360. 2023;4:e731–3. https://doi.org/10.34067/KID.0002502022.

47. Juncos LA, Wieruszewski PM, Kashani K. Pathophysiology of acute kidney injury in critical illness: a narrative review. Compr Physiol. 2022;12:3767–80. https://doi.org/10.1002/cphy.c210028.

48. Kellum JA, Prowle JR. Paradigms of acute kidney injury in the intensive care setting. Nat Rev Nephrol. 2018;14:217–30. https://doi.org/10.1038/nrneph.2017.184.

49. Karimzadeh I, Barreto EF, Kellum JA, et al. Moving toward a contemporary classification of drug-induced kidney disease. Crit Care. 2023;27:435. https://doi.org/10.1186/s13054-023-04720-2.

50. Ostermann M, Bellomo R, Burdmann EA, et al. Controversies in acute kidney injury: conclusions from a kidney disease: improving global outcomes (KDIGO) conference. Kidney Int. 2020a;98:294–309. https://doi.org/10.1016/j.kint.2020.04.020.

51. Perazella MA, Rosner MH. Drug-induced acute kidney injury. Clin J Am Soc Nephrol. 2022;17:1220–33. https://doi.org/10.2215/CJN.11290821.

52. Davenport MS, Perazella MA, Yee J, et al. Use of intravenous iodinated contrast media in patients with kidney disease: consensus statements from the American college of radiology and the national kidney foundation. Radiology. 2020;294:660–8. https://doi.org/10.1148/radiol.2019192094.

53. Vaara ST, Bhatraju PK, Stanski NL, et al. Subphenotypes in acute kidney injury: a narrative review. Crit Care. 2022;26:251. https://doi.org/10.1186/s13054-022-04121-x.

54. Meersch M, Schmidt C, Hoffmeier A, et al. Prevention of cardiac surgery-associated AKI by implementing the KDIGO guidelines in high risk patients identified by biomarkers: the PrevAKI randomized controlled trial. Intensive Care Med. 2017;43:1551–61. https://doi.org/10.1007/s00134-016-4670-3.

55. Göcze I, Jauch D, Götz M, et al. Biomarker-guided intervention to prevent acute kidney injury after major surgery: the prospective randomized BigpAK study. Ann Surg. 2018;267:1013–20. https://doi.org/10.1097/SLA.0000000000002485.

56. Zarbock A, Küllmar M, Ostermann M, et al. Prevention of cardiac surgery-associated acute kidney injury by implementing the KDIGO guidelines in high-risk patients identified by biomarkers: the PrevAKI-multicenter randomized controlled trial. Anesth Analg. 2021;133:292–302. https://doi.org/10.1213/ANE.0000000000005458.

57. Engelman DT, Crisafi C, Germain M, et al. Using urinary biomarkers to reduce acute kidney injury following cardiac surgery. J Thorac Cardiovasc Surg. 2020;160:1235–1246.e2. https://doi.org/10.1016/j.jtcvs.2019.10.034.

58. Brown JK, Shaw AD, Mythen MG, et al. Adult cardiac surgery-associated acute kidney injury: joint consensus report. J Cardiothorac Vasc Anesth. 2023;37:1579–90. https://doi.org/10.1053/j.jvca.2023.05.032.

59. Engelman DT, Ben Ali W, Williams JB, et al. Guidelines for perioperative care in cardiac surgery: enhanced recovery after surgery society recommendations. JAMA Surg. 2019;154:755–66. https://doi.org/10.1001/jamasurg.2019.1153.

60. von Groote TC, Ostermann M, Forni LG, et al. The AKI care bundle: all bundle components are created equal-are they? Intensive Care Med. 2022;48:242–5. https://doi.org/10.1007/s00134-021-06601-0.

61. Kane-Gill SL, Peerapornratana S, Wong A, et al. Use of tissue inhibitor of metalloproteinase 2 and insulin-like growth factor binding protein 7 [TIMP2]•[IGFBP7] as an AKI risk screening tool to manage patients in the real-world setting. J Crit Care. 2020;57:97–101. https://doi.org/10.1016/j.jcrc.2020.02.002.

62. Ali M, Naureen H, Tariq MH, et al. Rational use of antibiotics in an intensive care unit: a retrospective study of the impact on clinical outcomes and mortality rate. Infect Drug Resist. 2019;12:493–9. https://doi.org/10.2147/IDR.S187836.

63. Kane-Gill SL. Nephrotoxin stewardship. Crit Care Clin. 2021;37:303–20. https://doi.org/10.1016/j.ccc.2020.11.002.

64. Goldstein SL, Mottes T, Simpson K, et al. A sustained quality improvement program reduces nephrotoxic medication-associated acute kidney injury. Kidney Int. 2016;90:212–21. https://doi.org/10.1016/j.kint.2016.03.031.

65. Goldstein SL, Dahale D, Kirkendall ES, et al. A prospective multi-center quality improvement initiative (NINJA) indicates a reduction in nephrotoxic acute kidney injury in hospitalized children. Kidney Int. 2020;97:580–8. https://doi.org/10.1016/j.kint.2019.10.015.

66. Williams VL, Smithburger PL, Imhoff AN, et al. Interventions, barriers, and proposed solutions associated with the implementation of a protocol that uses clinical decision support and a stress biomarker test to identify ICU patients at high-risk for drug associated acute kidney injury. Ann Pharmacother. 2023;57:408–15. https://doi.org/10.1177/10600280221117993.

67. Parente DM, Cunha CB, Mylonakis E, Timbrook TT. The clinical utility of methicillin-resistant Staphylococcus aureus (MRSA) nasal screening to rule out MRSA pneumonia: a diagnostic meta-analysis with antimicrobial stewardship implications. Clin Infect Dis. 2018;67:1–7. https://doi.org/10.1093/cid/ciy024.

68. Diep C, Meng L, Pourali S, et al. Effect of rapid methicillin-resistant Staphylococcus aureus nasal polymerase chain reaction screening on vancomycin use in the intensive care unit. Am J Health Syst Pharm. 2021;78:2236–44. https://doi.org/10.1093/ajhp/zxab296.

69. Joannidis M, Druml W, Forni LG, et al. Prevention of acute kidney injury and protection of renal function in the intensive care unit: update 2017: expert opinion of the working group on prevention, AKI section, European society of intensive care medicine. Intensive Care Med. 2017;43:730–49. https://doi.org/10.1007/s00134-017-4832-y.

70. Bissell BD, Laine ME, Thompson Bastin ML, et al. Impact of protocolized diuresis for de-resuscitation in the intensive care unit. Crit Care. 2020;24:70. https://doi.org/10.1186/s13054-020-2795-9.

71. Amin AN, Menoyo J, Singh B, Kim CS. Efficacy and safety of sodium zirconium cyclosilicate in patients with baseline serum potassium level ≥5.5 mmol/L: pooled analysis from two phase 3 trials. BMC Nephrol. 2019;20:440. https://doi.org/10.1186/s12882-019-1611-8.

72. Packham DK, Kosiborod M. Pharmacodynamics and pharmacokinetics of sodium zirconium cyclosilicate [ZS-9] in the treatment of hyperkalemia. Expert Opin Drug Metab Toxicol. 2016;12:567–73. https://doi.org/10.1517/17425255.2016.1164691.

73. Peacock WF, Rafique Z, Vishnevskiy K, et al. Emergency potassium normalization treatment including sodium zirconium cyclosilicate: a phase II, randomized, double-blind, placebo-controlled study (ENERGIZE). Acad Emerg Med. 2020;27:475–86. https://doi.org/10.1111/acem.13954.

74. Bushinsky DA, Williams GH, Pitt B, et al. Patiromer induces rapid and sustained potassium lowering in patients with chronic kidney disease and hyperkalemia. Kidney Int. 2015;88:1427–33 https://doi.org/10.1038/ki.2015.270.

75. Di Palo KE, Sinnett MJ, Goriacko P. Assessment of patiromer monotherapy for hyperkalemia in an acute care setting. JAMA Netw Open. 2022;5:e2145236. https://doi.org/10.1001/jamanetworkopen.2021.45236.

76. Rafique Z, Liu M, Staggers KA, et al. Patiromer for treatment of hyperkalemia in the emergency department: a pilot study. Acad Emerg Med. 2020;27:54–60. https://doi.org/10.1111/acem.13868.

77. Rydell A, Thackrey C, Molki M, Mullins BP. Effectiveness of patiromer versus sodium zirconium cyclosilicate for the management of acute hyperkalemia. Ann Pharmacother. 2023;10600280231209968:790. https://doi.org/10.1177/10600280231209968.

78. Sullivan E, Ruegger M, Dunne I, et al. Comparison of effectiveness and safety of sodium polystyrene sulfonate and sodium zirconium cyclosilicate for treatment of hyperkalemia in hospitalized patients. Am J Health Syst Pharm. 2023;80:1238–46. https://doi.org/10.1093/ajhp/zxad137.

79. Cañas AE, Troutt HR, Jiang L, et al. A randomized study to compare oral potassium binders in the treatment of acute hyperkalemia. BMC Nephrol. 2023;24:89. https://doi.org/10.1186/s12882-023-03145-x.

80. Rafique Z, Budden J, Quinn CM, et al. Patiromer utility as an adjunct treatment in patients needing urgent hyperkalaemia management (PLATINUM): design of a multicentre, randomised, double-blind, placebo-controlled, parallel-group study. BMJ Open. 2023;13:e071311. https://doi.org/10.1136/bmjopen-2022-071311.

81. Chen S. Retooling the creatinine clearance equation to estimate kinetic GFR when the plasma creatinine is changing acutely. J Am Soc Nephrol. 2013;24:877–88. https://doi.org/10.1681/ASN.2012070653.

82. Kwong YD, Chen S, Bouajram R, et al. The value of kinetic glomerular filtration rate estimation on medication dosing in acute kidney injury. PLoS One. 2019;14:e0225601. https://doi.org/10.1371/journal.pone.0225601.

83. Pai MP, DeBacker KC. Modeling kinetic glomerular filtration rate in adults with stable and unstable kidney function: vancomycin as the motivating example. Pharmacotherapy. 2020;40:872–9. https://doi.org/10.1002/phar.2442.

84. Frazee E, Rule AD, Lieske JC, et al. Cystatin C-guided vancomycin dosing in critically ill patients: a quality improvement project. Am J Kidney Dis. 2017;69:658–66. https://doi.org/10.1053/j.ajkd.2016.11.016.

85. Frazee EN, Rule AD, Herrmann SM, et al. Serum cystatin C predicts vancomycin trough levels better than serum creatinine in hospitalized patients: a cohort study. Crit Care. 2014;18:R110. https://doi.org/10.1186/cc13899.

86. Behal ML, Flannery AH, Barreto EF. Medication Management in the Critically ill Patient with acute kidney injury. Clin J Am Soc Nephrol. 2023;18:1080–8. https://doi.org/10.2215/CJN.0000000000000101.

87. Barreto EF, Schreier DJ, May HP, et al. Incidence of serum creatinine monitoring and outpatient visit follow-up among acute kidney injury survivors after discharge: a population-based cohort study. Am J Nephrol. 2021;52:817–26. https://doi.org/10.1159/000519375.

88. Hsu C-Y, Chinchilli VM, Coca S, et al. Post-acute kidney injury proteinuria and subsequent kidney disease progression: the assessment, serial evaluation, and subsequent sequelae in acute kidney injury (ASSESS-AKI) study. JAMA Intern Med. 2020;180:402–10. https://doi.org/10.1001/jamainternmed.2019.6390.

89. Saran R, Robinson B, Abbott KC, et al. US renal data system 2016 annual data report: epidemiology of kidney disease in the United States. Am J Kidney Dis. 2017;69:A7–8. https://doi.org/10.1053/j.ajkd.2016.12.004.

90. Janse RJ, Fu EL, Clase CM, et al. Stopping versus continuing renin-angiotensin-system inhibitors after acute kidney injury and adverse clinical outcomes: an observational study from routine care data. Clin Kidney J. 2022;15:1109–19. https://doi.org/10.1093/ckj/sfac003.

91. Siew ED, Parr SK, Abdel-Kader K, et al. Renin-angiotensin aldosterone inhibitor use at hospital discharge among patients with moderate to severe acute kidney injury and its association with recurrent acute kidney injury and mortality. Kidney Int. 2021;99:1202–12. https://doi.org/10.1016/j.kint.2020.08.022.

92. Hall RK, Kazancıoğlu R, Thanachayanont T, et al. Drug stewardship in chronic kidney disease to achieve effective and safe medication use. Nat Rev Nephrol. 2024;20:386. https://doi.org/10.1038/s41581-024-00823-3.

93. Manley HJ, Aweh G, Weiner DE, et al. Multidisciplinary medication therapy management and hospital readmission in patients undergoing maintenance dialysis: a retrospective cohort study. Am J Kidney Dis. 2020;76:13–21. https://doi.org/10.1053/j.ajkd.2019.12.002.

94. May HP, Krauter AK, Finnie DM, et al. Acute kidney injury survivor care following hospital discharge: a mixed-methods study of nephrologists and primary care providers. Kidney Med. 2023b;5:100586. https://doi.org/10.1016/j.xkme.2022.100586.

95. Thanapongsatorn P, Chaikomon K, Lumlertgul N, et al. Comprehensive versus standard care in post-severe acute kidney injury survivors, a randomized controlled trial. Crit Care. 2021;25:322. https://doi.org/10.1186/s13054-021-03747-7.

96. Herges JR, May HP, Meade L, et al. Pharmacist-provider collaborative visits after hospital discharge in a comprehensive acute kidney injury survivor model. J Am Pharm Assoc (2003). 2023;63:909–14. https://doi.org/10.1016/j.japh.2022.12.029.

97. May HP, Griffin JM, Herges JR, et al. Comprehensive acute kidney injury survivor care: protocol for the randomized acute kidney injury in care transitions pilot trial. JMIR Res Protoc. 2023a;12:e48109. https://doi.org/10.2196/48109.

98. Giles C, Novakovic M, Hopman W, et al. The quality of discharge summaries after acute kidney injury. Can J Kidney Health Dis. 2023;10:20543581231199018. https://doi.org/10.1177/20543581231199018.

99. Kashani K, Rosner MH, Haase M, et al. Quality improvement goals for acute kidney injury. Clin J Am Soc Nephrol. 2019;14:941–53. https://doi.org/10.2215/CJN.01250119.

100. Watson KE, Dhaliwal K, Robertshaw S, et al. Consensus recommendations for sick day medication guidance for people with diabetes, kidney, or cardiovascular disease: a modified Delphi process. Am J Kidney Dis. 2023;81:564–74. https://doi.org/10.1053/j.ajkd.2022.10.012.

101. Stollings JL, Bloom SL, Wang L, et al. Critical care pharmacists and medication management in an ICU recovery center. Ann Pharmacother. 2018;52:713–23. https://doi.org/10.1177/1060028018759343.

102. Stollings JL, Poyant JO, Groth CM, et al. An international, multicenter evaluation of comprehensive medication management by pharmacists in ICU recovery centers. J Intensive Care Med. 2023;38:957–65. https://doi.org/10.1177/08850666231176194.

Chapter 27
Acid-Base Disorders

Haven Nisly, Elias H. Pratt, and Craig R. Rackley

27.1 Introduction

Cellular and physiologic processes within the human body are dependent on an internal environment with a pH tightly regulated between approximately 7.35 and 7.45. The maintenance of acid-base homeostasis in the body is essential to normal cellular function and is largely regulated through the work of the respiratory and renal systems. Assessment of acid-base status is a key skill required of any pharmacist working within the critical care environment.

Prompt evaluation of acid-base derangements in the critically ill patient is essential for making accurate diagnoses that require immediate treatment, such as septic shock, diabetic ketoacidosis, or acute hypercapnic respiratory failure. Acid-base derangements typically occur when the body's normal ability to clear excess acid or base is overwhelmed. This chapter explores the critical breakdown of acid-base analysis, identification of primary metabolic versus respiratory derangements, and how they overlap and compensate for each other and lists the potential diagnoses responsible for various acid-base disorders.

H. Nisly
Department of Medicine, Duke University School of Medicine, Durham, NC, USA

E. H. Pratt · C. R. Rackley (✉)
Division of Pulmonary Allergy, and Critical Care Medicine, Duke University School of Medicine, Durham, NC, USA
e-mail: craig.rackley@duke.edu

Y. Alzaidi, M. A. Gebily (eds.), *The Pharmacist's Expanded Role in Critical Care Medicine*, https://doi.org/10.1007/978-3-031-77335-8_27

27.2   Normal Acid-Base Equilibrium

Understanding how the body maintains a normal acid-base equilibrium is key to understanding and evaluating conditions where this equilibrium is altered. The normal pH of arterial blood is close to 7.40, with the normal range considered between 7.35 and 7.45. pH levels only slightly outside of this range can lead to derangements in normal physiologic functions and, if not promptly corrected, severe disability or death. A pH in the blood less than 7.35 is considered *acidemia*, while a pH greater than 7.45 is considered *alkalemia*. The terms *acidosis* and *alkalosis* specifically refer to the underlying processes that result in the state of *acidemia* or *alkalemia*.

Since pH measurement plays such a key role in identifying and defining acid-base states, it is important to review how it is measured. The pH scale is a negative logarithmic scale that represents the concentration of hydrogen ions [H$^+$] in a solution (Eq. 27.1):

$$pH = -\log\left[H^+\right] \tag{27.1}$$

The body contains a number of substances that act as buffers to regulate pH within the normal physiologic range. Key among these is the bicarbonate buffer system (Eq. 27.2). This reaction is catalyzed by carbonic anhydrase, an enzyme that primarily works in the red blood cells and renal tubules. In order to maintain balance, an increase in carbon dioxide (CO_2) shifts the equation to the right, where acid (H$^+$) is secreted by the kidneys, and increases in H$^+$ shift the equation to the left where CO_2 is expired by the lungs [1]:

$$CO_2 + H_2O \leftrightarrow H_2CO_3 \leftrightarrow H^+ + HCO_3^- \tag{27.2}$$

The Henderson-Hasselbalch equation can be used to relate the pH of the body to the concentration of the different components of the bicarbonate buffer system (Eq. 27.3):

$$pH = 6.1 + \log\left(\left[HCO_3^-\right]/\left(0.03 \times PCO_2\right)\right) \tag{27.3}$$

where [HCO_3^-] represents the concentration of dissolved bicarbonate and PCO_2 denotes the partial pressure of dissolved CO_2 in the blood. The normal range of bicarbonate concentration in arterial blood is 22–26 mEq/L. The normal range of PCO_2 in arterial blood is 35–45 mmHg. This equation illustrates how a disturbance in the ratio of bicarbonate to PCO_2 will lead to a change in pH.

27.3   Initial Assessment of Acid-Base Disturbances

The identification of acid-base disturbances requires laboratory evaluation of a blood gas, followed closely by a basic metabolic, blood chemistry, or renal function panel. The blood gas can be measured from either an arterial (ABG) or a venous (VBG) blood sample. There is overlap in information that these two tests provide, with some key differences, but for the evaluation of acid-base status in most patients, either is acceptable.

The ABG provides the most accurate assessment of arterial blood oxygenation, particularly the PaO_2, or partial pressure of oxygen dissolved in arterial blood. It is typically the test of choice for the assessment of respiratory conditions because it most accurately reflects gas exchange capabilities in the lungs. An ABG is performed on a sample typically taken from the patient's radial artery, but this can be obtained from any systemic artery that is accessed by an arterial catheter. In addition to the PaO_2, the ABG also reports arterial blood pH, $PaCO_2$, and serum bicarbonate. It is important to note that the bicarbonate reported on both the arterial and venous blood gas is calculated using the Henderson-Hasselbalch equation and is not measured directly. This calculated bicarbonate can be inaccurate, especially in cases of extreme pH or temperature. In contrast, a basic metabolic panel, blood chemistry, or renal function panel reports a measured serum bicarbonate in addition to information about other electrolytes and renal function, which helps further define the type of acid-base disturbance.

The VBG has the advantage of being performed on a standard venous sample, obviating the need for an arterial puncture, which must be performed by a trained clinician and is often painful for the patient. While the VBG does provide a measured venous serum pH and PCO_2 as well as a calculated serum bicarbonate, the PO_2 does not provide information about the lungs' gas transfer function. Therefore, like the ABG, the VBG has clinical utility in the evaluation of acid-base disturbances and hypercapnia and can be a valuable initial test in the evaluation of patients suspected to have metabolic or ventilatory derangements without concern for hypoxemia.

When venous and arterial blood gases have been directly compared to assess the degree to which they correlate, pH has typically correlated well between the two, with an average difference of approximately 0.03. Venous pH is generally slightly lower due to the higher concentrations of CO_2 in venous blood. Venous PCO_2 is generally 3–4 mmHg higher than $PaCO_2$, though considerable variability has been observed. Correlation is better at normal values, and a normal venous PCO_2 can predict a normal $PaCO_2$ fairly well. Venous and arterial bicarbonate also have a high degree of correlation, with venous bicarbonate approximately 1 mmol/L higher than arterial bicarbonate [2]. By convention, the terms PO_2 and PCO_2 refer to the partial pressure of oxygen and carbon dioxide, respectively, while the terms PaO_2 and $PaCO_2$ refer to these values when measured in arterial blood.

27.4   Simple Acid-Base Disturbances

Disturbances in the ratio of bicarbonate to PCO_2 occur in four primary ways: respiratory acidosis, respiratory alkalosis, metabolic acidosis, and metabolic alkalosis. They can easily be differentiated by the pH and PCO_2 (Fig. 27.1). While each of these conditions can occur simultaneously with others, presenting as a mixed

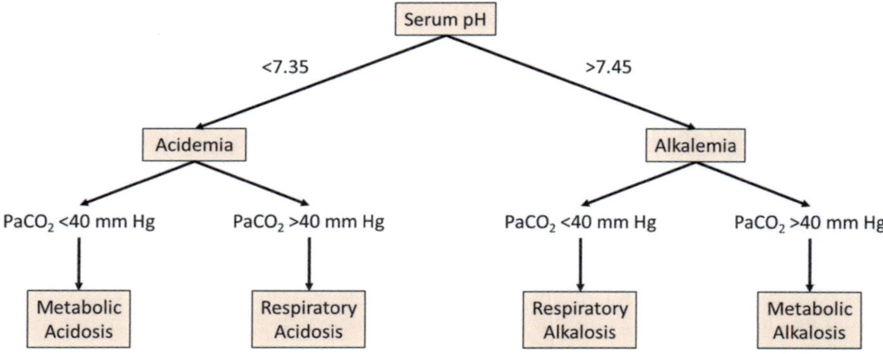

Fig. 27.1 Evaluation of acid-base status

acid-base disorder or as metabolic or respiratory compensation for a primary acid-base disturbance, we will first focus on simple disorders.

27.4.1 *Respiratory Acidosis*

The two physiologic functions of the respiratory system are oxygenation (which maintains an appropriate PaO_2) and ventilation (which maintains an appropriate $PaCO_2$). As previously mentioned, the normal range for the $PaCO_2$ is 35–45 mmHg. An abnormally high PCO_2 is referred to as hypercapnia. Thus, hypercapnia is understood as a failure of the respiratory system to provide adequate ventilation for the CO_2 clearance demands of the body, and as a clinical syndrome, it is identified by its chronicity (i.e., either acute, chronic, or acute on chronic). The increased PCO_2 associated with hypercapnic respiratory failure causes a shift of the bicarbonate buffer system toward carbonic acid production and results in increased production of H^+ ions, which lowers serum pH. Since the primary failure causing acidosis is the respiratory system, this scenario is termed a respiratory acidosis.

Respiratory acidosis can occur as a result of any process that decreases alveolar ventilation and is a common reason for patients to require invasive or noninvasive mechanical ventilation. Decreased alveolar ventilation can be caused by a number of etiologies (Table 27.1). Injuries, diseases, and medications can all impact the drive to breathe, the ability of the respiratory system to move air in and out, and/or the ability of the lungs to exchange gas.

Processes that depress the central respiratory centers in the medulla will decrease respiratory drive, impairing the patient's ability to initiate breaths. Sedatives, opioids, anesthetics, and any other medications that act on the central nervous system can have this effect. A stroke, severe anoxic brain injury, or brainstem herniation can also lead to an impaired or absent drive to breathe. If ventilation is not supported artificially, then respiratory acidosis will quickly ensue.

Table 27.1 Causes of respiratory acidosis

Depressed CNS drive to breathe
Sedating medications (e.g., opioids, benzodiazepines)
Brain death
Brainstem herniation
Stroke
Impaired nerve transmission
Guillain-Barre syndrome
Amyotrophic lateral sclerosis
High C-spine injury
Neuromuscular blocking medications
Muscle dysfunction
Critical illness myopathy
Muscular dystrophy
Upper airway obstruction
Angioedema
Laryngospasm
Vocal cord paralysis
Tracheal stenosis or obstructing tumor
Lower airway obstruction
Asthma
COPD
Bronchiolitis
Restrictive lung disease
Interstitial lung disease
Large pleural effusion
Restrictive chest wall disease
Kyphoscoliosis
Obesity
Scleroderma
Pleural scarring
Increased ventilatory demand
Overfeeding
Inadequate artificial ventilatory support

Disorders of the peripheral nerves or respiratory muscles diminish the ability of the patient to generate adequate inspiratory effort. Neuromuscular disorders that affect the respiratory muscles, such as Guillain-Barre syndrome, myasthenia gravis, amyotrophic lateral sclerosis, and injury to nerves or spinal cord, can also impair ventilation and lead to CO_2 accumulation. Other common findings in the intensive care unit that weaken or blunt the function of the respiratory muscles are the use of neuromuscular blocking agents and critical illness myopathy, which can occur following prolonged critical illness.

Two common causes of respiratory acidosis encountered in critical care are acute exacerbations of asthma or chronic obstructive pulmonary disease (COPD). Because of narrowed small airways in both of these diseases, patients have difficulty moving air through the obstructed airways, resulting in decreased alveolar ventilation and preventing adequate CO_2 clearance. Other processes such as laryngeal edema or tracheal stenosis can present similarly due to narrowed upper airways. Early signs and symptoms of acute hypercapnic respiratory failure due to airway obstruction commonly include dyspnea, tachypnea, and respiratory distress. This increased work of breathing causes excess energy expenditure and more CO_2 production, which subsequently can worsen the respiratory acidosis and precipitate rapid clinical deterioration. Eventually, unless this process is reversed, the patient will begin to fatigue, PCO_2 will rise even further, and the patient will develop a depressed level of consciousness and respiratory drive known as CO_2 narcosis.

Chronic restrictive lung disorders like chronic interstitial lung diseases and acute parenchymal lung disorders like pneumonia, acute respiratory distress syndrome, or pulmonary edema can all cause respiratory acidosis by reducing the volume of functional lung available for gas exchange. Restriction of the pleural space and/or chest wall, such as from pleural effusions, severe obesity, abdominal compartment syndrome, or kyphoscoliosis, similarly impairs ventilation.

In addition to addressing the underlying cause, treatment of hypercapnic respiratory failure often involves positive-pressure ventilation, through either noninvasive or invasive mechanical ventilation. It is also important to note that respiratory acidosis can result from minute ventilation that is too low in mechanically ventilated patients. Ventilator settings must be appropriately adjusted to respond to changes in a patient's clinical condition. Worsening in pulmonary function, and therefore alveolar ventilation; clinical changes resulting in increased CO_2 production, such as fever and agitation; or decreased respiratory drive, such as an increase in sedative or opioid administration, are all scenarios that may require adjustment of the minute ventilation provided by the ventilator.

27.4.2 *Respiratory Alkalosis*

In direct contrast to respiratory acidosis, respiratory alkalosis occurs as a result of alveolar hyperventilation. Alveolar hyperventilation decreases PCO_2 and raises pH. This requires a ventilatory stimulus that outpaces the rate of CO_2 production by the tissues (Table 27.2).

The brainstem contains the pacemaker for the lungs. Central nervous system causes of respiratory alkalosis include anxiety, pain, infection, and fever. Drugs including salicylates and progesterone can also stimulate the respiratory centers. Another driver of respiratory alkalosis is hypoxemia, of which a classic example is ascent to high elevation. As the oxygen concentration of ambient air decreases with ascending elevation, the body responds by increasing tidal volumes and then respiratory rate in an overall effort to increase ventilation, which helps to mitigate the fall in alveolar PO_2. This increases excretion of CO_2 and results in a respiratory alkalosis.

While not as common in critical illness as respiratory acidosis, respiratory alkalosis is frequently seen in critically ill patients, where it is associated with early sepsis and states of increased metabolic demand. In many disease states when respiratory alkalosis is initially present, the normalization of hypocapnia in a patient with

Table 27.2 Causes of respiratory alkalosis

Increased CNS drive to breath
Pain
Anxiety
Medications (salicylates, progesterone)
Increase intracranial pressure
Infection
Hypoxemia
Excess artificial ventilatory support

hyperventilation may herald respiratory fatigue and impending respiratory decompensation. In patients on mechanical ventilation, a respiratory alkalosis can result from minute ventilation (tidal volume, respiratory rate, or both) that is inappropriately high.

27.4.3 Metabolic Acidosis

In metabolic acidosis, the ratio of bicarbonate concentration to PCO_2 is decreased due to a fall in serum bicarbonate. This can occur as a result of increased acid ingestion or production, decreased acid secretion, or increased bicarbonate losses. When attempting to determine the etiology of a metabolic acidosis, assessment of the serum anion gap (AG) is the first critical step (Eq. 27.4):

$$AG = \left[Na^+ \right] - \left[Cl^- \right] + \left[HCO_3^- \right] \tag{27.4}$$

In extracellular fluid, the concentration of cations must always equal the concentration of anions to maintain neutrality [3]. The primary measured cation is sodium (Na^+), and the primary measured anions are chloride (Cl^-) and bicarbonate (HCO_3^-). Proteins and other minor anions fill the "gap" between the measured cations and anions, with an anion gap of 3–12 mEq/L considered normal. In certain disease states, accumulation of acid anions in the serum, such as lactic acid or ketoacids, raises the anion gap and is associated with metabolic acidosis.

Since albumin is a major contributor to the normal anion gap, any anion gap calculation must account for changes in serum albumin, especially hypoalbuminemia, which is extremely common in critically ill patients (Eq. 27.5). If a correction is not made, small changes in the anion gap may not be readily apparent as the calculated anion gap may underestimate the true anion gap [4]:

$$Corrected\ AG = AG_{Measured} + 2.5 \times \left(4 - albumin \right) \tag{27.5}$$

where albumin concentrations are in g/dL.

The causes of high anion gap metabolic acidosis include a variety of scenarios in which unmeasured anions accumulate in association with either increased acid production or decreased acid secretion (Table 27.3). Diabetic ketoacidosis (DKA) represents one common example of increased acid production associated with a high anion gap. DKA is caused by an insulin deficiency leading to increased lipolysis and subsequent generation of ketone bodies (acetoacetate, beta-hydroxybutyrate). These ketoacids accumulate, driving the anion gap higher. Ketoacidosis can also occur in settings of poor oral intake (starvation ketosis) or excessive alcohol consumption, which can impair hepatic metabolism and trigger ketogenesis.

Another highly relevant cause of a high anion gap metabolic acidosis in critically ill patients is lactic acidosis [5]. The most common form of lactic acidosis is that which occurs secondary to tissue hypoxia and is referred to as type A lactic acidosis. This results from inadequate tissue oxygenation leading to anaerobic metabolism and a subsequent accumulation of lactate. Lactate is an unmeasured anion, and its accumulation increases the anion gap. Lactate production is associated with equivalent production of H^+ from hydrolysis of ATP to ADP. If lactate consumption does not match production, the accumulation of H^+ will lead to a decrease in serum pH. Type A lactic acidosis is commonly seen in shock, which is understood at a

Table 27.3 Causes of high anion gap metabolic acidosis

Increased acid production
  Lactic acidosis
    Shock
    Sepsis
    Anemia
    Hypoxemia
    Carbon monoxide poisoning
    Cyanide poisoning
    Malignancy
    Medications
      Albuterol
      Epinephrine
      Metformin
      Antiretrovirals
      Propofol
    Liver disease
    Seizure
    Thiamine deficiency
  Ketoacidosis
    Diabetic
    Starvation
    Alcoholic
  Ingestions
    Methanol
    Ethylene glycol
    Salicylates
    Toluene
    Diethylene glycol
    Propylene glycol

Decreased acid secretion
  Uremia

fundamental level to be a state of tissue hypoperfusion. Septic, cardiogenic, hypovolemic, and other forms of shock can all cause tissue hypoxia and a resultant lactic acidosis, as can cardiac arrest, severe hypoxemia, severe anemia, and any other process that impairs oxygen delivery to tissues.

Type B lactic acidosis refers to conditions where tissue hypoxia is not the primary driver of lactate accumulation; however, the end result is similar: a high anion gap metabolic acidosis associated with the accumulation of lactate. Etiologies of type B lactic acidosis include processes that increase beta-2 agonism, such as administration of epinephrine or beta-2 agonists like albuterol in high doses. Cancer can also lead to a type B lactic acidosis via the Warburg effect, which describes the preference of some cancer cells for aerobic glycolysis. This preferentially produces lactate, even in the presence of oxygen and normal-functioning mitochondria [6]. A number of medications can interfere with oxidative phosphorylation and lead to a type B lactic acidosis, including metformin, propofol, reverse transcriptase inhibitors, and others. Additionally, liver disease can lead to a type B lactic acidosis due to impaired clearance of lactate. While it can be useful to differentiate lactic acidosis into types A and B, it is important to note that they are not exclusive of each other and can coexist in some clinical conditions.

Toxic ingestions such as methanol and ethylene glycol cause a high anion gap metabolic acidosis through the production of organic acids when metabolized to formic acid and glycolic acid, respectively. Uremia, caused by acute or chronic renal failure, is another cause of high anion gap metabolic acidosis. It involves the retention of urea and other nitrogenous waste products due to renal dysfunction. In this setting of decreased renal function, the kidney's abilities to excrete acids and retain bicarbonate are diminished. Additionally, unmeasured anions like sulfate and phosphate accumulate, contributing to the high anion gap.

In contrast to high anion gap metabolic acidosis, normal anion gap metabolic acidosis (NAGMA) typically results from the loss of alkali rather than the accumulation of acids (Table 27.4). In these processes, there are typically reciprocal changes in the concentrations of chloride and bicarbonate that result in a normal anion gap [7]. Normally, bicarbonate is secreted from the pancreas and duodenal mucosa to protect the small bowel from highly acidic contents entering from the stomach. Conditions that cause high output from the intestines, such as diarrhea or enteric

Table 27.4 Causes of normal anion gap metabolic acidosis

Renal tubular acidosis
Gastrointestinal loss
Diarrhea
Pancreatic fistula
Enteric fistula
Ureterosigmoidostomy
Jejunal loop
Medications (calcium chloride, magnesium sulfate, cholestyramine)
Miscellaneous
Rapid saline fluid expansion

fistulas, lead to a significant loss of bicarbonate from increased motility of the gut, causing a metabolic acidosis. Renal pathology is another common cause of a normal anion gap metabolic acidosis. Type 1 renal tubular acidosis (RTA) involves impaired hydrogen ion secretion in the distal tubules of the kidney, leading to decreased acid excretion. Type 2 RTA involves impaired bicarbonate reabsorption in the proximal tubules, resulting in bicarbonate wasting. Analysis of urine ammonium can aid in differentiating between renal and gastrointestinal causes of NAGMA. Levels of urine ammonium can be estimated by calculating the urine anion gap (UAG) (Eq. 27.6):

$$ UAG = \left[Na^+ \right] + \left[K^+ \right] - \left[Cl^- \right] \tag{27.6} $$

where [Na^+] is the concentration of Na^+ in the urine in mEq/L, [K^+] is the concentration of K^+ in the urine in mEq/L, and [Cl^-] is the concentration of Cl^- in the urine in mEq/L. When the UAG is negative, this indicates an increase in urine ammonium as the kidney is trying to excrete excess acid to compensate for gastrointestinal losses of bicarbonate. When the UAG is positive, it indicates a low urine ammonium level due to impaired urine excretion of acid and a likely renal etiology of the NAGMA.

27.4.4   Metabolic Alkalosis

In a metabolic alkalosis, the ratio of bicarbonate concentration to PCO_2 is increased. This results from processes that increase either the loss of acid or accumulation of bicarbonate within the extracellular fluid (Table 27.5). The acid loss typically occurs from the stomach or the kidney, whereas excess base intake may be via oral or parenteral routes.

Loss of acid via gastric secretions occurs with vomiting or gastric drainage or suctioning, creating a relative excess of bicarbonate in the body. Administration of loop or thiazide diuretics can also result in metabolic alkalosis by increasing urinary excretion of chloride, which results in a relative excess of bicarbonate as chloride depletion enhances bicarbonate reabsorption in the proximal tubule. Diuretic administration, along with other processes that decrease the extracellular fluid volume, such as dehydration, can also cause a metabolic alkalosis via contraction alkalosis. This refers to alkalosis that results from a decrease or "contraction" in extracellular fluid volume, which leads to activation of the renin-angiotensin-aldosterone (RAAS) system and an increase in reabsorption of Na^+, Cl^-, and bicarbonate ions. Bicarbonate is reabsorbed out of proportion to Na^+ and Cl^- ions, resulting in a metabolic alkalosis.

The kidney is equipped with sophisticated mechanisms to avert the generation or the persistence of metabolic alkalosis by enhancing bicarbonate excretion. These mechanisms include increased filtration as well as decreased absorption and enhanced secretion of bicarbonate by specialized transporters in specific nephron segments. Factors that interfere with these mechanisms will impair the ability of the

Table 27.5 Causes of metabolic alkalosis

Loss of gastric acid
Vomiting
Nasogastric suctioning
Gastric fistula
Loop or thiazide diuretics
Volume depletion
High aldosterone states
Exogenous mineralocorticoids
Primary hyperaldosteronism (Conn's syndrome)
Secondary hyperaldosteronism
Cushing's syndrome
Exogenous alkali loads
Bicarbonate administration or ingestion
Excessive calcium alkali ingestion
Milk-alkali syndrome
Post-hypercapnia
Genetic disorders
Bartter syndrome
Gitelman syndrome
Liddle syndrome
Cystic fibrosis
Adrenal enzyme deficiencies
Miscellaneous
Licorice

kidney to eliminate excess bicarbonate, thereby promoting the generation or impairing the correction of metabolic alkalosis. These factors include volume contraction, low glomerular filtration rate, potassium deficiency, hypochloremia, aldosterone excess, and elevated arterial carbon dioxide. Major clinical states are associated with metabolic alkalosis, including vomiting, aldosterone or cortisol excess, licorice ingestion, chloruretic diuretics, excess calcium alkali ingestion, and genetic diseases such as Bartter syndrome, Gitelman syndrome, and cystic fibrosis [8].

Excessive aldosterone activity leads to increased renal tubular absorption of sodium (Na^+) and bicarbonate. Additionally, ingestion of alkaline substances, such as antacids or sodium bicarbonate, can directly increase bicarbonate levels in the blood and lead to metabolic alkalosis. The rare genetic disorders Bartter syndrome and Gitelman syndrome affect the kidneys' ability to reabsorb certain electrolytes, and both characteristically cause a metabolic alkalosis. Post-hypercapnia metabolic alkalosis can occur in cases of chronic respiratory acidosis with appropriate metabolic compensation (elevation in serum bicarbonate levels) if the $PaCO_2$ is abruptly returned to normal (e.g., via initiation of noninvasive or invasive mechanical ventilation).

Measurement of urine chloride concentration can help determine the cause of metabolic alkalosis. If urine chloride concentration is low (<10–20 mEq/L), it suggests that the kidneys are conserving chloride in response to volume depletion or chloride depletion. Vomiting, diuretic administration, and contraction alkalosis are accompanied by a low urine chloride concentration. In these states, the alkalosis is often chloride responsive and may be corrected with infusion of sodium chloride. Conversely, if urine chloride is high (>40 mEq/L), it indicates that the kidneys are excreting chloride and are unable to conserve it adequately. High aldosterone states, Bartter and Gitelman syndromes, and post-hypercapnia metabolic alkalosis are associated with elevated urine chloride and are not chloride responsive.

27.5 Mixed and Compensated Acid-Base Disorders

Frequently, acid-base disorders do not exist in their simple form. Furthermore, a normal pH does not necessarily mean no acid-base disorder is present, as some mixed acid-base disturbances can result in a normal pH. Additionally, compensatory mechanisms exist to move the pH back toward a normal value in the presence of simple acid-base disorders, although they may fail to completely normalize pH [9].

In acute respiratory acidosis, a compensatory elevation in bicarbonate occurs rapidly due to cellular buffering mechanisms. This serves to increase serum bicarbonate by approximately 1 mEq/L for every 10 mmHg increase in $PaCO_2$. The main compensatory mechanism for respiratory acidosis is increased excretion of urinary acids and resorption of bicarbonate by the kidneys. This process is not immediate and often takes 3–6 days. This will ultimately result in an increase in serum bicarbonate by 4–5 mEq/L for every 10 mmHg increase in $PaCO_2$.

In the acute phase of respiratory alkalosis, the initial compensatory response is a buffering mechanism resulting in the release of intracellular H^+, and serum bicarbonate concentration will decrease by approximately 0.2 mEq/L for every 1 mmHg decrease in $PaCO_2$. Again, renal compensation may take several days to fully take effect. After that period, a chronic respiratory alkalosis is present, and renal bicarbonate excretion is increased in order to create a compensatory metabolic acidosis. In this state, the serum bicarbonate concentration will decrease by approximately 0.4 mEq/L for each 1 mmHg decrease in $PaCO_2$.

Differentiating between an acute versus chronic respiratory acidosis or alkalosis can be easily done by assessing the change in pH relative to the change in $PaCO_2$ from an expected normal value of 40 mm Hg. If the change in pH is 0.08 in the opposite direction for every 10 mm Hg change in $PaCO_2$ from 40 mm Hg, then the respiratory acidosis or alkalosis is purely acute. If the change in pH is 0.03 in the opposite direction for every 10 mm Hg change in $PaCO_2$ from 40 mm Hg, then the respiratory acidosis or alkalosis is purely chronic. If the value is somewhere in between, then this may represent an acute on chronic or inadequately compensated respiratory acidosis or alkalosis.

In a high anion gap metabolic acidosis, clinicians must assess for concomitant acid-base disturbances by calculating the delta-delta ratio. The delta-delta ratio compares the change in the anion gap (AG) to the change in the bicarbonate concentration relative to the normal range (Eq. 27.7):

$$\text{Delta} - \text{delta ratio} = \left(AG_{\text{Measured}} - AG_{\text{Normal}}\right) / \left(\left[HCO_3^-\right]_{\text{Normal}} - \left[HCO_3^-\right]_{\text{Measured}}\right)$$

$$(27.7)$$

The normal anion gap is typically considered to be between 3 and 12 mEq/L, and the normal bicarbonate concentration is usually around 24 mEq/L. A normal delta-delta ratio (approximately 1:1) suggests that the bicarbonate concentration has appropriately decreased in response to the increase in the anion gap. If the delta-delta ratio is greater than 1:1, it suggests the presence of an additional metabolic alkalosis (e.g., severe diabetic ketoacidosis with concomitant vomiting). Conversely, if the delta-delta ratio is less than 1:1, it suggests the presence of an additional non-anion gap metabolic acidosis (e.g., lactic acidosis and severe diarrhea).

Compensation for metabolic acidosis occurs via the respiratory system. Peripheral chemoreceptors in the carotid body and aortic arch sense a decrease in pH. As a result, the respiratory centers in the brainstem are stimulated to increase ventilation. This stimulation leads to an increase in the rate and depth of breathing, resulting in hyperventilation. The resulting rapid, deep respirations are often referred to as Kussmaul respirations and are characteristically associated with metabolic acidosis. The respiratory compensation response to metabolic disorders typically occurs within minutes to hours after the onset of the acid-base imbalance. Assessment of adequacy of respiratory compensation is done using Winter's formula, where the calculated $PaCO_2$ is the value that would be expected in appropriate compensation (Eq. 27.8) [10]:

$$\text{Expected } PaCO_2 = \left(1.5 \times \left[HCO_3^-\right]\right) + 8 \pm 2 \qquad (27.8)$$

where [HCO_3-] is the measured serum bicarbonate concentration.

Like in metabolic acidosis, compensation for metabolic alkalosis occurs via the respiratory system. Peripheral chemoreceptors are stimulated and, as a result, ventilation is decreased in order to raise $PaCO_2$. The increased $PaCO_2$ leads to the formation of carbonic acid (H_2CO_3) through the hydration of CO_2, which dissociates into bicarbonate ions (HCO_3^-) and hydrogen ions (H^+). The presence of additional hydrogen ions in the blood helps to lower the pH and counteract the alkalotic state caused by the excess bicarbonate. Appropriateness of respiratory compensation for a metabolic alkalosis can be calculated using the following formula, where the calculated $PaCO_2$ is that which would be expected in appropriate respiratory compensation:

$$\text{Expected } PaCO_2 = \left(0.7 \times \left[HCO_3^-\right]\right) + 20 \pm 5 \qquad (27.9)$$

27.6 Acid-Base Disturbances and Pharmacology

Many medications can contribute to acid-base disturbances [11], and this must be taken into account when evaluating a patient with an acid-base disturbance (Table 27.6). In addition to causing acid-base disorders, changes in pH can alter

Table 27.6 Drugs responsible for acid-base derangements

Drugs causing metabolic acidosis	Drugs causing metabolic alkalosis
Metformin	Loop diuretics
Propofol	Thiazide diuretics
Antiretrovirals	Mineralocorticoids
Albuterol	Glucocorticoids
Epinephrine	Calcium carbonate
Potassium-sparing diuretics	Sodium bicarbonate
Salicylates	Penicillins
Toluene	Aminoglycosides
Amphotericin B	
Ifosfamide	
Acetazolamide	
Propylene glycol (used as a solvent in some IV medications)	

medication function, as many drugs are optimized to interact with the body at a normal physiologic pH of 7.35–7.45. Acid-base disturbances can thus significantly influence the pharmacokinetics and pharmacodynamics of medications, impacting their effectiveness, distribution, metabolism, and elimination. pH affects the ionization state of drugs, which can influence their absorption in the gastrointestinal tract. Changes in ionization state can also impact a medication's ability to cross cell membranes and distribute into various body compartments. Enzymes involved in drug metabolism may be pH dependent, so alterations in pH levels can affect the rate and efficiency of drug metabolism, leading to variations in drug efficacy and risk of toxicity. Renal excretion of drugs can also be altered by changes in pH. Additionally, alterations in pH can compromise the stability of medications and influence drug-receptor interactions [12].

Acidosis can lead to endothelial dysfunction and contribute to vasoplegia, or widespread vasodilation and decreased systemic vascular resistance (SVR), which can exacerbate shock states. Moreover, acidosis can interfere with vascular smooth muscle tone and alter the response of blood vessels to vasopressors, which can make them less effective. In states of refractory shock with concomitant acidosis, administration of intravenous sodium bicarbonate may be used to raise the pH in an attempt to augment vasopressor efficacy. However, if the cause of refractory shock is not rapidly reversible, administration of sodium bicarbonate is unlikely to improve patient outcomes.

In addition to its impact on vasopressors, acidosis can also lead to decreased efficacy of inotropic agents. Acidosis can interfere with intracellular calcium handling within cardiomyocytes, leading to impaired myocardial contractility. It can also prolong the action potential duration and delay repolarization, increasing the risk of arrhythmias and reducing the effectiveness of inotropic agents. The aforementioned effects of acidosis on systemic vasodilation and SVR can combine with the impaired effects of inotropic agents on cardiac output and lead to total cardiovascular collapse and death.

27.7 Conclusion

A comprehensive understanding of acid-base disorders is paramount in the field of critical care medicine, where timely diagnosis and appropriate management can significantly impact patient outcomes. Arterial and venous blood gas assays provide valuable information about not only acid-base status but also disorders of oxygenation or ventilation. A systematic approach to assessment of acid-base derangements, including assessment for appropriate physiologic compensation, can aid in diagnosis and treatment of underlying etiologies. Acid-base derangements are particularly common in critical care medicine, and attention should be paid to their potential impact on pharmacokinetics and pharmacodynamics [4].

References

1. Berend K, de Vries AP, Gans RO. Physiological approach to assessment of acid-base disturbances. N Engl J Med. 2014;371(15):1434–45. https://doi.org/10.1056/NEJMra1003327.
2. Prasad H, Vempalli N, Agrawal N, Ajun UN, Salam A, Subhra Datta S, Singhal A, Ranjan N, Shabeeba Sherin PP, Sundareshan G. Correlation and agreement between arterial and venous blood gas analysis in patients with hypotension-an emergency department-based cross-sectional study. Int J Emerg Med. 2023;16(1):18. https://doi.org/10.1186/s12245-023-00486-0.
3. Seifter JL. Integration of acid-base and electrolyte disorders. N Engl J Med. 2014;371(19):1821–31. https://doi.org/10.1056/NEJMra1215672.
4. Figge J, Jabor A, Kazda A, Fencl V. Anion gap and hypoalbuminemia. Crit Care Med. 1998;26(11):1807–10. https://doi.org/10.1097/00003246-199811000-00019.
5. Kraut JA, Madias NE. Lactic acidosis. N Engl J Med. 2014;371(24):2309–19. https://doi.org/10.1056/NEJMra1309483.
6. Vander Heiden MG, Cantley LC, Thompson CB. Understanding the Warburg effect: the metabolic requirements of cell proliferation. Science. 2009;324(5930):1029–33. https://doi.org/10.1126/science.1160809.
7. Kraut JA, Madias NE. Differential diagnosis of nongap metabolic acidosis: value of a systematic approach. Clin J Am Soc Nephrol. 2012;7(4):671–9. https://doi.org/10.2215/CJN.09450911.
8. Do C, Vasquez PC, Soleimani M. Metabolic alkalosis pathogenesis, diagnosis, and treatment: core curriculum 2022. Am J Kidney Dis. 2022;80(4):536–51. https://doi.org/10.1053/j.ajkd.2021.12.016.
9. Adrogue HJ, Madias NE. Secondary responses to altered acid-base status: the rules of engagement. J Am Soc Nephrol. 2010;21(6):920–3. https://doi.org/10.1681/ASN.2009121211.
10. Albert MS, Dell RB, Winters RW. Quantitative displacement of acid-base equilibrium in metabolic acidosis. Ann Intern Med. 1967;66(2):312–22. https://doi.org/10.7326/0003-4819-66-2-312.
11. Kitterer D, Schwab M, Alscher MD, Braun N, Latus J. Drug-induced acid-base disorders. Pediatr Nephrol. 2015;30(9):1407–23. https://doi.org/10.1007/s00467-014-2958-5.
12. Liamis G, Milionis HJ, Elisaf M. Pharmacologically-induced metabolic acidosis: a review. Drug Saf. 2010;33(5):371–91. https://doi.org/10.2165/11533790-000000000-00000.

Chapter 28
Renal Replacement Therapy in the Intensive Care Unit

Fiorenza Ferrari, Giovanna Landi, Claudio Ronco, Alberto Zanella, and Giacomo Grasselli

28.1 Introduction

In critically ill patients, acute kidney injury (AKI) is a common clinical syndrome with a broad aetiological profile and a cause of increased morbidity and mortality. Within 1 week of admission to critical care units, approximately 57% of patients develop AKI of any KDIGO stage, with up to 39% showing severe AKI (stages 2 or 3). Among the patients with severe AKI, 13.5% require renal replacement therapy (RRT) [1]. The mortality rate among patients with AKI requiring RRT ranges from 40% to 55%, while survivors who show AKI during intensive care unit (ICU) stay face a heightened risk of developing chronic kidney disease, end-stage kidney disease (ESKD), or functional impairment with prolonged recovery periods [1].

Physiological metabolic processes continually release endogenous volatile, lipophilic, and hydrophilic toxins into the bloodstream. Hydrophilic and non-volatile toxins are eliminated through the kidneys, which play crucial roles not only in this context, but

F. Ferrari (✉)
Anestesia e Terapia Intensiva Adulti, Fondazione IRCCS Ca' Granda—Ospedale Maggiore Policlinico, Milan, Italy

International Renal research Institute of Vicenza (IRRIV), Vicenza, Italy

G. Landi
Department of Cardio-Thoracic Surgery, Maastricht University Medical Centre (MUMNC+), Maastricht, The Netherlands

C. Ronco
International Renal research Institute of Vicenza (IRRIV), Vicenza, Italy

A. Zanella · G. Grasselli
Anestesia e Terapia Intensiva Adulti, Fondazione IRCCS Ca' Granda—Ospedale Maggiore Policlinico, Milan, Italy

Department of Pathophysiology and Transplantation, University of Milan, Milan, Italy

Y. Alzaidi, M. A. Gebily (eds.), *The Pharmacist's Expanded Role in Critical Care Medicine*, https://doi.org/10.1007/978-3-031-77335-8_28

also in regulating electrolyte balance, acid-base equilibrium, and volaemia. Failure of a detoxifying organ necessitates alternative elimination methods, and if severe AKI occurs, RRT can partially substitute renal function. RRT primarily targets the plasma compartment and can only remove hydrophilic solutes not bound to proteins. The use of conventional RRT biosynthetic membranes with a cut-off value between 15,000 and 30,000 Da limits the passage of molecules with higher molecular weights. Furthermore, while RRT is lifesaving, it cannot fully replace the functions of the native kidney, especially the synthetic and reabsorptive functions of the renal tubules.

28.2 RRT Modalities

28.2.1 Mechanism of Solute Transport

During RRT, both water and solutes are removed from the patient's plasma. The transport mechanisms underlying this removal process are convection, diffusion, and adsorption [2].

(a) Convection: In convection, solute transport driven by a pressure gradient (transmembrane pressure, TMP) occurs across the membrane, leading to the removal of the fluid component of plasma. This process also selectively removes solutes that can cross the membrane pores based on their molecular size.
(b) Diffusion: Solute molecules cross the membrane based on differences in concentration and osmotic pressure, moving between the plasma and the dialysate.
(c) Adsorption: Solute molecules adhere to the membrane surface either through physical interactions with the protein layer or membrane pores or through biochemical interactions involving bonds between molecules of opposite charge.

Convection is the cornerstone of ultrafiltration (UF), wherein water is extracted. The volume of plasma liquid extracted by UF is called ultrafiltrate. The pressure gradient between the inner side of the hollow fibres, where blood from the RRT circuit is driven by the rotation of the roller pump, and the space between the fibres and their container is crucial for filtration through the pores. Consequently, UF is partially restrained by the oncotic pressure of plasma proteins. The result is a positive TMP that drives fluids through the hollow fibres based on their ultrafiltration coefficient (K_{uf}), which represents the membrane's permeability to water [2]. The K_{uf} depends on the membrane surface area, pore density, blood flow, and ultrafiltrate pump speed. UF can also yield solute removal since solutes are carried along with the solvent through the membrane pores. However, the pores are only traversed by solutes with dimensions, weight, and steric conformation that allow them to pass through the pores. The amount of solute crossing the membrane per unit of time with UF depends on the ultrafiltrate fluid flow rate multiplied by a coefficient called the sieving coefficient (Sc) [2], which is defined as the ratio of solute concentrations between the ultrafiltrate and the plasma.

When the ultrafiltrate is partially or entirely replaced by a reinfusion flow and the plasma, previously dehydrated by the ultrafiltration process, is consequently rehydrated, the process is called haemofiltration. UF involves a reduction in the body's water content without altering the solute concentration (e.g. urea, creatinine). Conversely, diluting the plasma through the replacement solution will affect the solute concentration. The composition of the reinfusion fluid determines the extent of alteration in the plasma composition, which is directed toward the solute concentration values of the reinfusion fluid.

Diffusion is the fundamental process underlying haemodialysis. The passage of solutes through the semi-permeable membrane occurs through a concentration gradient and is dependent on the solute's diffusion coefficient (K_d) [2]. Solute diffusion occurs when the dialysis fluid, which has a composition like the reinfusion fluid, circulates outside the hollow fibres. The blood flowing inside the fibres releases solutes with a higher plasma concentration than that in the dialysis fluid. Conversely, the dialysis fluid accumulates solutes with a concentration lower than in the plasma. The K_d of a solute depends on its molecular weight, membrane porosity, surface area, thickness, set flow rate, dialysis fluid flow rate, solute protein binding, electrical charge, and temperature at which the process occurs [2]. Unlike haemofiltration, dialysis does not require pressure gradients for fluid passage through the membrane, nor does it entail the infusion of fluid into the patient's plasma.

Absorption is a form of solute clearance whose extent is difficult to quantify during RRT, and its clinical effect is uncertain. The phenomenon of absorption can be quite relevant in specific treatments with membranes particularly endowed with absorbent properties. Absorption is the main mechanism of solute reduction when using absorbent cartridges in a technique called haemoperfusion.

28.2.2 Categorisation of Treatments

According to the Consensus Conference held in 2016 in Vicenza [2], treatment can be categorised according to session frequency and duration [3].

Continuous RRT (CRRT): Continuous therapies run for an extended period ($\geq$24 h/day). The KDIGO 2012 Guidelines on Acute Kidney Injury recommend the use of CRRT over standard intermittent RRT for haemodynamically unstable patients (grade 2B) [4]. They also suggest CRRT over intermittent RRT for AKI patients with acute brain injury or other causes of increased intracranial pressure or generalised brain oedema (grade 2B) [4].

Intermittent RRT (IRRT): Intermittent therapies are administered in sessions lasting 3–5 h per day. Since the treatment times are short, the depuration efficacy must be higher than that of CRRT. The most frequently prescribed intermittent therapies are intermittent haemodialysis (IHD), intermittent haemofiltration (IHF), intermittent haemodiafiltration (IHDF), and intermittent high-flux dialysis (IHFD), all of which require a higher depuration rate than CRRT. These techniques rely on diffusion (haemodialysis [HD]), convection (haemofiltration [HF]), or a combination of both (haemodiafiltration [HDF]).

Hybrid therapies: Hybrid therapies blend elements from both intermittent and continuous modalities [3]. They typically use conventional intermittent haemodialysis equipment (machine, filters, circuits) and involve sessions lasting 8–12 h per day [3]. These approaches aim to perfect the benefits while mitigating the limitations of each modality, thereby allowing effective solute removal, gradual ultrafiltration rates, and reduced exposure to anticoagulants due to a shorter treatment duration. Hybrid therapies encompass sustained low-efficiency dialysis (SLED), slow low-efficiency extended daily dialysis (SLEDD), prolonged intermittent RRT (PIRRT), extended daily dialysis (EDD), extended daily dialysis with filtration (EDDf), extended dialysis (ED), "go slow dialysis," and accelerated venovenous haemofiltration (AVVH).

The clinical parameters of continuous, hybrid, and intermittent RRT techniques are summarised in Table 28.1.

28.2.3   Continuous Therapies

CRRTs (Fig. 28.1) are currently performed using a double-lumen catheter for vascular access with a "venovenous" technique, whereby blood is driven from a vein and, after being purified, returned to the same vein. "Arteriovenous" circuits have been virtually abandoned [3].

Slow continuous ultrafiltration (SCUF): SCUF is a slow, isolated ultrafiltration technique in which fluids are removed without replacement. SCUF is used for patients with refractory fluid overload with or without renal dysfunction (e.g. acute pulmonary oedema in patients with congestive heart failure refractory to diuretic therapy). This therapy typically involves a net ultrafiltration rate (UF_{net}) of 100–1000 mL/h, depending on the need for fluid removal and the patient's clinical condition, for the time needed to achieve euvolaemia.

Continuous venovenous haemofiltration (CVVH): CVVH utilises the convection mechanism. The administration of the reinfusion fluid can occur before (predilution) or after (post-dilution) the filter or at both sites (pre- and post-dilution). In the pre-dilution method, the solute concentration of the ultrafiltrate will correspond to that of the plasma that has been diluted before entering the hollow fibres. Consequently, with all other flows being equal, the depurative capacity of predilution methods per unit of time is lower than that of post-dilution approaches. However, the pre-dilution of blood before encountering the haemofilter can help improve anticoagulation in the extracorporeal circuit by reducing the platelet count, fibrinogen and complement factor levels, and viscosity. Therefore, the reduction in depurative efficiency per unit of time may be balanced and potentially overcome by optimising the circuit's lifespan.

Continuous venovenous haemodialysis (CVVHD): CVVHD utilises the diffusion mechanism. In this technique, the dialysis fluid is circulated outside the hollow

Table 28.1 Parameters of continuous, hybrid, and intermittent RRT techniques

	CVVH	CVVHD	CVVHDF	SCUF	SLED/SLEED	IHD
Treatment duration (h/day)	24	24	24	Variable	6–18	3–6
Vascular access	Temporary/permanent CVC	Temporary/permanent CVC	Temporary/permanent CVC	Temporary/permanent CVC	Temporary/permanent CVC	Temporary/permanent CVC
Frequency	Daily	Daily	Daily	Variable	Three times per week plus additional treatments as indicated	Four times per week plus additional treatments as indicated
Mechanism of solute removal	Convection	Diffusion	Diffusion + convection	Ultrafiltration	Diffusion/convection/both	Diffusion/convection/both
Type of anticoagulation	RCA-UFH-LMWH	UFH-LMWH	RCA-UFH-LMWH	UFH-LMWH	RCA-UFH-LMWH	UFH-LMWH
Blood flow (mL/min) (Qb)	150–250	150–250	150–250	100–200	100–300	200–300
Dialysate flow (mL/h) (Qd)	0	1500–2000	1000–1500	0	100–300 mL/min	300–800 mL/min
Ultrafiltrate flow (mL/h)	1500–2000	Variable	1000–1500	100–300	Variable	Variable
Replacement fluid for zero balance (mL/h)	1500–2000	0	1000–1500	0	Variable	0
Effluent volume (L/d)	36–48	36–48	36–72	2–8	Variable	Variable

CVC central venous catheter; CVVH: continuous venovenous haemofiltration, *CVVHD* continuous venovenous haemodialysis, *CVVHDF* continuous venovenous haemodiafiltration, *IHD* intermittent haemodialysis, *LMWH* low-molecular-weight heparin, *RCA* regional citrate anticoagulation, *SCUF* slow continuous ultrafiltration, *SLED* sustained low-efficiency dialysis, *SLEED* sustained low-efficiency extended dialysis, *UFH* unfractionated heparin

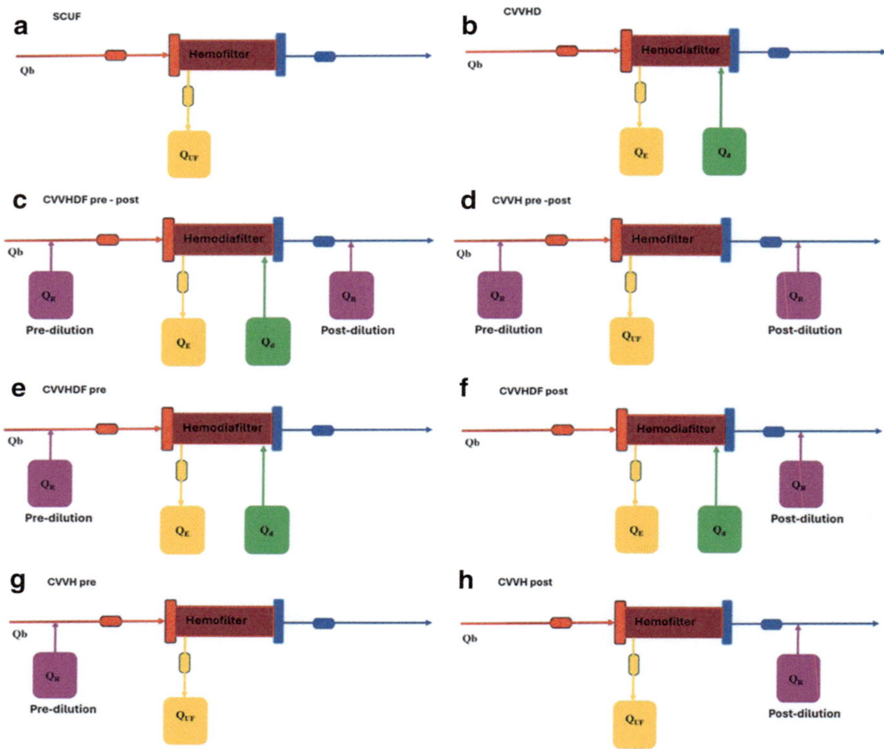

Fig. 28.1 Schemes of continuous RRT modalities. Blood is driven from a vein (red line) and, after being purified, returned to the same vein (blue line). *SCUF* slow continuous ultrafiltration (**a**); *CVVHD* continuous venovenous haemodialysis (**b**); *CVVH* continuous venovenous haemofiltration pre- and post-dilution (**d**), pre-dilution (**g**), and post-dilution (**h**); *CVVHDF* continuous venovenous haemodiafiltration pre- and post-dilution (**c**), pre-dilution (**e**), and post-dilution (**f**); Q_B blood flow, Q_D dialysate flow rate, Q_E effluent flow rate (spent dialysate or dialysate + ultrafiltrate), Q_R replacement fluid, Q_{UF} ultrafiltration flow rate

fibres of the filter to achieve solute clearance through diffusion. The dialytic fluid flow runs opposite to that of the blood (counter-current) to optimise the concentration gradient. With a counter-current flow, the blood entering the filter from the systemic circulation, with maximal solute concentrations, encounters a dialysate flow that is nearly saturated at the end of its path. While a diffusion gradient may still exist at this point in the circuit, it diminishes as the blood continues its depurative path, thus facing a progressively less saturated dialysate (e.g. at the end of the filter, blood will have minimal solute concentrations after being dialysed by fresh dialysis fluid).

Continuous venovenous haemodiafiltration (CVVHDF): CVVHDF involves the simultaneous use of haemofiltration and haemodialysis. In this technique, the blood flow is simultaneously subjected to diffusive and convective clearances, which act synergistically. While diffusive and convective clearances are conventionally considered to fully sum during the blood passage through the filter, the interaction between haemodialysis and haemofiltration introduces a series of phenomena within the filter, complicating calculations. However, from a clinical standpoint, particularly in CRRT, where depurative efficiency is expected to evolve over 24 h, this discrepancy is generally deemed insignificant.

Two relevant concepts are important to understand the CRRT prescription: net ultrafiltration (UF_{net}) and filtration fraction (FF).

UF_{net} refers to the negative balance of fluids within the device circuit (e.g. the difference between the fluids entering and leaving the RRT machine). UF_{net} does not fully reflect the potential weight loss of the patient, which also depends on other factors such as fluid intake and any type of water loss. In CVVH, UF_{net} is achieved when the total ultrafiltration is greater than the solutions reinfused (e.g. if the ultrafiltrate flow [Q_{uf}] is 2000 mL/h and the reinfusion flow is 1900 mL/h, UF_{net} will be 100 mL/h). In CVVHD, UF_{net} is achieved when the outgoing dialysate flow is greater than the incoming dialysis fluid flow (e.g. if the effluent flow is 2000 mL/h and dialysis flow is 1900 mL/h, the UF_{net} will be 100 mL/h). In CVVHD, UF_{net} is essentially achieved by adding a small convective component to the predominant diffusive mechanism of the treatment. In CVVHDF, UF_{net} is achieved when the sum of ultrafiltration and outgoing dialysate (effluent) (e.g. 2100 mL/h) is greater than the fluid reinfusion (e.g. 900 mL/h) plus the dialysis fluid (e.g. 1100 mL/h), resulting in a UF_{net} of 100 mL/h.

FF is defined as the ratio of net plasma water removal rate to the plasma flow rate delivered to the filter. To optimise the haemofiltration, an FF of 20% is considered ideal, like the FF in the renal glomerulus, and the safety threshold of 20–25% FF should not be exceeded. Thus, the blood flow should be five times greater than that of the ultrafiltrate. Post-dilution is more efficient than pre-dilution in terms of solute clearance, but it can raise filtration fraction leading to shorter lifespan of the circuit. Thus, FF in pre-dilution compared to post-dilution may be slightly lower, assuming equivalent flow rates. This is since the inflow rates into the filter, comprising both blood and pre-reinfusion solutions, have a higher denominator in relation to ultrafiltration. Moreover, during pre-dilution, there is a potential for the safety threshold of 20–25% FF to be exceeded due to the decrease in blood viscosity, oncotic pressure, and procoagulant activity in the pre-diluted blood, which may allow an elevated FF of up to 30%.

In summary, careful management of the FF is essential during haemofiltration to prevent adverse effects related to blood viscosity and coagulation. The ideal FF of 20% is comparable to the renal glomerulus, and the use of pre-dilution and post-dilution techniques may influence the actual FF achieved. These considerations are specific to haemofiltration and should not be extrapolated to diffusive techniques, since these methods rely on the passive diffusion of solutes across a semi-permeable membrane.

The term "multi-modality therapy" defines the application of >1 mechanism of extracorporeal therapies (EBP) (i.e. diffusion, convection, and/or adsorption) or >1 EBP therapy (i.e. CRRT plus plasmapheresis, or haemadsorption plus CRRT); specifically, Fig. 28.2 shows different configurations in which cartridge for haemadsorption could be inserted in the CRRT circuit [5].

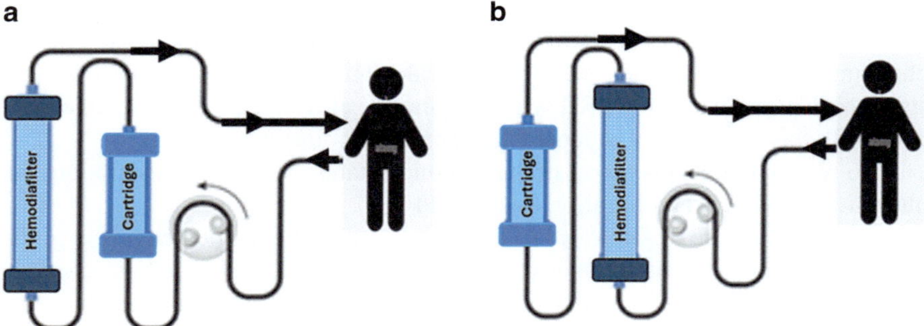

Fig. 28.2 Schemes of continuous renal replacement therapy (CRRT) combined with a cartridge for haemadsorption. The cartridge for haemadsorption can be inserted either before (**a**) or after (**b**) the haemodiafilter, depending on the features of the RRT machine

28.3 Indication and Dosing

The KDIGO guidelines categorise the potential application of RRT into two conditions: one where RRT replaces the failed kidney and another where RRT supports a partially functional kidney (Table 28.2) [4].

Furthermore, KDIGO guideline recommended urgent RRT start in the following life-threatening conditions:

- Hyperkalaemia refractory to medical treatment or rapidly increasing with ECG alterations: When therapeutic measures aimed at facilitating the intracellular shift of potassium (such as correction of acidosis with bicarbonate, glucose and insulin infusion, and beta-2 agonist administration) fail, emergent haemodialysis is the definitive treatment.
- Uremic complications, such as uremic pericarditis, pleuritis, encephalopathy, and coagulopathy (usually caused by uremic platelet dysfunction), are traditional indications of RRT.
- Progressive fluid accumulation and/or complication of fluid overload (e.g. pulmonary oedema): When fluid overload cannot be managed by pharmacologic treatment—by increasing loop diuretics dose or combining diuretics or by sequential nephron blockade—with persistent or worsening oliguria, RRT is required to achieve fluid balance.
- Poisoning with dialysable toxins (e.g. toxic alcohols, salicylates, lithium, metformin).
- Persistent or worsening acidosis that is refractory to medical management due to different causes.
- Metabolic acidosis is a common clinical issue in patients with AKI and is often aggravated by the underlying condition. Correction of metabolic acidosis with RRT in these conditions depends on the underlying disease process. While this guideline does not cover the timing for correcting metabolic acidosis in critically ill patients, it is generally manageable with bicarbonate in cases related to

Table 28.2 Potential indications for RRT

Renal replacement
(a) Life-threatening indications
Hyperkalaemia
Acidaemia
Pulmonary oedema
Uremic complications (pericarditis, bleeding, etc.)
(b) Nonemergent indications
Solute control
Fluid removal
Correction of acid-base abnormalities
Renal support
Volume control
Nutrition
Drug delivery
Regulation of acid-base and electrolyte status
Solute modulation

AKI. Urgent RRT is rarely needed unless there is concurrent volume overload or uraemia. Since there is no evidence-based consensus on the specific pH and bicarbonate levels that necessitate RRT for metabolic acidosis, no standardised criteria exist for initiating dialysis in these situations.

All previous conditions require urgent treatment, and RRT cannot be delayed [4].

However, recommendations consider the broader clinical context, presence of conditions that can be modified with RRT, and trends of laboratory tests, rather than single uraemia and creatinine thresholds alone, when making the decision to start RRT [4].

No urgent indication includes nonemergent indication (solute control, fluid removal, and acid-base control) and renal support, which is based on the utilisation of RRT techniques as an adjunct to enhance kidney function, modify fluid balance, and control solute levels. Fluid overload is emerging as an important factor associated with, and possibly contributing to, adverse outcomes in AKI. Recent studies have shown potential benefits from extracorporeal fluid removal in chronic heart failure and, intraoperatively, in paediatric cardiac surgery patients. Furthermore, restriction of fluid intake in AKI could limit the caloric intake and drug administration; RRT allows a better nutritional supplementation and control the plasma level of a drug in a therapeutic range, avoiding a toxic effect [4].

Regulation of acid-base and electrolyte status and solute modulation are other indications as renal support. Permissive hypercapnic acidosis in patients with lung injury can be corrected with RRT, without inducing fluid overload and hypernatraemia. Changes in solute burden should be anticipated (e.g. tumour lysis syndrome) [4].

In terms of intensity, randomised clinical trials did not prove the superiority of intensive vs. less intensive prescription of RRT [6].

The KDIGO guidelines suggest prescribing CRRT effluent flows of 20–25 mL/kg/h. This rate should be increased to 25–30 mL/kg/h to account for downtime (periods when the treatment is interrupted, such as during bag changes, out-of-ICU procedures, diagnostic tests, catheter malfunctions) [4]. No differences in terms of survival and renal recovery have been found when comparing standard dialysis doses to intensified dialysis doses in SLED. Regarding IHD treatment adequacy, there is no evidence that higher Kt/V values confer any benefits in terms of mortality or renal recovery. Therefore, the recommended Kt/V is 1.3 per session or a weekly Kt/V of 3.9 in AKI. Frequent assessment of the actual delivered dose to adjust the prescription is warranted based on changes in the patient's clinical condition or decreased efficiency of the RRT circuit [4].

28.4 Vascular Access

Dual-lumen temporary haemodialysis catheters are preferred, but tunnelled catheters may be used for prolonged therapy or may have been already placed in ESKD patients. In critically ill patients, a temporary central venous catheter (CVC) should be placed in aseptic conditions under ultrasound guidance by trained personnel. The right internal jugular (IJ) vein is preferred due to its direct route to the superior vena cava. Left IJ vein CVCs may malfunction due to a less direct route to the right atrium, while femoral veins are a secondary option despite infection risks. Subclavian vein use should be avoided due to stenosis-related concerns, especially for patients who will need arteriovenous fistula in the same arm. General recommendations advise changing femoral catheters within 7 days and jugular CVCs every 3–4 weeks.

RRT CVCs are typically made of polymers like polyurethane or silicone for durability, softness, and haemocompatibility. Semi-rigid CVCs are preferred to rigid CVCs to prevent venous wall trauma. Some newer polyurethane catheters are semi-rigid during insertion but soften inside the body, reducing vessel wall trauma. While antibiotic- or antiseptic-coated catheters and lock solutions may help certain patients, their widespread use has been limited by concerns regarding resistant organism colonisation and allergic reactions. Dual-lumen CVCs typically have an outer diameter ranging from 11 to 14 French, with side-by-side or coaxial arrangement of arterial and venous lumens. To minimise recirculation, the arterial port ends approximately 2–3 cm proximal to the venous port. The catheters are available in varying lengths: 15–16 cm for the right IJ vein, 19–20 cm for the left IJ vein, and 24 cm for the femoral veins. Triple-lumen temporary CVCs offer an extra distal port for medication or fluid administration.

28.5 Anticoagulation

Anticoagulation plays a crucial role in minimising clot formation in RRT circuits, thereby preventing premature treatment discontinuation. In IRRT, despite the risk of heparin-induced thrombocytopenia and the need for aPTT monitoring, administration of unfractionated or low-molecular-weight heparin is recommended. In CRRT, citrate is preferred over heparin in the absence of contraindications for citrate, while heparin-based options are considered otherwise [4]. For patients at risk of bleeding and not receiving anticoagulation, regional citrate anticoagulation is preferable over no anticoagulation and can help avoid the use of heparin. Hybrid RRT techniques can reduce anticoagulant exposure but require careful consideration due to the increased bleeding risks with heparin and the need for strict protocols with citrate. Monitoring unfractionated heparin levels during RRT involves maintaining aPTT between 35 and 45 s to balance clotting and bleeding risks. Regional citrate anticoagulation (RCA) can prolong circuit function and minimise downtime while potentially enhancing depuration. RCA also poses a lower bleeding risk, with manageable metabolic concerns like hypernatraemia, hypocalcaemia, and alkalosis through buffer or calcium infusion adjustments. Regular monitoring of blood ionised systemic calcium every 6 h (values between 1.0 and 1.2 mmol/L) and total plasma calcium levels is recommended. A total plasma-to-ionised calcium ratio exceeding 2.5 attenuates citrate accumulation and necessitates treatment adjustment or discontinuation.

References

1. Griffin BR, Liu KD, Teixeira JP. Critical care nephrology: core curriculum 2020. Am J Kidney Dis. 2020;75:435–52.
2. Neri M, Villa G, Garzotto F, et al. Nomenclature for renal replacement therapy in acute kidney injury: basic principles. Crit Care. 2016;20:318. https://doi.org/10.1186/s13054-016-1489-9.
3. Villa G, Neri M, Bellomo R, et al. Nomenclature for renal replacement therapy and blood purification techniques in critically ill patients: practical applications. Crit Care. 2016;20:283.
4. Kidney Disease: Improving Global Outcomes(KDIGO) Acute Kidney Injury Work Group. KDIGO clinical practice guideline for acute kidney injury. Kidney Inter. 2012;2:1–138.
5. Ostermann M, Ankawi G, Cantaluppi V, et al. Nomenclature of extracorporeal blood purification therapies for acute indications: the nomenclature standardization conference. Blood Purif. 2024;53:358–72.
6. Wald R, Beaubien-Souligny W, Chanchlani R, Clark EG, Neyra JA, Ostermann M, Silver SA, Vaara S, Zarbock A, Bagshaw SM. Delivering optimal renal replacement therapy to critically ill patients with acute kidney injury. Intensive Care Med. 2022;48:1368–81.